NUTRACEUTICALS IN OBESITY MANAGEMENT AND CONTROL

AAP Advances in Nutraceuticals

NUTRACEUTICALS IN OBESITY MANAGEMENT AND CONTROL

Raj K. Keservani, PhD, MPharm
Alka Lohani, PhD, MPharm
Editors

APPLE ACADEMIC PRESS

First edition published 2025

Apple Academic Press Inc.
1265 Goldenrod Circle, NE,
Palm Bay, FL 32905 USA

760 Laurentian Drive, Unit 19,
Burlington, ON L7N 0A4, CANADA

CRC Press
2385 NW Executive Center Drive,
Suite 320, Boca Raton FL 33431

4 Park Square, Milton Park,
Abingdon, Oxon, OX14 4RN UK

Apple Academic Press exclusively co-publishes with CRC Press, an imprint of Taylor & Francis Group, LLC

Library and Archives Canada Cataloguing in Publication

CIP data on file with Canada Library and Archives

Library of Congress Cataloging-in-Publication Data

CIP data on file with US Library of Congress

ISBN: 978-1-77491-766-4 (hbk)
ISBN: 978-1-77491-767-1 (pbk)
ISBN: 978-1-00355-788-3 (ebk)

ABOUT THE BOOK SERIES: AAP ADVANCES IN NUTRACEUTICALS

Series Editor:
Raj K. Keservani, PhD, MPharm
Faculty of B. Pharmacy, CSM Group of Institutions, Allahabad, India

Rajesh K. Kesharwani, PhD
Nehru Gram Bharati (Deemed to be University), Prayagraj, India

Anil K. Sharma, PhD, MPharm
Department of Pharmacy, School of Medical and Allied Sciences, GD Goenka University, Gurugram, India

In the modern era, mankind has witnessed a paradigm shift with respect to fundamental eating behavior. The lack of physical workouts and busy schedules at offices and in households have promoted the consumption of junk foods, which eventually results in numerous diseases and disorders since the nutritional content from fast food is inadequate. Plumpness and obesity have become a global health threat. The leading causes of death from most developing nations are noncommunicable diseases such as cardiovascular diseases, cancer, arthritis, osteoporosis, and liver toxicity. Patients suffering from such lifestyle ailments are a bit apprehensive towards prolonged use of costly modern therapeutics, which encourages instead the use of alternative approaches for management of such diseases and disorders.

The emerging sector of the nutraceutical industry encompasses products derived from nature, dietary supplements, and functional foods. Nutraceuticals are used for treatment and prevention of a broad range of diseases, such as the common cold, arthritis, sleep-related disorders, cancers, cardiovascular complications, metabolic disorders, and others.

The research on nutraceuticals is increasing day by day, considering the beneficial effects of food or food supplements in the management of diverse diseases. The issue of paramount concern is standardization and establishment of clinical efficacy of nutraceuticals, which is in fact a challenge for researchers around the globe.

This book series aims at realizing the significance of the variety of nutraceuticals for human well-being. The books in the series will also emphasize the role of dieticians and nutritionists for the prescription of judicious eating habits. The key food components such as carbohydrates, proteins, and lipids as well as micronutrients (vitamins, minerals) are demonstrated to maintain good health, obviating the need for medicines. Thus, nutraceuticals that are indeed derived from food ingredients are believed to be potential alternative therapeutics.

Asymptomatic diseases/disorders necessitate proper diagnosis. Stressed circumstances have been reported to cause weight loss. Workplace stress is a key variable in the genesis and propagation of metabolic disorders. The nuances of the underlying mechanisms are still to be deciphered. Poor lifestyle trends have been attributed along with the consumption of junk foods in several such instances. Sugar-rich carbonated beverages, the use of contraband drugs, and the consumption of liquor in excess are assigned as risk factors. This book series will cover advances and applications in addition to providing the basics of nutraceuticals.

The books in this series will be valuable resources for industry professionals to design and develop quality products for end users. In addition, the book series will be fortified by ideas of innovation, concept building, manufacturing aspects, quality control, and regulatory status of nutraceuticals.

Ostensibly, business has seen a rise in the nutraceutical consumption in recent years. Pure, safe, efficacious products are the need of the hour globally. There are a number of books on nutraceuticals in the market, yet these are only a few books presenting certain aspects of nutraceuticals therein. This book series aims to offer a holistic view of this promising strategy, which is picking up pace with time. This book series will be a unique endeavor to bring manufacturing, research and development, and marketing strategies under a single umbrella.

CURRENT BOOKS IN THE SERIES

- **Micronutrients and Macronutrients as Nutraceuticals**
  Editors: Prakash Chandra Gupta, PhD, Sayan Bhattacharyya, MBBS, MD, Nisha Sharma, PhD, MPharm, Rajesh K. Kesharwani, PhD, and Raj K. Keservani, PhD, MPharm
- **Formulations, Regulations, and Challenges of Nutraceuticals**
  Editors: Tingirikari Jagan Mohan Rao, PhD, Rajesh K. Kesharwani, PhD, Raj. K. Keservani, PhD, and Anil K. Sharma, PhD

- **Food Supplements and Dietary Fibers in Health and Disease**
  Editors: Bhushan R. Rane, PhD, MPharm, Raj K. Keservani, PhD, MPharm, Durgesh Singh, DPhil, Nayan A. Gujarathi, PhD, and Ashish S. Jain, PhD
- **Nutraceuticals in Cancer Prevention, Management, and Treatment**
  Editors: Raj K. Keservani, PhD, MPharm Bui Thanh Tung, PhD, Sippy Singh, DPhil, and Rajesh K. Kesharwani, PhD
- **Advances in Flavonoids for Human Health and Prevention of Diseases**
  Editors: Nisha Sharma, PhD, Deepika Saini, PhD, Rajesh K. Kesharwani, PhD, Prakash Chandra Gupta, and Raj. K. Keservani, PhD
- **The Flavonoids: Extraction and Applications**
  Editors: Deepika Saini, PhD, Rajesh K. Kesharwani, PhD, and Raj K. Keservani, PhD, MPharm
- **Immune-Boosting Nutraceuticals for Better Human Health: Novel Applications**
  Editors: Urmila Jarouliya, PhD, Raj K. Keservani, PhD, MPharm Rajesh K. Kesharwani, PhD, Virendra K. Patel, PhD, and Adi D. Bharti
- **Applications of Functional Foods in Disease Prevention**
  Editors: Raj K. Keservani, PhD, MPharm, and Eknath D. Ahire, MSPharm
- **Plant Metabolites and Vegetables as Nutraceuticals**
  Editors: Raj K. Keservani, PhD, MPharm, Bui Thanh Tung, PhD, Rajesh K. Kesharwani, PhD, MPharm, and Eknath D. Ahire
- **Preventive and Therapeutic Role of Vitamins as Nutraceuticals**
  Editors: Khemchand R. Surana, Eknath D. Ahire, Raj K. Keservani, PhD, MPharm, and Rajesh K. Kesharwani, PhD
- **Nutraceuticals and Bone Health**
  Editors: Deepak Sharma, PhD, Madan Mohan Gupta, PhD, Anil K. Sharma, PhD, MPharm, Raj K. Keservani, PhD, MPharm, and Rajesh K. Kesharwani, PhD
- **Flavonoids as Nutraceuticals**
  Editors: Rajesh K. Kesharwani, PhD, MTech, Deepika Saini, PhD, Raj K. Keservani, PhD, MPharm, and Anil Kumar Sharma, PhD
- **Herbals as Nutraceuticals: Their Role in Healthcare**
  Editors: Raj K. Keservani, PhD, MPharm, Rajeshwar Kamal Kant Arya, PhD, and Rajesh K. Kesharwani, PhD
- **Nutraceutical Fruits: Overview and Disease Prevention**
  Editors: Raj K. Keservani, PhD, MPharm

- **Nutrigenomics and Nutraceuticals**
  Editors: Raj K. Keservani, PhD, MPharm, Eknath D. Ahire, Shubham J. Khainar, PhD, Sanjay J. Kshirsagar, PhD, and Rajesh K. Kesharwani, PhD
- **Nutraceuticals in Cardiac Health Management**
  Editors: Raj K. Keservani, PhD, MPharm, Rajesh K. Kesharwani, PhD, Praveen Kumar Jain, PhD, Bhushan R. Rane, PhD, and Nayan A. Gujarathi, PhD
- **Nutraceuticals for the Treatment and Prevention of Sexual Disorders**
  Editors: Raj K. Keservani, PhD, MPharm, Sharangouda J. Patil, PhD, and Ivan Aranha, PhD
- **Nutraceuticals in Obesity Management and Control**
  Editors: Raj K. Keservani, PhD, MPharm, and Alka Lohani, PhD
- **Antioxidants as Nutraceuticals**
  Editors: Nayan A. Gujarathi, PhD, Raj K. Keservani, PhD, MPharm, Rajesh K. Kesharwani, PhD, Bhushan R. Rane, PhD, and Yogeeta Sameer Goyal, PhD
- **The Nature of Nutraceuticals: History, Properties, Sources, and Nanotechnology**
  Editors: Rajesh K. Kesharwani, PhD, Prashant Kumar, PhD, and Raj K. Keservani, PhD, MPharm
- **Nutraceuticals in Insomnia and Sleep Problems**
  Editors: Raj K. Keservani, PhD, MPharm, Sayan Bhattacharyya, PhD, and Rajesh K. Kesharwani, PhD
- **Nutraceuticals in Respiratory and Pulmonary Diseases**
  Editors: Deepika Saini, PhD, Rajesh K. Kesharwani, PhD, and Raj K. Keservani, PhD, MPharm
- **Nutraceuticals in Arthritis and Psoriasis**
  Editors: Meenakshi Jaiswal, PhD, Raj K. Keservani, PhD, MPharm Rajesh K. Kesharwani, PhD, and Swati G. Talele, PhD
- **Nutraceuticals for the Treatment and Prevention of Sexual Disorders**
  Editors: Raj K. Keservani, PhD, Sharangouda J. Patil, PhD, and Ivan Aranha, PhD
- **Antioxidants as Nutraceuticals**
  Editors: Nayan A. Gujaratih, PhD, Raj K. Keservani, PhD, Rajesh K. Kesharwani, PhD, Bhushan R. Rane, PhD, and Yogeeta Sameer Goyal, PhD

ABOUT THE EDITORS

Raj K. Keservani, PhD, MPharm
Associate Professor, Faculty of B. Pharmacy, CSM Group of Institutions, Prayagraj, Uttar Pradesh, India

Raj K. Keservani, PhD, MPharm, is working as Associate Professor in the Faculty of B. Pharmacy at CSM Group of Institutions, Prayagraj, India. He has more than 12 years of academic (teaching) experience from various institutes of India in pharmaceutical education. He has supervised more than 25 UG students for their research work, has published 31 peer-reviewed papers in the field of pharmaceutical sciences in national and international journals, one patent, 50 book chapters, three co-authored books, and 40 edited books. He is also active as a reviewer for several international scientific journals. Dr. Keservani graduated with a pharmacy degree from the Department of Pharmacy, Kumaun University, Nainital (Uttarakhand), India. He received his Master of Pharmacy (MPharm) (specialization in pharmaceutics) from the School of Pharmaceutical Sciences, Rajiv Gandhi Proudyogiki Vishwavidyalaya, Bhopal, India. He received his PhD degree from IKG Punjab Technical University, Jalandhar, Punjab, India. Dr. Keservani is a life member of Society of Pharmaceutical Education and Research (SPER). His research interests include nutraceutical and functional foods, novel drug delivery systems (NDDS), transdermal drug delivery/drug delivery, health science, cancer biology, and neurobiology.

Alka Lohani, PhD
Associate Professor, Amity Institute of Pharmacy, Amity University Uttar Pradesh, Noida, India

Dr. Alka Lohani is working as Associate Professor at Amity Institute of Pharmacy, Amity University, Noida, Uttar Pradesh, India. She obtained her BPharm and MPharm degree in Pharmacy (Pharmaceutics) from Kumaun University, Nainital, Uttarakhand, India, and her PhD. in Pharmacy from IFTM University, Moradabad (U.P.), India. Her area of research expertise is dermatology, development of cosmetic formulations, transdermal drug delivery systems, nanotechnology, and polymer-based drug delivery systems. Dr. Alka has gained international recognition and prestigious grants, including the IBRO-International Travel Grant to attend Neuroscience schools in Nepal (2024) and Hyderabad (2022). Her research excellence was acknowledged at the IBRO Neuroscience School Nepal-2024, where she received the 'Best Dream Project' award for her outstanding project. With over 12 years of teaching and research experience, Dr. Alka has made significant scholarly contributions. She has authored more than 30 research articles published with renowned international publishers like Elsevier, Wiley Publishers, Taylor and Francis, Hindawi, and MDPI. Dr. Alka has edited 2 books and published several book chapters with Elsevier, Nova publisher and Apple Academic Press. In addition, she holds three patent publications and one design patent. She serves as a reviewer for various prestigious journals including the *Journal of Cosmetic Dermatology, Cosmetics, Molecules, International Journal of Dermatology and Venereology*, and *Naunyn-Schmiedeberg's Archives of Pharmacology*.

CONTENTS

CONTRIBUTORS

Eknath D. Ahire
Department of Pharmaceutics, METs, Institute of Pharmacy, BKC, SPPU, Adgoan, Nashik, Maharashtra, India

Priyanka Arya
Galgotias College of Pharmacy, Knowledge Park II, Greater Noida, Uttar Pradesh, India

Sonia Bhatt
Lingaya's Vidyapeeth, Nachauli, Old Faridabad, Haryana, India

Mohit Chand
Bachelor of Technology, Lovely Professional University, Punjab, India

Monika Chand
Food Science and Technology, National Institute of Food Technology Entrepreneurship and Management (NIFTEM), Sonipat, Haryana, India

Pooja Chand
School of Health Sciences and Technology, University of Petroleum and Energy Studies, Energy Acre, Campus Bidholi, Dehradun, Uttarakhand, India

Kavita Gahlot
Department of Pharmacy, Shree Satya College of Higher Education, Moradabad, Uttar Pradesh, India

Praveen Kumar Gaur
Department of Pharmacy, Metro College of Health Sciences and Research, Greater Noida, Uttar Pradesh, India

Afreen Hashmi
Faculty of Pharmacy, Babu Banarasi Das Northern India Institute of Technology, Lucknow, Uttar Pradesh, India

Rahul Laxman Jadhav
Principal, Shivraj College of Pharmacy, Gadhinglaj, Kolhapur, Maharashtra, India

Poorvi Jain
Teerthanker Mahaveer College of Pharmacy, Teerthanker Mahaveer University, Moradabad, Uttar Pradesh, India

Priyansha Jain
Teerthanker Mahaveer College of Pharmacy, Teerthanker Mahaveer University, Moradabad, Uttar Pradesh, India

Lakshay Kapil
Department of Pharmacology, ISF College of Pharmacy Affiliated to I.K. Gujral Punjab Technical University, Jalandhar, Punjab, India

Maninderjit Kaur
School of Pharmaceutical Sciences, Lovely Professional University, Phagwara, Punjab, India

Tarnjot Kaur
School of Health Sciences and Technology, University of Petroleum and Energy Studies, Energy Acre, Campus Bidholi, Dehradun, Uttarakhand, India

Raj K. Keservani
Associate Professor, Faculty of B. Pharmacy, CSM Group of Institutions, Prayagraj, Uttar Pradesh, India

Shahbaz Khan
Pharmacy Academy, IFTM University, Lodhipur–Rajpoot, Moradabad, Uttar Pradesh, India

Kritika
Department of Pharmacy, School of Medical and Allied Sciences, Galgotias University, Greater Noida, Uttar Pradesh, India

Arvind Kumar
School of Pharmaceutical Sciences, IFTM University, Moradabad, Uttar Pradesh, India

Neeraj Kumar
Galgotias College of Pharmacy, Knowledge Park II, Greater Noida, Uttar Pradesh, India

Nitin Kumar
Galgotias College of Pharmacy, Knowledge Park II, Greater Noida, Uttar Pradesh, India

Vishal Kumar
Department of Pharmacology, ISF College of Pharmacy Affiliated to I.K. Gujral Punjab Technical University, Jalandhar, Punjab, India

Niharika Lal
Metro College of Pharmacy, Knowledge Park III, Greater Noida, Uttar Pradesh, India

Suman Lata Mehta
Department of Pharmacy, IEC College of Engineering and Technology, Greater Noida, Uttar Pradesh, India

Sakshi Minocha
Department of Pharmacy, Metro College of Health Sciences and Research, Greater Noida, Uttar Pradesh, India

Amrita Mishra
Delhi Pharmaceutical Science and Research University, New Delhi, India

Arun Kumar Mishra
Pharmacy Academy, IFTM University, Moradabad, Uttar Pradesh, India

Piyush Mittal
Teerthanker Mahaveer College of Pharmacy, Teerthanker Mahaveer University, Moradabad, Uttar Pradesh, India

Niharika
Department of Pharmacy, Metro College of Health Sciences and Research, Greater Noida, Uttar Pradesh, India

Rashmi Saxena Pal
School of Pharmaceutical Sciences, Lovely Professional University, Phagwara, Punjab, India

Yogendra Pal
Bharat College of Pharmacy, Nakodar, Jalandhar, Punjab, India

Yatender Singh Panwar
Food and Nutrition, GBPUAT, Pantnagar, Uttarakhand, India

Manisha Vyankatrao Patil
Professor, Adarsh College of Pharmacy, Vita, Sangli, Maharashtra, India

Sagar Patni
School of Pharmaceutical Sciences, C.S.J.M. University, Kanpur University, Uttar Pradesh, India

Pragya
Department of Pharmaceutics, Amity Institute of Pharmacy, Amity University Uttar Pradesh, Lucknow Campus, Uttar Pradesh, India

Sonima Prasad
Department of Pharmacology, ISF College of Pharmacy Affiliated to I.K. Gujral Punjab Technical University, Jalandhar, Punjab, India

Saranya Punniyakotti
School of Pharmaceutical Sciences, Lovely Professional University, Phagwara, Punjab, India

Garima Raj
Galgotias College of Pharmacy, Knowledge Park II, Greater Noida, Uttar Pradesh, India

Vaibhav Rastogi
Teerthanker Mahaveer College of Pharmacy, Teerthanker Mahaveer University, Moradabad, Uttar Pradesh, India

Ritika Saxena
School of Biotechnology, IFTM University, Moradabad, Uttar Pradesh, India

Alankar Shrivastav
Faculty of Pharmacy, IFTM University, Moradabad, Uttar Pradesh, India

Amrita Singh
Department of Pharmacy, IEC College of Engineering and Technology, Greater Noida, Uttar Pradesh, India

Arti Singh
Department of Pharmacology, ISF College of Pharmacy Affiliated to I.K. Gujral Punjab Technical University, Jalandhar, Punjab, India

Charan Singh
Department of Pharmaceutics, ISF College of Pharmacy Affiliated to I.K. Gujral Punjab Technical University, Jalandhar, Punjab, India

Gurdeep Singh
School of Pharmaceutical Sciences, Lovely Professional University, Phagwara, Punjab, India

Harpreet Singh
School of Pharmaceutical Sciences, IFTM University, Moradabad, Uttar Pradesh, India

Mukesh Kumar Singh
Faculty of Pharmacy, School of Pharmaceutical Sciences, IFTM University, Moradabad, Uttar Pradesh, India

Rashmi Singh
Department of Pharmacy, Metro College of Health Sciences and Research, Greater Noida, Uttar Pradesh, India

Snehil Singh
School of Pharmaceutical Sciences, C.S.J.M. University, Kanpur University, Uttar Pradesh, India

Shriyansh Srivastava
Department of Pharmacy, School of Medical and Allied Sciences, Galgotias University, Greater Noida, Uttar Pradesh, India

Jyoti Upadhyay
School of Health Sciences and Technology, University of Petroleum and Energy Studies, Energy Acre, Campus Bidholi, Dehradun, Uttarakhand, India

Anurag Verma
Teerthanker Mahaveer College of Pharmacy, Teerthanker Mahaveer University, Moradabad, Uttar Pradesh, India

Shweta Verma
Faculty of Pharmacy, IFTM University, Moradabad, Uttar Pradesh, India

PREFACE

Numerous easy solutions, short weight loss programs, and dubious medications have emerged as a result of increase in obesity worldwide. Risky side effects and rebound weight gain have made the treatment appear worse than the condition itself, leaving sufferers unsure of their next course of action. Creating planned therapeutic interventions using secure, all-natural supplements backed by reliable research is the only effective strategy to safely address the world's obesity problem.

Nutritional tactics that aim to reduce energy balance by lowering energy intake and increasing energy expenditures seem to be an alternate treatment for obesity. A substance known as a nutraceutical is one that has been refined from food and is typically used in medicines and sold on the market. Nutritional supplements demonstrate physiological function by offering protection from certain diseases. Administration of nutritional supplements together with saturated fats aids in the treatment of obesity and prevents the development of the disease by slowing the progression of oxidative stress and inflammation.

The purpose of this book is to clarify a number of key nutraceuticals based on a number of important factors, including source, extraction, chemistry, mechanism of action, pharmacology, bioavailability, safety, and various applications.

This book gives detailed information on nutraceuticals that can be helpful in the management of obesity. This book comprises four parts. In Part I, detailed information about nutrients, vegetables, and fruits in obesity is discussed. In Part II, antioxidants and vitamins helpful in the management of obesity are discussed. Part III contains information on spices and cereals in obesity. In Part IV, a detailed discussion on micronutrients, polyphenols, and others in obesity has been discussed.

The numerous chapters in this book, which is based on various chosen nutraceuticals, explore those elements that deserve consideration in many ways and need to be included in our diet on a regular basis. This book lays a solid foundation for examining the effectiveness and validity of various plant-derived nutraceuticals, which can be used as a crucial therapeutic tool in the prevention of chronic and degenerative diseases, such as cardiovascular diseases, cancer, obesity, and diabetes, as well as to advance good human health.

PART I: NUTRIENTS, VEGETABLES, AND FRUITS IN OBESITY

Chapter 1: Obesity and Nutraceuticals: Introduction and Overview, written by Gurdeep Singh and Mukesh Kumar Singh, provides a concise overview of the prevalence of obesity, complications related to obesity, current treatment regimen, and the significance of functional foods and nutraceuticals for the management of body weight and alleviating its co-morbid conditions.

Chapter 2: Supplementation of Nutrients for Weight Loss, written by Anurag Verma et al., discuss the effect of some of the most commonly and frequently used naturally occurring substances, along with their mechanism of action, in controlling the menace of obesity.

Chapter 3: Nutraceutical Fruits in Obesity Management, written by Jyoti Upadhyay and her colleagues, report that various nutraceuticals present in fruits are effective in the management of obesity.

Chapter 4: Role of Carotenoids in Obesity, written by Monika Chand and her associates, discusses the effect of carotenoids and their metabolites in the management of obesity.

PART II: ANTIOXIDANTS AND VITAMINS IN OBESITY

Chapter 5: Antioxidant-Rich Nutraceuticals in Obesity Management, written by Kavita Gahlot, examines current research on nutraceuticals and their role in managing obesity and body composition.

Chapter 6: Role of Vitamins and Supplements in the Treatment of Obesity, written by Shweta Verma and Alankar Shrivastav, reports on the possible role of dietary vitamins and supplements in body weight regulation and obesity.

Chapter 7: The Role of Green Tea in the Management of Obesity, written by Niharika and her coworker, examines the potential of green tea as a vital nutraceutical for the management of obesity. Additionally, the evidence for each of these proposed mechanisms is reviewed, with a focus on human studies.

PART III: SPICES AND CEREALS IN OBESITY

Chapter 8: Potential of Pseudocereals in the Management of Obesity, written by Harpreet Singh et al., delves in depth into the different kinds of pseudocereals, the dietary value of pseudocereals, the health benefits of eating them, and the role and importance of pseudocereals in the fight against obesity.

Chapter 9: Functional Foods and Spices in the Management of Metabolic Syndrome, written by Arti Singh and her associates, highlights the protective effects of several herbal remedies, spices, and functional foods against various metabolic diseases with evidence from preclinical as well as clinical trials conducted with functional foods and spices against different metabolic diseases.

PART IV: MICRONUTRIENTS, POLYPHENOLS, AND OTHERS IN OBESITY

Chapter 10: Role of Micronutrients in Obesity and Weight Management, written by Rashmi Saxena Pal et al., reviews the role of micronutrients, their importance, and their role in obesity and weight management.

The mechanisms of action of these polyphenols need to be confirmed in future research, which can then potentially contribute to the evidence-based use of these compounds in the field of human health, as discusssed in Chapter 11: Polyphenol Derivatives in Obesity Management, written by Pragya and her colleagues.

Another approach toward obesity is to reduce weight and slow down or to inhibit the absorption of carbohydrates and sugar by giving α-amylase inhibitors, with proper physical activity and fiber-rich diet simultaneously, which discussed by Snehil Singh et al., in Chapter 12: α-Amylase Inhibitors: A Safe Nutraceutical Approach for Obesity Management.

Chapter 13: Marine Nutraceuticals: A Potential Source for the Management of Obesity, written by Garima Raj and her associates, discusses the marine nutritional sources used in the management of obesity.

Functional foods that reduce appetite and enhance happiness and those that speed up the body's metabolism have been examined as obesity therapies, as discussed by Eknath D. Ahire and his associates in Chapter 14: The Role of Functional Foods to Combat Weight Gain and Obesity.

PART I

NUTRIENTS, VEGETABLES, AND FRUITS IN OBESITY

CHAPTER 1

OBESITY AND NUTRACEUTICALS: INTRODUCTION AND OVERVIEW

GURDEEP SINGH[1] and MUKESH KUMAR SINGH[2]

[1]*School of Pharmaceutical Sciences, Lovely Professional University, Phagwara, Punjab, India*

[2]*Faculty of Pharmacy, School of Pharmaceutical Sciences, IFTM University, Moradabad, Uttar Pradesh, India*

ABSTRACT

A significant public health issue is obesity, and environmental factors are involved in its development. Obesity has become a major problem in the world, increasing the risk of metabolic syndrome, which includes diabetes, heart disease, stroke, hypertension, and several types of cancer. Due to its associated complications, it has become the fifth leading cause of global mortality. However, obesity is difficult to control through diet and exercise alone, as they are hard to implement. Although recent advances in medical research have greatly aided in the treatment of obesity, it has recently come to light that dietary management may play a significant role in both prevention and treatment to some extent. Nutraceuticals are nutritional supplements that are used to improve health, postpone aging, fend against disease, and support normal bodily functions. Due to their potential for both nutrition and treatment, nutraceuticals are currently receiving a lot of attention. This comprehensive article provides a concise overview of the prevalence of obesity, complications related to obesity, current treatment regimens, and the significance of functional foods and nutraceuticals for the management of body weight and alleviation of its co-morbid conditions.

Nutraceuticals in Obesity Management and Control. Raj K. Keservani & Alka Lohani (Eds.)

1.1 INTRODUCTION

1.1.1 WHAT IS OBESITY?

In many nations around the world, obesity is a prevalent yet sometimes underappreciated illness with clinical and public health implications. Healthcare professionals and the general public alike deny that it is a disease in and of itself, which has contributed to its improper identification and management and the lack of efficient public health strategies to combat its rise to epidemic proportions. It is generally accepted by many societies as a sign of well-being or a symbol of high social status. The "New World Syndrome" can be used to characterize obesity. It is increasingly common across many of the wealthy countries around the world, in all age groups. According to statistics, during the past 10 years, the problem of obesity has grown among men (12–20%) and women (16–25%) (Flegal et al., 1998). Obesity is often defined as having an excessive amount of body weight for one's height; however, this straightforward description conceals a physiologically complex phenotype that is primarily caused by excessive body fatness (Crawford et al., 2008). Body mass index (BMI), which is calculated as body weight in kilograms divided by height in square meters (kg/m^2), is typically used in clinical practice to measure obesity, which is conventionally described as an excess of body fat that poses a health risk (González-Muniesa & Martínez, 2019). Cut-off points for straightforward anthropometric measurements including waist-hip ratio, total adiposity, and intra-abdominal fatness may serve as the foundation for new classifications of excessive weight. There is a link between higher BMI and mortality from related hazards. Despite significant research efforts devoted to understanding the biology of obesity and energy balance, it has become clear that the knowledge currently available has been of limited assistance to date in containing the obesity epidemic and that no region of the world has been spared from this phenomenon (Blüher, 2019). Various health associations published guidelines for the management of overweight and obese patients which were based on assessment, lifestyle interventions, and bariatric surgery but offered less insight into pharmacotherapy (Jensen et al., 2014). High-calorie consumption causes fat to accumulate in adipose tissue. An endocrine organ with blood capillaries surrounding it, adipose tissue controls the production of hormones, cytokines, and growth factors including tumor necrosis factor-alpha (TNF-α), interleukin-6 (IL-6), and adipokines that support the development of inflammation.

1.1.2 PREVALENCE OF OBESITY

More and more people are developing obesity, which is a concern for global health given that being overweight increases the chance of developing a number of illnesses, including cancer, diabetes, and cardiovascular disease (Wang et al., 2011). Due to a considerable change from undernutrition to overnutrition and an increase in sedentary lifestyle patterns, the incidence of obesity has been rising rapidly over the past two decades in many regions of the world, especially in developed and emerging countries (Wang et al., 2009). Particularly in underdeveloped nations, childhood obesity is a big worry since it has an impact on the next generation (Martorell et al., 2000).

Geographical location, race/ethnicity (gene), age, gender, socioeconomic level, physical activity/diet (accessibility of inexpensive unhealthy food), and lack of awareness all have a role in the prevalence of obesity (Schwartz, 2012). According to epidemiology, obesity primarily affects middle-aged individuals in low-income countries, but it affects people of all ages and genders in high-income countries (Swinburn et al., 2011). On the other side, rising obesity rates have a negative impact on everyone's health and economy worldwide (Rtveladze et al., 2014). Additionally, obesity is a prominent factor in many fatal illnesses/diseases such as cancer, non-alcoholic fatty liver disease, chronic renal disease, diabetes mellitus, cardiovascular disease, and hypertension (Huang et al., 2016). Nutritional stratagems target to decrease energy balance by reducing energy intake and elevating energy expenses appear to be an alternative medicine for illness treatment. A substance that has been extracted from food is referred to as a nutraceutical and is typically used in medicines and sold on the market (Keservani et al., 2016). Nutritional supplements demonstrate physiological function by offering protection from certain diseases. Administration of nutritional supplements together with saturated fats aids in the treatment of obesity and prevents the development of the disease by slowing the progression of oxidative stress and inflammation (Slavin et al., 2005).

1.2 NUTRACEUTICALS

Stephen De Felice first used the term "nutraceutical" in 1989. He united the terms nutrition and pharmaceuticals to describe how nutrition can be used for disease prevention (DeFelice et al., 1995). There isn't a single definition of a nutraceutical that is accepted worldwide, and several unclear definitions have been proposed. A nutraceutical, according to DeFelice, is a food or component of a food that has a medicinal or health advantage, such as the ability to prevent or treat disease. Various studies show that there is a rising consumer desire for health-promoting food and non-food products. In the last few decades, various food bioactive constituents have been commercialized in the form of pharmaceutical products that contain food extracts or phytochemical-enriched extracts that have been directly or indirectly linked to beneficial physiological functions. These items cannot be categorized as food, thus a new term between nutrients and pharmaceuticals called nutraceuticals has been coined to designate them (Keservani et al., 2017, 2020).

Nutraceuticals are functional foods that aid in the treatment and prevention of disease, according to several definitions and/or disorders. The nutraceuticals and functional foods have a small distinction. Food is referred to as a "functional meal" when it is prepared or cooked with "scientific intelligence," whether or not the cook is aware of how or why the food will be used. Thus, functional food (Keservani et al., 2010a, b) gives the body the precise ratio of vitamins, lipids, proteins, carbs, and other nutrients it needs to function properly. Nutraceuticals are functional foods that assist in the prevention and/or treatment of diseases and/or disorders other than anemia (Kalra et al., 2003).

Compounds obtained from fruits and vegetables are the most often utilized nutraceuticals. They frequently contain substances with antioxidant or anti-inflammatory qualities that are said to offer defense against long-term conditions like osteoporosis, cancer, diabetes, and cardiovascular disease (Weaver et al., 2012). The first countries to think that diet is more essential than exercise or inherited factors in achieving good health were the UK, Germany, and France. They are products made from foods but sold as pills, powders (potions), and other therapeutic forms not often associated with food, according to Canada. Nutraceuticals are food ingredients derived from herbal or botanical raw materials used in India to prevent or treat various acute and chronic illnesses.

1.3 CLASSIFICATION OF NUTRACEUTICALS

Traditional or natural nutraceuticals, such as nutrients, herbal ingredients, phytochemicals, probiotic microorganisms, and nutraceutical enzymes, are distinguished from non-traditional or artificial nutraceuticals (e.g., fortified and recombinant nutraceuticals) (Ruchi, 2017; Singh & Sinha, 2012).

1.3.1 TRADITIONAL NUTRACEUTICALS

Traditional nutraceuticals don't alter the diet in any way; they are just natural. In addition to providing basic nourishment, food contains a number of naturally occurring substances, such as lycopene in tomatoes, omega-3 fatty acids in salmon, and saponins in soy. Traditional nutraceuticals are grouped on the basis of (a) chemical constituents; (b) probiotic microorganisms; and (c) nutraceutical enzymes.

1.3.1.1 CHEMICAL CONSTITUENTS

Chemical constituents are further classified into functional foods, herbals, and phytochemicals.

1.3.1.1.1 Functional Foods

The Ministry of Health and Welfare defined the term functional food at the time of the establishment of a regulation system for foods that may have health advantages. Food can be deemed "functional" if it has positive impacts on target bodily processes, in addition to nutritional effects, with the goal of promoting health and wellbeing and/or preventing chronic diseases. Substances with well-established nutritional purposes, such as vitamins, minerals, amino acids, and fatty acids. Vitamins are found in the majority of vegetables, wholegrain cereals, dairy products, fruits, and animal products like meat and poultry. These foods can help prevent and treat diseases including cancer, diabetes, cataracts, heart disease, and stroke. These foods are made available for daily consumption for a specific population with a similar quality to other traditional foods in the market (Lau et al., 2013). The potential impact of functional foods and bioactive ingredients on weight management and the metabolic effects of obesity have been investigated in both animal research and human clinical trials.

1.3.1.1.2 Herbals

Not only in underdeveloped nations but also in rich nations, herbal therapies are widely used (Sharma et al., 2020; Rane et al., 2020a, b, c). Due to this, herbal compounds are one of the main types of anti-obesity drugs

(Sofowora et al., 2013). To treat obese patients, traditional herbalists today combine a number of herbs, such as mulberry leaf (Morus alba) and turmeric (Curcuma longa). A well-liked feature of the functional supplement market is the screening out of active ingredients from whatever people normally take every day. Products derived from vegetables, fruits (berries, citrus, etc.), grains (soybean), drinks (tea leaves), and grains are significantly safer and more well-liked by consumers.

1.3.1.1.3 Phytochemicals

Phytochemicals are non-nutritive plant compounds with either disease-prevention or defense mechanisms. They are optional nutrients that are mostly produced by plants as a form of defense. For instance, the isoprenoids known as carotenoids, which are found in many fruits, vegetables, and egg yolks, are anticarcinogenic, promote the activity of natural killer immune cells, and shield the cornea from UV rays. Non-carotenoids are found in grains, legumes (such as chickpeas and soybeans), and palm oil. These substances lower cholesterol and fight cancer. Berries, fruits, vegetables, and legumes contain flavonoid polyphenolics, which act as strong antioxidants and phytoestrogens, ward off breast and prostate cancer, and manage blood sugar.

1.3.1.2 PROBIOTIC MICROORGANISM

Probiotics are living microorganisms that promote human health. In essence, they promote healthy digestion. These are frequently referred to as "good bacteria" that support healthy gut flora. They aid in improving or restoring the gut microbiome's health. They are helpful bacteria that promote wholesome food digestion and nutrient absorption. As a nutritional supplement, probiotic products are conveniently available on the market. Milk (*L. lactis*), yogurt (*S. thermophilus*), and the digestive tract are a few possibilities (*L. johnsonii*).

1.3.1.3 NUTRACEUTICAL ENZYMES

Enzymes play a significant role in changing these proportions. Tableting or encapsulating enzymes to serve as digestive assistance is the simplest way to use enzymes in nutraceuticals. They work by breaking down indigestible substances like lactose in the stomach or gut. The structure of these enzymes is proteinous. By including enzymes in their daily diet, individuals who have blood sugar issues, hypoglycemia, obesity, etc., can alleviate their symptoms. These enzymes are produced by microorganisms, plants, and animals.

1.3.2 NON-TRADITIONAL OR ARTIFICIAL NUTRACEUTICALS

Non-traditional nutraceuticals are biotechnologically produced artificial foods. Bioactive ingredients found in food samples are used to create products for human wellness. These are further classified into fortified nutraceuticals and recombinant nutraceuticals.

1.3.2.1 FORTIFIED NUTRACEUTICALS

Nutraceuticals with agricultural breeding or additional nutrients are known as fortified foods. Some examples of fortified nutraceuticals include orange juice with calcium, cereals with extra vitamins or minerals, flour with added folic acid, and milk with cholecalciferol. For instance, milk is fortified with cholecalciferol to treat vitamin D deficiency, orange juice is fortified with calcium, and cereals are fortified with additional vitamins and minerals (Casey et al., 2010). In cases of iron shortage, bananas are supplemented using the soybean ferritin gene.

1.3.2.2 RECOMBINANT NUTRACEUTICALS

Biotechnology is used to make foods that provide energy, including bread, wine, fermented starches, yogurt, cheese, vinegar, and others. Biotechnology enables the creation of probiotics, the enzyme/fermentation-based extraction of bioactive components, and genetic engineering technology.

1.4 MECHANISMS OF ANTI-OBESITY DRUGS

Various research shows the mechanism of anti-obesity drugs and it is classified into two major categories namely peripheral and central mechanisms depending on their mechanism in the body (Figure 1.1).

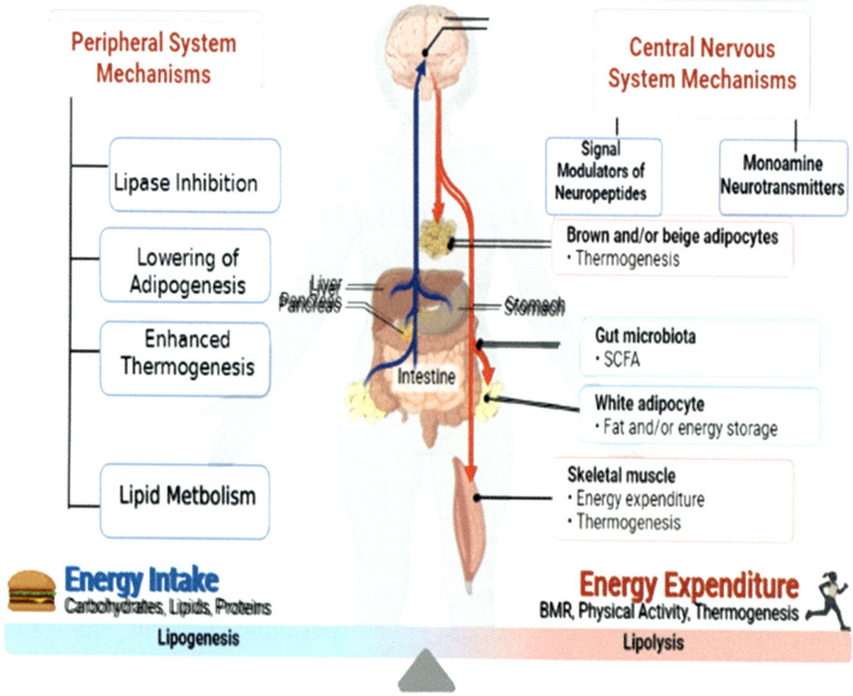

FIGURE 1.1 Mechanism of anti-obesity drugs.

1.4.1 PERIPHERAL MECHANISMS

Peripheral-acting drugs work by reducing gastrointestinal absorption of food or by changing the metabolic system. One way to reduce energy intake is to alter gastrointestinal mechanisms like food digestion and absorption. It is further classified into lipase inhibition, lowering of adipogenesis, enhanced thermogenesis, and lipid metabolism.

1.4.1.1 LIPASE INHIBITION

In today's world, obesity is frequently brought on by a diet high in fat and a lack of exercise due to poor lifestyles. Obesity is caused by excessive fat absorption and storage (Li et al., 2010). The primary organs for storing lipids are the liver and white adipose tissue (Marchesini et al., 2001). It is common knowledge that gastric lipase regulates pancreatic lipase secretion and serves as a support mechanism for lipolysis (Aloulou & Carriere, 2008). Anti-obesity medications block the breakdown of fats into absorbed monoglycerides and free fatty acids by forming a covalent link with the pancreatic lipase active site. Weight loss results from dietary fat absorption being lessened (Tsujita et al., 2006). The triglyceride-based lipid is first hydrolyzed by lipase to monoglyceride, glyceryl ester, and free fatty acid after the fat-containing food is consumed by the human body. As a result, the product has a larger level of 1,2-glycolide and fatty acids. Following hydrolysis into free fatty acids and monoacylglycerol in the small intestine and digestive tract by the lipase's gastric lipase and pancreatic lipase, the body subsequently produces cholesterol and lipoprotein. The small intestine absorbs lipid-mixed particles like bile acid, and the resynthesis of triacylglycerol stores energy as adipose tissue (Lie et al., 2020).

1.4.1.2 LOWERING OF ADIPOGENESIS

Obesity is characterized by an excessive buildup of adipose tissue. Excess energy is deposited as lipids in adipocytes. Adipocyte precursor cells in adult adipocytes proliferate and differentiate in a process known as adipocyte hyperplasia, or adipogenesis (Haider et al., 2019). Peroxisome Proliferator Activator Receptor (PPAR), C/EBP, and Sterol-Regulating Element-Binding Protein (SREBP) groups are linked to the main adipogenic transcription factors necessary for adipocyte proliferation. The process of adipogenesis in fat cells has been significantly influenced by PPAR expression in proliferation (Spiegelman et al., 1997). The signaling networks and transcriptional cascade firmly control adipogenesis. Transiently high levels of CCAAT/enhancer-binding proteins (C/EBP), C/EBP, and C/EBP are expressed in the early phases of development. The major transcriptional regulators of adipogenesis, C/EBP and peroxisome proliferator-activated receptor (PPAR), are stimulated by C/EBP during the intermediate stage of adipogenesis (Rosen et al., 2000).

1.4.1.3 ENHANCED THERMOGENESIS

The human body has a number of energy-wasting processes where energy is lost as heat instead of being used to power another cellular process. These processes are referred to as uncoupled when a considerable amount of energy is wasted. A fruitless cycle of the tricarboxylic acid is an illustration of exothermic uncoupled processes involving muscle and adipose tissue

(TCA). Human Brown Adipose Tissues (BAT) produce non-shivering heat production by releasing surplus energy as heat in order to regulate energy expenditure and body weight. Through the control of energy balance, BAT demonstrates strong involvement in the treatment of obesity (Tseng et al., 2010).

One of the key components in this process is a mitochondrial uncoupling protein (UCP). Brown adipose tissue (BAT) is the only place this protein is present, which is primarily used to insulate people from the cold, particularly infants. In order to produce ATP, UCP1 functions as a protonophore that modifies the normal flow of protons between the inner mitochondrial membrane and the intermembrane gap. This decouples oxidative phosphorylation, which results in the conversion of triglyceride energy into heat (Jimenez-Munoz et al., 2021).

1.4.1.4 LIPID METABOLISM

Triglyceride stimulation can cause lipolysis, which reduces reversible fat. By activating the β3-adrenergic receptor, this approach triggers the oxidation of freshly supplied fatty acids. Only Orlistat is available as a therapy for obesity in several nations. Orlistat has been linked to lower glycemic indices due to decreased lipid absorption and weight loss. Lipolysis is induced by protein kinase A activation, which phosphorylates hormone-sensitive lipase (HSL), or by G protein-coupled receptors and cyclic AMP-activated ERK, which phosphorylates HSL. Orlistat has been demonstrated to reduce sdLDL-C levels and increase LDL particle size when combined with rimonabant in obese patients, potentially improving their LDL phenotype (Stevanato et al). In order to reduce stored fat and prevent obesity, it is vital to target lipolysis when looking for anti-obesity drugs. One strategy is to increase triglyceride hydrolysis (lipolysis). It has been demonstrated that the protein perilipin, which controls access to the lipids they contain, influences weight loss, and prevents diet-induced obesity in animals.

1.4.2 CENTRAL NERVOUS SYSTEM MECHANISMS

Even while daily food consumption and energy expenditure can vary greatly, most people are able to keep their body weight relatively steady. Hypothalamic centers that receive signals from the peripheral and other CNS regions carry out this homeostatic regulation. These peripheral signals, which include nutrients, peptides produced from adipose tissue, the pancreas, and the gut, such as insulin, leptin, ghrelin, glucagon-like peptide-1, peptide YY, and cholecystokinin, might reflect body fat reserves and nutritional status. Energy homeostasis signals are integrated and processed by the hypothalamus, which also triggers the necessary adjustments in appetite and energy usage. The hypothalamus is made up of various distinct nuclei that communicate both with one another and with other regions of the brain by releasing particular neuropeptides. The neuropeptide systems in question are possible targets for weight-loss medications.

1.4.2.1 SIGNAL MODULATORS OF NEUROPEPTIDES

Weight fluctuates sporadically in humans despite periodic variations in dietary intake because net energy intake and utilization are long-term balanced using the energy balancing method (Morton et al., 2006). Leptin, insulin, and other adiposity-related hormones, as well as some gastrointestinal (GI) proteins like ghrelin, educate the central nervous system (CNS) about the state of the body's energy stores (Langin et al., 2006). The nucleus of the hypothalamus, which has an arch structure, releases hormones that control appetite. The two categories of neurons that make up the primary neural signaling location are as follows:

i. Anorexigenic (appetite-decreasing) neuropeptides amphetamine, cocaine, and controlled transcript (CART), and pro-opiomelanocortin (POMC); and
ii. Orexigenic (hunger-enhancing) neuropeptides, neuropeptide Y (NPY) (neuro peptide Y), and agouti-related peptide (AgRP).

Many NPY receptors, in addition to stimulating other catabolic pathways and melanocortins and the adipose hormones insulin and leptin, down-regulate anabolic neuropeptides (i.e., chronic NPY, and hypothalamic NPY) potentially increasing body weight and food intake. Hence, pharmacological blocking of NPY signaling is an important anti-obesity strategy.

1.4.2.2 MONOAMINE NEUROTRANSMITTERS

The intricate process of controlling body weight through controlling appetite is based on interactions between hormones and the nervous system. The results of the studies suggest that histamine, serotonin, and dopamine, together with the activity of the receptors for each, are involved in the regulation of the feeling of fullness. Serotonin, a monoaminergic neurotransmitter, acts through about 14 5-HT receptor subtypes to influence a variety of motor, behavioral, and sensing functions. Researchers have used these receptors to screen out medications that try to cure obesity by lowering caloric consumption (Nonogaki et al., 2009).

The stimulation of serotonin 2C (5-HT2C) receptors on pro-opiomelanocortin (POMC) neurons by serotonergic medications, such as meta-chlorophenyl piperazine (mCPP), has anorectic effects (Sohn et al., 2011). Leptin and other peripheral hormones' major targets, the arcuate POMC neurons, increase their activity after meals and during favorable energy balance. Melanocortins (MCs) and β-endorphin are released at POMC neuronal projections as a result of an increase in the firing rate of POMC neurons. Serotonin's influence on POMC neurons is thought to be mediated via secondary neurons that have their MC4 receptors activated (Lam et al., 2008). Common genetic variations near the MC4 receptor make it an appealing therapeutic target for treating obesity (Loos et al., 2008). The primary CNS hunger monoamine neurotransmitters may also change as a result of chemicals operating through peripheral satiety peptide networks, which is a useful prospect for medications that may reduce hunger. The hypothalamic malonyl-CoA signaling pathway may be suppressed by decoctions containing high fructose levels, thereby showing an anorexigenic effect (Wolfgang et al., 2011).

1.5 NUTRACEUTICALS AS ANTI-OBESITY AGENTS

Numerous research demonstrates how nutraceuticals can be used to control obesity. Some of them will be discussed here. The number of nutraceuticals that have been reported to have anti-obesity activities with similar and diverging mechanisms of action are given in Table 1.1.

1.5.1 CURCUMIN

Curcumin (1,7-bis(4-hydroxy-3-methoxyphenyl)-1,6-heptadien-3,5-dione)—the polyphenolic active ingredient of the spice turmeric (Curcuma longa L.)—which belongs to the ginger family Zingiberaceae (Meydani et al., 2010). It is a polyphenolic compound that represents the most important curcuminoid isolated from the rhizome of plants (Di Meo et al., 2019).

TABLE 1.1 Molecular Targets of Nutraceuticals Having Anti-Obesity Action

Sl. No.	Source	Active Compounds	Mechanism of Action	Molecular Targets	References
1.	Curcuma longa	Curcumin	• Inhibition of adipocytes. • Differentiation lipolysis.	Hormone-sensitive lipase.	Lee et al. (2009); Ejaz et al. (2009)
2.	Red wine grapes, peanuts, and blueberries.	Resveratrol	• Increased lipolysis. • Inhibition of adipogenesis and stimulation of apoptosis. • Modulating the expression of genes involved in lipogenesis and lipolysis.	PPARγ, C/EBP α, SREBP1c, FAS, HSL, LPL, SIRT3, UCP1, Mfn2 FDFT1, FASN, ALDH1B1	Rayalam et al. (2009)
3.	Citrus fruits, apples, onions, parsley, sage, tea, and red wine. Olive oil, grapes, dark cherries, and dark berries.	Quercetin	• Inhibition of adipogenesis.	AMPK ERK	Ahn et al. (2008)
4.	Camelia sinensis	Epigallocatechin gallate (EGCG)	• Inhibition of adipogenesis. • Increased lipolysis.	PPARα AMPK CTD-1 UCP C/CBPα	Yang et al. (2016)
5.	Caralluma fimbriata	Pregnane	• Suppress hunger. • Decrease NPY level. • Lipase inhibitor. • Decrease ORX peptide.	UCP CYP4A1 PPARα C/CBPα	Vitalone et al. (2017)
6.	Dairy products and beef.	Conjugated linoleic acid	• Lipolysis. • Energy expenditure.	UCP PPARα C/CBPα	Kennedy et al. (2010)
7.	Polyunsaturated fatty acids.	Alpha-linolenic acid. Docosapentaenoic acid. Eicosatetraenoic acid.	• Hepatic lipolysis. • Increased lipogenesis.	SREBP1c FAS	Silva et al. (2017)
8.	Amorphophallus konjac	Glucomannan	• Delaying gastric emptying • Adipogenesis	HMG-COA inhibitor	Devaraj et al. (2019)

Curcumin has been proven to improve lipoprotein metabolism by lowering LDL-C and TG and raising HDL-C in a rat model. Besides this, many possible mechanisms postulate the effect of curcumin on obesity management. One potential mechanism is that curcumin intake boosts p27 gene release, which prevents preadipocytes from maturing into adipocytes. Curcumin reduced the maturation of 3T3-L1 preadipocyte cells into mature adipocytes by accumulating the p27 gene (Ferguson et al., 2016). Other potential pathways include blocking wingless-related integration site/beta (Wnt/)-catenin signal activation, lipid oxidation, and the maturation of preadipocytes into mature adipocytes, boosting resting energy expenditure, and activating PPAR (Asai et al., 2001; Liu et al., 2015). Other research shows adding curcumin prevents adipocyte development by triggering the Wnt/-catenin signal (Ahn et al., 2010; Ross et al., 2000; Bennett et al., 2002). Aggarwal BB proposed Cyclo-oxygenase-2 (COX-2), DNA polymerase, lipoxygenase (LOX), glycogen synthase kinase-3b (GSK-3b), and cytokines are all directly impacted by curcumin connections (TNF-a). It has indirect connections with a lot of transcription factors, including peroxisome proliferator-activated receptor c (PPAR-c), signal transducer and activator of transcription (STAT) proteins, activator protein 1 (AP-1), and b-catenin (PPARc) (Aggarwal et al., 2010).

1.5.2 *CAMELLIA SINENSIS*

The consumption of green tea (*Camellia sinensis*, Theaceae), a favorite beverage, is second only to that of water globally. Chemically, green tea is distinguished by the presence of catechins, a type of polyphenol (1). The main catechins in green tea are (–)-epicatechin (EC), (–)-epigallocatechin (EGC), (–)-epicatechin-3-gallate (ECG), and (–)-epigallocatechin-3-gallate (EGCG). In contrast to high-fat-fed controls, Bose et al. discovered that treatment with 7.0 mmol/g dietary EGCG for 15 weeks reduced body weight gain (33–41%) in male C57bl/6J mice. Additionally, the EGCG-treated mice showed significantly decreased levels of plasma alanine aminotransferase, fasting blood glucose, fasting plasma cholesterol, and fat tissue weight. Fecal lipid concentrations were higher in the EGCG-treated mice than in the high-fat-fed animals, and there was a significant negative relationship between fecal lipid content and body weight growth. This suggests that the reduction in body weight seen in the EGCG-treated mice may be due to EGCG-mediated regulation of dietary fat (Bose et al., 2008). Premature adipocyte differentiation, adipocyte proliferation, adipocyte death, lipogenesis, lipolysis, and FA beta ()-oxidation are all inhibited by EGCG and GTE *in vitro* (Wang et al., 2014). A recent RCT study in overweight participants found that supplementing with EGCG (282 mg/day) for three days reduced skeletal muscle lactate levels and postprandial plasma glycerol concentration but had no appreciable effects on skeletal muscle lipolysis and whole-body fat oxidation (Most et al., 2015).

1.5.3 CONJUGATED LINOLEIC ACID

A category of conjugated linoleic acid is called CLA. Octadecadienoic acid isomers derived from linoleic acid, a fatty acid that contains 18 carbons and two double bonds in the cis configuration at the 9th and 12th carbons (i.e., cis-9, cis-12 octadecadienoic acid). Park et al. show a decrease in body fat mass (BFM) by using CLA. In this study, male and female mice administered a 0.5% (w/w) CLA combination exhibited lower BFM compared to controls by 57% and 60%, respectively (Park et al., 1997). Numerous studies have shown that giving a CLA combination to mice lowered obesity without altering calorie consumption. For instance, mice supplemented with a CLA mixture for 42 days experienced a drop in total body weight without a change in food intake (Terpstra et al., 2003). Wendel and colleagues investigated using ob/ob mice, a mouse model of spontaneous obesity (Jarouliya & Keservani, 2019) caused by leptin gene deletion, that CLA (1.5% mixed isomer) enhanced UCP1 expression in white adipose tissue (Wendel et al., 2009).

In hypercholesterolemic hamsters, dietary CLA lowers plasma lipoproteins and prevents the early onset of aortic atherosclerosis. This has been clinically proven to be anti-carcinogenic in rats. Additionally, it has been demonstrated that CLA controls lipid uptake and metabolism by preventing lipoprotein lipase activity. Additionally, it has been demonstrated that 9c11t-CLA increases the absorption of docosahexaenoic acid, 22:6n-3 (DHA), however, the exact mechanism is unknown (Lehnen et al., 2015). CLA increased β-oxidation in muscles but decreased lipid production, adipogenesis, and lipid storage in adipocytes (Dodson et al., 2011).

1.5.4 RESVERATROL

A natural polyphenol substance, resveratrol, is prevalent in a few plants, including the skin of red wine grapes, peanuts, and blueberries (Koushki et al., 2018). Rodent investigations have shown that resveratrol has positive impacts on obesity and associated metabolic abnormalities. In mice, resveratrol's anti-obesity properties were first investigated in 2006. In this study, C57BL/6 mice were given a standard or high-fat diet with or without resveratrol by researchers. In rats given a high-fat diet for 15 weeks, resveratrol (200 or 400 mg/kg/day) was found to significantly reduce body weight and the amount of inguinal, epididymal, and retroperitoneal WAT deposits. It shows that resveratrol significantly reduces the lipid level (Lagouge et al., 2006). Resveratrol ingestion under many other circumstances, aside from high-fat diets, also demonstrated anti-obesity effects. Intake of resveratrol (4 g/kg diet) had an impact on FVB/N mice fed a high-protein diet, as seen by noticeably reduced body weight and fat tissue weight (Mendes et al., 2016). Lasa and colleagues incubated pre-adipocyte cells with increasing doses of resveratrol (1, 10, and 25 μM) for 24 hours, reporting a decrease in triacylglycerol content and a lower expression of acetyl-CoA carboxylase (ACC) (Lasa et al., 2012). Another study found that daily resveratrol administration at a dose of 0.11 mg/kg of body weight for 12 months significantly decreased the amount of lipoprotein lipase mRNA in peripheral blood mononuclear cells (PBMC) of pigs (Azorín-Ortuño et al., 2012). Other animal investigations, mostly in rats, have demonstrated a decrease in belly fat, lipoprotein lipase, and ACC activity following resveratrol therapy (Nagao et al., 2013).

1.5.5 POLYUNSATURATED FATTY ACIDS

Alpha-linolenic acid as well as other dietary omega-3 polyunsaturated fatty acids (ω-3 PUFAs) (ALA), docosapentaenoic acid (DHA), and eicosapentaenoic acid (EPA) are mostly attractive as nutraceuticals for the management of obesity. Saturated FAs induce inflammation by regulating toll-like receptor 4 (TLR4) on fat cells. ω-3 polyunsaturated fatty acids (PUFAs) present in fish oils, such as docosahexaenoic acid (DHA), are known as anti-inflammatory factors that inhibit obesity (Sekiya et al., 2003). PUFAs ameliorate obesity-associated symptoms by downregulating the stimulation of PPAR alpha (Kris-Etherton et al., 2002). *In vivo* tests on rodents indicate that DHA and EPA also enhance FA oxidation in the liver and small intestine. Hepatic lipogenesis is inhibited by DHA and EPA in a way that is dependent on AMPK and PPAR (Siriwardhana et al., 2013). Their anti-obesity effects may be due to the EPA and DHA-mediated increase in FA oxidation and decrease in lipogenesis. Both omega-3 and omega-6 PUFAs have the ability to bind to and/or influence transcription factors that affect the expression of genes involved in pre-adipocyte development. In order to differentiate fat cells and hasten maturation, AA and its derivatives primarily serve as ligands for PPAR and PPAR by upregulating lipoprotein lipase expression *in vitro* (Martínez-Fernández et al., 2015).

1.5.6 QUERCETIN

The first *in vitro* study investigation of quercetin revealed the anti-obesity effect on primary adipose. Kuppusamy and Das discovered that quercetin increased cyclic adenosine monophosphate (cAMP) levels and hormone-sensitive lipase (HSL) activity, which in turn caused lipolysis of primary rat adipocytes in both time and dose-dependent manners (Kuppusamy et al., 1992). By lowering the gene expression of the important adipogenic proteins peroxisome proliferator-activated receptor (PPAR) and CCAAT/enhancer binding protein (C/EBP), quercetin can also prevent adipogenesis (Ahn et al., 2011). Herranz-López et al. showed that quercetin can rapidly lower the intracellular ROS levels, which were correlated with the higher levels of quercetin metabolite by using hypertrophied 3T3-L1 adipocyte model (Herranz-López et al., 2017). Quercetin (50 M) activated AMP-activated protein kinase, which led to the production of brown adipocyte-specific genes such as UCP-1 and cell death-inducing DNA fragmentation factor-alpha-like effector A (CIDEA) in 3T3-L1 adipocytes (AMPK) (Lee et al., 2017). In another study, quercetin also prevents preadipocytes from differentiating into adipocytes by altering a network of transcription adipogenesis-related variables and biochemical processes. By triggering the adenosine 5′-monophosphate-activated protein kinase (AMPK) pathway and specifically increasing the levels of phosphorylated AMPK and its substrate, acetyl-CoA carboxylase, quercetin (10–100 μM) exerts an anti-adipogenic effect in 3T3-L1 preadipocytes (ACC) (Ahn et al., 2008). The effects of quercetin on lipolysis have also been studied in the mouse OP9 stromal cells, which rapidly differentiate into adipocytes. In this model, 10 μM quercetin suppresses adipogenesis by upregulating the expression of adipose triglyceride lipase (ATGL) and hormone-sensitive lipase while downregulating the expression of FA synthase (FAS), LPL, and aP2 (HSL) (Seo et al., 2015). Furthermore, Dong et al. discovered that in mice fed a high-fat diet (HFD), quercetin reduced mast cell and macrophage infiltration into epididymal adipose tissues (EATs) via the AMPK-1-silent information regulator (SIRT) 1 pathway (Dong et al., 2014). Quercetin reduced the expression of inflammatory and oxidative stress markers in Wistar rats, such as nuclear factor kappa B (NF-κB), nuclear factor erythroid 2-related factor (Nrf2), and heme oxygenase-1 (HO-1) (Panchal et al., 2012). Currently, a phase II clinical experiment is being conducted to determine whether quercetin affects how the body absorbs glucose in obese people. Future studies should look more closely at quercetin's bioactive properties and bioavailability (Trials, 2003).

1.5.7 CARALLUMA FIMBRIATA

C. fimbriata is a plant that can be consumed, in the Apocynaceae family, native to India. *C. fimbriata* has been utilized as a portable food for hunting and for its ability to reduce hunger. Since hunting tribes have used chewable pieces or chunks of the *C. fimbriata* to sate their thirst and control their appetite. Pregnane glycosides, which are known to reduce appetite and boost endurance, are present in it. Pregnancy affects lipid metabolism and inhibits the synthesis of fatty acids (Qayyum et al., 2018). They also have an impact on the hypothalamus and the hormone cortisol, which leads to a feeling of fullness that reduces hunger and is most likely the root of appetite control (Kell et al., 2019). *C. fimbriata* may inhibit the production of ghrelin in the stomach and neuropeptide-Y in the hypothalamus, which would lower appetite (Gardiner et al., 2005). The anti-obesogenic and anti-atherosclerotic activities of *C. fimbriata* extract were reported by Kamalakkannan and colleagues. Oral administration of the extract revealed a significant decrease in food consumption in this study, and the extract also prevented increases in body weight, liver weight, and fat pad mass (Gardiner et al., 2010). According to a study, hyperphagia in a 14-year-old girl with Prader-Willi syndrome (PWS) was successfully treated. The youngster started taking a supplemented *C. fimbriata* extract (CFE) for appetite management when he was two years old. For appetite suppression, the CFE was administered as a drink once a day, and the dosage was gradually raised (Griggs et al., 2019). Another study explained how giving CFE supplements to kids and teenagers with PWS decreased hyperphagia. At the highest dose of CFE supplementation, 1,000 mg/day, hyperphagia significantly decreased. The results indicate that CFE might have an advantageous effect on PWS management (Griggs et al., 2015).

1.5.8 GLUCOMANNAN

Glucomannan is a commonly promoted dietary supplement, and some reports have confirmed prolonging the time of gastric emptying with the use of glucomannan, which improves satiety and decreases body weight (Keithley et al., 2013). Different mechanisms, such as promoting satiety through greater mastication attempts, delaying gastric emptying, and reducing small bowel transit, have been postulated to explain the benefits of glucomannan on weight loss. Because soluble fibers decrease the absorption of fat and protein, fecal energy loss has also been hypothesized as a mechanism. Glucomannan was linked to decreases in body weight (BW) and blood lipid and glucose levels in adults (Wood et al., 2007). Glucomannan helps to facilitate weight reduction by transferring energy from other nutrients and producing satiety and satiation as it absorbs water and expands throughout the gastrointestinal tract. By transferring energy from other nutrients and causing fullness and satiation as it absorbs water and swells throughout the gastrointestinal tract, glucomannan aids in weight loss (Gallaher et al., 2000). Zhai and colleagues studied the effects of bacterial cellulose (BC) and Glucomannan (GM) on HFD-induced obesity in C57BL/6J mice. Compared with adding BC or Glucomannan to the diet alone, the combined addition of BC/GM could more effectively reduce the weight of mice and inhibit the secretion of adipocytokines and adipogenesis-related proteins (Zhai et al., 2018).

1.6 CONCLUSION

Obesity is a serious metabolic disorder caused by the interactivity of several causative factors, including lifestyle, diet-related, environmental, and genetic factors. Proper lifestyle and conduct alterations are the basics of positive weight reduction theory, but sustaining such healthful living styles can prove difficult. Researchers have recognized the significance of nutraceuticals and their positive effects on health in order to stop the widespread spread of these disorders. To further understand the mechanisms underlying the possible nutraceuticals' therapeutic effects on metabolic syndrome, more research needs to be done on them. Functional foods and nutraceuticals are always used as adjuvant therapy with traditional anti-obesity medications for improved weight management since they cannot be prescribed alone to treat obesity. Anti-obesity therapeutic treatment should be dispensed when recommended as safe and beneficial for obese patients. Over the last three decades, fewer obesity-therapeutic drugs have been approved or screened. Natural substances offer anti-obesity actions accompanied by extra health advantages, such as controlling diabetes and hyperlipidemia. It is predicted that the use of various natural resources will pave the way for screening new anti-obesity agents. The current review focused on the prevalence of obesity, co-morbid conditions (obesity-related complications), mechanism of anti-obesity drugs, and current treatment plans for managing body weight with particular attention to standard oral anti-obesity medications, complementary therapy, and functional foods/nutraceuticals and their anti-obesity mechanisms.

KEYWORDS

- **adipogenesis**
- **dietary supplements**
- **mortality**
- **nutraceuticals**
- **obesity**
- **prevalence**
- **weight loss**

REFERENCES

Aggarwal, B. B. (2010). Targeting inflammation-induced obesity and metabolic diseases by curcumin and other nutraceuticals. Annual Review of Nutrition, 30, 173.

Ahn, J., Lee, H., Kim, S., & Ha, T. (2010). Curcumin-induced suppression of adipogenic differentiation is accompanied by activation of Wnt/β-catenin signaling. American Journal of Physiology-Cell Physiology, 298(6), C1510–C1516.

Ahn, J., Lee, H., Kim, S., Park, J., & Ha, T. (2008). The anti-obesity effect of quercetin is mediated by the AMPK and MAPK signaling pathways. Biochemical and Biophysical Research Communications, 373(4), 545–549.

Ahn, J., Lee, H., Kim, S., Park, J., & Ha, T. (2011). The anti-obesity effect of quercetin is mediated by the AMPK and MAPK signaling pathways. Biochemical and Biophysical Research Communications, 404(1), 579–579.

Aloulou, A., & Carriere, F. (2008). Gastric lipase: An extremophilic interfacial enzyme with medical applications. Cellular and Molecular Life Sciences, 65(6), 851.

Asai, A., & Miyazawa, T. (2001). Dietary curcuminoids prevent high-fat diet-induced lipid accumulation in rat liver and epididymal adipose tissue. Journal of Nutrition, 131(11), 2932–2935.

Azorín-Ortuño, M., Yáñez-Gascón, M. J., González-Sarrías, A., Larrosa, M., Vallejo, F., Pallarés, F. J., & Espín, J. C. (2012). Effects of long-term consumption of low doses of resveratrol on diet-induced mild hypercholesterolemia in pigs: A transcriptomic approach to disease prevention. Journal of Nutritional Biochemistry, 23(7), 829–837.

Bennett, C. N., Ross, S. E., Longo, K. A., Bajnok, L., Hemati, N., Johnson, K. W., & MacDougald, O. A. (2002). Regulation of Wnt signaling during adipogenesis. Journal of Biological Chemistry, 277(34), 30998–31004.

Blüher, M. (2019). Obesity: Global epidemiology and pathogenesis. Nature Reviews Endocrinology, 15(5), 288–298. https://doi.org/10.1038/s41574-019-0176-8.

Bose, M., Lambert, J. D., Ju, J., Reuhl, K. R., Shapses, S. A., & Yang, C. S. (2008). The major green tea polyphenol, (–)-epigallocatechin-3-gallate, inhibits obesity, metabolic syndrome, and fatty liver disease in high-fat–fed mice. Journal of Nutrition, 138(9), 1677–1683.

Casey, C., Slawson, D. C., & Neal, L. R. (2010). Vitamin D supplementation in infants, children, and adolescents. American Family Physician, 81(6), 745–748.

Crawford, D., Jeffery, R., Ball, K., & Brug, J. (2008). Obesity Epidemiology. Oxford University Press.

DeFelice, S. L. (1995). The nutraceutical revolution: Its impact on food industry R&D. Trends in Food Science and Technology, 6(2), 59–61.

Devaraj, R. D., Reddy, C. K., & Xu, B. (2019). Health-promoting effects of konjac glucomannan and its practical applications: A critical review. International Journal of Biological Macromolecules, 126, 273–281.

Di Meo, F., Margarucci, S., Galderisi, U., Crispi, S., & Peluso, G. (2019). Curcumin, gut microbiota, and neuroprotection. Nutrients, 11(10), 2426.

Dodson, M. V., Mir, P. S., Hausman, G. J., Guan, L. L., Du, M., Jiang, Z., & Bergen, W. G. (2011). Obesity, metabolic syndrome, and adipocytes. Journal of Lipids, 2011, 1–5.

Dong, J., Zhang, X., Zhang, L., Bian, H. X., Xu, N., Bao, B., & Liu, J. (2014). Quercetin reduces obesity-associated ATM infiltration and inflammation in mice: A mechanism including AMPKα1/SIRT1. Journal of Lipid Research, 55(3), 363–374.

Ejaz, A., Wu, D., Kwan, P., & Meydani, M. (2009). Curcumin inhibits adipogenesis in 3T3-L1 adipocytes and angiogenesis and obesity in C57/BL mice. Journal of Nutrition, 139(5), 919–925.

Ferguson, B. S., Nam, H., & Morrison, R. F. (2016). Curcumin inhibits 3T3-L1 preadipocyte proliferation by mechanisms involving post-transcriptional p27 regulation. Biochemical and Biophysical Reports, 5, 16–21.

Flegal, K. M., Carroll, M. D., Kuczmarski, R. J., & Johnson, C. L. (1998). Overweight and obesity in the United States: Prevalence and trends, 1960–1994. International Journal of Obesity, 22(1), 39–47. https://doi.org/10.1038/sj.ijo.0800541.

Gallaher, C. M., Munion, J., Hesslink, R., Jr., Wise, J., & Gallaher, D. D. (2000). Cholesterol reduction by glucomannan and chitosan is mediated by changes in cholesterol absorption and bile acid and fat excretion in rats. Journal of Nutrition, 130(11), 2753–2759.

Gardiner, J. V., Kong, W. M., Ward, H., Murphy, K. G., Dhillo, W. S., & Bloom, S. R. (2005). AAV-mediated expression of anti-sense neuropeptide Y cRNA in the arcuate nucleus of rats results in decreased weight gain and food intake. Biochemical and Biophysical Research Communications, 327(4), 1088–1093.

González-Muniesa, P., & Martínez, J. A. (2019). Precision nutrition and metabolic syndrome management. Nutrients, 11(10), 2411.

Griggs, J. (2019). Single-case study of appetite control in Prader-Willi syndrome, over 12 years by the Indian extract Caralluma fimbriata. Genes, 10(6), 447.

Griggs, J. L., Su, X. Q., & Mathai, M. L. (2015). Caralluma fimbriata supplementation improves the appetite behavior of children and adolescents with Prader-Willi syndrome. North American Journal of Medical Sciences, 7(11), 509.

Haider, N., & Larose, L. (2019). Harnessing adipogenesis to prevent obesity. Adipocyte, 8(1), 98–104.

Herranz-López, M., Borrás-Linares, I., Olivares-Vicente, M., Gálvez, J., Segura-Carretero, A., & Micol, V. (2017). Correlation between the cellular metabolism of quercetin and its glucuronide metabolite and oxidative stress in hypertrophied 3T3-L1 adipocytes. Phytomedicine, 25, 25–28.
Huang, W. H., Hwang, L. C., Chan, H. L., Lin, H. Y., & Lin, Y. H. (2016). Study of seven single-nucleotide polymorphisms identified in East Asians for association with obesity in a Taiwanese population. BMJ Open, 6(8), e011713.
Jarouliya, U., & Keservani, R. K. (2019). Pathways leading to child obesity. In D. Bagchi (Ed.), Global Perspectives on Childhood Obesity: Current Status, Consequences and Prevention (2nd ed., pp. 137–146). Academic Press. ISBN: 9780128128404.
Jensen, M. D., Ryan, D. H., Apovian, C. M., Ard, J. D., Comuzzie, A. G., Donato, K. A., & Yanovski, S. Z. (2014). 2013 AHA/ACC/TOS'S guideline for the management of overweight and obesity in adults: A report of the American College of Cardiology/American Heart Association Task Force on Practice Guidelines and The Obesity Society. Journal of the American College of Cardiology, 63(25 Part B), 2985–3023.
Jimenez-Munoz, C. M., López, M., Albericio, F., & Makowski, K. (2021). Targeting energy expenditure—Drugs for obesity treatment. Pharmaceuticals, 14(5), 435.
Kalra, E. K. (2003). Nutraceutical definition and introduction. AAPS PharmSci, 5(3), 27–28.
Kamalakkannan, S., Rajendran, R., Venkatesh, R. V., Clayton, P., & Akbarsha, M. A. (2010). Antiobesogenic and antiatherosclerotic properties of Caralluma fimbriata extract. Journal of Nutrition and Metabolism, 2010, 1–6.
Keithley, J. K., Swanson, B., Mikolaitis, S. L., DeMeo, M., Zeller, J. M., Fogg, L., & Adamji, J. (2013). Safety and efficacy of glucomannan for weight loss in overweight and moderately obese adults. Journal of Obesity, 2013, 1–7.
Kell, G., Rao, A., & Katsikitis, M. (2019). A randomized placebo-controlled clinical trial on the efficacy of Caralluma fimbriata supplement for reducing anxiety and stress in healthy adults over eight weeks. Journal of Affective Disorders, 246, 619–626.
Kennedy, A., Martinez, K., Schmidt, S., Mandrup, S., La Point, K., & McIntosh, M. (2010). Antiobesity mechanisms of action of conjugated linoleic acid. Journal of Nutritional Biochemistry, 21(3), 171–179.
Keservani, R. K., Kesharwani, R. K., Sharma, A. K., Gautam, S. P., & Verma, S. K. (2016). Nutraceutical formulations and challenges. In D. Bagchi & S. Nair (Eds.), New Product Development in Nutraceuticals & Functional Foods: From Concept to Market (pp. 161–177). Academic Press. ISBN: 9780128128404.
Keservani, R. K., Kesharwani, R. K., Sharma, A. K., Vyas, N., & Chadoker, A. (2010b). Nutritional supplements: An overview. International Journal of Current Pharmaceutical Review and Research, 1(1), 59–75.
Keservani, R. K., Kesharwani, R. K., Vyas, N., Jain, S., Raghuvanshi, R., & Sharma, A. K. (2010a). Nutraceutical and functional food as future food: A review. Der Pharmacia Lettre, 2(1), 106–116.
Keservani, R. K., Sharma, A. K., & Kesharwani, R. K. (2017). An overview and therapeutic applications of nutraceutical and functional foods. In Recent Advances in Drug Delivery Technology (pp. 160–201). ISBN: 9781522507543.
Keservani, R. K., Sharma, A. K., & Kesharwani, R. K. (Eds.). (2020). Nutraceuticals and Dietary Supplements: Applications in Health Improvement and Disease Management. pp. 1–344. CRC Press. ISBN: 9781771888738.

Koushki, M., Amiri-Dashatan, N., Ahmadi, N., Abbaszadeh, H. A., & Rezaei-Tavirani, M. (2018). Resveratrol: A miraculous natural compound for disease treatment. Food Science & Nutrition, 6(8), 2473–2490.

Kris-Etherton, P. M., Taylor, D. S., Smiciklas-Wright, H., Mitchell, D. C., Bekhuis, T. C., Olson, B. H., & Slonim, A. B. (2002). High-soluble-fiber foods in conjunction with a telephone-based, personalized behavior change support service result in favorable changes in lipids and lifestyles after 7 weeks. Journal of the American Dietetic Association, 102(4), 503–510.

Kuppusamy, U. R., & Das, N. P. (1992). Effects of flavonoids on cyclic AMP phosphodiesterase and lipid mobilization in rat adipocytes. Biochemical Pharmacology, 44(7), 1307–1315.

Lagouge, M., Argmann, C., Gerhart-Hines, Z., Meziane, H., Lerin, C., Daussin, F., & Auwerx, J. (2006). Resveratrol improves mitochondrial function and protects against metabolic disease by activating SIRT1 and PGC-1α. Cell, 127(6), 1109–1122.

Lam, D. D., Przydzial, M. J., Ridley, S. H., Yeo, G. S., Rochford, J. J., O'Rahilly, S., & Heisler, L. K. (2008). Serotonin 5-HT2C receptor agonist promotes hypophagia via downstream activation of melanocortin 4 receptors. Endocrinology, 149(3), 1323–1328.

Langin, D. (2006). Adipose tissue lipolysis is a metabolic pathway to define pharmacological strategies against obesity and metabolic syndrome. *Pharmacological Research, 53*(6), 482–491.

Lasa, A., Churruca, I., Eseberri, I., Andrés-Lacueva, C., & Portillo, M. P. (2012). Delipidating effect of resveratrol metabolites in 3T3-L1 adipocytes. *Molecular Nutrition & Food Research, 56*(10), 1559–1568.

Lau, T. C., Chan, M. W., Tan, H. P., & Kwek, C. L. (2013). Functional food: A growing trend among the health conscious. *Asian Social Science, 9*(1), 198.

Lee, S. G., Parks, J. S., & Kang, H. W. (2017). Quercetin, a functional compound of onion peel, remodels white adipocytes to brown-like adipocytes. *Journal of Nutritional Biochemistry, 42*, 62–71.

Lee, Y. K., Lee, W. S., Hwang, J. T., Kwon, D. Y., Surh, Y. J., & Park, O. J. (2009). Curcumin exerts an anti-differentiation effect through AMPKα-PPAR-γ in 3T3-L1 adipocytes and an antiproliferatory effect through AMPKα-COX-2 in cancer cells. *Journal of Agricultural and Food Chemistry, 57*(1), 305–310.

Lehnen, T. E., da Silva, M. R., Camacho, A., Marcadenti, A., & Lehnen, A. M. (2015). A review on effects of conjugated linoleic fatty acid (CLA) upon body composition and energetic metabolism. *Journal of the International Society of Sports Nutrition, 12*(1), 36.

Li, T., Owsley, E., Matozel, M., Hsu, P., Novak, C. M., & Chiang, J. Y. (2010). Transgenic expression of cholesterol 7α-hydroxylase in the liver prevents high-fat diet-induced obesity and insulin resistance in mice. *Journal of Hepatology, 52*(2), 678–690.

Liu, B. L., Chen, Y. P., Cheng, H., Wang, Y. Y., Rui, H. L., Yang, M., & Dong, J. (2015). The protective effects of curcumin on obesity-related glomerulopathy are associated with inhibition of Wnt/β-catenin signaling activation in podocytes. *Journal of Evidence-Based Complementary & Alternative Medicine, 2015*, 1–12.

Liu, T. T., Liu, X. T., Chen, Q. X., & Shi, Y. (2020). Lipase inhibitors for obesity: A review. *Biomedicine & Pharmacotherapy, 128*, 110314.

Loos, R. J., Lindgren, C. M., Li, S., Wheeler, E., Zhao, J. H., Prokopenko, I., & Barroso, I. (2008). Common variants near MC4R are associated with fat mass, weight, and risk of obesity. *Nature Genetics, 40*(6), 768–775.

Marchesini, G., Brizi, M., Bianchi, G., Tomassetti, S., Bugianesi, E., Lenzi, M., & Melchionda, N. (2001). Nonalcoholic fatty liver disease: A feature of the metabolic syndrome. *Diabetes, 50*(8), 1844–1850.

Martínez-Fernández, L., Laiglesia, L. M., Huerta, A. E., Martínez, J. A., & Moreno-Aliaga, M. J. (2015). Omega-3 fatty acids and adipose tissue function in obesity and metabolic syndrome. *Prostaglandins & Other Lipid Mediators, 121*, 24–41.

Martorell, R., Khan, L. K., Hughes, M. L., & Grummer-Strawn, L. M. (2000). Overweight and obesity in preschool children from developing countries. *International Journal of Obesity, 24*(8), 959–967.

Mendes, K. L., de Pinho, L., Andrade, J. M. O., Paraíso, A. F., Lula, J. F., Macedo, S. M., & Santos, S. H. S. (2016). Distinct metabolic effects of resveratrol on lipogenesis markers in mice adipose tissue treated with high-polyunsaturated fat and high-protein diets. *Journal of Life Sciences, 153*, 66–73.

Meydani, M., & Hasan, S. T. (2010). Dietary polyphenols and obesity. *Nutrients, 2*(7), 737–751.

Morton, G. J., Cummings, D. E., Baskin, D. G., Barsh, G. S., & Schwartz, M. W. (2006). Central nervous system control of food intake and body weight. *Nature, 443*(7109), 289–295.

Most, J., van Can, J. G., van Dijk, J. W., Goossens, G. H., Jocken, J., Hospers, J. J., & Blaak, E. E. (2015). A 3-day EGCG supplementation reduces interstitial lactate concentration in the skeletal muscle of overweight subjects. *Scientific Reports, 5*(1), 1–9.

Nagao, K., Jinnouchi, T., Kai, S., & Yanagita, T. (2013). Effect of dietary resveratrol on the metabolic profile of nutrients in obese OLETF rats. *Lipids in Health and Disease, 12*(1), 1–6.

Nonogaki, K., Ohba, Y., Wakameda, M., & Tamari, T. (2009). Fluvoxamine exerts an anorexic effect in 5-HT2C receptor mutant mice with heterozygous mutation of the β-endorphin gene. *International Journal of Neuropsychopharmacology, 12*(4), 547–552.

Panchal, S. K., Poudyal, H., & Brown, L. (2012). Quercetin ameliorates cardiovascular, hepatic, and metabolic changes in diet-induced metabolic syndrome in rats. *Journal of Nutrition, 142*(6), 1026–1032.

Park, Y., Albright, K. J., Liu, W., Storkson, J. M., Cook, M. E., & Pariza, M. W. (1997). Effect of conjugated linoleic acid on body composition in mice. *Lipids, 32*(8), 853–858.

Qayyum, N., Rani, H., Mir, K. B., & Khan, A. Q. (2018). Caralluma pharmacological attributes. *Journal of Nutrition and Health, 2*(2), 1–13.

Rane, B. R., Bharath, M. S., Patil, R. R., Keservani, R. K., & Jain, A. S. (2020b). Novel approaches in nutraceuticals. In R. K. Kesharwani, R. K. Keservani, & A. K. Sharma (Eds.), *Enhancing the Therapeutic Efficacy of Herbal Formulations through Novel Drug Delivery Systems* (pp. 241–266). IGI Global. ISBN: 9781799844532.

Rane, B. R., Patil, A. S., Keservani, R. K., & Jain, A. S. (2020a). Novel approaches in herbal formulation. In R. K. Kesharwani, R. K. Keservani, & A. K. Sharma (Eds.), *Enhancing the Therapeutic Efficacy of Herbal Formulations through Novel Drug Delivery Systems* (pp. 43–68). IGI Global. ISBN: 9781799844532.

Rane, B. R., Tadavi, S. A., & Keservani, R. K. (2020c). Naturopathy. In A. K. Sharma, R. K. Keservani, & S. P. Gautam (Eds.), Herbal Product Development (pp. 321–347). Apple Academic Press, CRC Press, Taylor & Francis Group. ISBN: 9781771888776.

Rayalam, S., Yang, J. Y., Ambati, S., Della-Fera, M. A., & Baile, C. A. (2008). Resveratrol induces apoptosis and inhibits adipogenesis in 3T3-L1 adipocytes. Phytotherapy Research:

International Journal of Pharmacology, Toxicology and Evaluation of Natural Products Derivatives, 22(10), 1367–1371.
Rosen, E. D., Walkey, C. J., Puigserver, P., & Spiegelman, B. M. (2000). Transcriptional regulation of adipogenesis. Genes & Development, 14(11), 1293–1307.
Ross, S. E., Hemati, N., Longo, K. A., Bennett, C. N., Lucas, P. C., Erickson, R. L., & MacDougald, O. A. (2000). Inhibition of adipogenesis by Wnt signaling. Science, 289(5481), 950–953.
Rtveladze, K., Marsh, T., Barquera, S., Romero, L. M. S., Levy, D., Melendez, G., & Brown, M. (2014). Obesity prevalence in Mexico: impact on health and economic burden. Journal of Public Health Nutrition, 17(1), 233–239. doi: 10.1017/S1368980013000086.
Ruchi, S. (2017). Role of nutraceuticals in health care: A review. International Journal of Green Pharmacy, 11(03), S385–S394.
Schwartz, M. W. (2012). An inconvenient truth about obesity. Molecular Metabolism, 1(1–2), 2–4.
Sekiya, M., Yahagi, N., Matsuzaka, T., Najima, Y., Nakakuki, M., Nagai, R., & Shimano, H. (2003). Polyunsaturated fatty acids ameliorate hepatic steatosis in obese mice by SREBP-1 suppression. Hepatology, 38(6), 1529–1539.
Seo, Y. S., Kang, O. H., Kim, S. B., Mun, S. H., Kang, D. H., Yang, D. W., & Kwon, D. Y. (2015). Quercetin prevents adipogenesis by regulating transcriptional factors and lipases in OP9 cells. International Journal of Molecular Medicine, 35(6), 1779–1785.
Singh, J., & Sinha, S. (2012). Classification, regulatory acts, and applications of nutraceuticals for health. International Journal of Pharma and Bio Sciences, 2(1), 177–187.
Siriwardhana, N., Kalupahana, N. S., Cekanova, M., LeMieux, M., Greer, B., & Moustaid-Moussa, N. (2013). Modulation of adipose tissue inflammation by bioactive food compounds. Journal of Nutritional Biochemistry, 24(4), 613–623.
Slavin, J. L. (2005). Dietary fiber and body weight. Nutrition, 21(3), 411–418. doi: 10.1016/j.nut.2004.08.018.
Sofowora, A., Ogunbodede, E., & Onayade, A. (2013). The role and place of medicinal plants in the strategies for disease prevention. African Journal of Traditional, Complementary and Alternative Medicines, 10(5), 210–229.
Sohn, J. W., Xu, Y., Jones, J. E., Wickman, K., Williams, K. W., & Elmquist, J. K. (2011). The Serotonin 2C receptor activates a distinct population of arcuate pro-opiomelanocortin neurons via TRPC channels. Neuron, 71(3), 488–497.
Spiegelman, B. M., Hu, E., Kim, J. B., & Brun, R. (1997). PPARγ and the control of adipogenesis. Biochimie, 79(2–3), 111–112.
Stevanato, J., Bertolla, R. P., Barradas, V., Spaine, D. M., Cedenho, A. P., & Ortiz, V. (2008). Semen processing by density gradient centrifugation does not improve sperm apoptotic deoxyribonucleic acid fragmentation rates. Fertility and Sterility, 90(3), 889–890.
Swinburn, B. A., Sacks, G., Hall, K. D., McPherson, K., Finegood, D. T., Moodie, M. L., & Gortmaker, S. L. (2011). The global obesity pandemic: shaped by global drivers and local environments. The Lancet, 378(9793), 804–814.
Terpstra, A. H. M., Javadi, M., Beynen, A. C., Kocsis, S., Lankhorst, A. E., Lemmens, A. G., & Mohede, I. C. M. (2003). Dietary conjugated linoleic acids as free fatty acids and triacylglycerols similarly affect body composition and energy balance in mice. Journal of Nutrition, 133(10), 3181–3186.

Trials.gov C. (2003–2020). Investigating the use of quercetin on glucose absorption in obesity, and obesity with type 2 diabetes. Retrieved from: http://clinicaltrials.gov/show/NCT00065676 (accessed on 15 June 2024).

Tseng, Y. H., Cypess, A. M., & Kahn, C. R. (2010). Cellular bioenergetics as a target for obesity therapy. Nature Reviews Drug Discovery, 9(6), 465–482.

Tsujita, T., Takaichi, H., Takaku, T., Aoyama, S., & Hiraki, J. (2006). Antiobesity action of ε-polylysine, a potent inhibitor of pancreatic lipase. Journal of Lipid Research, 47(8), 1852–1858.

Vitalone, A., Di Sotto, A., Mammola, C. L., Heyn, R., Miglietta, S., Mariani, P., & Mazzanti, G. (2017). Phytochemical analysis and effects on ingestive behavior of a Caralluma fimbriata extract. Food and Chemical Toxicology, 108, 63–73.

Wang, S., Moustaid-Moussa, N., Chen, L., Mo, H., Shastri, A., Su, R., & Shen, C. L. (2014). Novel insights of dietary polyphenols and obesity. Journal of Nutritional Biochemistry, 25(1), 1–18.

Wang, Y. C., McPherson, K., Marsh, T., Gortmaker, S. L., & Brown, M. (2011). Health and economic burden of the projected obesity trends in the USA and the UK. The Lancet, 378(9793), 815–825. doi: 10.1016/S0140-6736(11)60814-3.

Wang, Y., Chen, H. J., Shaikh, S., & Mathur, P. (2009). Is obesity becoming a public health problem in India? Examine the shift from under to overnutrition problems over time. *Obesity Reviews, 10*(4), 456–474.

Weaver, C. M., Alekel, D. L., Ward, W. E., & Ronis, M. J. (2012). Flavonoid intake and bone health. *Journal of Nutrition in Gerontology and Geriatrics, 31*(3), 239–253.

Wendel, A. A., Purushotham, A., Liu, L. F., & Belury, M. A. (2009). Conjugated linoleic acid induces uncoupling protein 1 in white adipose tissue of ob/ob mice. *Lipids, 44*(11), 975–982.

Wolfgang, M. J., & Lane, M. D. (2011). Hypothalamic malonyl-CoA and CPT1c in the treatment of obesity. *FEBS Journal, 278*(4), 552–558.

Wood, R. J., Fernandez, M. L., Sharman, M. J., Silvestre, R., Greene, C. M., Zern, T. L., & Volek, J. S. (2007). Effects of a carbohydrate-restricted diet with and without supplemental soluble fiber on plasma low-density lipoprotein cholesterol and other clinical markers of cardiovascular risk. *Metabolism, 56*(1), 58–67.

Yang, C. S., Zhang, J., Zhang, L., Huang, J., & Wang, Y. (2016). Mechanisms of body weight reduction and metabolic syndrome alleviation by tea. *Molecular Nutrition & Food Research, 60*(1), 160–174.

Zhai, X., Lin, D., Zhao, Y., Li, W., & Yang, X. (2018). Enhanced anti-obesity effects of bacterial cellulose combined with konjac glucomannan in high-fat diet-fed C57BL/6J mice. *Food & Function, 9*(10), 5260–5272.

CHAPTER 2

SUPPLEMENTATION OF NUTRIENTS FOR WEIGHT LOSS

ANURAG VERMA, PIYUSH MITTAL, PRIYANSHA JAIN, and POORVI JAIN

Teerthanker Mahaveer College of Pharmacy, Teerthanker Mahaveer University, Moradabad, Uttar Pradesh, India

ABSTRACT

These days, obesity is a medical condition that raises the risk of several illnesses, including heart disease, diabetes, high blood pressure, and some malignancies. Besides the above, obesity also negatively impacts educational outcomes and reduces employment and workers' productivity. The problem of obesity can be solved by changing one's lifestyle, which includes eating healthier, consuming fewer calories, and exercising more. However, altering one's diet and way of life can be challenging; many people turn to dietary supplements, which are advertised as aids in weight loss, in the hopes that these items will make it easier for them to reach their objectives. Dietary supplements that help weight loss can include a wide range of compounds that are produced from plants, animals, or minerals. The claims made by the manufacturers of these products are that they enhance metabolism and thermogenesis while decreasing hunger, body fat, and weight by absorption of macronutrients. The current chapter reviews the effect of some most commonly and frequently used naturally occurring substances, along with their mechanism of action, in controlling the menace of obesity.

Nutraceuticals in Obesity Management and Control. Raj K. Keservani & Alka Lohani (Eds.)

2.1 INTRODUCTION

Overweight or obese refers to a person's weight that is greater than what is deemed healthy for their height. Body weight is caused by a variety of variables, including poor dietary choices, metabolism, heredity, overeating, and culture (Gavin et al., 2010). Obesity is connected to a variety of health issues and disorders, including diabetes, cardiovascular disease, some cancers, and stroke. Numerous epidemiological studies have demonstrated a high prevalence of cardiovascular mortality and complications in individuals with obesity, metabolic syndrome, T2DM (Okamura et al., 2019), and hypertension (Mariani et al., 2012). Clinical guidelines have set strict targets for blood pressure, dyslipidemia, and glycemia control for "risk groups" inclined to target organ damage; however, clinical trials and actual proof suggest that these targets are challenging to achieve and maintain. Weight loss is the primary recommendation for obesity and its related conditions. Recent decades have seen a significant rise in the prevalence of obesity across different age groups, which results from receiving more energy than one is using. Additionally, the greatest preventive cause of death is obesity. Even though these illnesses can have detrimental effects on one's health, there are now more overweight and obese people than ever before. In fact, most regions of the world consider obesity to be a modern epidemic. Since 1975, global obesity has roughly tripled. The World Health Organization (WHO) estimates that 1.9 billion people under the age of 18 were overweight (39%) and 650 million of them (13%) were obese in 2016.

One of the most widely used metrics to assess obesity is body mass index or BMI. It is calculated by dividing a person's weight (in kg) by their height (in meters) squared. A body mass index of 30 kg/m^2 or higher indicates obesity, while a BMI of 25 to 30 kg/m^2 indicates overweight.

2.1.1 GLOBAL OBESITY PREVALENCE

The 10 Most Obese Countries in the World – the Cook Islands is the most obese nation in terms of average BMI, with a BMI of 32.9. Nauru comes in second with 32.5, followed by Niue with 32.4. Both Samoa and Tonga possess average BMIs of 32.2. Tuvalu (30.8), Kiribati (30.1), Saint Lucia (30.0), Micronesia (29.7), and Egypt round out the top 10 most obese countries (29.6). The South Pacific is shared by eight of these countries.

The 10 Least Obese Countries in the World – Eritrea, Madagascar, and Ethiopia all rank among the least obese nations on the planet in terms of average BMI, each having a BMI of 21.1. Japan (21.8), Burundi (21.6), Timor-Leste (21.3), China, and India (21.9) are the five other countries with average BMIs less than 22. The ranking is completed by Bangladesh (22.0) and Burkina Faso (22.1) (World Population Review, 2022).

2.2 WAYS OF WEIGHT LOSS

Eating healthy foods, reducing calories, and being physically active are all tried and true methods for losing weight. Making these lifestyle adjustments, however, is difficult, so you may wonder if using a weight reduction dietary supplement (Keservani et al., 2020) could assist. The supplement sector has primarily concentrated on dosage extracts of thermogenic or metabolic herbs. In order to lose weight, dietary supplements have been used for two reasons: (a) to supplement any nutrients that might be missing from a constrained diet; and (b) because of their capability to accelerate weight loss. Planning a diet for weight loss should aim to ensure that total nutrient intake via meals and additions complies with dietary recommendations for optimal consumption levels while not considerably surpassing them for any nutrients apart from energy. If the reducing diet's nutrient intake via protein sources is insufficient, nutritional supplements (Keservani et al., 2010a, b, 2017, 2020) using one element or a vitamin supplement complex may be beneficial (WHO fact sheets). These medicines decrease hunger, provide short-term energy boosts, and may alter glucose metabolism. Caffeine, pseudoephedrine, and phenylephrine are commonly found in these products.

There are many different weight loss programs, each with its own subcategories and commercial plans. The majority focus on a certain range of macronutrients and typically entail some kind of calorie restriction. Due to the problematic loss of lean body mass associated with conventional weight loss procedures, recent weight reduction research has concentrated on body composition alterations in addition to overall weight loss (Dwyer et al., 2005).

Weight loss medications are classified as either those that suppress appetite (such as diethylpropion and phentermine) or those that block calorie absorption (orlistat). For weight loss, serotonin and norepinephrine reuptake inhibitors (bupropion and fluoxetine), sympathomimetic agents (diethylpropion), GABAergic agents (topiramate), and cannabinoid antagonists have all been used (rimonabant). Appetite-suppressing drugs typically have an impact on the CNS's appetite centers and may also cause headaches, nervousness, excitability, insomnia, mood swings, and mood changes. Other gastrointestinal side effects of drugs that affect nutrient absorption include diarrhea, flatulence, and abdominal bloating. All of the currently approved weight-loss medications are unlikely to cause liver damage but serious hepatotoxicity has been associated with several over-the-counter and weight-loss supplements (Koithan et al., 2010).

Historically, plants have been a reliable source of cutting-edge potential and all-natural treatments for illnesses, including body weight management products. Although the proportion of the use of botanicals and nutraceuticals is unknown, a study conducted in 6 European nations found that, with the exception of herbal products, 18.8% of the 2,358 consumers chosen for this research have used one or more dietary supplements. Around 9.6% of people in Finland, Germany (16.9%), Italy (22.7%), Romania (17.9%), Spain (18.0%), and the United Kingdom (19.1%) were consumers of plant food supplements (Willoughby et al., 2018).

2.3 CONJUGATED LINOLEIC ACID

Conjugated linoleic acid (CLA) consists of a polyunsaturated fatty acid with distinct characteristics (Alvarez et al., 2014) So far, at least 28 CLA isomers have been identified, each defined by two conjugated double bonds in distinct geometric and positional places. CLA has been examined in rats, mice, pigs, chickens, and hamsters to see how it affects body composition. CLAs are derived from the biohydrogenation of linoleic acid by bacteria that express linoleic acid isomerase, which includes many ruminant microorganisms. All of these studies reveal a decrease in body fat and an increase in lean body mass (Bethesda, 2012).

CLA, which was originally classified as an anti-carcinogenic fatty acid, has now been proven to have anti-atherosclerotic capabilities in addition to its anti-obesogenic benefits (Alvarez et al., 2014) CLA is found naturally in ruminant foods such as lamb, and beef, and butter, and dairy products (Thom et al., 2001) CLA supplementation may improve immunological function, aid in glycogen resynthesis, and increase bone mineralization. CLA supplementation may potentially promote lipolysis and decrease fatty acid build-up in adipose tissue. However, studies in humans have shown some advantages to taking CLA supplements for fat loss, although the outcomes are still unclear (Hartigh, 2019).

In studies with a shorter length than eight weeks, CLA supplementation may be able to lower circulating leptin levels, particularly in overweight and male patients (Lehnen et al., 2015).

The potential mechanisms by which CLA alters body composition include metabolic adjustments that favor a decrease in lipogenesis and an upregulation of lipolysis, along with the oxidation of fatty acids in skeletal muscle, as a result of increased carnitine palmitoyl transferase-1 activity and action or perhaps due to the inhibition of adipocyte differentiation.

2.4 SPIRULINA POWDER

The blue-green algae spirulina is a fantastic source of proteins, vitamins, and antioxidants (Figure 2.1). In 1 M HCl medium, the effectiveness of *Sunova spirulina* powder as a green corrosion inhibitor against mild steel was assessed. *S. platensis* is a member of the Oscillatoriaceae family, which possesses numerous medicinal qualities like hypocholesterolemia, immunological, antiviral, and antimutagenic capabilities. This alga is said to include amino acids including methionine and c-linoleic acid, as well as peptides, proteins, carbohydrates, and phycocyanins. In particular, the manufacture of nutraceuticals uses *S. platensis* as an antioxidant (Haghighatdoosp et al., 2018).

This alga is a crucial component of the human diet and has been utilized in humans as a safe source of additional high-quality protein. Additionally, having a high protein content (up to 70%), vitamins including B12 and provitamin A (β-carotenes), and minerals, particularly iron, are also present. Spirulina's lack of cellulose cell walls makes it simple to digest (Kamal et al., 2012).

Numerous toxicological studies have confirmed spirulina's safety. Spirulina is currently one of the substances that the US Food and Drug Administration has designated as Generally Recognized as Safe (GRAS). *Spirulina* is relatively simple to grow, however, it grows best in alkaline lakes with exceptionally high pH levels and huge outside ponds under regulated conditions. With "extraordinary components" that help create high energy levels, spirulina has been hailed as "the meal of the future."

Although spirulina can be used to reduce cholesterol, its value as a nutritious food supplement for treating hyperlipidemia should not be overlooked when used in conjunction with other therapeutic measures (Haghighatdoosp et al., 2018).

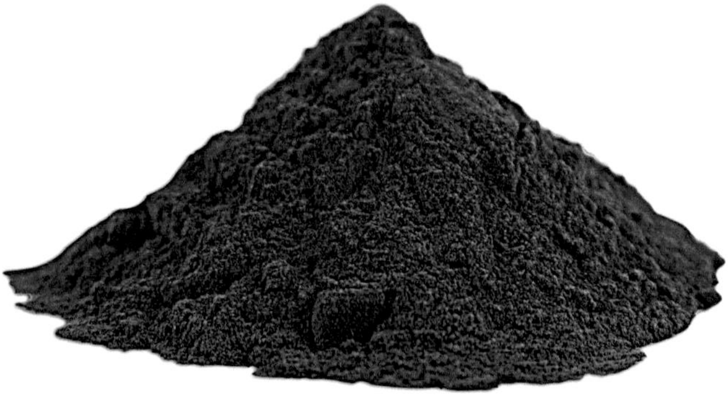

FIGURE 2.1 Spirulina.

Image credit: Music4thekids. https://creativecommons.org/licenses/by-sa/3.0/

2.5 *COLEUS FORSKOHLII*

Forskohlii Coleus, synonym *Plectranthus barbatus*, is a well-known medicinal plant from the Lamiaceae family and order Lamiales. *C. forskohlii* is thought to have originated in the Indian subcontinent (Figure 2.2). In India, Nepal, Burma, Sri Lanka, and Thailand's subtropical temperate climates, it naturally flourishes (Karkos, 2010).

Bronchitis, asthma, hay fever, angina, and stomach disorders are just a few of the conditions that can be treated with the use of leaf and root extracts.

Forskolin, a key metabolite found solely within cork cells of the root of *C. forskohlii*, is used commercially to treat glaucoma, asthma, and various heart problems. Additionally, the plant's essential oil with its antimicrobial qualities is derived from its tubers (Mitra et al., 2020).

Three-phase partitioning (TPP), a method that relies on the fragmentation of proteins, lipophobic parts, and lipophilic parts in three phases composed of H_2O, $(NH_4)_2SO_4$, and organic solvent, has been investigated for the purpose of extracting the diterpene forskolin from *Coleus forskohlii* roots.

The procedure that involves adding t-butanol and ammonium sulfate to the aquatic slurry of *C. forskohlii* roots at the same time has been optimized with regard to the proportion of t-butanol to the slurry and the quantity of ammonium sulfate injection (Harde et al., 2012).

According to Henderson et al. (2005), *C. forskohlii* appears to have no clinically relevant adverse effects but may help overweight females avoid gaining weight instead of promoting weight loss. When *C. forskohlii* extracts were administered to ovariectomized rats, body weight, food intake, and fat buildup decreased, indicating that *C. forskohlii* might be effective in the treatment of obesity (Kavitha et al., 2010).

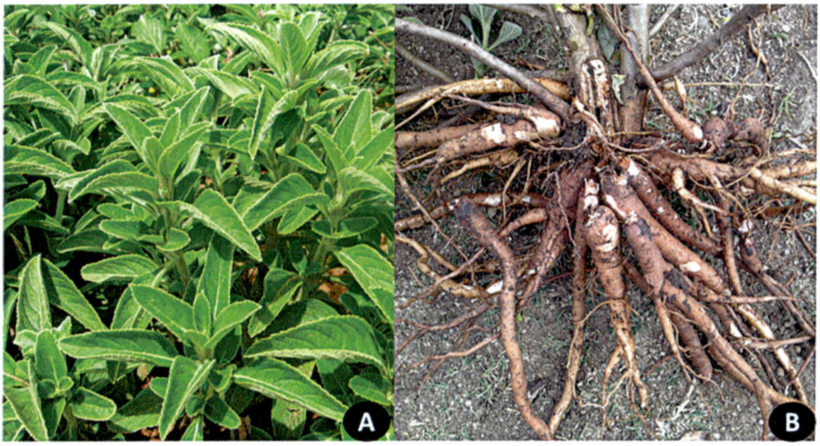

FIGURE 2.2 *Coleus forskohlii* plant and root.

Source: Majeed et al., 2021. Copyright: © 2021 by the authors.Licensee MDPI, Basel, Switzerland. https://creativecommons.org/licenses/by/4.0/

2.6 *IRVINGIA GABONENSIS*

African Mango, or *Irvingia gabonensis* (Aubry-Le Comte ex O'Rorke) Bail, is a part of the Irvingiaceae family (Figure 2.3). Other popular names for it are bread tree, African wild mango, wild mango, and bush mango. It is also known locally as goron or biri, Apon (Yoruba, Southwest Nigeria), Ogbono (Igbo, Southeast Nigeria), and Yoruba (Southwest Nigeria; in Hausa, Northern Nigeria).

According to reports, *Irvingia gabonensis* seeds provide medical and nutritional benefits, including antidiabetic, weight-loss, antihyperlipidemic, and antioxidant properties. The ongoing fall in physical activity is one of the many factors contributing to overweight and obesity (Olorundare et al., 2020).

Similar to other types of water-soluble dietary fibers, the fiber found in *Irvingia gabonensis* seed is a bulk-forming laxative. *Irvingia gabonensis* seeds slow abdomen evacuation, resulting in more gradual sugar absorption, which can lessen the regular post-meal rise in blood sugar levels. *Irvingia gabonensis* seed fiber, like other soluble fibers, binds to bile acids in the gut and conveys them out of the body through feces, necessitating the body to increase the conversion of cholesterol into bile acids.

Given that *Irvingia gabonensis* is commonly used in Cameroonian cuisine, increased promotion of its use for dietary cholesterol control and weight loss goals is necessary (Ngondi et al., 2005).

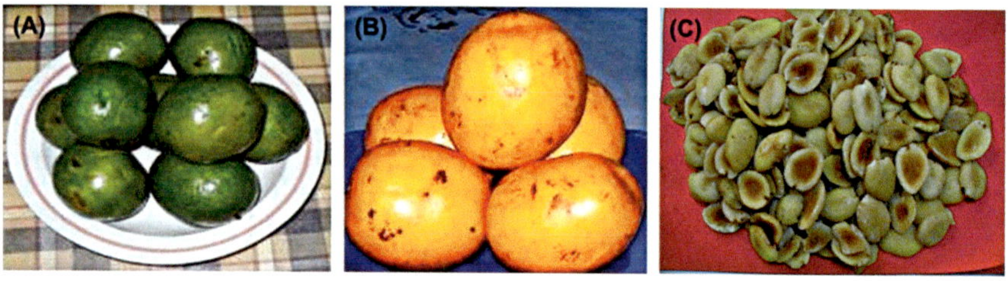

FIGURE 2.3 *Irvingia gabonensis* fruits and seeds.

Source: Reprinted with permission from Preedy et al., 2011. Copyright © 2011 Elsevier Inc.

2.7 *GARCINIA CAMBOGIA*

The fruit of the Malabar tamarind tree, also known as *Garcinia gummi-gutta*, which is indigenous to Nepal, India, and Sri Lanka, is the source of the herbal supplement *Garcinia cambogia* (Figure 2.4; National Institute of Diabetes and Digestive and Kidney Diseases, 2019).

Garcinia cambogia is a high calcium source, of thiamine, phosphorus, riboflavin, iron, and niacin, and each of these compounds has been linked to the health benefits of *Garcinia cambogia* (Landim et al., 2018).

Garcinia cambogia has recently been promoted as an appetite suppressant that aids in weight loss. Xanthones, benzophenones, amino acids, and organic acids are among the chemicals found in Garcinia extracts, but hydroxy citric acid (HCA), the substance thought to be responsible for the extract's anti-inflammatory and appetite-suppressing effects, is the most significant. Garcinia fruit contains 10% to 30% HCA, and HCA inhibits ATP citrate lyase, an enzyme involved in the synthesis of fatty acids. Although HCA and Garcinia derivatives have been demonstrated to lessen hunger and encourage weight reduction in rats, there is conflicting evidence regarding their effects on humans (Figure 2.5; National Institute of Diabetes and Digestive and Kidney Diseases, 2019).

Garcinia cambogia may act as an appetite suppressant, making meals more filling and satisfying. Hydroxy citric acid can help to reduce citrate lyase levels in the body, which is an enzyme that aids in the formation of fat cells from dietary carbohydrates. As a result, Dr. Oz promoted *Garcinia cambogia* as a fantastic aid in weight loss in 2012, and consumer demand for it has skyrocketed. The vast majority of studies recommend taking the supplement about 1 hour before meals. It has also been demonstrated that splitting HCA doses is more efficient than administering the same quantity as a single dose (Andueza et al., 2021).

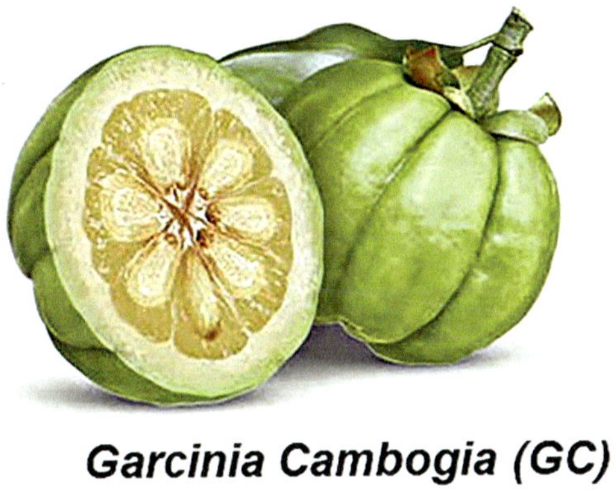

FIGURE 2.4 *Garcinia cambogia* fruits.

Source: Reprinted from Hanse et al., 2023.

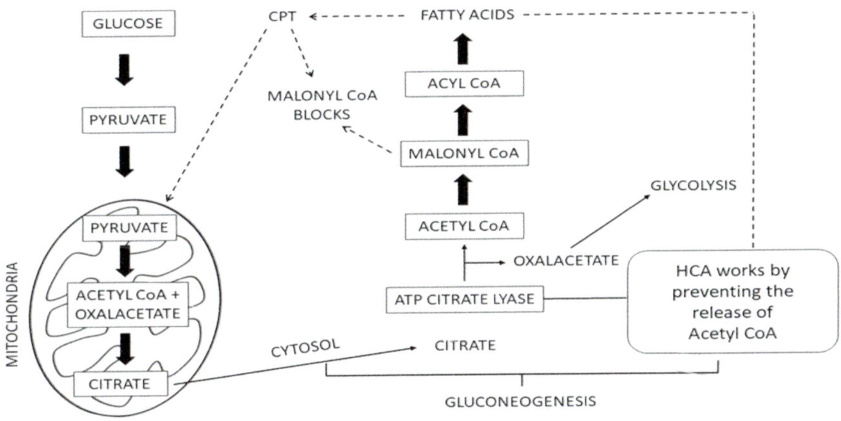

FIGURE 2.5 Hydroxycitric acid (HCA) – mechanism of action [CPT: Carnitine palmitoyl transferase].

Source: Adapted from Andueza et al., 2021

In recent studies conducted, it was observed that in patients with overweight or obesity, administration of GC and GNN reduces weight and enhances lipid and glucose blood profiles, though the presence of polymorphisms PLIN4, FTO, and ADRB3 may partially offset these effects (Landim et al., 2018). Numerous human studies have established the safety of garcinia-based supplements, but an increase in cases reporting serious side effects, primarily linked to liver damage and to a minimal extent, serotonin toxicity and mania, may cause researchers to reevaluate these products' safety profile. It should be emphasized that although HCA has usually been cited as the primary component generating the harmful effects of Garcinia pills. *Garcinia cambogia* fruit has been consumed for centuries in Southeast Asia and is a significant source of HCA. It is generally regarded as safe (Stohs et al., 2009; Haber et al., 2018). Many Garcinia supplements contain a large number of ingredients. As a result, the toxicity cannot be causally linked to Garcinia, and drawing conclusions is challenging without raising questions or concerns. Additionally, it is impossible to rule out the possibility of any negative effects brought on by taking the Garcinia supplementation with other nutritional supplements or even with various drugs that the user takes (Andueza et al., 2021).

2.8 CHROMIUM PINCOLATE

Chromium is a trace element that is required for protein, carbohydrate, and fat metabolism. Chromium supplementation significantly improved overall health, insulin sensitivity, and glucose metabolism in human trials. An essential cofactor for insulin's function is chromium (Drake et al., 2012).

It is widely believed that chromium influences weight reduction by reducing body composition, improving insulin sensitivity, and influencing neurotransmitters that control mood, eating habits, and food cravings. Some people may experience weight loss and an improved body composition as a result of chromium, as well as improvements in blood lipid levels, impaired glucose tolerance, and impaired body composition.

2.9 CURCUMIN (TURMERIC)

Continuous work is being done to identify and assess natural substances for weight loss that have few negative effects. Curcumin (1,7-bis(4-hydroxy-3-methoxyphenyl)-1,6-heptadien-3,5-dione), the polyphenolic active component of the spice turmeric (Curcuma longa L.), a member of the ginger family (Zingiberaceae), is one such chemical (Kasprzak et al., 2022).

The most significant curcuminoid to be extracted from plant rhizomes is curcumin, a polyphenolic substance.

An indigenous of Southeast Asia, turmeric is a member of the ginger family and is largely farmed there for commercial purposes in India. Traditional medicines and food both use the rhizome, or subterranean stem, of the plant (Figure 2.6; Kasprzak et al., 2022).

Curcumin has been demonstrated to be efficient in boosting weight reduction and lowering the prevalence of disorders linked to obesity, according to experimental data. Phytochemicals (Keservani & Sharma, 2014) with anti-inflammatory properties like curcumin are being thoroughly studied in light of the finding that obesity is differentiated by persistent low-grade metabolic inflammation. Curcumin directly interacts with white adipose tissue, according to recent scientific studies, to reduce chronic inflammation. Curcumin prevents inflammatory agents' induction of nuclear factor κb (NF-κB) and macrophage infiltration in adipose tissue. The potent proinflammatory adipokines tumor necrosis factor-α (TNF-α), plasminogen activator inhibitor type 1 (PAI-1), and monocyte chemoattractant protein-1 (MCP-1) are all decreased by curcumin and adiponectin, the main adipocyte-secreted anti-inflammatory protein, is increased (Peter, 2013).

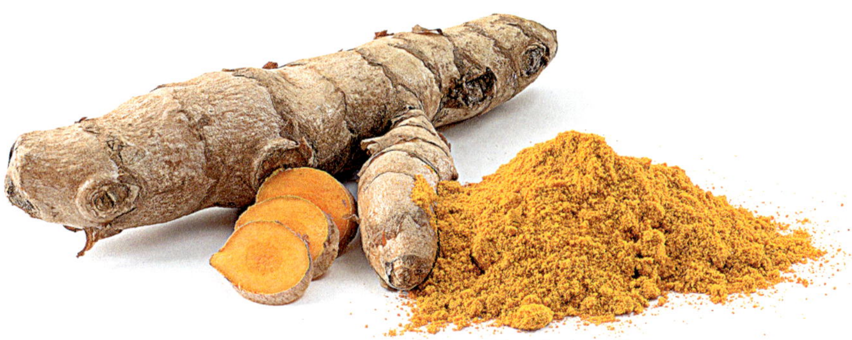

FIGURE 2.6 Turmeric rhizome and powder.

Image credit: Simon A. Eugster. https://creativecommons.org/licenses/by-sa/3.0/deed.en

2.10 FIBER COMPLEX

Proteins and dietary fiber aid in the binding of fat, lowering the intake of dietary fat, and as a result, weight loss (Kumar et al., 2013). IQP G-002AS, a natural fiber complex made from Opuntia ficus-indica and enhanced with extra soluble fiber, has the ability to bind fat. The lipophilic activity of IQP G-002AS has been standardized, and studies have shown that it lowers dietary fat absorption by GI fat binding. In order to prevent dietary fat from being absorbed by the intestine and being excreted, the lipophilic IQP G-002AS binds to it. It has been shown to lower the amount of dietary fat absorbed and increase fecal fat excretion, which lowers the amount of calories the body absorbs from the diet and promotes weight loss (Bakre, 2009). According to a randomized, double-blind, placebo-controlled experiment including obese patients, IQP-AE-103 is a reliable and secure weight reduction treatment (Uebelhack et al., 2019). With a standard deviation of 2.4 kg between trial groups, IQ-treated participants dropped considerably more body composition than placebo; 35.4% of IQ-treated individuals lost at least 5% of their starting body weight. This result may have clinical significance as it decreased the likelihood of metabolic syndrome (as determined by the Adult Treatment Panel III criteria of the National Cholesterol Education Program) by 59% when 5% or more of the initial body weight was lost (Phelam et al., 2007; Grube et al., 2013).

2.11 WHITE KIDNEY BEAN

Phaseolus vulgaris L., sometimes known as white kidney beans or common beans, is a species that evolved in South American nations like Mexico and Argentina (Figure 2.7). PVE derivatives, extracts, and components have been shown to significantly reduce appetite, carbohydrate metabolism, weight gain, lipid accumulation, food intake, glycated hemoglobin, and blood sugar absorption, as well as gut microbiota regulation in both thin and obese animals following acute or chronic administration (Wang & Chen, 2020). There are currently a number of commercially marketed white kidney bean extracts (WKBEs) that are said to contain significant levels of α-amylase inhibitors obtained from white kidney beans. These WKBEs are frequently offered in powder form, making it possible to encapsulate or include them in meals (Nolan et al., 2020). These supplements assert that by inhibiting the enzyme α-amylase, they can decrease the absorption and digestion of carbohydrates, improving metabolic health and body weight.

Obesity-related oxidative stress is a crucial modulator of how obesity affects health outcomes and the onset of co-morbidities (Manna & Jain, 2015). A constrained number of creatures have explored the effects of WKBE organization on the markers of oxidative push (Uebelhack et al., 2019). Although nicotinamide adenine dinucleotide hydrogen (NADH) dehydrogenase was not enhanced, WKBE anticipated lipid penetration inside the aortic tissue and raised the levels of two myocardial antioxidant compounds, peroxide synthase, and reduced glutathione. There was also a trend toward a reduction in elevated diet-induced peptide carbonylation as a biomarker of myocardial oxidative strain, despite the fact that this was not objectively significant (Nolan et al., 2020) Significant amounts of peptides, including the α-amylase antagonist phaseolin, polyphenols, exopolysaccharides, and lectins are present in white kidney beans. Moreover, they contain a lot of carbohydrates (39–47% of seed weight) and proteins (22–27% of seed weight). Interestingly, the high concentration of lectins raised some questions because, in addition to their potential anti-cancer and anti-obesity effects, these peptides may potentially have toxic and allergic effects (Kumar et al., 2013; He et al., 2018). There are numerous reports about clinical side effects following consumption of white kidney beans (Nciri et al., 2015). Phaseolin is an α-amylase inhibitor (α-AI) that can bind to α-amylase non-covalently and prevent the degradation of complex carbohydrates, which reduces the uptake of such nutrients through the gut wall. PVE has been developed to separate the activity of phaseolin (Layer et al., 1985; Barrett, 2011). PVE is known for its antioxidant, anti-inflammatory, anticarcinogenic, cardioprotective, glucose-lowering, and possibly weight-loss qualities (Ganesan, 2017; Obiro et al., 2008; Oseguera et al., 2011). Notably, a number of PVE products have been created to maximize α-AI activity, which is extremely reliant on temperature, pH, incubation period, and the presence of certain elements, such as Phase2® aqueous extracts of Phaseolus vulgaris calibrated to alpha-amylase (8; 12; 15; 39) inhibitory units. Barrett et al. carefully examined 10 trials between 2000 and 2010 investigating the impact of Phase 2® products on body mass and glycemic management in people with overweight and obesity and found that the product significantly reduced weight when taken along with meals high in carbohydrates (Santimone et al., 2004; Udani et al., 2018). PVE supplementation might be promoted as a weight-reduction aid (Mikiko et al., 2020).

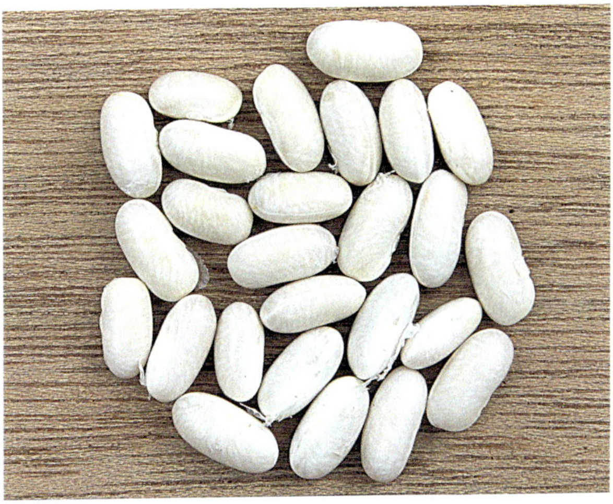

FIGURE 2.7 White kidney beans.

Image credit: Rasbak. https://creativecommons.org/licenses/by-sa/3.0/

2.12 GINSENG

For more than 1,000 years, Asian nations like Korea, China, and Japan have utilized ginseng (the root of *Panax ginseng* Meyer, Araliaceae) as a general tonic to promote health (Figure 2.8; Nuri et al., 2016). Ginsenosides, also known as steroid saponins, are present in ginseng extracts and are thought to have the pharmacological characteristics of ginseng (Dong-Hyun, 2012). Inflammation, immunity, and cancer have all been reported to be affected by the pharmacological actions of ginseng extracts and ginsenosides (Joh et al., 2011; Chang et al., 2003; Cang et al., 2012). There have also been reports of ginseng's impact on metabolic diseases like hypertension, diabetes, hyperlipidemia, and obesity (Gu et al., 2013; Lee et al., 2009; Seohee et al., 2011; So Young Hong et al., 2012; Matt et al., 2013). The gut microbiota is one of the main etiological variables that affect body weight control, thus medications or other substances that support the balance of the gut microbiota's composition can have an increased anti-obesity effect (Song et al., 2014). Though ginseng has been shown to have anti-obesity properties, its impact on the gut microbiota is still unknown (Han et al., 2005).

Because of its high saponin content, ginseng is thought to aid in weight loss by slowing intestinal dietary fat absorption by suppressing pancreatic lipase activity (Liu et al., 2008; Kwon et al., 2012). In addition, obese mice given Korean ginseng extract (8–18 g/kg) for 8 weeks demonstrated that its use could affect leptin, adiponectin, and ghrelin blood levels (Watanabe et al., 2020).

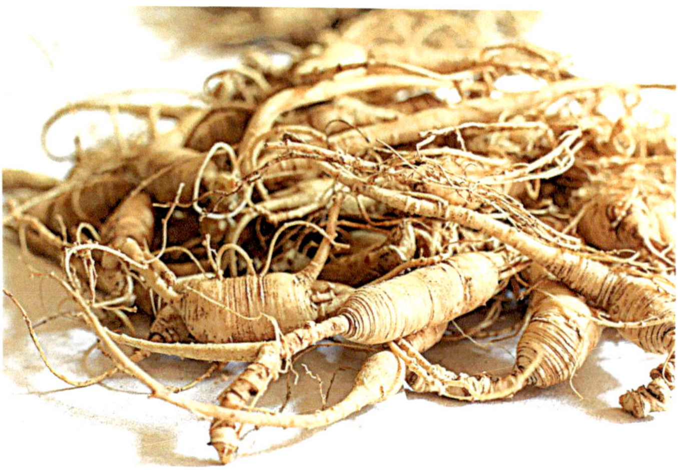

FIGURE 2.8 Ginseng roots.

Image credit: Priya Jaishanker. https://creativecommons.org/licenses/by-nd/2.0/

24 obese women were given 18 g of Korean red ginseng (KRG) for 8 weeks as part of a randomized controlled trial. The results show a reduction in BMI, food intake, aspartate aminotransferase, and improved quality of life (Woolston, 2012).

As a result of the low evidence quality and wide dose range (100 mg–18 g/day) supporting ginseng's usage as a weight reduction aid, the clinical value of the herb is yet unknown.

2.13 CAFFEINE

Caffeine is the most widely used stimulant and a xanthine alkaloid. It is abundant in nature and can be extracted from the foliage, seeds, and berries of many different plants (Ishak et al., 2012). The well-known plant sources for caffeine are yerba mate, kola nuts, guarana, tea leaves, and coffee seeds (Figure 2.9; Mattioli et al., 2017). Although caffeine is toxic in high doses, regular, moderate consumption has more positive effects than negative ones (Davoodi et al., 2014). Caffeine has a diuretic effect in addition to being a centrally active stimulant (Kennedy et al., 2008). As a result, it might encourage water loss. When treating edema or losing water weight, this effect is necessary, but it can also lead to dehydration.

Frequent consumption of large amounts of caffeine has the potential to convert resistance into cognitive and emotional dependence. Acute caffeine withdrawal can cause symptoms like irritation, loss of mental clarity, headache, sleeplessness, sleepiness, body aches, and gastrointestinal problems when dependence develops (Sung et al., 1990, 1995; Boekema et al., 1999; Pickering et al., 2019). These signs and symptoms could deteriorate and turn into anxiety, depression, motion sickness, and strong caffeine cravings (Kennedy et al., 2008).

To summarize the effects of caffeine consumption on weight reduction, a systematic review and meta-analysis of randomized controlled trials (RCTs) were conducted. The results showed that caffeine consumption may promote weight, BMI, and body fat reduction (Tabrizi et al., 2019).

Many studies focus on three main theories on fat loss mechanisms via caffeine intake, with the first being fat burning. The most frequently cited explanation for the weight loss that regular caffeine users experience is fat burning. Being thermogenic in nature, it is specifically known to promote the metabolism of fat and the mobilization of free fatty acids to produce the energy required to counteract the stimulatory effects it has on the body (Westerterp et al., 2005). Caffeine enhances epinephrine secretion, sharpens the mind, and lessens fatigue (Pickering et al., 2019). It uses fat instead of glycogen to burn off all of this energy. The second reason is appetite suppression; caffeine has also been shown to reduce appetite. Although it is unclear whether it will be sufficient to aid in weight loss, this effect is fleeting. Many studies also consider the diuretic effect of caffeine to be the source of the reduction of water weight in the body. However, some studies also focus on weight reduction due to decaffeinated coffee, which has shown modest results in weight reduction and further puts the role of caffeine in fat loss into question.

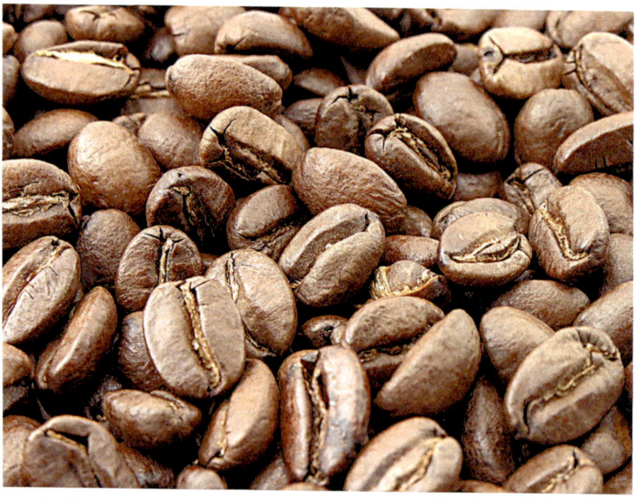

FIGURE 2.9 Coffee seeds.

Source: Public domain

2.14 GREEN TEA

Since ancient times, people have sipped on green tea, a naturally occurring product produced from the dried, unfermented leaves of the *Camellia sinensis* plant, as a social beverage and to sharpen their minds (Figure 2.10; Filippini et al., 2020). Epigallocatechin-3-gallate (EGCG), a type of catechin, and caffeine, the primary ingredient in tea, have been shown to have a wide range of biological effects, including the ability to reduce body weight, improve metabolic syndrome, prevent cancer, cardiovascular disease, and neurodegenerative diseases, among others (Yang et al., 2013). Recently, green tea concoctions have been utilized as a treatment for a variety of disorders, from osteoarthritis to weight reduction, along with preventive measures for cancer, despite the fact that the medical evidence for the bulk of the following conditions is inadequate or missing (Jurgens et al., 2012).

Green tea preparations can contain a wide range of chemicals, both in terms of type and quantity. The pharmacological activities of green tea preparations may be directly impacted by this variation in chemical composition. Therefore, it is crucial to understand the precise composition of the particular green tea preparation being tested when assessing trials on the effects of green tea on weight management (Rothenberg et al., 2018).

The literature extensively discusses how well green tea works to reduce body weight and fat. The vast majority of research, as per a recent analysis and meta-analysis, shows that green tea produced EGCG in varied doses (100–460 mg/day) demonstrates measurable weight-loss benefits, especially during trial durations of 3 or more months (Vazquez et al., 2017; Jurgens et al., 2012). Numerous studies have documented how green tea extract has positive effects on a person's health, including weight loss. In a randomized clinical trial, the patients who received green tea extract treatment showed significantly increased leptin levels and decreased LDL-C levels (Huang et al., 2018).

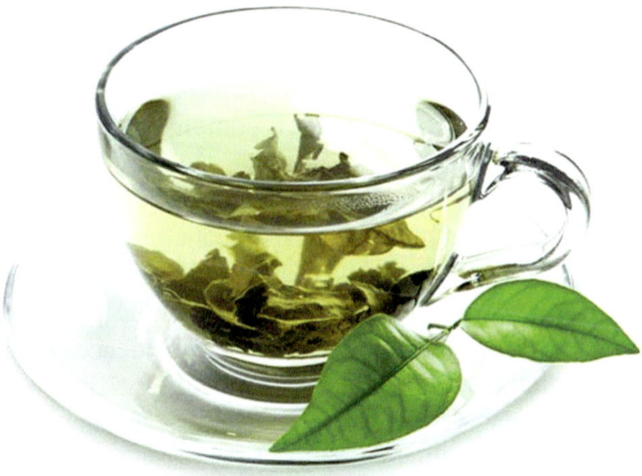

FIGURE 2.10 Green tea leaf extract.

Image credit: Toxic Free Foundation. https://thetoxicfreefoundation.com/database/ingredient/camellia-sinensis-green-tea-leaf-extract

2.15 DISCUSSION

Changing one's lifestyle, which includes eating a balanced diet, consuming fewer calories, and exercising regularly, is the key to attaining long-term weight loss, according to health experts. However, since altering one's diet and way of life may be challenging, many individuals resort to dietary supplements that are advertised as aids in weight reduction in the hopes that these items will make it easier for them to achieve their objectives. However, certain supplements have been linked to the possibility of bodily risk. It is determined that there is less information regarding whether weight reduction pills are useful. Consumers are drawn to the guarantee of taking something "natural" to aid in weight loss. Customers who have tried numerous treatments may find new hope in a natural substitute that they have not previously tried and is simply accessible. An increasing number of overweight adults are using weight loss products obtained from natural ingredients like caffeine, green tea, ginseng, curcumin, *Garcinia cambogia*, white kidney beans, spirulina, and *Coleus forskohlii* in the hopes that they will be safer in comparison to prescription medications and effective in losing weight. Some of the chemicals in many expensive weight-loss pills may conflict with or interfere with some medicines. Therefore, before utilizing any dietary supplement, it is crucial to take into account what is known and what is unknown regarding each of its ingredients. Before deciding whether these products are a suitable option for weight loss therapy, healthcare professionals and users need to be aware of how effective these products are in managing weight. The presence of adverse events and decreased compliance is the main problem, even though it often results in improvement. Due to the widespread belief that natural substances are synonymous with health and balance, so-called superfoods and food supplements have become increasingly popular in recent years. The truth is that many of the commercially available dietary supplements have very few, if any, significant side effects, despite the fact that this is only partly false given the numerous negative incidences that might result from ingesting natural compounds. For people who suffer from illnesses like high blood pressure, diabetes, liver, or heart disease, this is extremely crucial. The ideal strategy for weight loss and weight maintenance is to stick to a reasonable regimen that includes a calorie-reduced diet, moderate physical exercise, and supervision from a healthcare professional. Doctors may recommend supplementary therapy, such as FDA-approved prescription drugs or bariatric surgery, in addition to lifestyle changes for those people with high BMIs who also have other health concerns. We draw the conclusion that more credible evidence is urgently required despite many of the products under investigation appearing to be useful even though they have limited clinical utility when used alone. As a result, combinations that aim to target multiple mechanisms of action must be sufficiently studied from an efficacy and safety perspective in order to determine whether they will have additive or synergistic effects in the absence of serious adverse events.

KEYWORDS

- **antiobesity**
- **body mass**
- **healthcare**
- **nutrients**
- **supplementation**
- **synergistic effects**
- **weight loss**

REFERENCES

Andueza, N., Giner, R. M., & Portillo, M. P. (2021). Risks associated with the use of Garcinia as a nutritional complement to lose weight. *Nutrients, 13*(2), 450.

Bakre, L. G., & Jaiyeoba, K. T. (2009). Studies on the physicochemical properties of Abelmuscus esculentus L. (Okra) pods: a potential tablet excipient. *International Journal of Biological and Chemical Sciences, 3*(3), 448–456.

Barrett, M. L., & Udani, J. K. (2011). A proprietary alpha-amylase inhibitor from white bean (Phaseolus vulgaris): A review of clinical studies on weight loss and glycemic control. *Nutrition Journal, 10*, 24.

Boekema, P. J., Samsom, M., van Berge Henegouwen, G. P., & Smout, A. J. (1999). Coffee and gastrointestinal function: facts and fiction. A review. *Scandinavian Journal of Gastroenterology Supplement, 230*, 35–39.

Bradford, P. G. (2013). Curcumin and obesity. *Biofactors, 39*(1), 78–87.

Chang, Y. S., Seo, E. K., Gyllenhaal, C., & Block, K. I. (2003). Panax ginseng: A role in cancer therapy? *Integrative Cancer Therapies, 2*(1), 13–33.

Davoodi, S. H., Hajimiresmaiel, S. J., Ajami, M., Mohseni-Bandpei, A., Ayatollahi, S. A., Dowlatshahi, K., Javedan, G., & Pazoki-Toroudi, H. (2014). Caffeine treatment prevented weight regain after calorie-shifting diet-induced weight loss. *Iranian Journal of Pharmaceutical Research, 13*(2), 707–718.

Den Hartigh, L. J. (2019). Conjugated linoleic acid effects on cancer, obesity, and atherosclerosis: A review of pre-clinical and human trials with current perspectives. *Nutrients, 11*(2), 370.

Drake, T. C., Rudser, K. D., Seaquist, E. R., & Saeed, A. (2012). Chromium infusion in hospitalized patients with severe insulin resistance: a retrospective analysis. *Endodontic Practice, 31*, 1–17.

Dwivedi, A. K., Dubey, P., Cistola, D. P., & Reddy, S. Y. (2020). Association between obesity and cardiovascular outcomes: Updated evidence from meta-analysis studies. *Current Cardiology Reports, 22*, 25.

Dwyer, J. T., Allison, D. B., & Coates, P. M. (2005). Dietary supplements in weight reduction. *Journal of the American Dietetic Association, 105*(5–1), 80–86.

Filippini, T., Malavolti, M., Borrelli, F., Izzo, A. A., Fairweather-Tait, S. J., Horneber, M., & Vinceti, M. (2020). Green tea (Camellia sinensis) for the prevention of cancer. *Cochrane Database of Systematic Reviews, 3*(3), CD005004.

Ganesan, K., & Xu, B. (2017). Polyphenol-rich dry common beans (Phaseolus vulgaris L.) and their health benefits. *International Journal of Molecular Sciences, 18*, 2331.

Garcia-Alvarez, A., Egan, B., de Klein, S., Dima, L., Maggi, F. M., Isoniemi, M., Ribas-Barba, L., Raats, M. M., Meissner, E. M., Badea, M., Bruno, F., Salmenhaara, M., Milà-Villarroel, R., Knaze, V., Hodgkins, C., Marculescu, A., Uusitalo, L., Restani, P., & Serra-Majem, L. (2014). Usage of plant food supplements across six European countries: Findings from the PlantLIBRA consumer survey. PLoS One, 9(3), e92265.

Grube, B., Chong, P. W., Lau, K. Z., & Orzechowski, H. D. (2013). A natural fiber complex reduces body weight in the overweight and obese: A double-blind, randomized, placebo-controlled study. Obesity (Silver Spring), 21(1), 58–64.

Gu, J., Li, W., Xiao, D., Wei, S., Cui, W., Chen, W., Hu, Y., Bi, X., Kim, Y., Li, J., Du, H., Zhang, M., & Chen, L. (2013). Compound K, a final intestinal metabolite of ginsenosides, enhances insulin secretion in MIN6 pancreatic β-cells by upregulation of GLUT2. Fitoterapia, 87, 84–88.

Haber, S. L., Awwad, O., Phillips, A., Park, A. E., & Pham, T. M. (2018). Garcinia cambogia for weight loss. American Journal of Health-System Pharmacy, 75(2), 17–22.

Haghighatdoost, F., & Hariri, M. (2018). Effect of conjugated linoleic acid supplementation on serum leptin concentration: A systematic review and meta-analysis. Endocrine, Metabolic & Immune Disorders – Drug Targets, 18(3), 185–193.

Han, L. K., Zheng, Y. N., Yoshikawa, M., Okuda, H., & Kimura, Y. (2005). Anti-obesity effects of chikusetsusaponins isolated from Panax japonicus rhizomes. BMC Complementary and Alternative Medicine, 5(1), 9.

Hanse, M.; Akbar, S.; Layeghkhavidaki, H.; Yen, F.T. Garcinia cambogia Extract Increased Hepatic Levels of Lipolysis-Stimulated Lipoprotein Receptor and Lipids in Mice on Normal Diet. Int. J. Mol. Sci. 2023, 24, 16298. https://doi.org/10.3390/ijms242216298

Harde, S. M., & Singhal, R. S. (2012). Extraction of forskolin from Coleus forskohlii roots using three-phase partitioning. Separation and Purification Technology, 96, 20–25.

He, S., Simpson, B. K., Sun, H., Ngadi, M. O., Ma, Y., & Huang, T. (2018). Phaseolus vulgaris lectins: A systematic review of characteristics and health implications. Critical Reviews in Food Science and Nutrition, 58(1), 70–83.

Hong, S. Y., Kim, J. Y., Ahn, H. Y., Shin, J. H., & Kwon, O. (2012). Panax ginseng extract rich in ginsenoside protopanaxatriol attenuates blood pressure elevation in spontaneously hypertensive rats by affecting the Akt-dependent phosphorylation of endothelial nitric oxide synthase. Journal of Agricultural and Food Chemistry, 60(12), 3086–3091.

Huang, L. H., Liu, C. Y., Wang, L. Y., Huang, C. J., & Hsu, C. H. (2018). Effects of green tea extract on overweight and obese women with high levels of low-density lipoprotein cholesterol (LDL-C): A randomized, double-blind, and crossover placebo-controlled clinical trial. BMC Complementary and Alternative Medicine, 18(1), 294.

Ishak, W. W., Ugochukwu, C., Bagot, K., Khalili, D., & Zaky, C. (2012). Energy drinks: Psychological effects and impact on well-being and quality of life—A literature review. Innovations in Clinical Neuroscience, 9(1), 25–34.

Joh, E. H., Lee, I. A., Jung, I. H., & Kim, D. H. (2011). Ginsenoside Rb1 and its metabolite compound K inhibit IRAK-1 activation—The key step of inflammation. Biochemical Pharmacology, 82(3), 278–286.

Jurgens, T. M., Whelan, A. M., Killian, L., Doucette, S., Kirk, S., & Foy, E. (2012). Green tea for weight loss and weight maintenance in overweight or obese adults. Cochrane Database of Systematic Reviews, 12, CD008650.

Kamal, C., & Sethuraman, M. G. (2012). Spirulina platensis – A novel green inhibitor for acid corrosion of mild steel. Arabian Journal of Chemistry, 5(2), 155–161.

Kang, S., & Min, H. (2012). Ginseng, the 'Immunity Boost': The effects of Panax ginseng on the immune system. Journal of Ginseng Research, 36(4), 354–368.

Karkos, P. D., Leong, S. C., Karkos, C. D., Sivaji, N., & Assimakopoulos, D. A. (2011). Spirulina in clinical practice: Evidence-based human applications. Evidence-Based Complementary and Alternative Medicine, 2011, 531053.

Kasprzak-Drozd, K., Oniszczuk, T., Gancarz, M., Kondracka, A., Rusinek, R., & Oniszczuk, A. (2022). Curcumin and weight loss: Does it work? International Journal of Molecular Sciences, 23(2), 639.

Kavitha, C., Rajamani, K., & Vadivel, E. (2010). Coleus forskohlii: A comprehensive review on morphology, phytochemistry, and pharmacological aspects. Journal of Medicinal Plant Research, 4(4), 278–285.

Kennedy, M. D., Galloway, A. V., Dickau, L. J., & Hudson, M. K. (2008). The cumulative effect of coffee and a mental stress task on heart rate, blood pressure, and mental alertness is similar in caffeine-naïve and caffeine-habituated females. Nutrition Research, 28(9), 609–614.

Keservani, R. K., & Sharma, A. K. (2014). Flavonoids: Emerging trends and potential health benefits. Journal of Chinese Pharmaceutical Sciences, 23(12), 815.

Keservani, R. K., Kesharwani, R. K., Sharma, A. K., Vyas, N., & Chadoker, A. (2010b). Nutritional supplements: An overview. International Journal of Current Pharmaceutical Review and Research, 1(1), 59–75.

Keservani, R. K., Kesharwani, R. K., Vyas, N., Jain, S., Raghuvanshi, R., & Sharma, A. K. (2010). Nutraceutical and functional food as future food: A review. Der Pharmacia Lettre, 2(1), 106–116.

Keservani, R. K., Sharma, A. K., & Kesharwani, R. K. (2017). An overview and therapeutic applications of nutraceutical and functional foods. In Recent Advances in Drug Delivery Technology (pp. 160–201). ISBN: 9781522507543.

Keservani, R. K., Sharma, A. K., & Kesharwani, R. K. (Eds.). (2020). Nutraceuticals and Dietary Supplements: Applications in Health Improvement and Disease Management. pp.1–344. CRC Press. ISBN: 9781771888738.

Kim, D. H. (2012). Chemical diversity of Panax ginseng, Panax quinquifolium, and Panax notoginseng. *Journal of Ginseng Research, 36*(1), 1–15.

Koithan, M., & Niemeyer, K. (2010). Using herbal remedies to maintain optimal weight. Journal of the American Association of Nurse Practitioners, 6(2), 153–154.

Kumar, D. S., Tony, D. E., Kumar, A. P., Kumar, K. A., Rao, D. B. S., & Nadendla, R. (2013). A review on Abelmoschus esculentus (okra). International Research Journal of Pharmacy and Applied Sciences, 3(4), 129–132.

Kumar, S., Verma, A. K., Das, M., Jain, S. K., & Dwivedi, P. D. (2013). Clinical complications of kidney bean (Phaseolus vulgaris L.) consumption. Nutrition, 29, 821–827.

Kwon, D. H., Bose, S., Song, M. Y., Lee, M. J., Lim, C. Y., Kwon, B. S., & Kim, H. J. (2012). Efficacy of Korean Red Ginseng by single nucleotide polymorphism in obese women: Randomized, double-blind, placebo-controlled trial. Journal of Ginseng Research, 36, 176–189.

Lambert, G. W., Kazuko, M., & John, B. D. (2010). Weight loss in obesity and metabolic syndrome. Current Hypertension Reviews, 6(2), 130–138.

Layer, P., Carlson, G. L., & DiMagno, E. P. (1985). Partially purified white bean amylase inhibitor reduces starch digestion in vitro and inactivates intraduodenal amylase in humans. Gastroenterology, 88, 1895–1902.

Lee, H. J., Lee, Y. H., Park, S. K., Kang, E. S., Kim, H. J., Lee, Y. C., Choi, C. S., Park, S. E., Ahn, C. W., Cha, B. S., Lee, K. W., Kim, K. S., Lim, S. K., & Lee, H. C. (2009). Korean red ginseng (Panax ginseng) improves insulin sensitivity and attenuates the development of diabetes in Otsuka Long-Evans Tokushima fatty rats. Metabolism, 58(8), 1170–1177.

Lee, S. H., Lee, H. J., Lee, Y. H., Lee, B. W., Cha, B. S., Kang, E. S., Ahn, C. W., Park, J. S., Kim, H. J., Lee, E. Y., & Lee, H. C. (2012). Korean red ginseng (Panax ginseng) improves insulin sensitivity in high fat fed Sprague-Dawley rats. Phytotherapy Research, 26(1), 142–147.

Lehnen, T. E., da Silva, M. R., Camacho, A., Marcadenti, A., & Lehnen, A. M. (2015). A review on effects of conjugated linoleic fatty acid (CLA) upon body composition and energetic metabolism. Journal of the International Society of Sports Nutrition, 12, 36.

Liu, W., Zheng, Y., Han, L., Wang, H., Saito, M., Ling, M., Kimura, Y., & Feng, Y. (2008). Saponins (ginsenosides) from stems and leaves of Panax quinquefolium prevented high-fat diet-induced obesity in mice. Phytomedicine, 15, 1140–1145.

Maia-Landim, A., Ramírez, J. M., Lancho, C., Poblador, M. S., & Lancho, J. L. (2018). Long-term effects of Garcinia cambogia/Glucomannan on weight loss in people with obesity, PLIN4, FTO, and Trp64Arg polymorphisms. BMC Complementary and Alternative Medicine, 18(1), 26.

Majeed, Muhammed & Majeed, Shaheen & Nagabhushanam, Kalyanam & Gnanamani, Muthuraman & Mundkur, Lakshmi. (2021). Lesser Investigated Natural Ingredients for the Management of Obesity. Nutrients. 13. 510. 10.3390/nu13020510.

Manna, P., & Jain, S. K. (2015). Obesity, oxidative stress, adipose tissue dysfunction, and the associated health risks: Causes and therapeutic strategies. Metabolic Syndrome and Related Disorders, 13, 423–444.

Mariani, S., Fiore, D., Varone, L., Basciani, S., Persichetti, A., Watanabe, M., Saponara, M., Spera, G., Moretti, C., & Gnessi, L. (2012). Obstructive sleep apnea and bone mineral density in obese patients. Diabetes Metabolic Syndrome and Obesity, 5, 395–401.

Mattioli, A. V., Pennella, S., Farinetti, A., & Manenti, A. (2018). Energy drinks and atrial fibrillation in young adults. Clinical Nutrition, 37(3), 1073–1074.

Million, M., & Raoult, D. (2013). The role of the manipulation of the gut microbiota in obesity. Current Infectious Disease Reports, 15(1), 25–30.

Mitra, M., Gantait, S., & Mandal, N. (2020). Coleus forskohlii: Advancements and prospects of in vitro biotechnology. Applied Microbiology and Biotechnology, 104(6), 2359–2371.

National Institute of Diabetes and Digestive and Kidney Diseases. (2012–2019). Clinical and research information on drug-induced liver injury. [Internet].

Nciri, N., Cho, N., El Mhamdi, F., Ben Ismail, H., Ben Mansour, A., Sassi, F. H., & Ben Aissa-Fennira, F. (2015). Toxicity assessment of common beans (Phaseolus vulgaris L.) widely consumed by Tunisian population. Journal of Medicinal Food, 18, 1049–1064.

Ngondi, J. L., Oben, J. E., & Minka, S. R. (2005). The effect of Irvingia gabonensis seeds on body weight and blood lipids of obese subjects in Cameroon. Lipids in Health and Disease, 4, 12.

Nolan, R., Shannon, O. M., Robinson, N., Joel, A., Houghton, D., & Malcomson, F. C. (2020). It's no having bean: A review of the effects of white kidney bean extract on body composition and metabolic health. Nutrients, 12(5), 1398.

Nuri, T. H., Yee, J. C., Gupta, M., Khan, M. A., & Ming, L. C. (2016). A review of Panax ginseng as an herbal medicine. Archives of Pharmacy Practice, 7, 61–65.

Obesity and Overweight, (2021). Available at: https://www.who.int/en/news-room/fact-sheets/detail/obesity-and-overweight (accessed on 15 June 2024).

Obesity Rates by Country, (2022); World Population Review. Available at: https://worldpopulationreview.com/country-rankings/obesity-rates-by-country (accessed on 15 June 2024).

Obiro, W. C., Zhang, T., & Jiang, B. (2008). The nutraceutical role of the Phaseolus vulgaris alpha-amylase inhibitor. British Journal of Nutrition, 100, 1–12.

Okamura, T., Hashimoto, Y., Hamaguchi, M., Obora, A., Kojima, T., & Fukui, M. (2019). Ectopic fat obesity presents the greatest risk for incident type 2 diabetes: A population-based longitudinal study. International Journal of Obesity, 43, 139–148.

Olorundare, O., Adeneye, A., Akinsola, A., Kolo, P., Agede, O., Soyemi, S., Mgbehoma, A., Okoye, I., Albrecht, R., & Mukhtar, H. (2020). Irvingia gabonensis seed extract: An effective attenuator of doxorubicin-mediated cardiotoxicity in Wistar rats. Oxidative Medicine and Cellular Longevity, 2020, 1602816.

Oseguera-Toledo, M. E., de Mejia, E. G., Dia, V. P., & Amaya-Llano, S. L. (2011). Common bean (Phaseolus vulgaris L.) hydrolysates inhibit inflammation in LPS-induced macrophages through suppression of NF-kappaB pathways. Food Chemistry, 127, 1175–1185.

Phelan, S., Wadden, T. A., Berkowitz, R. I., Sarwer, D. B., Womble, L. G., Cato, R. K., & Rothman, R. (2007). Impact of weight loss on the metabolic syndrome. International Journal of Obesity, 31(9), 1442–1448.

Pickering, C., & Grgic, J. (2019). Caffeine and exercise: What next? Sports Medicine, 49(7), 1007–1030.

Rothenberg, D. O., Zhou, C., & Zhang, L. (2018). A review on the weight-loss effects of oxidized tea polyphenols. Molecules, 23, 1176.

Santimone, M., Koukiekolo, R., Moreau, Y., Le Berre, V., Rougé, P., Marchis-Mouren, G., & Desseaux, V. (2004). Porcine pancreatic alpha-amylase inhibition by the kidney bean (Phaseolus vulgaris) inhibitor (alpha-AI1) and structural changes in the alpha-amylase inhibitor complex. Biochimica et Biophysica Acta (BBA) – General Subjects, 1696(2), 181–190.

Song, M. Y., Kim, B. S., & Kim, H. (2014). Influence of Panax ginseng on obesity and gut microbiota in obese middle-aged Korean women. Journal of Ginseng Research, 38(2), 106–115.

Stohs, S. J., Preuss, H. G., Ohia, S. E., Kaats, G. R., Keen, C. L., Williams, L. D., & Burdock, G. A. (2009). No evidence demonstrating hepatotoxicity associated with hydroxycitric acid. World Journal of Gastroenterology, 15(32), 4087–4089.

Sung, B. H., Lovallo, W. R., Pincomb, G. A., & Wilson, M. F. (1990). Effects of caffeine on blood pressure response during exercise in normotensive healthy young men. American Journal of Cardiology, 65(13), 909–913.

Sung, B. H., Lovallo, W. R., Whitsett, T., & Wilson, M. F. (1995). Caffeine elevates blood pressure response to exercise in mild hypertensive men. American Journal of Hypertension, 8(12.1), 1184–1188.

Tabrizi, R., Saneei, P., Lankarani, K. B., Akbari, M., Kolahdooz, F., Esmaillzadeh, A., Nadi-Ravandi, S., Mazoochi, M., & Asemi, Z. (2019). The effects of caffeine intake on weight loss: A systematic review and dose-response meta-analysis of randomized controlled trials. Critical Reviews in Food Science and Nutrition, 59(16), 2688–2696.

Thom, E., Wadstein, J., & Gudmundsen, O. (2001). Conjugated linoleic acid reduces body fat in healthy exercising humans. The Journal of International Medical Research, 29, 392–396.

Udani, J., Tan, O., & Molina, J. (2018). Systematic review and meta-analysis of a proprietary alpha-amylase inhibitor from white bean (Phaseolus vulgaris L.) on weight and fat loss in humans. Foods, 7(4), 63.

Uebelhack, R., Bongartz, U., Seibt, S., Bothe, G., Chong, P. W., De Costa, P., & Wszelaki, N. (2019). Double-blind, randomized, three-armed, placebo-controlled, clinical investigation to evaluate the benefit and tolerability of two dosages of IQP-AE-103 in reducing body weight in overweight and moderately obese subjects. Journal of Obesity, 2019, 3412952.

Vázquez Cisneros, L. C., López-Uriarte, P., López-Espinoza, A., Navarro Meza, M., & Espinoza-Gallardo, A. C. (2017). Efectos del té verde y su contenido de galato de epigalocatequina (EGCG) sobre el peso corporal y la masa grasa en humanos. Una revisión sistemática [Effects of green tea and its epigallocatechin (EGCG) content on body weight and fat mass in humans: A systematic review]. Nutrición Hospitalaria, 34(3), 731–737.

Victor R. Preedy, Ronald Ross Watson, Vinood B. Patel, 2011. Chapter 32 - Seed Extract of the West African Bush Mango (Irvingia Gabonensis) and its Use in Health, Nuts and Seeds in Health and Disease Prevention, Academic Press, 271-278, https://doi.org/10.1016/B978-0-12-375688-6.10032-5.

Wang, S., Chen, L., Yang, H., Gu, J., Wang, J., & Ren, F. (2020). Regular intake of white kidney beans extract (Phaseolus vulgaris L.) induces weight loss compared to placebo in obese human subjects. Food Science & Nutrition, 8(3), 1315–1324.

Watanabe, M., Risi, R., Masi, D., Caputi, A., Balena, A., Rossini, G., Tuccinardi, D., Mariani, S., Basciani, S., Manfrini, S., Gnessi, L., & Lubrano, C. (2020). Current evidence to propose different food supplements for weight loss: A comprehensive review. *Nutrients, 12*(9), 2873. https://doi.org/10.3390/nu12092873.

Westerterp-Plantenga, M. S., Lejeune, M. P., & Kovacs, E. M. (2005). Body weight loss and weight maintenance in relation to habitual caffeine intake and green tea supplementation. *Obesity Research, 13*(7), 1195–1204. https://doi.org/10.1038/oby.2005.142.

Willoughby, D., Hewlings, S., & Kamlan, D. (2018). Body composition changes in weight loss: Strategies and supplementation for maintaining lean body mass, a brief review. *Nutrients, 10*(12), 1876. https://doi.org/10.3390/nu10121876.

Woolston, C. (2012). Current evidence to propose different food supplements for weight loss: a comprehensive review. *Nutrients, 12*(9), 2873.

Yang, C. S., & Hong, J. (2013). Prevention of chronic diseases by tea: Possible mechanisms and human relevance. *Annual Review of Nutrition, 33*, 161–181. https://doi.org/10.1146/annurev-nutr-071812-161120.

CHAPTER 3

NUTRACEUTICAL FRUITS IN OBESITY MANAGEMENT

JYOTI UPADHYAY, TARNJOT KAUR, and POOJA CHAND

School of Health Sciences and Technology, University of Petroleum and Energy Studies, Energy Acre, Campus Bidholi, Dehradun, Uttarakhand, India

ABSTRACT

There is a high prevalence of obesity worldwide. Obesity is a complex disorder and is a result of the consumption of calories exceeding the energy requirements of the body. Fruits are an essential part of a diet and are rich in polyphenols such as phenolic acid and flavonoids. Phenolic compounds are associated with regulating appetite, lipid metabolism, gut bacteria, and energy expenditure. So, they help in the management of obesity. Flavonoids effectively treat obesity by increasing lipolysis and energy expenditure and stimulating β-oxidation of fatty acid and carbohydrate metabolism. Some fruits contain pancreatic lipase and α-amylase inhibitors and help manage obesity by decreasing fat absorption in the diet. Hence, various nutraceuticals present in fruits are effective in the management of obesity.

3.1 INTRODUCTION

Obesity is one of the most significant factors contributing to ill health. It increases the incidence of diabetes mellitus, hypertension, coronary heart diseases, sleep apnea, depression, certain cancers, chronic disorders such as kidney and liver disorders, and osteoarthritis (Kopelman, 2000). The leading cause of obesity is the imbalance between energy consumption

Nutraceuticals in Obesity Management and Control. Raj K. Keservani & Alka Lohani (Eds.)

and expenditure. The excess energy is stored in the form of fat cells, which results in hypertrophy, hyperplasia of fat cells, and clinical problems related to obesity (Bray, 2004). Lifestyle modifications and environmental and genetic factors are the leading causes of obesity and continue to rise globally. Food is the main environmental factor causing obesity. Consuming dietary fat in excess amounts leads to an increase in the number of fat cells and their size. An increase in fat cells causes an inability to store triglycerides and metabolic dysfunctions. This activates the secretion of proinflammatory cytokines and inflammatory and apoptotic pathways. In obesity, infiltration of inflammatory cells occurs in various target organs, causing the interaction of several stromal and substantial cells, ultimately leading to organ dysfunction (Xiong et al., 2019).

Dr. Stephen DeFelice coined nutraceuticals by combining two terms, 'Nutrition' and 'Pharmaceutical,' in 1989. A nutraceutical is any substance considered as a food or part of the food that can be used to provide health benefits and prevent or treat diseases. Nutraceuticals have nutritional and therapeutic potential (Sachdeva, Roy, & Bharadvaja, 2020; Keservani et al., 2010a, b). Nutraceuticals can be used as an alternative therapy that cannot be categorized as per the existing regulations and are defined as food supplements with useful properties for maintaining health, especially during pathological conditions. Therefore, nutraceutical-based therapeutic approaches for maintaining health cause a "nutraceutical revolution" globally (Quagliariello et al., 2018). Fruits have a beneficial effect on health as they contain a considerable amount of bioactive constituents, vitamins, and minerals. Their lipidic arrangements have antioxidant, anti-inflammatory, and anticoagulant properties that prevent oxidative stress, thrombogenesis, and hypercholesterolemia activated by obesity (Vij & Prashar, 2015). Fruits have the potential for prophylaxis and treatment of obesity. Fruits are a rich source of phenolic compounds, flavonoids, carotenes, and antioxidants. Therefore, this helps reduce the size and number of fat cells. Hence, it can be used in the prevention and treatment of obesity (Jarouliya & Keservani, 2019). Various nutraceutical fruits (Keservani et al., 2016), that are helpful in obesity management, are citrus fruits, berries, watermelon, muskmelon, and amla.

3.2 FRUITS IN NUTRACEUTICALS

3.2.1 PAPAYA

Carica papaya is a widely available plant used either in its natural form or processed as pulp, sweets, and other parts of the plant like seeds and leaves are added to enhance its nutritional value and used in products like flours and teas (Ojimelukwe, Nwofia, Ojimelukwe, & Eji, 2012). The papaya pulp contains antioxidants and three critical sources of vitamins A, C, and E, in addition to B-Complex vitamins (pantothenic acid), folate, and mineral ions like potassium, magnesium, as well as dietary fibers (Marfo, Oke, & Afolabi, 1986; Shivananda et al., 2007). Furthermore, it also contains the enzyme papain, which helps in peristaltic movement, increases transit time and is utilized in treating lesions, allergies, and trauma (Vij & Prashar, 2015). Many studies have revealed the presence of the enzyme chymopapain in papaya, a proteolytic enzyme with antibacterial, antiviral, and anti-inflammatory properties (Bhat & Surolia, 2001). The phenolic compounds in papaya seeds include benzyl isothiocyanate, glucosinolates, α and δ tocopherols, beta-carotene, beta-cryptoxanthin, and carotenoids (Kermanshai et al., 2001). Papaya seed oil contains oleic fatty acid, stearic acid, palmitic acid, and linoleic acid (van Breemen & Pajkovic, 2008). Table 3.1 represents the nutritional value of micronutrients, fibers, minerals, and vitamins present in 100 gm of ripe fruit pulp and seeds of *Carica papaya*.

TABLE 3.1 Nutritional Value of Micronutrients, Fibers, Minerals, and Vitamins Present in 100 Gm of Ripe Fruit Pulp and Seeds of *Carica papaya*

Sl. No.	Component	Pulp	Seed
1.	Carbohydrates	7.2 g	43.6 g
2.	Proteins	0.6 g	2.6 g
3.	Lipid	0.1 g	3.1 g
4.	Energy	32.1 Kcal	212.7 Kcal
5.	Fiber	0.8 g	2.1 g
6.	Sodium	3 mg	ND
7.	Potassium	257 mg	344 mg
8.	Phosphorus	5 mg	241.5 mg
9.	Magnesium	10 mg	10.4 mg
10.	Iron	0.1 mg	0.2 mg
11.	Calcium	24 mg	54.4 mg
12.	Vitamin C	61.8 mg	11.7 mg
13.	Vitamin B6	0.1 mg	ND
14.	Vitamin B9	38 mg	ND
15.	Vitamin B2	0.05 mg	0.05 mg
16.	Vitamin A	328 mg	ND
17.	Beta carotene	888 IU	65.64 IU

Source: Santana et al. (2019).

The main phytochemical components present in the fruit pulp of *Carica papaya* are glutathione peroxidase, glutathione transferase, glutathione reductase, catalase, glucose-6-phosphate, total phenols, terpenols alkaloids, flavonoids, and saponins (Santana et al., 2019). Obesity is caused by various etiological factors involving social, environmental, behavioral, psychological, genetic, and metabolic factors. It is characterized by visceral fat accumulation, a significant risk factor in developing metabolic syndrome like dyslipidemia, hypertension, and insulin resistance (Samson & Garber, 2014). Adipose tissue contains many adipokines, including interleukin-6, tumor necrosis factors, chemokine ligands like MCP-1/CCL-2 (monocyte attractant protein), adiponectin, resistin, and leptin (Anderson et al., 2009). An excessive amount of adipose tissue causes a more significant production of adipokines that leads to elevated levels of proinflammatory cytokines and a reduction in inflammatory adipokines activating the inflammatory process, thus causing insulin resistance (Feillet-Coudray et al., 2019). These processes connect metabolic syndrome and fat accumulation in ectopic tissues in excess (like the liver) that further stimulate inflammation and stress in the endoplasmic reticulum (Ottaiano et al., 2016). Papaya fruit contains a high amount of bioactive compounds, vitamins, and lipidic composition that help reduce inflammatory markers and oxidative stress, thus preventing hypercholesterolemia and hyperglycemia triggered by obesity (Santana et al., 2019). Ezekwe et al. (2017) investigated the antidiabetic effect of *C. papaya* in an albino rat model by inducing alloxan 120 mg/kg/body weight. They gave pulp of green *C. papaya* to the treatment group for 28 days. Their study reported a reduction in the level of glycosylated hemoglobin, the weight of animals, and the lipidic profile of the treatment group. Another study reported the antioxidant property of *C. papaya* seed on human hepatoma cell strains, HepG2. They have observed that polyphenolic components are responsible for this antioxidant activity (Salla, Sunkara, Ogutu, Walker, & Verghese, 2016).

3.2.2 CITRUS FRUITS

Genus Citrus consists of various orange fruits such as *Citrus aurantium, Citrus sinensis*, and *Citrus reticulata* belonging to the family *Rutaceae* (Saini et al., 2022). *Citrus* fruits are cultivated worldwide. Citrus fruits are cultivated in the tropical and subtropical areas near the equator at 35°S and 35°N latitudes. The Northern Hemisphere is the central region for its cultivation and production (Liu, Heying, & Tanumihardjo, 2012). Various bioactive components of citrus fruits are flavonoids such as flavones (Vitegin, rhoifolin, and diosmin), flavanones (narirutin, naringin, and hesperidin), flavanols (rutin, quercetin, and kaempferol), anthocyanins (cyanidin 3-(6″-malonyl) glucoside, cyanidin 3-glucoside, and peonidin 3-(6″-malonyl) glucoside), polymethoxyflavone (tangeretin, nobiletin, and 5-demethylnobiletin), and isoflavonols. Other chemical constituents of citrus fruits are apocarotenoids and carotenoids such as xanthophylls (lutein, violaxanthin, 9Z-violaxanthin, β-cryptoxanthin), xanthophyll esters (violaxanthin ester and 9Z-violaxanthin ester), carotenes (α-carotene and β-carotene), apocarotenoids (β-citraurin and β-citraurin palmitate). Various essential oils like terpenes, namely monoterpene hydrocarbons (D-limonene, γ-terpinene, p-cymene, β-phellandrene, and β-pinene), oxygenated monoterpenes (geranial, nonanal, (Z)-neral), terpene alcohol (linalool, geraniol, α-terpineol), aldehyde (decanal), ester (ethyl cinnamate and ethyl p-methoxycinnamate), and limonoid (limonin and nomilin) (Saini et al., 2022). *In vitro* studies showed that polyphenols present in citrus fruits reduce the differentiation of adipocytes and the lipid content of the cells and induce apoptosis of adipocytes. Citrus fruits also promote β-oxidation of fatty acids and help improve glycemia and lipid profile. Few studies showed that citrus fruits could reduce proinflammatory cytokines, so helpful in reducing complications related to obesity. Citrus fruits also reduce adiposity (Nakajima, Macedo, & Macedo, 2014). Table 3.2 represents the nutritional value of micronutrients, fibers, minerals, and vitamins in 100 gm of ripe fruit pulp of *Citrus aurantium*.

Flavonoid glycoside and hesperidin isolated from citrus peel showed antioxidative and anti-inflammatory activity, helped lower blood pressure and cholesterol levels, and had anti-obesity activity (Xiong et al., 2019). It activates cholecystokinin secretion (CCK), which maintains appetite-regulating hormones in enteroendocrine cells, thus used in treating obesity (Kim, Park, Kim, Lee, & Rhyu, 2013). Some studies also found that dietary bioflavonoid hesperidin reduces triglyceride and cholesterol levels in pectoral muscle and broiler serum. It also improves lipid metabolism dose-dependently in broiler breasts (Kamboh & Zhu, 2013). Naringin and naringenin are flavanone glycosides in citrus fruits that possess antioxidant properties. However, naringin is less potent than naringenin because of the sugar moiety, which causes steric hindrance of scavenging radicals. Naringin gets broken down into naringenin, which is aglycone in nature in the intestine and thus reabsorbed in the gut. Differentiating adipocytes is the foremost step involved in fat deposition in fat cells. Some studies reported

TABLE 3.2 Nutritional Value of Micronutrients, Fibers, Minerals, and Vitamins Present in 100 Gm of Ripe Fruit Pulp of *Citrus aurantium*

Sl. No.	Component	Pulp
1.	Carbohydrates	11.75 g
2.	Proteins	0.94 g
3.	Lipid	0.12 g
4.	Energy	47 Kcal
5.	Fiber	2.40 g
6.	Folate, total	30 μg
7.	Sodium	0
8.	Potassium	181 mg
9.	Calcium	40 mg
10.	Copper	45 μg
11.	Iron	0.10 mg
12.	Calcium	24 mg
13.	Magnesium	10 mg
14.	Manganese	0.025 mg
15.	Zinc	0.07 mg
16.	Niacin	0.282 mg
17.	Pantothenic acid	0.250 mg
18.	Pyridoxine	0.060 mg
19.	Riboflavin	0.040 mg
20.	β-Carotene	71 μg
21.	α-Carotene	11 μg
22.	β-Cryptoxanthin	116 μg
23.	Xanthophyll	129 μg

Source: Liu et al. (2012).

that naringenin promotes the expression of genes and secretion of protein adiponectin from adipocytes, i.e., 3T3-L1, thus improving adipocyte function and enhancing adiponectin production (Horiba et al., 2013). Dietary supplementation with naringin lowered the elevated level of plasma lipid concentration in a high-fat diet-fed animal model. This hypolipidemic effect was observed in low-density lipoprotein receptors (LDLR) in knockout mice (Li, Zheng, Bukuru, & De Kimpe, 2004). Some studies reported a reduction in the level of liver enzyme HMG CoA (3-hydroxy-3-methyl Coenzyme A) in the naringin-supplemented group, and no effect was observed in cholesterol acyl transferase (ACAT) activity in LDLR knockout mice (Li et al., 2004).

3.2.3 MULBERRY

Mulberry (*Morus alba*) belongs to the family *Moraceae*. Mulberry is cultivated all over the world wherever silkworm grows, as it is the primary food source of the silkworm. It is a tree or shrub in countries like China, India, and Japan. Occasionally, it is cultivated in North America, Africa, and Europe (Jambheshwar, Jeet, Devi, Sharma, & Kumar, 2013). It contains various nutrients such as carbohydrates, lipids, proteins, and vitamins (Bhattacharjya et al., 2021). Other chemical constituents in mulberry are alkaloids, phenolic compounds such as gallic acid, flavonoids such as caffeic acid and rutin, anthocyanins, flavonols, and resveratrol (Yuan & Zhao, 2017). It helps in obesity management in many ways, such as inhibiting the digestive enzyme pancreatic lipase and inhibiting carbohydrate-hydrolyzing enzymes. It also inhibits the differentiation of adipocytes and regulates lipid metabolism. It controls appetite and stimulates energy expenditure (Mahboubi, 2019). Table 3.3 represents the nutritional value of micronutrients, fibers, minerals, and vitamins present in 100 gm of ripe fruit pulp of *Mulberry* fruit.

TABLE 3.3 Nutritional Value of Micronutrients, Fibers, Minerals, and Vitamins Present in 100 Gm of Ripe Fruit Pulp of *Mulberry* Fruit

Sl. No.	Component	Pulp
1.	Carbohydrates	15.30 g
2.	Proteins	1.46 g
3.	Lipid	0.58 g
4.	Energy	72.30 Kcal
5.	Crude fiber	1.2 g
6.	Vitamin A IU	25
7.	Vitamin E	0.80 mg
8.	Vitamin K	7.60 µg
9.	Malic acid	0.090 mg
10.	Tartaric acid	0.0014 mg
11.	Fumaric acid	0.0021 mg
12.	Lactic acid	0.0066 mg
13.	Citric acid	0.018 mg
14.	Oxalic acid	0.0066 mg
15.	Succinic acid	0.02836 mg
16.	Thiamine (B1)	0.026 mg
17.	Riboflavin (B2)	0.900 mg

TABLE 3.3 *(Continued)*

Sl. No.	Component	Pulp
18.	Nicotinic acid	0.700 mg
19.	Ascorbic acid	36 mg
20.	Niacin	0.600 mg

Source: Manzoor et al. (2022).

Mulberry fruits are rich in alkaloids and anthocyanins and have antioxidant, anti-atherosclerotic, antidiabetic, hepatoprotective, and anti-obesity activities. Research studies depicted the beneficial effect of fruit extract of *M. alba* on obesity in mice models. Their results reported that fruit extract ameliorates the level of cholesterol transfer proteins, and oxidative stress gets reduced in the obese mice model (Valacchi, Belmonte, Miracco, Eo, & Lim, 2014). Wu et al. (2013) identified the impact of Mulberry juice in obese mice model C57BL/6. Their result indicated that a high-fat diet-fed mice model treated with mulberry juice inhibits body weight gain, less cholesterol, reduced insulin resistance, reduced leptin secretion, and lipid accumulation. Another study investigated that mulberry fruit extract increases AMPK (adenosine monophosphate-activated protein kinase) activity and downregulates microRNA in adipocytes that ameliorate adipogenesis (Lee & Kim, 2020).

3.2.4 BLACK CHOKEBERRY

The biological name of the chokeberry is *Aronia melanocarpa*. It belongs to the *Rosaceae* family. It is a shrub with high antioxidant properties. Its origin and center are the Northeastern states of the USA. It is also cultivated in parts of Europe such as Russia, Siberia, Poland, Finland, Germany, Norway, the Czech Republic, Denmark, and Hungary (Jurikova et al., 2017). The chemical constituents in black chokeberry are carbohydrates, phenolic compounds such as anthocyanins, flavonols, hydroxycinnamic acids and procyanidins, amygdalin, and carotenoids such as β-carotene, β-Cryptoxanthin, and Violaxanthin (Kulling & Rawel, 2008). Many studies show the chokeberry fruit's anti-obesity activity in various cell and animal models. It was found that black chokeberry extract inhibits the expression of lipoprotein lipase (LPL), fatty acid binding protein 4 (FABP4), and PPARγ, as well as adipokine secretion in cell line studies (Shin & Jung, 2016). Chokeberry was also found to alter the gut microbiota, changing mRNA expression for lipolysis and lipogenesis in rats' liver and bile acid metabolism (Lee et al., 2021). Table 3.4 represents the nutritional value of micronutrients, fibers, minerals, and vitamins present in 100 gm ripe fruit of Black Chokeberry.

TABLE 3.4 Nutritional Value of Micronutrients, Fibers, Minerals, and Vitamins Present in 100 Gm of Ripe Fruit of Black Chokeberry

Sl. No.	Component	Pulp
1.	Carbohydrates	14.37 g
2.	Proteins	0.7 g
3.	Lipid	0.15 g
4.	Energy	50 Kcal
5.	Crude fiber	56.2 mg
6.	Vitamin C	0.137 mg
7.	Vitamin B1	0.18 mg
8.	Vitamin K	0.242 μg
9.	Vitamin B2	0.02 μg
10.	Vitamin B6	0.28 μg
11.	Malic acid	0.13 g
12.	Citric acid	0.021 g
13.	Folate	0.03 μg
14.	Niacin	3 μg
15.	Chromium	0.029 μg
16.	Sodium	26 μg
17.	Potassium	2,180 μg
18.	Magnesium	162 μg
19.	Calcium	322 μg
20.	Iron	9.3 μg

Source: Zhang et al. (2021).

The chokeberry fruit is consumed in juice form as a dietary supplement, and there is one study conducted on 20 postmenopausal women aged 50–58 years having a BMI of 30–36 kg/m^2 and a waist circumference of 100–110 cm. They were allowed to consume glucomannan-enriched chokeberry juice. After 4 weeks, they observed a decrease in waist circumference and biochemical parameters such as HDL cholesterol. It is also reported that long-term consumption of chokeberry juice and its other products has beneficial effects on metabolic parameters including fasting plasma glucose, blood pressure level, and fasting plasma glucose (Broncel et al., 2010).

3.2.5 MUSKMELON

The biological name of muskmelon is *Cucumis melo*. It belongs to the family *Cucurbitaceae*. It is grown worldwide. The origin of muskmelon is believed to be East Africa; however, some literature also states it originates from Asia. It is cultivated in East Asia to the Mediterranean Sea, central as well as Southeast Asia, China, the Iberian Peninsula, the Philippines, India, Japan, Australia, the USA, and Korea (Manchali & Murthy, 2020). Chemical constituents present in muskmelon are volatile and non-volatile. Volatile oils include ethanol, ethyl acetate, methyl acetate, benzyl acetate, benzaldehyde, ethyl butanol, phenylmethyl acetate, benzyl alcohol, and eugenol. Non-volatile constituents are carbohydrates, amino acids, phospholipids, glycolipids, flavonoids, β-carotene, linoleic acid, and phenolic glycosides (Asif et al., 2014). Muskmelon improves lipid profile in rat models. It increases the level of high-density lipoproteins (HDL) and decreases the level of low-density lipoproteins (LDL), very low-density lipoprotein (VLDL), triglycerides, and total cholesterol. It significantly reduces food intake and body weight (Cucumis, Linn, & Rats, 2021) (Table 3.5).

TABLE 3.5 Nutritional Value of Micronutrients, Fibers, Minerals, and Vitamins Present in 100 Gm of the Edible Portion of Muskmelon Fruit

Sl. No.	Component	Pulp
1.	Carbohydrates	8.2 gm
2.	Fat	0.2 gm
3.	Energy	34 Kcal
4.	Fiber	0.9 gm
5.	Calcium	9 mg
6.	Magnesium	12 mg
7.	Phosphorus	15 mg
8.	Iron	0.2 mg
9.	Zn	0.2 mg
10.	Vitamin A	3,382 IU
11.	Vitamin C	37 mg

Source: USDA (2002).

3.2.6 WATERMELON

Watermelon (*Citrullus lanatus*) belongs to the *Cucurbitaceae* family. Watermelon is consumed almost all over the world. It is cultivated in China,

Brazil, Costa Rica, Ecuador, Santa Romania, and Italy (Casacchia et al., 2020). Various chemical constituents in watermelon are carotenoids such as xanthophylls and carotene (β-carotene and lycopene), amino acids such as L-citrulline, polyphenols (flavonoids and non-flavonoids), and fatty acids (Zamuz et al., 2021). Watermelon contains α-amylase and pancreatic lipase inhibitory properties (Ajithadas & Vijayalakshmi, 2014; Jibril et al., 2019). This property is believed to control diet-induced obesity by decreasing the absorption of fats (Lowet, 2002; Mahmood, 2016).

According to Healthline, watermelon consists of 92% water and contains a modest amount of potassium and some of the highest levels of lycopene, a red pigment responsible for the color of the watermelon. It consists of Arginine, which helps to improve the blood flow in the body and may help reduce the accumulation of excess fat. The rind and seeds of the watermelon fruit are also edible.

In the year 2019, one of the studies indicated that watermelon helps improve the functions of metabolic syndrome, including cardiovascular and obesity measures. In that study, 33 people under the overweight and obesity category were advised to take 2 cups of watermelon or cookies made up of low fat for four weeks. The result of this study reported that the people who ate watermelon were feeling less hungry and were more satisfied than those who ate low-fat cookies. Along with that, those who ate watermelon had a higher level of antioxidants in their blood, lower systolic blood pressure, and lower body weight and BMI (Lum et al., 2019) (Table 3.6).

TABLE 3.6 Nutritional Value of Micronutrients, Fibers, Minerals, and Vitamins Present in 100 Gm of the Edible Portion of Watermelon Fruit

Sl. No.	Components	Pulp
1.	Carbohydrates	8 gm
2.	Protein	0.61 gm
3.	Fat	0.2 gm
4.	Energy	30 Kcal
5.	Fiber	0.4 gm
6.	Folates	3 mcg
7.	Niacin	0.178 mg
8.	Pantothenic acid	0.221 mg
9.	Pyridoxin	0.045 mg
10.	Thiamine	0.033 mg
11.	Vitamin A	569 IU
12.	Vitamin C	8.1 mg

TABLE 3.6 *(Continued)*

Sl. No.	Components	Pulp
13.	Vitamin E	0.05 mg
14.	Sodium	1 mg
15.	Potassium	112 mg
16.	Calcium	7 mg
17.	Copper	42 mcg
18.	Iron	0.24 mg
19.	Magnesium	10 mg
20.	Manganese	0.038 mg
21.	Zinc	0.10 mg

Source: USDA (2019).

3.2.7 AMLA

Amla (*Emblica Officinalis/Phyllanthus Emblica*) belongs to the family *Euphorbiaceae*, also called Indian gooseberry, and has been used in the traditional system of medicine since ancient times. It is used as a medicine as well as a tonic. Amla is a deciduous tree cultivated in the subtropical and tropical areas of countries like India, China, Pakistan, Malaysia, Indonesia, Sri Lanka, the Malay Peninsula, and Uzbekistan (Kaur, Masih, & Khan, 2013). Amla contains many beneficial chemical constituents such as alkaloids, glycosides (phenolic, flavone, and flavonols), tannins, amino acids, mucic acid, and terpenoids (sesquiterpenoids and norsesquiterpenoids), phenolic acid, and carbohydrates. Amla is also a great source of vitamin C. Other chemical constituents present in amla are gallic acid, ellagic acid, chlorogenic acid, and quercetin (Variya, Bakrania, & Patel, 2016). It also plays a significant role in diabetes as it activates the small group of cells that produce the insulin hormone, which reduces the blood sugar level in diabetic patients (Bhattacharya et al., 1999).

Various studies have demonstrated the potential of amla in the management of obesity. Extract of amla can inhibit lipid accumulation in mice. It assimilates the peroxisome proliferator-associated receptor gamma (PPARγ) and the nuclear transcription factor expression of adipose mRNA (Sato, Buesa, & Nerurkar, 2010). Anti-obesity activity of amla by downregulation of Tumor necrosis factor-α (TNF-α), leptin, and gene expression of PPARγ2 has also been reported in rats (Nazish & Ansari, 2018) (Table 3.7).

TABLE 3.7 Nutritional Value of Micronutrients, Fibers, Minerals, and Vitamins Present in 100 Gm of Amla Fruit

Sl. No.	Component	Pulp
1.	Carbohydrates	10 gm
2.	Protein	1 gm
3.	Fat	0.5 gm
4.	Energy	48 Kcal
5.	Phenolic compound (gallic acid)	3012.5 mg
6.	Vitamin A	290 IU
7.	Vitamin C	478 mg
8.	Vitamin E (α-tocopherol)	2,450 mg*
9.	Vitamin B6	0.1 mg
10.	Folate	6 mcg
11.	Pantothenic acid	0.3 mg
12.	Calcium	25 mg
13.	Iron	0.9 mg
14.	Magnesium	10 mg
15.	Phosphorus	27 mg
16.	Potassium	198 mg
17.	Sodium	1 mg
18.	Zinc	0.12 mg
19.	Copper	0.1 mg
20.	Manganese	0.1 mg

Source: Sachan, Gangwar, & Kumar (2013).

3.3 CONCLUSION

Obesity is a chronic disorder that affects the global public health sector. Nutraceutical fruits have high potential in preventing, controlling, treating, and mitigating this disorder. They act by inhibiting pancreatic and α-amylase lipase, promoting apoptosis of adipocytes, and regulating lipid metabolism. Various types of fruits available worldwide contain active nutraceutical agents that can help reduce the prevalence of obesity. Clinical trial studies are required to explore the effectiveness of various nutraceutical fruits in obesity management. Moreover, various nutritional and chemical constituents present in nutraceutical fruits are attractive targets for researchers to develop anti-obesity nutraceuticals to prevent life-threatening diseases.

KEYWORDS

- **global public health sector**
- **life-threatening diseases**
- **nutraceutical agents**
- **nutraceutical fruits**
- **nutritional value**
- **obesity**
- **obesity management**
- **polyphenols**

REFERENCES

Aruna, A., Vijayalakshmi, K. V., & Ajithadas, K. (2014). Pancreatic lipase inhibitory screening of Citrullus lanatus leaves. *The Pharma Innovation Journal, 3*(7), 44–52.

Asif, H. M., Akhtar, N., Sultana, S., Rehman, S. U., Akram, M., & Rehman, U. J. (2014). Medicinal properties of Cucumis melo Linn. *Journal of Pharmacy and Pharmaceutical Sciences, 2*(1), 58–62.

Bhat, G. P., & Surolia, N. (2001). In vitro antimalarial activity of extracts of three plants used in the traditional medicine of India. *The American Journal of Tropical Medicine and Hygiene, 65*(4), 304–308. https://doi.org/10.4269/AJTMH.2001.65.304.

Bhattacharjya, D., Sadat, A., Dam, P., Buccini, D. F., Mondal, R., Biswas, T., & Mandal, A. K. (2021). Current concepts and prospects of mulberry fruits for nutraceutical and medicinal benefits. *Current Opinion in Food Science, 40*, 121–135. https://doi.org/10.1016/j.cofs.2021.03.009.

Bray, G. A. (2004). Medical consequences of obesity. *The Journal of Clinical Endocrinology & Metabolism, 89*(6), 2583–2589. https://doi.org/10.1210/JC.2004-0535.

Broncel, M., Koziróg, M., Duchnowicz, P., Koter-Michalak, M., Sikora, J., & Chojnowska-Jezierska, J. (2010). Aronia melanocarpa extract reduces blood pressure, serum endothelin, lipid, and oxidative stress marker levels in patients with metabolic syndrome. *Medical Science Monitor, 16*(1), 28–34.

Casacchia, T., Sofo, A., Claudia-Crinatoma, Drăgănescu, D., Tița, B., & Statti, G. A. (2020). Nutraceutical properties and health-promoting biological activities of fruits of watermelon cultivars with different origins. *Farmacia, 68*(4), 679–686. https://doi.org/10.31925/farmacia.2020.4.13.

Cucumis, O. F., Linn, M., & Rats, I. N. (2021). Pharmacological Investigation of Anti-Obesity Activity of Seeds. International Pharmaceutical Research, 5(4), 313–319.

Ezekwe, S. A., & Chikezie, P. C. (2017). GC-MS Analysis, Hypoglycemic Activity of Aqueous Root Extract of Carica papaya and Its Effects on Blood Lipid Profile and Hepatorenal

Tissues Biomarkers of Diabetic Rats. Journal of Diabetes & Metabolism, 8(1), 1–9. https://doi.org/10.4172/2155–6156.1000740.

Feillet-Coudray, C., Fouret, G., Vigor, C., Bonafos, B., Jover, B., Blachnio-Zabielska, A., & Coudray, C. (2019). Long-term measures of dyslipidemia, inflammation, and oxidative stress in rats fed a high-fat/high-fructose diet. *Lipids, 54*(1), 81–97. https://doi.org/10.1002/LIPD.12128.

Jambheshwar, G., Jeet, K., Devi, B., Sharma, N., & Kumar, D. (2013). Morus alba Linn: A phytopharmacological review Pharmacognostical and Phytopharmacological Studies of Argyreia nervosa View project Neha Sharma Morus Alba Linn: A Phytopharmacological Review. Retrieved from: https://www.researchgate.net/publication/237180712 (accessed on 15 June 2024).

Jarouliya, U., & Keservani, R. K. (2019). Pathways leading to child obesity. In D. Bagchi (Ed.), *Global Perspectives on Childhood Obesity: Current Status, Consequences and Prevention* (2nd ed., pp. 137–146). Academic Press, Elsevier. ISBN: 9780128128404.

Jibril, M. M., Abdul-Hamid, A., Ghazali, H. M., Sabri, M., Dek, P., Ramli, N. S., & Profile, P. (2019). Antidiabetic antioxidant and phytochemical profile of yellow-fleshed seeded watermelon (*Citrullus lanatus*) extracts. *Journal of Food and Nutrition Research, 7*(1), 82–95. https://doi.org/10.12691/JFNR-7-1-10.

Jurikova, T., Mlcek, J., Skrovankova, S., Sumczynski, D., Sochor, J., Hlavacova, I., & Orsavova, J. (2017). Fruits of black chokeberry (*Aronia melanocarpa*) in the prevention of chronic diseases. *Molecules, 22*(6), 944. https://doi.org/10.3390/MOLECULES22060944.

Kamboh, A. A., & Zhu, W. Y. (2013). Effect of increasing levels of bioflavonoids in broiler feed on plasma anti-oxidative potential, lipid metabolites, and fatty acid composition of meat. *Poultry Science, 92*(2), 454–461. https://doi.org/10.3382/PS.2012-02584.

Kaur, J., Masih, M., & Khan, U. (2013). *Emblica officinalis*: A meritocratic drug for treating various disorders. Retrieved from: www.iajpr.com (accessed on 15 June 2024).

Kermanshai, R., McCarry, B. E., Rosenfeld, J., Summers, P. S., Weretilnyk, E. A., & Sorger, G. J. (2001). Benzyl isothiocyanate is the chief or sole anthelmintic in papaya seed extracts. Phytochemistry, 57(3), 427–435. https://doi.org/10.1016/S0031-9422(01)00077-2.

Keservani, R. K., Kesharwani, R. K., Sharma, A. K., Vyas, N., & Chadoker, A. (2010b). Nutritional supplements: An overview. International Journal of Current Pharmaceutical Review and Research, 1(1), 59–75.

Keservani, R. K., Kesharwani, R. K., Vyas, N., Jain, S., Raghuvanshi, R., & Sharma, A. K. (2010a). Nutraceutical and functional food as future food: A review. Der Pharmacia Lettre, 2(1), 106–116.

Keservani, R. K., Sharma, A. K., & Kesharwani, R. K. (2016). Nutraceutical and functional foods for cardiovascular health. In A. K. Sharma & R. K. Kesharwani (Eds.), Food Process Engineering (pp. 291–312). Apple Academic Press, CRC Press. ISBN: 9781771884020.

Kim, H. Y., Park, M., Kim, K., Lee, Y. M., & Rhyu, M. R. (2013). Hesperetin stimulates cholecystokinin secretion in enteroendocrine STC-1 cells. Biomolecules & Therapeutics, 21(2), 121. https://doi.org/10.4062/BIOMOLTHER.2012.077.

Kopelman, P. G. (2000). Obesity as a medical problem. Nature, 404(6778), 635–643. https://doi.org/10.1038/35007508.

Kulling, S. E., & Rawel, H. M. (2008). Chokeberry (Aronia melanocarpa)– A review on the characteristic components and potential health effects. Planta Medica, 74(13), 1625–1634. https://doi.org/10.1055/S-0028-1088306.

Lee, H. Y., Suh, K. S., Kim, Y. I., Jang, B. K., Kim, B. H., & Yim, S. V. (2021). Bioactive fraction of Aronia melanocarpa fruit inhibits adipogenic differentiation of cultured 3T3-L1 cells. Applied Sciences, 11(19), 9224. https://doi.org/10.3390/APP11199224.

Lee, M. S., & Kim, Y. (2020). Mulberry fruit extract ameliorates adipogenesis via increasing AMPK activity and downregulating microRNA-21/143 in 3T3-L1 adipocytes. Journal of Medicinal Food, 23(3), 266–272. https://doi.org/10.1089/JMF.2019.4654.

Li, W. L., Zheng, H. C., Bukuru, J., & De Kimpe, N. (2004). Natural medicines used in the traditional Chinese medical system for therapy of diabetes mellitus. Journal of Ethnopharmacology, 92(1), 1–21. https://doi.org/10.1016/J.JEP.2003.12.031.

Liu, Y., Heying, E., & Tanumihardjo, S. A. (2012). History, global distribution, and nutritional importance of citrus fruits. Comprehensive Reviews in Food Science and Food Safety, 11(6), 530–545. https://doi.org/10.1111/J.1541-4337.2012.00201.X.

Lowet, M. E. (2002). The triglyceride lipases of the pancreas. Journal of Lipid Research, 43(12), 2007–2016. https://doi.org/10.1194/JLR.R200012-JLR200.

Lum, T., Connolly, M., Marx, A., Beidler, J., Hooshmand, S., Kern, M., & Hong, M. Y. (2019). Effects of fresh watermelon consumption on the acute satiety response and cardiometabolic risk factors in overweight and obese adults. Nutrients, 11(3), 595. https://doi.org/10.3390/NU11030595.

Mahboubi, M. (2019). Morus alba (mulberry), a natural potent compound in management of obesity. Pharmacological Research, 146, 104341. https://doi.org/10.1016/j.phrs.2019.104341.

Mahmood, N. (2016). A review of α-amylase inhibitors on weight loss and glycemic control in pathological state such as obesity and diabetes. Comparative Clinical Pathology, 25(6), 1253–1264. https://doi.org/10.1007/S00580-014-1967-X.

Manchali, S., & Murthy, K. N. C. (2020). Muskmelon. In V. R. Preedy (Ed.), Nutritional Composition and Antioxidant Properties of Fruits and Vegetables (pp. 533–546). https://doi.org/10.1016/B978-0-12-812780-3.00033-7.

Marfo, E. K., Oke, O. L., & Afolabi, O. A. (1986). Chemical composition of papaya (Carica papaya) seeds. Food Chemistry, 22(4), 259–266. https://doi.org/10.1016/0308-8146(86)90084-1.

Nakajima, V. M., Macedo, G. A., & Macedo, J. A. (2014). Citrus bioactive phenolics: Role in the obesity treatment. LWT – Food Science and Technology, 59(2), 1205–1212. https://doi.org/10.1016/J.LWT.2014.02.060.

Nazish, I., & Ansari, S. H. (2018). Emblica officinalis – Anti-obesity activity. Journal of Complementary and Integrative Medicine, 15(2), 1–11. https://doi.org/10.1515/jcim-2016-0051.

Ojimelukwe, P., Nwofia, E., Ojimelukwe, P., & Eji, C. (2012). Chemical composition of leaves, fruit pulp and seeds in some Carica papaya (L) morphotypes an aspect of my BSc work View project Presentations for Capacity Building in Research View project Chemical composition of leaves, fruit pulp and seeds in some Cari. Int. J. Med. Arom. Plants, 2(1), 200–206.

Ottaiano, A., Nappi, A., Tafuto, S., Nasti, G., De Divitiis, C., Romano, C., & Iaffaioli, V. R. (2016). Diabetes and body mass index are associated with neuropathy and prognosis in colon cancer patients treated with capecitabine and oxaliplatin adjuvant chemotherapy. Oncology, 90(1), 36–42. https://doi.org/10.1159/000442527.

Quagliariello, V., Vecchione, R., Coppola, C., Di Cicco, C., De Capua, A., Piscopo, G., & Maurea, N. (2018). Cardioprotective effects of nanoemulsions loaded with anti-inflammatory nutraceuticals against doxorubicin-induced cardiotoxicity. Nutrients, 10(9), 1304. https://doi.org/10.3390/NU10091304.

Sachan, N. K., Gangwar, S. S., Sharma, R., & Kumar, Y. (2013). An investigation into phytochemicals profile and nutraceutical value of amla (Emblica officinalis) fruits. International Journal of Modern Pharmaceutical Research, 2, 1–12.

Sachdeva, V., Roy, A., & Bharadvaja, N. (2020). Current prospects of nutraceuticals: A review. Current Pharmaceutical Biotechnology, 21(10), 884–896. https://doi.org/10.2174/1389201021666200130113441.

Saini, R. K., Ranjit, A., Sharma, K., Prasad, P., Shang, X., Gowda, K. G. M., & Keum, Y. S. (2022). Bioactive Compounds of Citrus Fruits: A Review of Composition and Health Benefits of Carotenoids, Flavonoids, Limonoids, and Terpenes. Antioxidants (Basel, Switzerland), 11(2), 239. https://doi.org/10.3390/antiox11020239.

Salla, S., Sunkara, R., Ogutu, S., Walker, L. T., & Verghese, M. (2016). Antioxidant activity of papaya seed extracts against H2O2 induced oxidative stress in HepG2 cells. LWT – Food Science and Technology, 66, 293–297. https://doi.org/10.1016/J.LWT.2015.09.008.

Samson, S. L., & Garber, A. J. (2014). Metabolic syndrome. Endocrinology and Metabolism Clinics, 43(1), 1–23. https://doi.org/10.1016/J.ECL.2013.09.009.

Santana, L. F., Inada, A. C., Santo, B. L. S. do E., Filiú, W. F. O., Pott, A., Alves, F. M., & Hiane, P. A. (2019). Nutraceutical potential of Carica papaya in metabolic syndrome. Nutrients, 11(7), 1608. https://doi.org/10.3390/NU11071608.

Sato, R., Buesa, L. M., & Nerurkar, P. V. (2010). Anti-obesity effects of Emblica officinalis (Amla) are associated with inhibition of nuclear transcription factor, peroxisome proliferator-activated receptor gamma (PPARγ). The FASEB Journal, 24(S1), 661.4–661.4. https://doi.org/10.1096/FASEBJ.24.1_SUPPLEMENT.661.4.

Shin, J., & Jung, J. (2016). Reduction of adipogenesis by chokeberry (Aronia melanocarpa) extract in 3T3-L1 preadipocytes. Journal of Food and Nutrition Research, 4(4), 210–215. https://doi.org/10.12691/JFNR-4-4-3.

Shivananda Nayak, B., Sivachandra Raju, S., Orette, F. A., & Chalapathi Rao, A. V. (2007). Effects of Hibiscus rosa sinensis L (Malvaceae) on wound healing activity: A preclinical study in a Sprague Dawley rat. International Journal of Lower Extremity Wounds, 6(2), 76–81. https://doi.org/10.1177/1534734607302840.

Valacchi, G., Belmonte, G., Miracco, C., Eo, H., & Lim, Y. (2014). Effect of combined mulberry leaf and fruit extract on liver and skin cholesterol transporters in high fat diet-induced obese mice. Nutrition Research and Practice, 8(1), 20–26. https://doi.org/10.4162/NRP.2014.8.1.20.

van Breemen, R. B., & Pajkovic, N. (2008). Multitargeted therapy of cancer by lycopene. Cancer Letters, 269(2), 339–351. https://doi.org/10.1016/J.CANLET.2008.05.016.

Variya, B. C., Bakrania, A. K., & Patel, S. S. (2016). Emblica officinalis (Amla): A review for its phytochemistry, ethnomedicinal uses and medicinal potentials with respect to molecular mechanisms. Pharmacological Research, 111, 180–200. https://doi.org/10.1016/j.phrs.2016.06.013.

Vij, T., & Prashar, Y. (2015). A review on medicinal properties of Carica papaya Linn. Asian Pacific Journal of Tropical Disease, 5(1), 1–6. https://doi.org/10.1016/S2222-1808(14)60617-4.

Wu, T., Tang, Q., Gao, Z., Yu, Z., Song, H., Zheng, X., & Chen, W. (2013). Blueberry and mulberry juice prevent obesity development in C57BL/6 mice. PLOS ONE, 8(10), e77585. https://doi.org/10.1371/JOURNAL.PONE.0077585.

Xiong, H., Wang, J., Ran, Q., Lou, G., Peng, C., Gan, Q., & Huang, Q. (2019). Hesperidin: A therapeutic agent for obesity. Drug Design, Development and Therapy, 13, 3855–3866. https://doi.org/10.2147/DDDT.S227499.

Yuan, Q., & Zhao, L. (2017). The mulberry (Morus alba L.) fruit – A review of characteristic components and health benefits. Journal of Agricultural and Food Chemistry, 65(48), 10383–10394. https://doi.org/10.1021/ACS.JAFC.7B03614.

Zamuz, S., Munekata, P. E. S., Gullón, B., Rocchetti, G., Montesano, D., & Lorenzo, J. M. (2021). Citrullus lanatus as source of bioactive components: An up-to-date review. Trends in Food Science and Technology, 111, 208–222. https://doi.org/10.1016/J.TIFS.2021.03.002.

CHAPTER 4

ROLE OF CAROTENOIDS IN OBESITY

MONIKA CHAND,[1] YATENDER SINGH PANWAR,[2] and MOHIT CHAND[3]

[1]*Food Science and Technology, National Institute of Food Technology Entrepreneurship and Management (NIFTEM), Sonipat, Haryana, India*

[2]*Food and Nutrition, GBPUAT, Pantnagar, Uttarakhand, India*

[3]*Bachelors of Technology, Lovely Professional University, Punjab, India*

ABSTRACT

Obesity has become a serious health issue worldwide, and more than 1.9 billion adults are obese. Diet plays a crucial role in decreasing obesity. This chapter discusses the effect of carotenoids and their metabolites in the management of obesity. According to many clinical and pre-clinical studies, there is a relationship between carotenoids and obesity. Since adipose tissues are a storage site for carotenoids and an important organ in obesity, in this chapter we discuss carotenoid metabolism and its effect on biological processes in adipose tissues, resulting in obesity and other disorders like insulin resistance, diabetes, cardiovascular disease, etc. It is also well established that the brain and genetics may also be involved in obesity processes.

4.1 INTRODUCTION

In 2015–2016, the US recorded a 39.8% prevalence of obesity (Hales et al., 2017) and $2 trillion in medical expenses on the treatment of obesity in 2014 (Tremmel et al., 2017). From a basic perspective, obesity results from excessive energy intake with less energy expenditure, which leads to the

Nutraceuticals in Obesity Management and Control. Raj K. Keservani & Alka Lohani (Eds.)

accumulation of a positive energy balance in the body (Church et al., 2018; Hill et al., 2012). Obesity is characterized by an excessive production of triglycerides in adipocytes, which are the primary biological components of white adipose tissue (Cinti, 2012). Obesity can be caused by a variety of variables, including genetic or epigenetic susceptibility (Jirtle, 2007), but learned behaviors like eating patterns and a lack of physical activity are what ultimately lead to the disease (Cohen & Spiegelman, 2016; Spiegelman & Flier, 2001). For example, ingesting just 5% more calories than what is consumed in one year could result in the accumulation of about 5 kg of fat tissue (Klein, 2002). Obesity, once established, becomes challenging to reverse. The current obesity epidemic and the realization that traditional approaches focused only on dietary restriction and increased physical activity are failing to combat it and are accelerating research into adjuvant therapies that could successfully support lifestyle changes. This implies a significant public health concern in the near future; obesity and overweight are now becoming epidemics not just in Western nations but especially in low- and middle-income nations.

4.2 OBESITY AND ITS MECHANISM

The excess fat mass that defines obesity is supported by the growth of adipose tissue as a consequence of adipocyte hypertrophy and/or hyperplasia (Arner et al., 2010), which is connected to complex, tightly regulated adipogenesis. This process has been studied in depth; both the transcriptional regulators and temporal sequences are now known. These include the nuclear receptor peroxisome proliferator-activated receptor gamma (PPARγ) and other members of the CCAAT enhancer binding protein (CEBP) family, which are believed to regulate adipogenesis through transcription (Farmer, 2006). This mechanism allows adipose tissue to contribute to energy balance by enabling the accumulation of surplus energy as triglycerides (lipogenesis) and fatty acids (lipolysis) for the release of energy. A disturbance in this balanced process could cause an increase or decrease in body weight.

4.2.1 OBESITY AND ADIPOCYTES

Free fatty acids and a number of other hormones are produced by adipose tissue, also referred to as endocrine tissue. Adipose tissue secretes about 50 physiologically active proteins that work in an autocrine, paracrine, or endocrine way. Among the most extensively investigated are leptin (Friedman,

2014) and adiponectin (Ruhl et al., 2015). Adipocytes and stromal vascular fraction cells, primarily macrophages, in adipose tissue have the capacity to secrete and synthesize adipokines.

According to Gregor & Hotamisligi et al. (2011), obesity acts as a catalyst for the development of chronic low-grade inflammation, which is characterized by abnormal secretion of cytokines, chemokines, and miRNA, acute phase proteins, and other immune response mediators linked to the activation of inflammatory signaling pathways. Adipose tissues have a crucial role in the development of chronic inflammation. The regulation of the molecules generated by adipose tissue is associated with a variety of pathophysiological diseases, including increased levels of circulating free fatty acids, hypertrophic adipose tissue hypoxia, local and systemic oxidative stress, endoplasmic reticulum stress, and the generation of inflammatory cytokines are only a few examples. These strains all exhibit IKK- and c-Jun amino-terminal kinase-dependent signaling pathways (JNK). Increased numbers of infiltrating macrophages during adipose tissue expansion reduce a variety of inflammatory diseases. This invasion has links to insulin resistance, obesity, and the growth of fat cells. By releasing pro-inflammatory cytokines like interleukin (IL)-1, tumor necrosis factor (TNF), and IL-6, macrophages impair adipocyte function. This results in changed adipokines, insulin resistance, an excess of free fatty acids secreted through enhanced lipolysis, and decreased lipogenesis.

Inflammatory circumstances have been shown to affect the function of adipocytes and adipose tissue in addition to metabolic inflammation, which has been linked to neuroinflammation. It is widely thought that central inflammation controls energy homeostasis, which contributes to the etiology of obesity (both at the level of energy expenditure and food intake). Neuronal and endocrine processes that balance calorie intake and expenditure control the homeostasis of energy.

4.2.2 ROLE OF THE CENTRAL NERVOUS SYSTEM IN OBESITY

The central nervous system (CNS) continuously controls changes in hormones (leptin, insulin, and ghrelin) or metabolic parameters (free fatty acid levels or blood glucose) and activates adaptive responses, such as food intake (Derghal et al., 2006; Morton et al., 2006). Leptin is essential for maintaining both appropriate body weight and food behavior by acting in multiple sections of the hypothalamus, including the paraventricular, arcuate, or ventromedial nuclei, and lateral hypothalamus. It acts in these regions of the hypothalamus through unique neural networks. More specifically, peripheral signals are detected by hypothalamic arcuate neurons that express the orexigenic peptides neuropeptide Y (NPY)/Agouti-related peptide (AgRP) or the anorexigenic peptide proopiomelanocortin (POMC). The melanocortin 3 and 4 receptor-expressing neurons in the hypothalamus and other regions of the brain receive signals from these neurons. By activating the autonomic nervous system (ANS) and higher brain structures, these neurons, collectively known as the melanocortin pathway, play a role in regulating feeding behavior, glucose homeostasis, and energy expenditure. Metabolic syndrome is a condition that can arise from a breakdown in the brain's ability to communicate with peripheral organs, which affects fat gain.

Increased inflammatory mediators and immune cells in peripheral tissues and brain regions, which are essential for regulating energy homeostasis and maintaining energy balance, are brought on by obesity. Adipose tissue's production of inflammatory cytokines and the activation of microglia, which are the brain's resident immune cells, and astrocytes in the hypothalamus may interfere with leptin transmission, which can result in hyperphagia and many other obesity-related diseases. In this situation, maintaining normal endocrine function is crucial for maintaining weight.

4.2.3 OBESITY AND DIET

The cornerstone of weight reduction therapy is an effective dietary intervention since it is simpler for most obese persons to generate a negative energy balance by reducing food consumption than it is by just increasing physical activity (Hall et al., 2011; Westerterp, 2010). So, changing to a healthy diet is a great approach to fighting obesity, and a key sign of a healthy diet is the amount of plant-based foods it contains (Tian et al., 2018). We cannot discount the presence of micronutrients with bioactive properties, some of which have effects on energy metabolism that have been scientifically proven, even though fruits and vegetable aid in weight loss because of their macronutrient makeup (high fiber, water, and complex carbohydrates, for example) (Maria et al., 2015; Williams et al., 2013). Among all of these micronutrients, carotenoids seem to be a potential alternative for treating and preventing obesity (Bonet et al., 2016). Carotenoids and the products made from them have been shown to have anti-obesity characteristics in recent years by a number of pre-clinical trials. These chemicals may be very beneficial in the prevention and treatment of obesity because the molecular processes underlying these activities have begun to become understood.

Significant evidence also suggests that the metabolism of endogenous carotenoid and retinoid molecules may change physiological processes involved in the control of body fat.

4.3 CAROTENOIDS

Carotenoids are lipophilic C-40-based isoprenoid pigments usually red, orange, or yellow in color, which are produced by plants and certain photosynthetic microorganisms. They contain in their molecule a polyene backbone with a variable number of conjugated double bonds. A few carotenoid structures are mentioned in Figures 4.1–4.4.

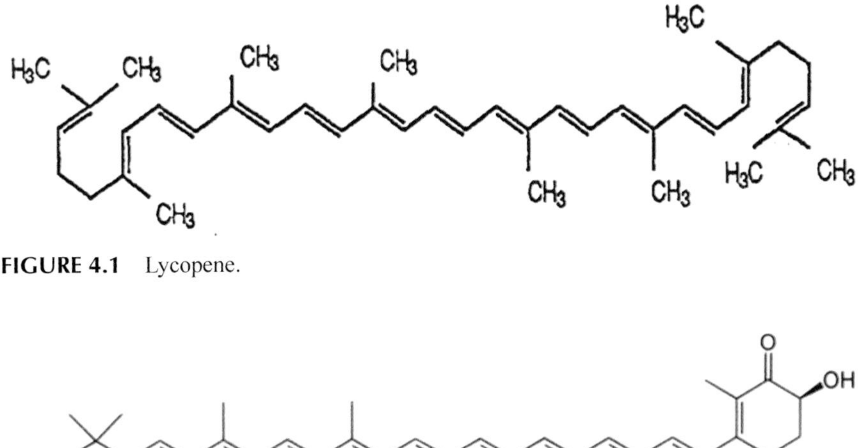

FIGURE 4.1 Lycopene.

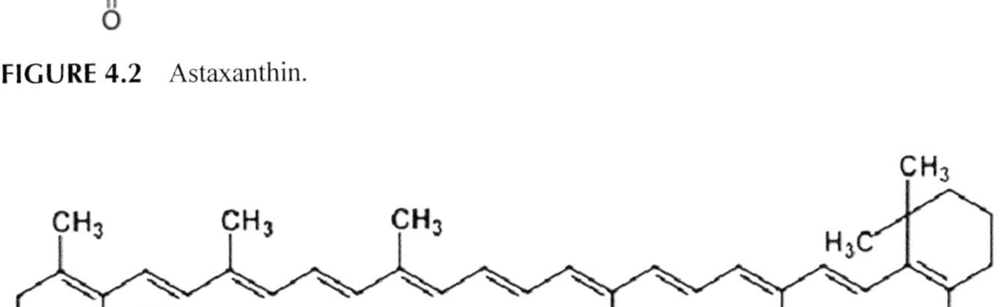

FIGURE 4.2 Astaxanthin.

FIGURE 4.3 Beta-carotene.

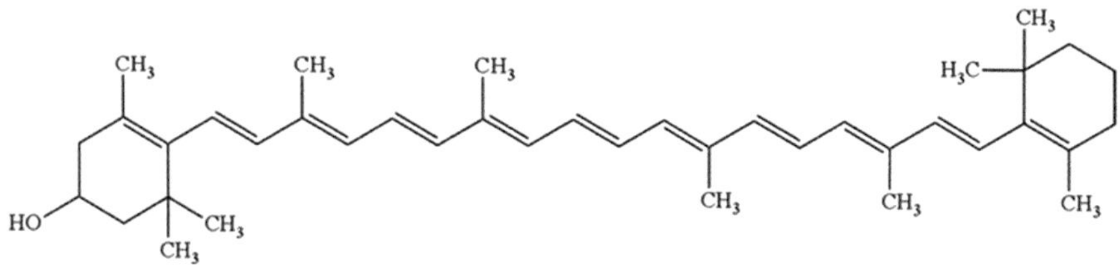

FIGURE 4.4 Beta-cryptoxanthin.

Primary dietary sources are fruits and vegetables, though they can also be obtained from bread, eggs, milk, beverages, fats, and oils. Of the 600 carotenoids in nature, 50 are present in the human diet, but only six are ubiquitous in human serum, namely β-carotene (BC), α-carotene, β-cryptoxanthin, lycopene, lutein, and zeaxanthin (Rodriguez et al., 2018). Carotenes and xanthophylls, which also include oxygen and are less apolar than carotenes, are two types of carotenoids that can be classified as cyclic or acyclic based on whether or not their chemical structures contain end rings (Figure 4.1). The double bond structure of the carotenoids gives them the ability to absorb light in the visible range and antioxidant characteristics. Carotenoids are precursors for light harvesting and photoprotectants in photosynthetic organisms (Rodriguez-Concepcio et al., 2018). Animals consume carotenoids mostly through vegetables and fruits, and certain of them have uses for the animals, either as intact molecules or after metabolism. The polyene backbone must first go through an oxidative cleavage, either enzymatic or nonenzymatic, at central or eccentric sites, in order to create shorter derivatives known as apocarotenoids. Terminal group alterations are just one example of additional reactions that may be present. Only around 10 of the more than 600 known chemicals are detected in significant concentrations in human plasma, of which 50 are found in the human diet (Paetau et al., 1998). Because they can be broken down by animals to release retinal, which can then be converted to retinol, carotenoids with an unsubstituted-ionone ring are referred to as provitamin A. Because they contain at least one unsubstituted-ionone ring, which is necessary to make vitamin A, only a few carotenoids have been shown to exhibit provitamin A activity. Only one of these carotenoids, β-cryptoxanthin, is a xanthophyll, while the other three, β-carotene (β-carotene), α-carotene (α-carotene), and γ-carotene, are carotenes. The three provitamin A carotenoids that are most prevalent in the human diet are β-carotene, β-cryptoxanthin, and α-carotene (Table 4.1).

TABLE 4.1 List of Food Sources Abundant on Provitamin A Carotenoids and Retinyl Esters [RAE: Retinol Activity Equivalent]

Sl. No.	Source	β-Carotene	α-Carotene	β-Cryptoxanthin	Vitamin A, RAE
1.	Carrots	33,954	14,251	–	3,423
2.	Lettuce	5,226	–	–	532
3.	Paprika	26,162	595	6,186	2,463
4.	Grape leaves	16,194	629	9	1,376
5.	Sweet potatoes	12,498	47	–	1,043
6.	Chili powder	15,000	2,090	3,490	1,483
7.	Peppers	42,891	6,931	-	3,863
8.	Pumpkins	6,940	4,795	-	778
9.	Liver	–	–	–	28,318
10.	Duck liver	–	–	–	11,984

Source: USDA Food Composition Database; Data expressed in μg/100 g food.

4.3.1 FUNCTIONS OF CAROTENOIDS

Carotenoids have been given several roles by scientists, the majority of which are beneficial to human health. Retinaldehyde and the regulation of gene expression, which are both important for many physiological and developmental processes, are both functions of vitamin A retinoids (majorly retinoic acid). By consuming the preformed vitamin A found in foods of animal origin, retinoids can be synthesized independently of carotenoids. Preformed vitamin A is thought to make up close to 65% of the total quantity of vitamin A consumed by people in developed nations, with carotenoids making up the remaining 35% (Weber et al., 2012). However, according to Wang et al. (2015), all naturally occurring retinoids identified in mammals originate from provitamin A carotenoids, either directly or indirectly via a lower-order animal in the food chain. As a result, retinoids are regarded as a class of apocarotenoids. Carotene-9′,10′-oxygenase is a second carotenoid cleavage enzyme that is expressed in mammals (BCO2). This mitochondrial enzyme cleaves cis lycopene, the xanthophylls lutein, zeaxanthin, provitamin A carotenoids, as well as other carotenoids eccentrically to create apo-10′-carotene. In addition to retinoids, non-retinoid apocarotenoids may potentially influence cellular functions and have an effect on the health of mammals, according to accumulating research. According to accumulated data, nonretinoid apo-carotenoids can also have an impact on cellular processes and have a bearing on mammal health in addition to these retinoids (Harrison et al., 2018).

It is commonly believed that β-carotene is one of the prominent sources of vitamin A among mammals, as the two β-ionone rings consist of two vitamin A molecules. However, this has not been characterized in detail to date. Other factors, such as transport and differential absorption, cell type specificity, enzymatic accessibility, or tissue storage, could determine which provitamin A source is preferred for production in humans specifically. Some researchers report that β-cryptoxanthin might prove to be a better source of vitamin A compared to β-carotene, most probably due to the presence of a hydroxyl group in its structure, which also affects its absorption and solubility. Whereas β-carotene, the conversion of β-cryptoxanthin into vitamin A is a multi-step enzymatic process (Amengual et al., 2013) and involves an extra layer of complexity that includes substrate partitioning and enzymatic activities. Moreover, genetic variations are localized in both the coding and promoter regions of transporters and enzymes involved in carotenoid metabolism, as carotenoid metabolism has a tremendous impact on human health (Farook et al., 2017; Meyers et al., 2013) (Figure 4.5).

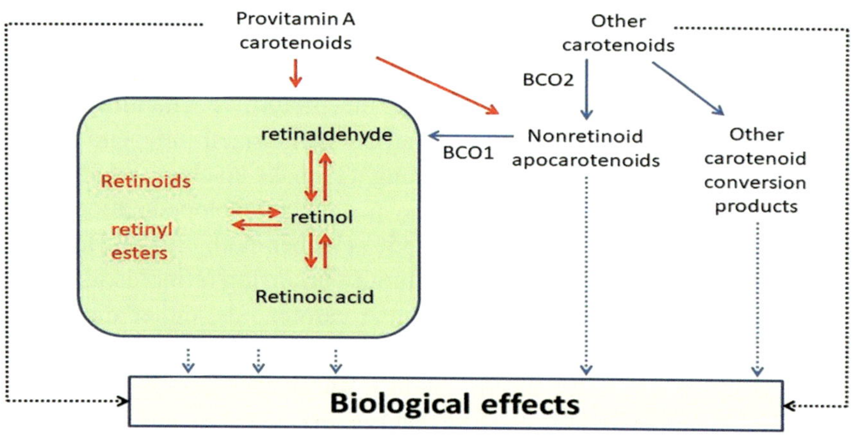

FIGURE 4.5 Simplified overview of interactions between carotenoids and their metabolites in vertebrate tissues.

Source: Adapted from Bonet et al., 2020

Carotenoids and Apocarotenoids are derivatives created when molecular oxygen cleaves a double bond inside the polyene backbone, releasing an aldehyde or ketone group in their place. The vitamin A retinoid apocarotenoids are created by the central cleavage of the provitamin A carotenoids, which is mediated by BCO1 (retinaldehyde, retinol, retinoic acid). Provitamin A carotenoids are enzymatically broken down by BCO2 to create non-retinoid apocarotenoids, among which apo-10′-carotenal can be transformed into retinaldehyde by the action of BCO1. Some non-provitamin A carotenoids are recognized by BCO2 as substrates, and from them, other non-retinoid apocarotenoids are generated. Carotenoids can undergo additional changes in animal tissues in addition to oxidative breakage of the polyene backbone, resulting in more carotenoid conversion products (CCPs). However, nonretinoid apocarotenoids and nonapocarotenoid CCPs may also have biological action in animal tissues, as revealed in recent studies. Retinoids and other carotenoids in intact form are better documented for their biological effects in animals. Beta-carotene (BC) is the main provitamin A carotenoid in the human diet. Key to retinoid production from BC in mammals is the activity of β-carotene-15,15′-oxygenase (BCO1), a cytosolic enzyme that cleaves BC centrally into two molecules of retinal (also named retinaldehyde, Rald), which can be oxidized irreversibly to retinoic acid or reduced reversibly to retinol (Figure 4.6).

Cell and animal studies suggest that adipose tissue is an important target of carotenoid action, despite the fact that effects on body fat content can relate to action in various tissues, including the liver, which serves as the primary reservoir for carotenoids and vitamin A and whose lipid metabolism is impacted by retinoids. Animals can get their vitamin A from sources other than carotenoids. Once vitamin A, a fat-soluble vitamin, is produced from eaten carotenoids, it is then deposited in the form of retinyl esters among different organs, like the adipose tissue and fat-soluble. As a result, consuming specific organs like animal liver may serve as a substantial source of vitamin A for people (*see* Table 4.1). Additionally, milk contains vitamin A, giving the newborn this necessary ingredient (Haskell et al., 1999). Vitamin A deficiency continues to be a major public health issue that affects more than half of the world's nations. Many governments today use fortification techniques, such as the inclusion of retinyl esters, as a preventive tactic. Both provitamin A carotenoids and non-provitamin A carotenoids have demonstrated adiposity-reducing effects, primarily in animal trials (reviewed in Bonet et al., 2015; Mounien, et al., 2019). Carotene's provitamin A activity in rodents is correlated with its antiobesity action (Amengual et al., 2011), which proves retinoids' anti-adiposity activities.

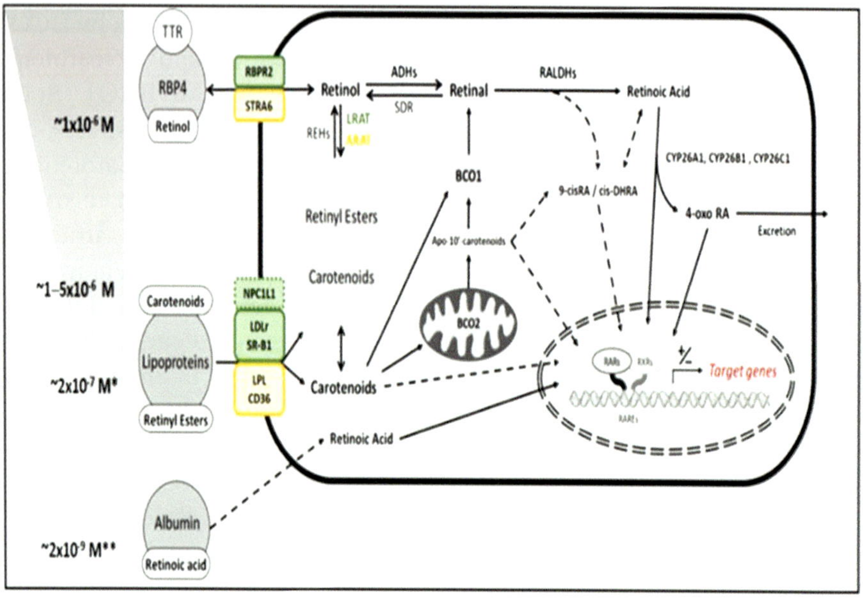

FIGURE 4.6 Schematic diagram of carotenoid: Vitamin A uptake: Metabolism.

Note: Left: Extracellular sources for provitamin A carotenoids and vitamin A and their relative concentration. It indicates that depending on the fasting vs. fed conditions, these sources can vary more than one order of magnitude. The data show fasting values. Right: It shows the major proteins and conversion pathways associated with catabolism and conversion of vitamin A and carotenoids. The proteins present in adipocytes and the hepatocytes are yellow and green, respectively. Dotted arrows represent pathways not fully established.

Abbreviations: Transthyretin, RBP4: retinol-binding protein 4; RBPR2: retinol-binding protein 4-receptor 2; STRA6: stimulated retinoic acid gene 6; LDLr: low-density lipoprotein receptor; SR-B1: scavenger receptor class B type 1; LPL: lipoprotein lipase; CD36: a cluster of differentiation 36; LRAT: lecithin:retinol acyltransferase; SDR: short-chain dehydrogenase/reductase; RALDH: retinaldehyde dehydrogenase; CYP26: cytochrome P450; 9-cisRA: 9-cis-retinoic acid; cis-DHRA: 9-cis-13,14-dihydroretinoic acid; RARs: retinoic acid receptors; and RAREs: retinoic acid-response elements.

Source: Reprinted from Coronel et al., 2019. Copyright ©2019 by the authors. Licensee MDPI, Basel, Switzerland.

4.3.2 CAROTENOIDS AND ADIPOSE TISSUE

The anti-obesity activity of carotenoids and carotenoid derivatives has been connected to activities in various tissues that are most likely related effects due to the substantial connection among tissues in mammals through metabolism and neuroendocrine signaling. Since there is frequently tissue-to-tissue crosstalk in mammals due to neuroendocrine signaling and metabolism, it is possible that the anti-obesity activity of carotenoids and carotenoid derivatives is connected to effects in several tissues. White and brown adipose tissue (BAT) are both significant targets in the anti-obesity activity of carotenoids and CCPs, though (WAT). Adipose tissues are critical locations for carotenoid and retinoid storage and metabolism in animals and play important pathological and physiological functions in lipid and energy metabolism (Figure 4.7).

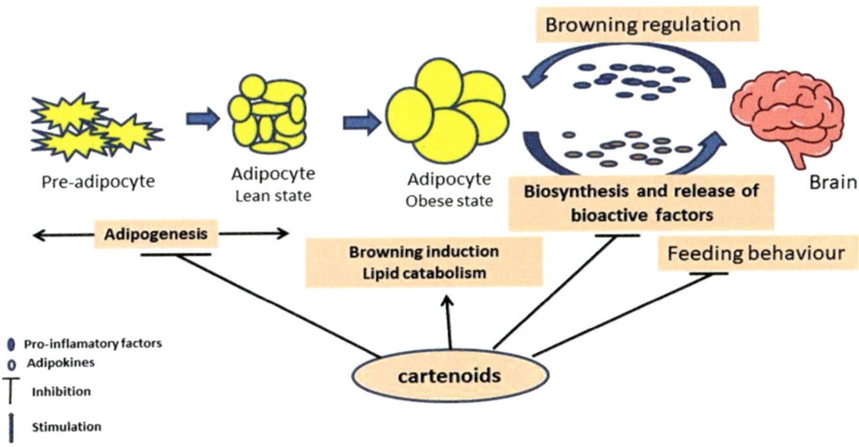

FIGURE 4.7 Carotenoids affect on brain and adipose tissue.

Source: Adapted from Mounien et al., 2019. Copyright ©2019 by the authors. Licensee MDPI, Basel, Switzerland.

White adipose tissue is skilled at storing excess ingested energy as triglycerides as well as delivering regulated energy to other tissues as needed in the form of fatty acids created by the lipolysis of stored triglycerides (beyond the energy needed to meet continuing expenses). White adipose tissue is skilled at both the controlled delivery of energy to other tissues as required in the form of fatty acids produced by the lipolysis of stored triglycerides and the storage of excess ingested energy (beyond the energy needed to fulfill ongoing expenses) as triglycerides. Both adipocyte hypertrophy (increased size) and adipocyte hyperplasia (increased number) are outcomes of progenitor cell proliferation within adipocytes and their differentiation into adipocytes (adipogenesis). WAT growth is brought on by an increase in lipid deposition in their cytoplasm. Contrarily, BAT concentrates on the regulated release of energy as heat (adaptive thermogenesis). Brown adipose tissue's ability to generate heat depends on the inner mitochondrial membrane protein known as uncoupling protein 1 (UCP1). Substrate oxidation generates a proton gradient across the inner mitochondrial membrane, and UCP1 activity encourages proton re-entry. By entering the mitochondrial matrix without the aid of ATP synthase, substrate oxidation decouples from ATP generation.

The phenomenon known as WAT browning or beiging occurs when several stimuli and signals stimulate BAT thermogenesis and encourage the formation of thermogenically capable, UCP1m-expressing "beige" cells in WAT depots. Browned WAT and BAT thermogenesis fight fat. Additionally, it is possible to increase mitochondrial oxidative metabolism in WAT *in vivo* without inducing UCP1, which favors a leaner phenotype and a reduction in body fat (Flachs et al., 2013). Known collectively as batokines for BAT and adipokines for WAT, respectively, both BAT and WAT are crucial secretory tissues that play a role in the production and secretion of a wide variety of signaling proteins as well as non-protein molecules like free fatty acids, miRNAs, and other lipids. These products influence significant procedures such as whole-body energy balance, inflammation, and metabolism by acting locally or on distant targets (Ouchi et al., 2011). Obesity alters the secretory activity of adipose tissues, especially visceral fat, which promotes the onset of prediabetes, insulin resistance, and other metabolic disorders. This alteration in adipose tissue secretion in obesity may be due, at least in part, to macrophage infiltration of the cells/tissue. In actuality, low-grade adipose tissue and chronic, systemic inflammation are now thought to be the main components of obesity (Maurizi et al., 2018).

Carotenoids are known to accumulate in adipose tissue. The two main carotenoids present in human adipose tissue are lycopene and beta-carotene. Lycopene is found to be the most prevalent carotenoid in adipose tissue, accounting for more than half of all carotenoids, followed by beta-carotene, which makes up around 1/3 of all carotenoids, zeaxanthin, lutein, cryptoxanthin, and alpha-carotene. The total carotenoid concentration appears to vary depending on the area, with the belly having a higher concentration than the thigh or buttocks. The levels of carotenoids in adipose tissue are remarkably similar in men and women. It is believed that during obesity, carotenoids are cloistered in adipose tissue since the plasma levels of key carotenoids are inversely associated with fat mass and both central and overall adiposity. In contrast, weight loss is connected to an increase in zeaxanthin and lutein serum concentration (Kirby et al., 2011).

Even while the concentration of β-carotene in adipose tissue is lower in obese people, the total pool of β-carotene in both groups is equivalent when total fat mass is taken into account. According to several studies, lutein and lycopene uptake by adipocytes and adipose tissue occurs independently of the carotenoids' chemical and physical properties, suggesting the involvement of putative facilitators or transporters or possibly a cluster of differentiation (CD36) (Moussa et al., 2011). Although it can also be found in plasma and nuclear membranes, lycopene is primarily kept in the form of lipid droplets in adipocytes. In addition to food, various tissue concentrations are also linked with adipose tissue carotenoid levels. Thus, it has also been noted that the amount of lutein in adipose tissue is positively connected with macular pigment density in males but not in women. With the exception of lycopene and lutein-zeaxanthin, the total carotenoid concentration in adipose tissue is also significantly correlated with blood levels. Similarly, the carotenoid content of breast adipose tissue corresponds with plasma levels, with the exception of β-cryptoxanthin, with a correlation coefficient of 0.20. Carotenoids target cells to control metabolic health and overall body obesity (Figure 4.8).

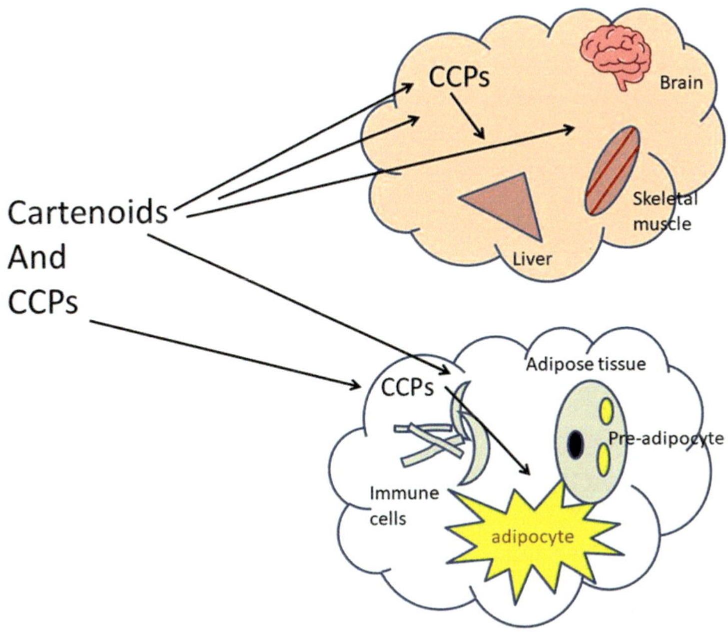

FIGURE 4.8 Adipocytes and other pertinent cell types within the adipose tissue depots, such as preadipocytes, adipose progenitor cells, endothelial cells, and immune cells, and the effect of carotenoids and CCPs on non-adipose tissues. (Additionally shown here are adipose-driven effects on non-adipose tissues that are mediated by metabolites or released signals.)

4.3.3 CAROTENOIDS AND GENE EXPRESSION

Numerous molecular mechanisms that have been implicated in mediating the effects of carotenoids on gene expression have been documented to have an impact on adipocyte biology. Provitamin A carotenoids are particular signaling targets for RARs and retinoid X receptors (RXRs), which are involved in the production of retinoic acid. Two families of receptors mediate the effects of retinoids (Germain et al., 2006). Each subtype has three different descriptions (RAR, RAR, RXR, RXR, and RXR). With specific DNA sequences known as retinoic acid response elements (RARE) or RXR-RXR dimers, these receptors perform as ligand-dependent transcriptional regulators.

Retinoid target genes contain retinoid X response elements (RXRE) in the promoter region. Every cell type contains RXR and RAR subtypes. RARs, thyroid hormone receptors (TR), farnesoid X receptors (FXR), pregnane X receptors (PXR), liver X receptors (LXR), farnesoid-activated receptors (PPARs), farnesoid X receptors (FXR), pregnane X receptors (PXR), RARs, and vitamin D receptors (VDR) are dimerization partners for other nuclear receptors. Additionally, retinoic acid (Yasmeen et al., 2002) modulates a number of other transcription factors and signaling pathways, including PPAR. Lycopene (Aydemir et al., 2012) and apo-10′-lycopenoic acid are also capable of activating RAR. Numerous carotenoids use common signaling pathways like nuclear factor-kappa B (NF-B) and mitogen-activated proteins to control gene expression. MAP) kinases or through detoxification-related transcription factors such as the aryl hydrocarbon receptor (AhR), nuclear factor erythroid-2-related factor 2 (NRF2), or PXR (Ben-Dor et al., 2005).

4.4 CAROTENOIDS METABOLITES ARE INVOLVED IN BODY WEIGHT MANAGEMENT: PRECLINICAL STUDIES

Numerous research studies have suggested a connection between obesity and low levels of circulating carotenoids in both epidemiological and observational investigations (Kimmons et al., 2006; Garcia et al., 2009). Body mass index (BMI) and all tested carotenoids in plasma—aside from lycopene—have strong inverse relationships, according to the CARDIA study (Andersen et al., 2006). Furthermore, there is a strong inverse relationship between blood carotenoid concentrations and a number of obesity-related diseases, including insulin resistance and low-grade inflammation (Beydoun et al., 2011).

4.5 INTERVENTION STUDIES

Numerous important studies have been done to determine how beta-carotene affects energy metabolism and how obesity is affected by it (Coronel et al., 2019). In the majority of research, vitamins and carotenoids were combined in a natural matrix, including plant extracts or fruit juices (Bonet et al.). Canas et al. (2017) observed that children who received a variety of carotenoids (beta-carotene, alpha-carotene, zeaxanthin, lutein, lycopene, alpha-tocopherol, and astaxanthin) for six months experienced a reduction in their waist-to-height ratio, subcutaneous adipose tissue, and BMI z-score. These positive outcomes were closely related to a rise in plasma levels of beta-carotene in children. In a different study, healthy overweight participants received a mixture of xanthophylls, paprika, and carotenoids for 12 weeks. When compared to the placebo group, this supplementation decreased subcutaneous fat area, visceral fat area, total fat area, and BMI in the treated group (Kakutani et al., 2018). According to one of these studies, it had an anti-obesity effect that was connected to a provitamin A effect. Since mice lacked the enzyme beta-carotene (Amengua et al., 2010), the weight of adipose tissue did not change when 15,15′-monooxygenase (BCO) was measured. This effect was discovered to be connected to decreased PPAR expression in adipose tissue as well as retinoid X receptor (RAR) signaling's involvement in the regulation (Lobo et al., 2010).

Through limiting the growth of adipose tissue, astaxanthin assisted in preventing obesity in mice fed a high-fat diet (Ikeuchi et al., 2007). Similar anti-obesity outcomes have been observed in mice fed a high-fat, high-fructose diet, where astaxanthin also reduced inflammation and increased insulin sensitivity. In studies using mice models of non-alcoholic steatohepatitis (NASH) and diet-induced obesity (DIO), astaxanthin was found to have a protective effect against hepatic steatosis (Kim et al., 2007) as well as fibrosis and inflammation in the liver (Kim et al., 2007). Anti-adiposity properties for β-cryptoxanthin have also been reported, but their mechanism is still unknown. Additionally, β-cryptoxanthin restored insulin resistance and hepatic steatosis. The anti-inflammatory properties of this carotenoid in the liver may be responsible for this impact in DIO mice.

Fucoxanthin has been thoroughly examined and reviewed for its ability to help people manage their weight (Maeda, 2015). In KK-Ay mice, this carotenoid decreased the expression of several pro-inflammatory cytokines, which in turn reduced weight gain and hyperglycemia (Hosokawa et al., 2010). Similar outcomes have been reported in DIO mice, possibly by modulation of adiponectin production, lipogenesis, and adipose tissue inflammation. Zeaxanthin inhibits lipogenesis in adipose tissue and induces AMP-activated protein kinase (AMPK) activation to reduce obesity in mice fed high-fat diets (Liu et al., 2017).

Lycopene has been shown to have a similar anti-obesity effect in mice fed a high-fat diet, where adiposity was decreased after treatment. The severity of several co-occurring diseases, including steatosis, glucose intolerance, and insulin sensitivity, was decreased. This positive impact of lycopene and/or tomato powder rich in lycopene on glucose homeostasis, obesity, adipose tissue steatosis, and liver inflammation was seen by Fennie et al. (2017) in a DIO mouse model. All of these findings suggest that carotenoids may act on the biology of adipocytes and adipose tissue in order to modify a number of factors related to obesity and/or associated co-occurring conditions, in addition to providing strong support for the beneficial effect of carotenoids on the management of obesity. Due to the fact that carotenoids are stored, metabolized, and bioactive in adipocytes and adipose tissue, this hypothesis was strongly supported by the available data.

The anti-obesity activity of carotenoids and carotenoid derivatives has been related to activities in various tissues that are most likely connected effects due to the considerable connection across tissues in mammals through metabolism and neuroendocrine signaling. However, the adipose tissues, including brown adipose tissue (BAT) and white adipose tissue, are significant targets in the anti-obesity activity of carotenoids and CCPs (WAT). This is understandable given that adipose tissues are relevant locations of retinoid and carotenoid metabolism and storage in animals and play significant pathological and physiological roles in energy and lipid metabolism and obesity.

4.6 CONCLUSION

All of this research points to the provitamin A (carotenoids) diet's positive benefits on obesity and its related metabolic problems, including insulin resistance, hepatic steatosis, metabolic inflammation, diabetes, and atherosclerosis. The primary precursor to vitamin A and retinoic acid, which supports fatty acid oxidation in adipocytes and other tissues, lowers obesity. Additionally, carotenoids aid in controlling changes to the hormones leptin, insulin, and ghrelin. These findings are supported by observational and interventional studies, which also offer a molecular explanation for how eating foods high in provitamin A carotenoids can stop the onset of obesity. However, there is still much to understand about how genetic variations affect the biological activity and metabolism of these substances at the level of adipose tissue. To support preclinical and observational studies, some pure carotenoid-based randomized clinical trials are urgently required. Implementing policies and tactics that encourage the consumption of foods high in provitamin A carotenoids may also help to avoid the onset of metabolic disorders like obesity.

KEYWORDS

- **adipocytes**
- **adipose tissue**
- **brain**
- **carotenoids**
- **genetic variations**
- **metabolic disorders**
- **obesity**
- **provitamin A**

REFERENCES

Agarwal, A. V., & Rao, A. V. (1998). Tomato lycopene and low-density lipoprotein oxidation: A human dietary intervention study. *Lipids, 33*, 981–984.

Amengual, J., Widjaja-Adhi, M. A., Rodriguez-Santiago, S., Hessel, S., Golczak, M., Palczewski, K., & von Lintig, J. (2013). Two carotenoid oxygenases contribute to mammalian provitamin A metabolism. *Journal of Biological Chemistry, 288*, 34081–34096. https://doi.org/10.1074/jbc.M113.501049.

Andersen, L. F., Jacobs, D. R., Jr., Gross, M. D., Schreiner, P. J., Dale Williams, O., & Lee, D. H. (2006). Longitudinal associations between body mass index and serum carotenoids:

The CARDIA study. *British Journal of Nutrition, 95*, 358–365. https://doi.org/10.1079/BJN20051638.

Beydoun, M. A., Shroff, M. R., Chen, X., Beydoun, H. A., Wang, Y., & Zonderman, A. B. (2011). Serum antioxidant status is associated with metabolic syndrome among U.S. adults in recent national surveys. *Journal of Nutrition, 141*, 903–913. https://doi.org/10.3945/jn.110.136580.

Bonet, M. L., Canas, J. A., Ribot, J., & Palou, A. (2015). Carotenoids and their conversion products in the control of adipocyte function, adiposity and obesity. *Archives of Biochemistry and Biophysics, 572*, 112–125. https://doi.org/10.1016/j.abb.2015.02.022.

Bonet, M. L., Canas, J. A., Ribot, J., & Palou, A. (Eds.). (2016). *Carotenoids in Nature* (Vol. 79). Springer. Carotenoids in Adipose Tissue Biology and Obesity, pp. 377–414.

Bonet, M. Luisa & Ribot, Joan & Galmés, Sebastià & Serra, Francisca & Palou, Andreu. (2020). Carotenoids and carotenoid conversion products in adipose tissue biology and obesity: Pre-clinical and human studies. Biochimica et Biophysica Acta (BBA) - Molecular and Cell Biology of Lipids. 1865. 158676. 10.1016/j.bbalip.2020.158676.

Canas, J. A., Lochrie, A., McGowan, A. G., Hossain, J., Schettino, C., & Balagopal, P. B. (2017). Effects of mixed carotenoids on adipokines and abdominal adiposity in children: A pilot study. *Journal of Clinical Endocrinology & Metabolism, 102*, 1983–1990. https://doi.org/10.1210/jc.2017-00185.

Chung, H. Y., Ferreira, A. L., Epstein, S., Paiva, S. A., Castaneda-Sceppa, C., & Johnson, E. J. (2009). Site-specific concentrations of carotenoids in adipose tissue: Relations with dietary and serum carotenoid concentrations in healthy adults. *American Journal of Clinical Nutrition, 90*, 533–539. https://doi.org/10.3945/ajcn.2009.27712.

Church, T., & Martin, C. K. (2018). The obesity epidemic: A consequence of reduced energy expenditure and the uncoupling of energy intake? *Obesity, 26*, 14–16. https://doi.org/10.1002/oby.22072.

Cinti, S. (2012). The adipose organ at a glance. *Disease Models & Mechanisms, 5*, 588–594. https://doi.org/10.1242/dmm.009662.

Cohen, P., & Spiegelman, B. M. (2016). Cell biology of fat storage. *Molecular Biology of the Cell, 27*, 2523–2527. https://doi.org/10.1091/mbc.e15-10-0749.

Coronel, Johana & Pinos Cabezas, Iván & Amengual, Jaume. (2019). β-carotene in Obesity Research: Technical Considerations and Current Status of the Field. Nutrients. 11. 842. 10.3390/nu11040842.

Derghal, A., Djelloul, M., Trouslard, J., & Mounien, L. (2017). The role of microRNA in the modulation of the melanocortinergic system. *Frontiers in Neuroscience, 11*, 181. https://doi.org/10.3389/fnins.2017.00181.

El-Sohemy, A., Baylin, A., Kabagambe, E., Ascherio, A., Spiegelman, D., & Campos, H. (2002). Individual carotenoid concentrations in adipose tissue and plasma as biomarkers of dietary intake. American Journal of Clinical Nutrition, 76(1), 172–179. https://doi.org/10.1093/ajcn/76.1.172.

Farook, V. S., Reddivari, L., Mummidi, S., Puppala, S., Arya, R., Lopez-Alvarenga, J. C., Fowler, S. P., Chittoor, G., Resendez, R. G., Kumar, B. M., et al. (2017). Genetics of serum carotenoid concentrations and their correlation with obesity-related traits in Mexican American children. American Journal of Clinical Nutrition, 106, 52–58. https://doi.org/10.3945/ajcn.116.144006.

Fenni, S., Hammou, H., Astier, J., Bonnet, L., Karkeni, E., Couturier, C., Tourniaire, F., & Landrier, J. F. (2017). Lycopene and tomato powder supplementation similarly inhibit high-fat diet induced obesity, inflammatory response, and associated metabolic disorders. Molecular Nutrition & Food Research, 61, 1601083 https://doi.org/10.1002/mnfr.201601083.

Friedman, J. (2014). 20 years of leptin: Leptin at 20: An overview. Journal of Endocrinology, 223, T1–T8. https://doi.org/10.1530/JOE-14-0405.

Garcia, O. P., Long, K. Z., & Rosado, J. L. (2009). Impact of micronutrient deficiencies on obesity. Nutrition Reviews, 67, 559–572. https://doi.org/10.1111/j.1753-4887.2009.00228.x.

Germain, P., Chambon, P., Eichele, G., Evans, R. M., Lazar, M. A., Leid, M., De Lera, A. R., Lotan, R., Mangelsdorf, D. J., & Gronemeyer, H. (2006). International Union of Pharmacology. LXIII. Retinoid X receptors. Pharmacological Reviews, 58, 760–772. https://doi.org/10.1124/pr.58.4.7.

Gregor, M. F., & Hotamisligil, G. S. (2011). Inflammatory mechanisms in obesity. Annual Review of Immunology, 29, 415–445. https://doi.org/10.1146/annurev-immunol-031210-101322.

Hales, C. M., Carroll, M. D., Fryar, C. D., & Ogden, C. L. (2017). Prevalence of obesity among adults and youth: United States, 2015–2016. Centers for Disease Control and Prevention, National Center for Health Statistics; Hyattsville, MD, USA: 1–8. NCHS Data Brief No. 288.

Hall, K. D., Sacks, G., Chandramohan, D., Chow, C. C., Wang, Y. C., Gortmaker, S. L., & Swinburn, B. A. (2011). Quantification of the effect of energy imbalance on bodyweight. The Lancet, 378, 826–837. https://doi.org/10.1016/S0140-6736(11)60812-X.

Harrison, E. H., & Quadro, L. (2018). Apocarotenoids: Emerging roles in mammals. *Annual Review of Nutrition, 38*, 153–172. https://doi.org/10.1146/annurev-nutr-071816-064608.

Haskell, M. J., & Brown, K. H. (1999). Maternal vitamin A nutriture and the vitamin A content of human milk. Journal of Mammary Gland Biology and Neoplasia, 4, 243–257. https://doi.org/10.1023/A:1018745812512.

Hill, J. O., Wyatt, H. R., & Peters, J. C. (2012). Energy balance and obesity. Circulation, 126, 126–132. https://doi.org/10.1161/CIRCULATIONAHA.111.087213.

Johnson, E. J., Suter, P. M., Sahyoun, N., Ribaya-Mercado, J. D., & Russell, R. M. (1995). Relation between beta-carotene intake and plasma and adipose tissue concentrations of carotenoids and retinoids. American Journal of Clinical Nutrition, 62(3), 598–603. https://doi.org/10.1093/ajcn/62.3.598.

Kakutani, R., Hokari, S., Nishino, A., Ichihara, T., Sugimoto, K., Takaha, T., Kuriki, T., & Maoka, T. (2018). Effect of oral paprika xanthophyll intake on abdominal fat in healthy overweight humans: A randomized, double-blind, placebo-controlled study. Journal of Oleo Science, 67, 1149–1162. https://doi.org/10.5650/jos.ess18076.

Kardinaal, A. F., van't Veer, P., Brants, H. A., van den Berg, H., van Schoonhoven, J., & Hermus, R. J. (1995). Relations between antioxidant vitamins in adipose tissue, plasma, and diet. American Journal of Epidemiology, 141, 440–450. https://doi.org/10.1093/oxfordjournals.aje.a117446.

Kim, B., Farruggia, C., Ku, C. S., Pham, T. X., Yang, Y., Bae, M., Wegner, C. J., Farrell, N. J., Harness, E., Park, Y. K., et al. (2017). Astaxanthin inhibits inflammation and fibrosis in the liver and adipose tissue of mouse models of diet-induced obesity and nonalcoholic steatohepatitis. Journal of Nutritional Biochemistry, 43, 27–35. https://doi.org/10.1016/j.jnutbio.2016.01.006.

Kirby, M. L., Beatty, S., Stack, J., Harrison, M., Greene, I., McBrinn, S., Carroll, P., & Nolan, J. M. (2011). Changes in macular pigment optical density and serum concentrations of lutein and zeaxanthin in response to weight loss. British Journal of Nutrition, 105, 1036–1046. https://doi.org/10.1017/S0007114510004721.

Klein, S., Wadden, T., & Sugerman, H. J. (2002). AGA technical review on obesity. Gastroenterology, 123, 882–932. https://doi.org/10.1053/gast.2002.35514.

Li, B., Vachali, P. P., Gorusupudi, A., Shen, Z., Sharifzadeh, H., Besch, B. M., Nelson, K., Ben-Dor, A., Steiner, M., Gheber, L., Danilenko, M., Dubi, N., Linnewiel, K., Zick, A., Sharoni, Y., & Levy, J. (2005). Carotenoids activate the antioxidant response element transcription system. *Molecular Cancer Therapeutics, 4*, 177–186.

Liu, M., Liu, H., Xie, J., Xu, Q., Pan, C., Wang, J., Wu, X., Zheng, M., & Liu, J. (2017). Anti-obesity effects of zeaxanthin on 3T3-L1 preadipocyte and high fat induced obese mice. *Food Function, 8*, 3327–3338. https://doi.org/10.1039/C7FO00486A.

Makris, A., & Foster, G. D. (2011). Dietary approaches to the treatment of obesity. *Psychiatric Clinics of North America, 34*, 813–827. https://doi.org/10.1016/j.psc.2011.08.004.

Maria, A. G., Graziano, R., & Nicolantonio, D. O. (2015). Carotenoids: Potential allies of cardiovascular health? *Food & Nutrition Research, 59*, 26762. https://doi.org/10.3402/fnr.v59.26762.

Meyers, K. J., Johnson, E. J., Bernstein, P. S., Iyengar, S. K., Engelman, C. D., Karki, C. K., Liu, Z., Igo, R. P., Jr., Truitt, B., Klein, M. L., et al. (2013). Genetic determinants of macular pigments in women of the Carotenoids in Age-Related Eye Disease Study. *Investigative Ophthalmology & Visual Science, 54*, 2333–2345. https://doi.org/10.1167/iovs.12-10867.

Morton, G. J., Cummings, D. E., Baskin, D. G., Barsh, G. S., & Schwartz, M. W. (2006). Central nervous system control of food intake and body weight. *Nature, 443*, 289–295. https://doi.org/10.1038/nature05026.

Mounien, L., Tourniaire, F., & Landrier, J. F. (2019). Anti-obesity effect of carotenoids: Direct impact on adipose tissue and adipose tissue-driven indirect effects. *Nutrients, 11*(4), 761–766. https://doi.org/10.3390/nu11040761.

Moussa, M., Gouranton, E., Gleize, B., Yazidi, C. E., Niot, I., Besnard, P., Borel, P., & Landrier, J. F. (2011). CD36 is involved in lycopene and lutein uptake by adipocytes and adipose tissue cultures. *Molecular Nutrition & Food Research, 55*, 578–584. https://doi.org/10.1002/mnfr.201000399.

Obesity and overweight. (2021, June 9). *World Health Organization*. Retrieved from: https://www.who.int/news-room/fact-sheets/detail/obesity-and-overweight (accessed on 15 June 2024).

P.C., Ahluwalia, N., Brouns, F., Buetler, T., Clement, K., Cunningham, K., Esposito, K., Jonsson, L. S., Kolb, H., Lansink, M., et al. (2011). Dietary factors and low-grade inflammation in relation to overweight and obesity. *British Journal of Nutrition, 106*(Suppl), S5–S78. https://doi.org/10.1017/S0007114511005460.

Paetau, I., Khachik, F., Brown, E. D., Beecher, G. R., Kramer, T. R., Chittams, J., & Clevidence, B. A. (1998). Chronic ingestion of lycopene-rich tomato juice or lycopene supplements significantly increases plasma concentrations of lycopene and related tomato carotenoids in humans. *American Journal of Clinical Nutrition, 68*, 1187–1195. https://doi.org/10.1093/ajcn/68.6.1187.

Razny, U., Lietz, A., Wyss, A., Dembinska-Kiec, A., Palou, A., Keijer, J., Landrier, J. F., & Bonet, M. L. (2011). Beta-carotene reduces body adiposity of mice via BCMO1. *PLoS One, 6*(6), e20644. https://doi.org/10.1371/journal.pone.0020644.

Rodríguez-Concepción, M., Avalos, J., Bonet, M. L., Boronat, A., Gómez-Gómez, L., Hornero-Méndez, D., Limón, M. C., Meléndez-Martínez, A. J., Olmedilla-Alonso, B.,

Palou, A., Ribot, J., Rodrigo, M. J., Zacarías, L., & Zhu, C. (2018). A global perspective on carotenoids: Metabolism, biotechnology, and benefits for nutrition and health. *Progress in Lipid Research, 70*, 62–93. https://doi.org/10.1016/j.plipres.2018.07.001.
Ruhl, R., & Landrier, J. F. (2015). Dietary regulation of adiponectin by direct and indirect lipid activators of nuclear hormone receptors. *Molecular Nutrition & Food Research, 60*, 175–184. https://doi.org/10.1002/mnfr.201500619.
S.A. Lee, H. Jiang, C.M. Trent, J.J. Yuen, S. Narayanasamy, R.W. Curley, Jr., E.H. Harrison, Spiegelman B.M., Flier J.S. (2001). Obesity and the regulation of energy balance. *Cell, 104*, 531–543. https://doi.org/10.1016/S0092-8674(01)00240-9.
Tian, Y., Su, L., Wang, J., Duan, X., & Jiang, X. (2018). Fruit and vegetable consumption and risk of the metabolic syndrome: A meta-analysis. *Public Health Nutrition, 21*, 756–765. https://doi.org/10.1017/S136898001700310X.
Tourniaire, F., Romier-Crouzet, B., Lee, J. H., Marcotorchino, J., Gouranton, E., Salles, J., Malezet, C., Astier, J., Darmon, P., Blouin, E., et al. (2013). Chemokine expression in inflamed adipose tissue is mainly mediated by NF-kappaB. *PLoS ONE, 8*(6), e66515. https://doi.org/10.1371/journal.pone.0066515.
Tremmel, M., Gerdtham, U. G., Nilsson, P. M., & Saha, S. (2017). Economic burden of obesity: A systematic literature review. *International Journal of Environmental Research and Public Health, 14*(4), 435. https://doi.org/10.3390/ijerph14040435.
Walfisch, Y., Walfisch, S., Agbaria, R., Levy, J., & Sharoni, Y. (2003). Lycopene in serum, skin and adipose tissues after tomato-oleoresin supplementation in patients undergoing haemorrhoidectomy or peri-anal fistulotomy. *British Journal of Nutrition, 90*, 759–766. https://doi.org/10.1079/BJN2003955.
Wang, C. X., Jiang, H., Yuen, J. J., Lee, S. A., Narayanasamy, S., Curley, R. W., Jr., Harrison, E. H., & Blaner, W. S. (2015). Actions of beta-apo-carotenoids in differentiating cells: Differential effects in P19 cells and 3T3-L1 adipocytes. *Archives of Biochemistry and Biophysics, 572*, 2–10.
Weber, D., & Grune, T. (2012). The contribution of beta-carotene to vitamin A supply of humans. *Molecular Nutrition & Food Research, 56*, 251–258. https://doi.org/10.1002/mnfr.201100229.
Westerterp, K. R. (2010). Physical activity, food intake, and body weight regulation: Insights from doubly labeled water studies. *Nutrition Reviews, 68*, 148–154. https://doi.org/10.1111/j.1753-4887.2010.00270.x.
Williams, D. J., Edwards, D., Hamernig, I., Jian, L., James, A. P., Johnson, S. K., & Tapsell, L. C. (2013). Vegetables containing phytochemicals with potential anti-obesity properties: A review. *Food Research International, 52*, 323–333. https://doi.org/10.1016/j.foodres.2013.03.015.
World Health Organization. (2012). *Obesity and Overweight*. WHO Media Center; Geneva, Switzerland. Retrieved from https://www.who.int/news-room/fact-sheets/detail/obesity-and-overweight (accessed on 15 June 2024).

PART II

ANTIOXIDANTS AND VITAMINS IN OBESITY

CHAPTER 5

ANTIOXIDANT-RICH NUTRACEUTICALS IN OBESITY MANAGEMENT

KAVITA GAHLOT

Department of Pharmacy, Shree Satya College of Higher Education, Moradabad, Uttar Pradesh, India

ABSTRACT

Nutrition and exercise are essential to preventing and treating obesity, which is becoming more prevalent throughout the world. Currently, extensive research is being done on natural product (nutraceutical) interventions as prospective treatments for obesity and weight management. Because of their safety and notable nutritional and therapeutic properties, nutraceuticals have drawn a lot of attention. Important nutraceutical ingredients include nutrients, natural remedies, and dietary supplements that work to prevent and treat various diseases, thereby promoting health. Chronic, excessive adipose tissue development raises the risk for cardiovascular disease (CVD), type 2 diabetes mellitus, and cancer, according to extensive research on obesity that has been conducted for more than 10 years. It is speculated that the decreased plasma concentrations of vitamins and antioxidants in obese people compared to non-obese people may have a negative impact on the occurrence of inflammation and disease. Nutraceuticals have been discovered to have good impacts on various elements of pathogenic obesity as well as the activity of adipocyte cell lines, according to research. This chapter looks at recent studies on dietary supplements and how they affect body composition and obesity.

Nutraceuticals in Obesity Management and Control. Raj K. Keservani & Alka Lohani (Eds.)

5.1 INTRODUCTION

5.1.1 OBESITY

Obesity is a condition resulting from the lack of body energy balance. Despite numerous initiatives to lower obesity prevalence, obesity remains the main cause of public health concerns. Around 17% of children and one-third of adults in the United States are obese, according to a study (Ogden et al., 2014). Obesity in infants and preschoolers has decreased from 13.8% to 8.1% during the past 10 years. Other age groups, however, continue to have the same level of obesity. Overnutrition and undernutrition are problems in developing nations. In developing nations, the number of overweight people increased in the last 30 years, reaching more than 900 million by 2008. However, within the same time span, developed countries' overweight rates increased by 1.7 times (Keats & Wiggins, 2014). Growth in overweight or obesity is worrying; however, there have been issues with the efficacy and application of a tight regimen (Berthoud, 2011; Davidson & Swithers, 2004). The search for alternate tactics to meet the need for secure anti-obesity medications has resulted. Over the past 10 years, research has concentrated on assessing the effectiveness of dietary and natural bioactive ingredients that may modify the pathophysiology of obesity. Due to increased awareness of illness prevention through adopting a healthy eating pattern, the food sector has an enormous opportunity to develop functional meals to fulfill the demands of consumers who are health conscious.

5.2 ETIOLOGY OF OBESITY

5.2.1 INFLAMMATION AS A PROGENITOR IN OBESITY

Obesity is characterized by hyperplasia and hypertrophy of adipocytes. It is accompanied by the infiltration of macrophages and the consequent liberation of cytokines, namely IL-1, TNF-α, leptin, and macrophage inflammatory protein (MIP) (Sethi & Hotamisligil, 1999). This results in insulin resistance and dysregulation of thermogenesis. Adipose tissue is an endocrine organ enclosed by blood capillaries that regulate the generation of hormones, vascular endothelial growth factors, and interleukin-6, which endorse the progression of inflammation (Koh-Banerjee et al., 2004). Enlargements of adipocytes are characterized by elevated plasma, hypoxia, hyperplasia, and inflammation infiltration of macrophages. Formation of de novo blood vessels from the parent blood vessels and stimulation and relocation of endothelial cells result in angiogenesis (Schenk, 2008). Angiogenesis plays a significant role in healing, organ restoration, and the development of the female reproductive system. The event of angiogenesis is regulated by pro-angiogenic agents, namely leptin, resistin, TNF-α, interleukin-6, and anti-angiogenic agents such as endostatin, thrombospondin (TSP-1), and Kalistatin. However, overexpression of pro-angiogenic factors dysregulates endothelial function and results in angiogenesis. Consequently, if anti-angiogenic molecules predominate over the angiogenic molecules, then the event of angiogenesis is diminished. Also, the plasma volume of antioxidants is decreased in obese people, which deleteriously affects the progression of inflammation.

5.2.2 AFFERENT SIGNALS

Swelling in the gastric through stimulation of vagal afferents is a cascade for satiety, with gastric retrenchment signaling for appetite. The afferent process is initiated by nutrients, neural impulses, and hormones that regulate energy intake and spending. Captivating glucose by nutrients induces satiety while decreasing glucose levels initiates hunger. This process is regulated by several neurotransmitters, hormones, and peptides (Campfield, 1985). Leptin is a hormone produced by adipose tissue that decreases food uptake, whereas the secretion increases as fat storage increases (Considine et al., 1996). Growth hormone-releasing hormone is secreted by the duodenum and stomach and it controls GH production. It increases food intake, and food consumption inhibits its secretion. The hindbrain receives afferent impulses for a variety of functions (Berthoud, 2002). Neural inputs are processed in the hindbrain in the nucleus of the tractus solitarius. Leptin impulses travel to the hypothalamus arcuate nucleus, which promotes the production and release of neuropeptide Y (NPY), hence increasing appetite.

5.2.3 PATHOGENIC OBESITY

Chronic, excessive adipose tissue development raises the risk of CVD, type 2 diabetes mellitus, and cancer, according to extensive research on obesity that has been conducted for more than 10 years. Due to the fact that obese people use healthcare services far more frequently than non-obese people (Bertakis & Azari, 2005), the load on healthcare systems will grow as prevalence rises. The development of obesity-related diseases is assumed to be influenced by the chronic, low-grade, systemic inflammatory response that is associated with obesity and results from increased adipose tissue (AT) depots (Trayhurn & Wood, 2004). Additionally, obese people have decreased plasma levels of vitamins and antioxidants (Aasheim et al., 2008; Panagiotakos et al., 2005). Research also indicates the modulatory effects of vitamins and antioxidants on the immune system (Wintergerst et al., 2008), and it may be that reduced levels have a role in the development of inflammation and ultimately disease in obesity, and an inverse relationship between serum total antioxidant capacity and waist circumference (Chrysohoou et al., 2007). Orlistat and sibutramine are the main medications used in the current pharmacotherapy for obesity, but due to their adverse effects and the unknown long-term effects of their use, research into alternatives has become necessary. In order to prevent the start of obesity comorbidities, it is intended to observe the ability of nutraceuticals to reduce (Conroy et al., 2011) the development of oxidative stress and inflammation in obesity.

5.3 WHAT ARE NUTRACEUTICALS?

The terms "nutritional supplements" and "pharmaceuticals" were combined to form the term "nutraceuticals" (a medical drug). Dr. Stephen De Felice, the founder and head of the Foundation for Innovation in Medicine (FIM), invented the word "nutraceutical" in 1989 (De Felice, 1995; Mannion, 1998). He defines nutraceuticals as a product or component of food that has health advantages, such as the ability to prevent or treat disease (Sarin, 2012; Kalra, 2003; Keservani et al., 2010a, b, 2017, 2020). Nutraceuticals include a variety of foods that have been processed, such as cereals, soups, and beverages, as well as separated nutrients, dietary supplements, and special diets (Biesalski, 2007). The use of nutraceuticals is rapidly gaining popularity around the world (Childs, 1999). According to a recent BCC research analysis, the global market for nutraceuticals is growing at a compound annual growth rate (CAGR) of 7.5% and is expected to reach US $285.0 billion by 2021 from US $198.7 billion in 2016 (Golla, 2018; Brower, 1998).

5.3.1 NUTRACEUTICALS' ADVANTAGES

Several advantages of dietary supplements include:

- Might improve the nutritional value of our diet.
- It might lengthen our lives.
- It might aid us in preventing specific medical conditions.

- Taking care of oneself could be beneficial psychologically.
- It might be thought of as more "natural" and less likely to have negative side effects than conventional treatment.
- Might provide food for special needs populations (e.g., nutrient-dense foods for the elderly).
- It might be easily accessible and reasonably priced (Pandey et al., 2010).

The health benefits of using nutraceutical products are well known and include lowering the risk of cancer and heart disease, as well as preventing or treating headaches, high blood pressure, high cholesterol, obesity, osteoporosis, diabetes, arthritis, digestive problems, and constipation (Rajasekaran, 2008; Packer, 2001; Maddi, 2007). In concentrated forms, such as pills, capsules, powders, and tinctures, nutraceuticals can be purchased as a single ingredient or in combination with other ingredients.

5.3.2 CATEGORIES OF NUTRACEUTICALS

The term "nutraceutical" is broad. There are numerous things that can be categorized as nutraceuticals (Dureja et al., 2003).

5.3.2.1 NUTRITIONAL SUPPLEMENT

- Vitamins, minerals, amino acids, fatty acids, and antioxidants are among the nutrients.
- Herbals: Extracts and concentrates made from herbs or other botanical items.
- Phytochemicals include glucosinolates, polysaccharides, anthocyanidins, phytoestrogens, terpenoids, carotenoids, limonoids, polyphenols, and isoflavonoids.
- Live microbial feed supplements known as probiotics are used to balance the bacteria in the gut. The two most significant probiotics are bifidobacteria and lactobacillus bacteria.
- Prebiotics: A fermented food component that enables certain alterations in the gut microbiota's composition and/or activity that confer advantages on the host's well-being and health.
- Enzymes used in nutraceuticals.
- Non-starchy polysaccharides like cellulose, hemicelluloses, gum and pectin, lignin, and resistant dextrin are included in dietary fiber.

5.3.2.2 NUTRACEUTICALS AND FORTIFIED/FUNCTIONAL FOODS

It is a food that has been supplemented with extra nutrients or ingredients. For instance, calcium-fortified orange juice, vitamin D-fortified milk, and folic acid- and fiber-fortified cereal flour.

5.3.2.3 RECOMBINANT PHARMACEUTICALS AND NUTRACEUTICALS

Farm and pharmaceuticals combine to form the word "farmaceuticals." Medically beneficial substances derived from genetically altered crops typically employ biotechnological techniques.

5.3.2.4 THERAPEUTIC FOOD

The medical evaluation establishes the specialized dietary management of a certain disease or condition for specific nutritional requirements, and the medicinal foods are meant to be ingested under the guidance of a physician.

5.4 OBESE AND NUTRACEUTICALS

A current global public health issue affecting 315 million people is obesity. Numerous illnesses, including hypertension, congestive heart failure, angina pectoris, hyperlipidemia, respiratory problems, osteoarthritis, cancer, renal vein thrombosis, and decreased fertility, are risk factors for obesity (Caterson & Gill, 2002). The increased accessibility of meals heavy in fat and calories is one of the main factors contributing to obesity. In order to prevent and treat obesity, which has a relatively high incidence worldwide, nutrition and exercise are essential. Large-scale nutritional interventions are currently being researched as possible treatments for obesity and weight management. Nutraceuticals with possible anti-obesity benefits include capsaicin-conjugated linoleic acid, *Momordica charantia*, and psyllium fiber (Rubin & Levin, 1994).

Even while excessive consumption of calorie-dense meals such as processed foods, drinks, and snacks can make people gain weight, calorie restriction and increased physical activity have only sporadic efficacy in treating obesity. In order to prevent or treat obesity, researchers and obese people turn to nutraceuticals and medications. For body weight loss, an efficient dietary supplement that can raise energy expenditure while lowering calorie consumption is preferred (Boozer et al., 2001).

5.5 CURRENTLY AVAILABLE NUTRACEUTICALS FOR THE TREATMENT OF OBESITY

Several nutraceuticals possess anti-obese properties. A blend of galactomannan and Sylvester, in the diet, promotes fat loss in obese individuals.

5.5.1 TURMERIC

A naturally occurring phenolic substance called curcumin, which is an active component of turmeric and is known to provide health advantages, is obtained from the spice *Curcuma longa* L of the Zingiberaceae family. It is understood that chronic inflammation plays a key role in the etiology of diabetes and obesity. Cytokines and cyclooxygenase-2 (COX-2) are affected by curcumin (TNF-a). TNF and interleukins 1, 6, which are involved in obesity-induced insulin resistance, are produced by adipose tissue (Iyer et al., 2009). The safety and effectiveness of curcumin have been reported. According to Shehzad et al. (2012), curcumin also inhibits CYP-450 and UDP-glucuronosyltransferase. It can be applied to a variety of businesses, including those in the food, textile, and pharmaceutical sectors. Curcumin has a wide spectrum of medicinal effects, but due to its extremely limited bioavailability, it must be enhanced using pharmaceutical methods. In numerous disorders, including cancer, diabetes, autoimmune diseases, and neurological diseases, curcumin has been shown to be helpful (Watanabe et al., 2020; Borges-Canha et al., 2015; Shen & Ji, 2016; Shen et al., 2017). Numerous studies have demonstrated that curcumin can alter the composition of the gut microbiota in a beneficial way.

5.5.2 INULIN

A carbohydrate called inulin is made by numerous plants, primarily chicory. Chemically speaking, it is a member of the inulin-type fructans family (ITFs), which also includes inulin itself and (2→1) linear fructose polymers like oligofructose and fructooligosaccharides (FOS). The consumption of inulin at 12 g/day was correlated with specific changes in the relative amount of Anaerostipes, Bilophila, and *Bifidobacterium* spp., associated with improvement in gut function, in a clinical study involving 44 healthy adults with mild constipation, in the absence of significant differences in the uniformity or diversity of the microbiota (Vandeputte et al., 2017).

5.5.3 CURRY TREE

Murraya koenigii is an ancient plant used by Indians as a spice for preparing food and treating numerous ailments, belonging to Rutaceae (Vijayanand & Wesely, 2010). Traditionally, different parts of the *Murraya koenigii* plant have been used in the management and prevention of hypertension, hepatitis, cough, hysteria, and skin infections. Moreover, it exhibits antioxidant, anti-inflammatory, anti-hyperglycemic, and hypoglycemic properties. In a clinical study, the leaves of *Murraya koenigii* were tested for hypoglycemic activity. From the study, it has been revealed that leaves can be used as an alternative for a number of disorders (Yankuzo et al., 2011). *Murraya koenigii* elevates hepatic glycogen levels and reduces gluconeogenic enzymatic activity. It scavenges free radicals by producing antioxidant properties.

5.5.4 FLAXSEED

Linum usitatissimum L. is a well-known medicinal plant that is also used as a source of food, textile fiber, and other nutrients. The flaxseed seed (semen), which is rich in oil (consisting of polyunsaturated fatty acids (PUFAs), particularly ω-3), lignans like linustatin, neolinustatin, and linamarin, as well as soluble and insoluble complex polysaccharides, is part of the plant that is of interest for medical applications (EMA assessment). Flaxseed is primarily used to alleviate constipation and relieve gastrointestinal pain, according to the WHO and EMA monographs (Watanabe et al., 2020). The effectiveness of flaxseed in promoting weight loss has been studied, and certain clinical trials have shown that oil and ground seed have positive effects.

5.5.5 FENUGREEK

Fenugreek (*Trigonella foenum-graecum*) belongs to the family Leguminosae and is used in food as a spice. It is used in the treatment of wound healing and initiates lactation in mothers. Medicinal values are present in steroidal sapogenins, galactomannans, and isoleucine. They show their action synergistically to produce health benefits; hence, fenugreek is known to be a "nutraceutical." Fenugreek seed is a source of diosgenin. Diosgenin is a pioneer in manufacturing many drugs, namely testosterone and progesterone.

Polysaccharides such as galactomannans are the main compounds present in fenugreek seeds. They help absorb water and make viscous solutions that decrease glucose absorption in the stomach. Fenugreek helps in lowering the glucose in plasma. The seeds of fenugreek (sapogenins) decrease serum

TGs, total cholesterol, and LDL cholesterol (Basch et al., 2003). Although fenugreek is safe, several adverse effects accompany it. It is to be avoided in pregnant women due to their uterine-stimulating properties.

5.5.6 CHILI PEPPERS

Pure capsaicin is a colorless and crystalline substance. Capsaicin is present in red chili peppers. Chili peppers produce several secondary metabolites known as capsaicinoids, perhaps as a restraint against fungi. It has been investigated that capsaicin exhibits therapeutic potential for preventing obesity in animal models (Kim et al., 2003; Manjunatha & Srinivasan, 2006; Park et al., 2004). Daily intake of capsaicin between 8 and 25 μmol results in the prevention of obesity.

5.5.7 GREEN TEA

Green tea (*Camellia sinensis)* is a beverage consumed by people globally. The active component is catechin epigallocatechin-3-gallate (EGCG). In China, it is consumed to reduce weight gain, as it washes out excessive fat from the body. *Camellia sinensis* consists of three major components: xanthine bases, essential oils, and polyphenolic compounds that are beneficial for humans.

i. Consumption of green tea for one year decreases the risk of hypertension (Bose et al., 2008).
ii. Green tea results in the reduction of cardiovascular-related disorders. Scientists studied the effect of green tea on body weight in people. It was recorded that about 2.4% of body weight was reduced in obese women after consumption of green tea for 3 months.
iii. Oolong tea, a rich source of catechins when included in a dietary regime for obese people for 12 weeks, showed a significant decline in body weight. Thus, it has been concluded that catechins help in weight management, whereas green tea catechins produce a notable decrease in weight (Sae-Tan et al., 2001).

Due to polyphenols, which are its main bioactive constituents and have shown numerous capabilities, including antioxidant, anti-aging, and anti-inflammatory action (Saeed et al., 2017), it has a number of beneficial health impacts. Green tea use was observed to increase the relative abundance of Firmicutes and Actinobacteria in humans and reduce the concentration of the phylum Bacteroidetes using 16S rRNA sequencing. Additionally, green tea raised the number of short-chain fatty acid (SCFA)-producing bacteria such as *Roseburia* spp., *Faecalibacterium* spp., *Eubacterium rectale group, Blautia* spp., *Coprococcus* spp., *Bifidobacterium longum* while decreasing the number of other Prevotella species (Yuan et al., 2018).

5.5.8 BLACK GRAM

Black gram is known as *Vigna mungo* and black lentil, belonging to the family of Dicotyledonae, rich in proteins (Champ, 2002). They are effective in the management of a number of diseases.

1. **Cardiovascular Disease:** The administration of black gram with saturated food reduces the risk of congestive heart failure by manifesting lipid homeostasis.
2. **Diabetes:** Due to low glycemic and a large number of indigestible fibers, black grams uphold the glycemic index in diabetes and inhibit insulin resistance.
3. **Obesity:** Black gram helps regulate normal body weight by producing satiety effects. Black grams act by inhibiting α-amylase protein inhibitors by delaying carbohydrate absorption, thus inhibiting the progression of obesity.

5.5.9 GUAR GUM

Guar gum is a fiber made from *Cyamopsis tetragonolobus* (L.) Taub, a leguminous plant native to India. Galactomannan is a D-galactose and D-mannose polymer that is (Watanabe et al., 2020). Guar gum consumption was linked to an increase in *Ruminococcus, Fusicatenibacter, Faecalibacterium,* and *Bacteroides* spp., and a decrease in *Roseburia, Lachnospiracea,* and *Blautia* spp., which improved defecation frequency, stool consistency, and the abundance of metabolites like butyrate, acetate, and amino acids (Reider et al., 2020). Data were evaluated on a broader scale of samples, and results showed that in one instance, guar gum consumption increased the growth of *Bifidobacterium*, *Ruminococcus*, and *Megasphaera* spp. while inhibiting Bacteroides *and Phascolarctobacterium spp*. Without changing the frequency of the hives, this impact changed the consistency of the stools (Yasukawa et al., 2019).

5.5.10 FLAVONOIDS

Flavonoid (Keservani & Sharma, 2014; Keservani et al., 2016a, b) is a polyphenol found in plants, fruits, and vegetables and induces a number of health benefits. The anti-inflammatory property of flavonoids has been used in the treatment of disorders. Consumption of green tea by an individual has been conversely interrelated with liver dysfunction (Steptoe et al., 2007). Citrus flavonoids in animals reduce plasma lipid levels and improve plasma lipid levels (Nichols et al., 2011).

5.5.11 PLANTAGO OVATA

Psyllium fiber is a water-soluble fiber that can create a viscous gel and is obtained from the husks of *Plantago ovata* Forsk.fr seeds. According to Watanabe et al. (2020), it is used to control intestinal regularity, suppress hunger, and obstruct the absorption of carbs, fats, and bile salt. Its consumption in both healthy subjects and patients with constipation revealed subtle but important changes in the microbiota. In healthy subjects, it increases Veillonella and decreases *Subdoligranulum spp.*, while in patients with constipation, it increases *Lachnospira, Faecalibacterium, Phascolarctobacterium*, *Veillonella,* and *Sutterella* spp. Additionally, it has been found that the change in the fecal levels of acetate and propionate has resulted in a decrease in Coriobacteria and Christensenella species (Jalanka et al., 2019). Additional research supports the positive effects of psyllium on hive frequency, microbiome level, and SCFA concentration (Rasmussen et al., 2017). It is involved in decreasing LDL levels in individuals (Tai et al., 1999). Minolest is a combination of psyllium fiber and guar gum and was taken in the clinical trial. Subjects who were administered Minolest improved LDL levels in contrast with the placebo (Jenkins et al., 2002).

5.5.12 MOMORDICA CHARANTIA

Momordica charantia (MC) is cultivated in Asia. The active constituents contain antiviral activity. Momordica has been induced to decrease adipose tissue expansion in mice (Senanayake et al., 2004; Miura et al., 2004). When Momordica is taken during exercise, it increases insulin sensitivity (Baur & Sinclair, 2006). However, the drug's therapeutic effect can be used as a preventative measure to counteract the progression of obesity.

5.5.13 AMLA

Amla (*Emblica officinalis*) is a widely used plant in India for medicinal purposes. The whole plant is used for medical health benefits. The Amla fruit is used in the treatment of a number of illnesses viz. diuretic, liver tonic, stomachic, and digestive. Intake of *E. officinalis* decreased the level of cholesterol and triacylglyceride in the liver. It mitigates the production of oxidative stress by counteracting age-related hyperlipidemia (Baquer et al., 2011). Also, oral administration of Amla indicates a substantial decrease in total cholesterol (TC) and a subsequent increase in high-density lipoprotein levels.

5.5.14 GINSENG

The dried roots of *Panax ginseng* C.A. Meyer are used to make ginseng. Triterpene saponins, also known as ginsenosides and polysaccharides, are the primary phytochemical components of ginseng. Asian ginseng is the most well-known kind. In contrast, *Panax quinquefolius* L., also referred to as American ginseng, varies from Asian ginseng primarily in terms of the qualitative and quantitative profile of various ginsenosides (Flagg, 2021). American and Asian ginseng have both been studied for their involvement in weight loss and the improvement of gluco-lipidemic profiles in both animal models and clinical trials (Governa et al., 2018). Due to the variety of administered preparations, herbal combinations, and dosages (Kim et al., 2011; Sharma et al., 2020), even the majority of clinical trials fail to address the clear effectiveness of ginseng. However, recent studies have noted the high potential of ginseng in body weight control through the modulation of gut microbiota. According to a clinical exploratory study involving 10 obese women between the ages of 40 and 60, taking 8 grams of a chemically characterized *P. ginseng* extract daily for eight weeks caused them to lose weight and slightly altered their gut microbiota species compared to the untreated healthy obese participants. Before ginseng was administered, the altered gut microbiota structure was linked to the treatment's anti-obesity effects.

5.5.15 CARALLUMA FIMBRIATA

Caralluma fimbriata is a traditional food used by the Indian population to suppress hunger. The chemical constituents are pregnane glycosides, flavone glycosides, and flavonoids (Kuriyan et al., 2007). Hunger is suppressed by the pregnane glycosides constituent. Intake of 1 g daily of *Caralluma fimbriata* results in a 20% decrease in hunger (Kamalakkannan et al., 2010). Food intake is inhibited by *Caralluma fimbriata*, and increases in body weight, liver weight, and fat deposition are reduced in a dose-dependent manner. Additionally, it offers a defense against atherogenesis.

5.5.16 GINGER COMPONENTS

The ginger components 6-gingerol and 6-shogaol exhibit anti-inflammatory properties (Han et al., 2005). In a study conducted on rats, it was seen that weight loss occurs by inhibiting dietary lipids (Kamal & Aleem, 2009). Therefore, it has been concluded that ginger exhibits properties to inhibit inflammation and associated complications.

5.5.17 RESVERATROL

The stilbenoid family of polyphenols includes resveratrol, which is frequently found in its trans-isomer form in many different plants, including *Polygonum cuspidatum* Siebold & Zucc., fruits such as grapes and berries, peanuts, and red wine. Its bioavailability is extremely poor because of substantial glucuronidation in the liver and gut and sulfation in the liver (Watanabe et al., 2020; Walle, 2011). Both animal studies and human clinical trials have been used to investigate the effects of resveratrol supplementation. Resveratrol appears to have a number of health advantages, including the prevention of cancer, obesity, and type 2 diabetes (Rauf et al., 2018), as well as anti-aging properties (Li et al., 2018) and the promotion of cardiovascular health (Li & Xia, 2019).

5.5.18 GLUCANS

The cell walls of fungi, yeast, and grains contain glucose polymers called glucans. They are extensively distributed in everyday foods such as seaweed, barley, mushrooms, and oats. Beta-glucans have been shown to have a number of beneficial effects, including those that are anti-inflammatory, anti-cancer, and immune-modulating (Daou & Zhang, 2012; Hong et al., 2005; Tosh, 2013). Around 52 healthy volunteers participated in multiple clinical trials where the prebiotic benefit of beta-glucans was proven. In fact, a glucan-enriched diet was able to raise the concentrations of *Ruminococcus* spp., *Clostridium orbiscindens,* and *Roseburia hominis* while lowering the concentrations of Firmicutes and Fusobacteria. The primary SCFAs, such as 2-methyl-propanoic, acetic, butyric, and propionic acids, exhibited a noticeable increase in levels as well (De Angelis et al., 2015). In addition, numerous *in vivo* and *in vitro* studies have demonstrated that beta-glucans have a significant prebiotic effect because of their capacity to modify gut microbiota.

5.5.19 CALCIUM-RICH FOOD

Calcium-rich foods such as milk, yogurt, and cheese play a vital role in body weight regulation. Daily intake reduces adipose tissue mass (Blankson et al., 2000). Conjugated linolenic acid is present in fish and eggs. It is not to be cooked as it is temperature-sensitive, so it should be consumed as a supplement or in a salad. Administration of Conjugated linolenic acid decreases the fat mass of overweight people (Lavigne et al., 2001).

5.5.20MBOTTLE GOURD

Bottle gourd (*Lagenaria siceraria*) belongs to the *Cucurbitaceae* family and originated in India and other tropical parts of the world. Bottle gourd comprises chemical constituents such as minerals, vitamins, fiber, etc. It is used in managing various ailments, namely headache, baldness, anti-hyperglycemic, analgesic, immunomodulatory, and hepatoprotective actions in humans (Katare et al., 2012). Several varieties are known; the sweet bottle gourd is used as a vegetable, whereas the wild variety is used to prevent disorders. Also, drinking a glass of bottled gourd juice on an empty stomach helps in managing obesity and related complications. It has been reported in a study that bottle gourd decreases LDL levels. The study consisted of 50 individuals aged 40–60 years, and they were asked to drink fresh *L. siceraria* juice for 90 days on an empty stomach. Regularly, individuals were observed for kidney functioning, body weight, and BMI. After 90 days, it was observed that there was progress in HDL and a decrease in LDL was observed (Katare et al., 2011). However, there was no variation in the BMI of the individuals.

5.5.21 WHEY PROTEIN

In comparison to other proteins like casein and soy, whey protein can induce a higher degree of muscle protein synthesis because of its high content of branched-chain amino acids (Watanabe et al., 2020; van Vliet et al., 2015). It is therefore consumed or supplemented to support the development of muscle mass and to improve body composition in athletes. Additionally, whey protein has a number of positive health effects and may help fight obesity by regulating hunger and the plasma levels of satiety hormones such as insulin, ghrelin, cholecystokinin, and glucagon-like peptide.

5.5.22 CHLOROGENIC ACID

One of the most prevalent dietary polyphenols, chlorogenic acid is a key ingredient in coffee and some other plant species. Other properties have recently been described in basic and clinical research investigations, with an apparent reduced risk of a variety of disorders (Watanabe et al., 2020). It shares antioxidant and anti-inflammatory effects with other polyphenols. It has been found that chlorogenic acid plays crucial roles in the control of glucose and lipid metabolism, which has an impact on linked disorders including diabetes and obesity, and reduces the risk of cardiovascular diseases, cancer, and fatty liver disease (Tajik et al., 2017). These findings are primarily based on animal studies. Numerous studies have suggested that the microbiota is responsible for these benefits, although no pattern of microbial alteration in response to chlorogenic acid supplementation has been found (McAllan et al., 2014).

5.5.23 L. CARNITINE

Widely found in animal tissues, L-carnitine is an amino acid derivative made from the amino acids lysine and methionine (Watanabe et al., 2020). The function of *L. carnitine* in the augmentation of endogenous levels of trimethylamine-N-oxide (TMAO), a factor connected with a considerable rise in cardiovascular risk, has been examined in a number of research. Numerous bacteria, including those in the Deferribacteraceae, Enterobacteriaceae, Anaeroplasmataceae, Prevotellaceae, Ruminococcaceae, and Lachnospiraceae families, as well as those belonging to specific genera, including Mitsuokella, Fusobacterium, Desulfovibrio, and *Methanobrevibacter smithii*, have been implicated in TMAO production or the level (Koeth et al., 2013).

5.5.24 CHITOSAN

Two derivatives of the polysaccharide chitin, which is a common component of arthropod and insect exoskeletons and fungal cell walls, are chitosan and chitosan oligosaccharide (COS). Deacetylated N-acetyl glucosamine polymers, such as chitosan, are produced from chitin. An oligomer of β-(1→4)-linked d-glucosamine is called chitosan oligosaccharide (COS). Due to COS's high water solubility and ease of absorption via the human colon, it has lately been investigated as a nutraceutical, enteric coating for cells, and a means of improving medication and DNA delivery. Chitosan has demonstrated lipid-binding capabilities *in vivo*, lowering serum cholesterol and diminishing gastrointestinal absorption (Muanprasat & Chatsudthipong, 2017; Naveed et al., 2019). There is still disagreement on whether the therapeutic qualities of chitosan and COS result from a different microbiome.

5.5.25 POLYUNSATURATED FATTY ACIDS

Saturated fatty acids control the toll-like receptor 4 (TLR4) on fat cells, which causes inflammation. Docosahexaenoic acid (DHA), one of the W-3 polyunsaturated fatty acids (PUFAs) found in fish oils, is recognized as an anti-inflammatory agent that prevents obesity (Sekiya et al., 2003).

5.6 CONCLUSION

With the modern regimen, people are more susceptible to a number of ailments. Obesity is a worldwide issue, affecting a large number of the population. Cost-effective treatments have been made to counteract weight loss. It has been reported that functional food has emerged to be a nutritional addition to elevate satiety. They seem like conventional food, but they exhibit more nutritional properties. They have been investigated in the treatment of various diseases. Now, they should be used in the management of obesity, as it is a global epidemic nowadays. Caloric restriction may increase energy expenditure to manifest weight loss. The word nutraceutical comprises nutritional and pharmaceutical that are portrayed in the treatment of obesity. Today, dietary nutrients seem to be the most promising agent for their effects on weight management. More people will be able to regulate their obesity and lessen the burden it could have on them physically, socially, and psychologically if health is optimized through the use of nutraceuticals. Therefore, obesity is not limited to being treated in only one manner; rather, it is now being treated via a multidisciplinary approach. Diet, exercise, nutritional awareness, and a sound psychological state provide an excellent environment by which this disease will one day be controlled. Studies should concentrate on figuring out the best dosage, effectiveness, and safety of products for long-term consumption.

KEYWORDS

- **antioxidants**
- **disease modifiers**
- **functional foods**
- **long-term consumption**
- **nutraceuticals**
- **obesity**
- **oxidative stress**
- **weight management**

REFERENCES

Aasheim, E. T., Hofso, D., & Hjelmesaeth, J. (2008). Vitamin status in morbidly obese patients: A cross-sectional study. *American Journal of Clinical Nutrition, 87*(2), 362–369.

Basch, E., Ulbricht, C., Kuo, G., Szapary, P., & Smith, M. (2003). Therapeutic applications of fenugreek. *Alternative Medicine Review, 8*(1), 20–27.

Basciani, S., Manfrini, S., Watanabe, M., Risi, R., Masi, D., Caputi, A., Balena, A., Rossini, G., Tuccinardi, D., Mariani, S., Gnessi, L., & Lubrano, C. (2020). Current evidence to propose different food supplements for weight loss: A comprehensive review. *Nutrients, 12*(10), 2873.

Baur, J. A., & Sinclair, D. A. (2006). Therapeutic potential of resveratrol: The in vivo evidence. *Nature Reviews Drug Discovery, 5*(6), 493–506.

Berthoud, H. R. (2002). Multiple neural systems controlling food intake and body weight. *Neuroscience and Biobehavioral Reviews, 26*(4), 393–428.

Berthoud, H. R., Lenard, N. R., & Shin, A. C. (2011). Food reward, hyperphagia, and obesity. *American Journal of Physiology-Regulatory, Integrative and Comparative Physiology, 300*(6), R1266–R1277.

Biesalski, H. K. (2002). Nutraceuticals: The link between nutrition and medicine. In K. Kramer & P. P. Hoppe (Eds.), *Proceedings of the Nutraceuticals 2000 Conference*. 9–30; CRC Press, Taylor & Francis.

Blankson, H., Stakkestad, J. A., Fagertun, H., Thom, E., Wadstein, J., & Gudmundsen, O. (2000). Conjugated linoleic acid reduces body fat mass in overweight and obese humans. *Journal of Nutrition, 130*(12), 2943–2948.

Boozer, C. N., Nasser, J. A., Heymsfield, S. B., Wang, V., Chen, G., & Solomon, J. L. (2001). An herbal supplement containing Ma Huang-Guarana for weight loss: A randomized, double-blind trial. *International Journal of Obesity and Related Metabolic Disorders, 25*(3), 316–324.

Borges-Canha, M., Portela-Cidade, J. P., Dinis-Ribeiro, M., Leite-Moreira, A. F., & Pimentel-Nunes, P. (2015). Role of colonic microbiota in colorectal carcinogenesis: A systematic review. *Revista Española de Enfermedades Digestivas, 107*(11), 659–671.

Bose, M., Lambert, J. D., Ju, J., Reuhl, K. R., Shapses, S. A., & Yang, C. S. (2008). The major green tea polyphenol, (–)-epigallocatechin-3-gallate, inhibits obesity, metabolic syndrome, and fatty liver disease in high-fat-fed mice. *Journal of Nutrition, 138*(9), 1677–1683.

Brower, B. (1998). Nutraceuticals: Poised for a healthy slice of the market. *Nature Biotechnology, 16*(8), 728–731.

Campfield, L. A., Brandon, P., & Smith, F. J. (1985). On-line continuous measurement of blood glucose and meal pattern in free-feeding rats; the role of glucose in meal initiation. *Brain Research Bulletin, 14*(6), 605–616.

Caterson, I. D., & Gill, T. P. (2002). Obesity: Epidemiology and possible prevention. *Best Practice & Research Clinical Endocrinology & Metabolism, 16*(4), 595–610.

Champ, M. M. (2002). Non-nutrient bioactive substances of pulses. *British Journal of Nutrition, 88*(Suppl. 3), S307–S319.

Chaplin, A., Carpéné, C., & Mercader, J. (2018). Resveratrol, metabolic syndrome, and gut microbiota. *Nutrients, 10*(11), 1651.

Childs, N. M. (1999). Nutraceutical industry trends. *Journal of Nutraceuticals, Functional & Medical Foods, 2*(1), 73–85.

Chrysohoou, C., Panagiotakos, D. B., & Pitsavos, C. (2007). The implication of obesity on total antioxidant capacity in apparently healthy men and women: The ATTICA study. *Nutrition, Metabolism, and Cardiovascular Diseases, 17*(8), 590–597.

Conroy, K. P., Davidson, I. M., & M. (2011). Pathogenic obesity and nutraceuticals. *Proceedings of the Nutrition Society, 70*, 426–438.

Considine, R. V., Sinha, M. K., Heiman, M. L., Kriauciunas, A., Stephens, T. W., Nyce, M. R., Ohannesian, J. P., Marco, C. C., McKee, L. J., Bauer, T. L., & Caro, J. F. (1996). Serum immune reactive-leptin concentrations in normal weight and obese humans. *New England Journal of Medicine, 334*(5), 292–295.

Craciun, S., & Balskus, E. P. (2012). Microbial conversion of choline to trimethylamine requires a glycyl radical enzyme. *Proceedings of the National Academy of Sciences USA, 109*(52), 21307–21312.

Daou, C., & Zhang, H. (2012). Oat Beta-Glucan: Its role in health promotion and prevention of diseases. *Comprehensive Reviews in Food Science and Food Safety, 11*(4), 355–365.

Davidson, T. L., & Swithers, S. E. (2004). A Pavlovian approach to the problem of obesity. *International Journal of Obesity, 28*, 933–935.

De Angelis, M., Montemurno, E., Vannini, L., Cosola, C., Cavallo, N., Gozzi, G., Maranzano, V., Di Cagno, R., Gobbetti, M., & Gesualdo, L. (2015). Effect of whole-grain barley on the human fecal microbiota and metabolome. *Applied and Environmental Microbiology, 81*(22), 7945–7956.

De Felice, S. L. (1995). The nutraceutical revolution, its impact on food industry. *Trends in Food Science & Technology, 6*(2), 59–61.
Dolgin, E. (2012). A history of drugs on the weight list. *Nature Medicine, 18*, 843.
Dureja, H., Kaushik, D., & Kumar, V. (2003). Developments in nutraceuticals. *Indian Journal of Pharmacology, 35*, 363–372.
Flagg, A. J. (2021). Traditional and current use of ginseng. *Nursing Clinics of North America, 56*, 109–121.
Fu, B. C., Hullar, M. A. J., Randolph, T. W., Franke, A. A., Monroe, K. R., Cheng, I., Wilkens, L. R., Shepherd, J. A., Madeleine, M. M., Le Marchand, L., et al. (2020). Associations of plasma trimethylamine N-oxide, choline, carnitine, and betaine with inflammatory and cardiometabolic risk biomarkers and the fecal microbiome in the Multiethnic Cohort Adiposity Phenotype Study. *American Journal of Clinical Nutrition, 111*(6), 1226–1234.
Golla, U. (2018). Emergence of nutraceuticals as the alternative medications for pharmaceuticals. *International Journal of Complementary & Alternative Medicine, 11*(3), 155–158.
Governa, P., Baini, G., Borgonetti, V., Cettolin, G., Giachetti, D., Magnano, A. R., Miraldi, E., & Biagi, M. (2018). Phytotherapy in the management of diabetes: A review. *Molecules, 23*, 105.
Han, L. K., Gong, X. J., Kawano, S., Saito, M., Kimura, Y., & Okuda, H. (2005). Antiobesity actions of Zingiber officinale Roscoe. *Yakugaku Zasshi, 125*(3), 213–217.
Hong, K. H., Jang, K. H., Lee, J. C., Kim, S. H., Kim, M. K., Lee, I. Y., Kim, S. M., Lim, Y. H., & Kang, S. A. (2005). Bacterial β-glucan exhibits potent hypoglycemic activity via decrease of serum lipids and adiposity, and increase of UCP mRNA expression. *Journal of Microbiology and Biotechnology, 15*(5), 823–830.
Jalanka, J., Major, G., Murray, K., Singh, G., Nowak, A., Kurtz, C., Silos-Santiago, I., Johnston, J. M., De Vos, W. M., & Spiller, R. (2019). The effect of psyllium husk on intestinal microbiota in constipated patients and healthy controls. *International Journal of Molecular Sciences, 20*(2), 433.
Jenkins, D. J., Kendall, C. W., Vuksan, V., Vidgen, E., Parker, T., Faulkner, D., Mehling, C., Garsetti, M., Testolin, G., Cunnane, C., Ryan, M., & Corey, P. N. (2002). Soluble fiber intake at a dose approved by the US Food and Drug Administration for a claim of health benefits: Serum lipid risk factors for cardiovascular disease assessed in a randomized controlled crossover trial. *American Journal of Clinical Nutrition, 75*(5), 834–839.
Kalagi, N. A., Abbott, K. A., Alburikan, K. A., Alkofide, H. A., Stojanovski, E., & Garg, M. L. (2019). Modulation of circulating trimethylamine N-oxide concentrations by dietary supplements and pharmacological agents: A systematic review. *Advances in Nutrition, 10*(5), 876–887.
Kalra, E. K. (2003). Nutraceutical—Definition and introduction. *AAPS PharmSci, 5*(3), 25.
Kamal, R., & Aleem, S. (2009). Clinical evaluation of the efficacy of a combination of zanjabeel (Zingiber officinale) and Amla (Emblica officianalis) in hyperlipidemia. *Indian Journal of Traditional Knowledge, 8*, 413–416.
Kamalakkannan, S. (2010). Antiobesogenic and antiatherosclerotic properties of Caralluma fimbriata extract. *Journal of Nutrition and Metabolism, 28*, 5301.
Katare, C., Agrawal, S., Jain, M., Rani, S., Saxena, S., Bisen, P., & Godavarthi, P. (2011). Lagenaria siceraria: A potential source of anti-hyperlipidemia and other pharmacological agents. *Current Nutrition & Food Science, 7*, 1–7.

Katare, C., Agrawal, S., Rana, S., Sharma, S., Chauhan, S., & Prasad, G. B. (2012). Lagenaria siceraria: A nutraceutical for good health. *International Journal of Green Pharmacy, 6*, 253–256.

Keats, S., & Wiggins, S. (2014). The Overseas Development Institute (ODI). Future diets: Implications for agriculture and food prices. https://cdn.odi.org/media/documents/8773.pdf.

Keservani, R. K., Kesharwani, R. K., Sharma, A. K., Vyas, N., & Chadoker, A. (2010b). Nutritional supplements: An overview. *International Journal of Current Pharmaceutical Review and Research, 1*(1), 59–75.

Keservani, R. K., Kesharwani, R. K., Vyas, N., Jain, S., Raghuvanshi, R., & Sharma, A. K. (2010a). Nutraceutical and functional food as future food: A review. *Der Pharmacia Lettre, 2*(1), 106–116.

Keservani, R. K., Sharma, A. K., & Kesharwani, R. K. (2016). Nutraceutical formulations and challenges. In D. Bagchi & S. Nair (Eds.), *New Product Development in Nutraceuticals & Functional Foods: From Concept to Market* (pp. 161–177). Academic Press, Elsevier.

Keservani, R. K., Sharma, A. K., & Kesharwani, R. K. (Eds.). (2020). *Nutraceuticals and Dietary Supplements: Applications in Health Improvement and Disease Management*. pp.1–344. CRC Press. ISBN: 9781771888738.

Kim, C. S., Kawada, T., Kim, S. B., Han, I. S., Choe, S. Y., Kurata, T., & Yu, R. (2003). Capsaicin exhibits anti-inflammatory property by inhibiting IkB-a degradation in LPS-stimulated peritoneal macrophages. *Cellular Signalling, 15*, 299–306.

Kim, S., Shin, B. C., Lee, M. S., Lee, H., & Ernst, E. (2011). Red ginseng for type 2 diabetes mellitus: A systematic review of randomized controlled trials. *Chinese Journal of Integrative Medicine, 17*(12), 937–944.

Koeth, R. A., Wang, Z., Levison, B. S., Buffa, J. A., Org, E., Sheehy, B. T., Britt, E. B., Fu, X., Wu, Y., Li, L., et al. (2013). Intestinal microbiota metabolism of l-carnitine, a nutrient in red meat, promotes atherosclerosis. *Nature Medicine, 19*, 576–585.

Koh-Banerjee, P., Wang, Y., Hu, F. B., Spiegelman, D., Willett, W. C., & Rimm, E. B. (2004). Changes in body weight and body fat distribution as risk factors for clinical diabetes in US men. *American Journal of Epidemiology, 159*, 1150–1159.

Kuriyan, R., Raj, T., Srinivas, S. K., Vaz, M., Rajenfran, R., & Kurpad, A. V. (2007). Effect of Caralluma fimbriata extract on appetite, food intake and anthropometry in adult Indian men and women. *Appetite, 48*, 338–344.

Lavigne, C., Tremblay, F., Asselin, G., Jacques, H., & Marette, A. (2001). Prevention of skeletal muscle insulin resistance by dietary cod protein in high fat-fed rats. *American Journal of Physiology-Endocrinology and Metabolism, 281*(1), E62–E71.

Li, H., Xia, N., Hasselwander, S., & Daiber, A. (2019). Resveratrol and vascular function. *International Journal of Molecular Sciences, 20*(9), 2155.

Li, Y. R., Li, S., & Lin, C. C. (2018). Effect of resveratrol and pterostilbene on aging and longevity. *BioFactors, 44*, 69–82.

Maddi, V. S., Aragade, P. D., Digge, V. G., & Nitaliker, M. N. (2007). Importance of nutraceuticals in health management. *Pharmacognosy Reviews, 1*, 377–379.

Manjunatha, H., & Srinivasan, K. (2006). Protective effect of dietary curcumin and capsaicin on induced oxidation of low-density lipoprotein, iron induced hepatotoxicity, and carrageenan induced inflammation in experimental rats. FEBS Journal, 273(20), 4528–4537.

Mannion, M. (1998). Nutraceutical revolution continues at Foundation for Innovation in Medicine Conference. American Journal of Natural Medicine, 5, 30–33.

McAllan, L., Skuse, P., Cotter, P. D., Connor, P. O., Cryan, J. F., Ross, R. P., Fitzgerald, G., Roche, H. M., & Nilaweera, K. N. (2014). Protein quality and the protein to carbohydrate ratio within a high fat diet influences energy balance and the gut microbiota in C57BL/6J mice. PLoS ONE, 9(2), e88904.

Miller, L. E. (2013). Lorcaserin for weight loss: Insights into US Food and Drug Administration approval. Journal of the Academy of Nutrition and Dietetics, 113(1), 25–30.

Miura, T., Itoh, Y., Iwamoto, N., Kato, M., & Ishida, T. (2004). Suppressive activity of the fruit of Momordica charantia with exercise on blood glucose in type-2 diabetic mice. Biological and Pharmaceutical Bulletin, 27(2), 248–250.

Muanprasat, C., & Chatsudthipong, V. (2017). Chitosan oligosaccharide: Biological activities and potential therapeutic applications. Pharmacology & Therapeutics, 170, 80–97.

Naveed, M., Phil, L., Sohail, M., Hasnat, M., Baig, M. M. F. A., Ihsan, A. U., Shumzaid, M., Kakar, M. U., Khan, T. M., & Akbar, M. D. (2019). Chitosan oligosaccharide (COS): An overview. International Journal of Biological Macromolecules, 129, 827–843.

Nichols, L. A., Jackson, D. E., Manthey, J. A., & Shukla, S. D. (2011). Citrus flavonoids repress the mRNA for stearoyl-CoA desaturase, a key enzyme in lipid synthesis and obesity control, in rat primary hepatocytes. Lipids in Health and Disease, 10, 36.

Oellgaard, J., Winther, S. A., Hansen, T. S., Rossing, P., & Von Scholten, B. J. (2017). Trimethylamine N-oxide (TMAO) as a new potential therapeutic target for insulin resistance and cancer. Current Pharmaceutical Design, 23(24), 3699–3712.

Ogden, C. L., Carroll, M. D., Kit, B. K., & Flegal, K. M. (2014). Prevalence of childhood and adult obesity in the United States. JAMA, 311(8), 806–814.

Packer, L., & Weber, S. U. (2001). The role of vitamin E in the emerging field of nutraceuticals. Nutraceuticals in Health and Disease Prevention. 15, 43–62.

Panagiotakos, D. B., Pitsavos, C., & Yannakoulia, M. (2005). The implication of obesity and central fat on markers of chronic inflammation: The ATTICA study. Atherosclerosis, 183(2), 308–315.

Pandey, M., Verma, R. K., & Shubhini, S. (2010). Nutraceuticals: New era of medicine and health. Asian Journal of Pharmaceutical and Clinical Research, 3(1), 11–15.

Park, J. Y., Kawada, T., Han, I. S., Kim, B. S., Goto, T., Takahashi, N., Fushiki, T., Kurata, T., & Yu, R. (2004). Capsaicin inhibits the production of tumor necrosis factor by LPS stimulated murine macrophages, RAW 264.7: A PPAR ligand-like action as a novel mechanism. FEBS Letters, 572(1–3), 266–270.

Rajasekaran, G. S., & Rathinam, X. (2008). Nutraceuticals as therapeutic agents – Review. Research Journal of Pharmacy and Technology, 1(4), 328–340.

Rasmussen, H. E., Hamaker, B., Rajan, K. B., Mutlu, E., Green, S. J., Brown, I., Kaur, A., & Keshavarzian, A. (2017). Starch-entrapped microsphere fibers improve bowel habit but do not exhibit prebiotic capacity in those with unsatisfactory bowel habits: A phase I, randomized, double-blind, controlled human trial. Nutrition Research, 44, 27–37.

Rauf, A., Imran, M., Butt, M. S., Nadeem, M., Peters, D. G., & Mubarak, M. S. (2018). Resveratrol as an anti-cancer agent: A review. Critical Reviews in Food Science and Nutrition, 58(14), 1428–1447.

Reider, S. J., Moosmang, S., Tragust, J., Trgovec-Greif, L., Tragust, S., Perschy, L., Przysiecki, N., Sturm, S., Tilg, H., Stuppner, H., & Carballido, J. M. (2020). Prebiotic effects of partially hydrolyzed guar gum on the composition and function of the human microbiota – Results from the PAGODA trial. Nutrients, 12(5), 1257.

Romano, K. A., Vivas, E. I., Amador-Noguez, D., & Rey, F. E. (2015). Intestinal microbiota composition modulates choline bioavailability from diet and accumulation of the proatherogenic metabolite trimethylamine-N-oxide. mBio, 6(2), e02481–e02514.

Rubin, S. A., & Levin, E. R. (1994). Clinical review: The endocrinology of vasoactive peptides: Synthesis to function. The Journal of Clinical Endocrinology & Metabolism, 78(1), 6–10.

Saeed, M., Naveed, M., Arif, M., Kakar, M. U., Manzoor, R., El-Hack, M. A., Alagawany, M., Tiwari, R., Khandia, R., Munjal, A., & Karthik, K. (2017). Green tea (Camellia sinensis) and l-theanine: Medicinal values and beneficial applications in humans – A comprehensive review. Biomedicine & Pharmacotherapy, 95, 1260–1275.

Sae-tan, S. (2011). Weight control and prevention of metabolic syndrome by green tea. Pharmacological Research, 64(2), 146–154.

Sarin, R. (2012). Nutraceuticals: A review. International Research Journal of Pharmacy, 3(4), 95–99.

Schenk, S., Saberi, M., & Olefsky, J. M. (2008). Insulin sensitivity: Modulation by nutrients and inflammation. The Journal of Clinical Investigation, 118(9), 2992–3002.

Sekiya, M., Yahagi, N., Matsuzaka, T., Najima, Y., Nakakuki, M., Nagai, R., Ishibashi, S., Osuga, J., Yamada, N., & Shimano, H. (2003). Polyunsaturated fatty acids ameliorate hepatic steatosis in obese mice by SREBP-1 suppression. Hepatology, 38(6), 1529–1539.

Senanayake, G. V., Maruyama, M., Shibuya, K., Sakono, M., Fukuda, N., Morishita, T., Yukizaki, Y., Kawano, M., & Ohta, H. (2004). The effects of bitter melon (Momordica charantia) on serum and liver triglyceride levels in rats. Journal of Ethnopharmacology, 91(2–3), 257–262.

Sethi, J. K., & Hotamisligil, G. S. (1999). The role of TNF-alpha in adipocyte metabolism. *Seminars in Cell & Developmental Biology, 10*(1), 19–29.

Sharma, A. K., Keservani, R. K., & Gautam, S. P. (2020). Herbal Product Development. Apple Academic Press, CRC Press, Taylor & Francis Group.

Shehzad, A., Khan, S., & Lee, Y. S. (2012). Curcumin molecular targets in obesity and obesity-related cancers. *Future Oncology, 8*(2), 179–190.

Shen, L., Liu, L., & Ji, H.-F. (2017). Alzheimer's disease histological and behavioral manifestations in transgenic mice correlate with specific gut microbiome state. *Journal of Alzheimer's Disease, 56*(1), 385–390.

Steptoe, A., Gibson, E. L., Vounovirta, R., Hamer, M., Wardley, J., Ryecroft, J. A., Martin, J. F., & Erusalimsky, J. D. (2007). The effects of chronic tea intake on platelet activation and inflammation: A double-blind placebo-controlled trial. *Atherosclerosis, 193*(2), 277–282.

Tai, E. S. (1999). A study to assess the effect of dietary supplementation with soluble fiber (Minolest) on lipid levels in normal subjects with hypercholesterolemia. *Annals of the Academy of Medicine, Singapore, 28*(2), 209–213.

Tajik, N., Tajik, M., Mack, I., & Enck, P. (2017). The potential effects of chlorogenic acid, the main phenolic components in coffee, on health: A comprehensive review of the literature. *European Journal of Nutrition, 56*(7), 2215–2244.

Tosh, S. M. (2013). Review of human studies investigating the post-prandial blood-glucose lowering ability of oat and barley food products. *European Journal of Clinical Nutrition, 67*(4), 310–317.

Trayhurn, P., & Wood, I. S. (2004). Adipokines: Inflammation and the pleiotropic role of white adipose tissue. *British Journal of Nutrition, 92*(3), 347–355.

Van Vliet, S., Burd, N. A., & van Loon, L. J. (2015). The skeletal muscle anabolic response to plant- versus animal-based protein consumption. *Journal of Nutrition, 145*(8), 1981–1991.

Vandeputte, D., Falony, G., Vieira-Silva, S., Wang, J., Sailer, M., Theis, S., Verbeke, K., & Raes, J. (2017). Prebiotic inulin-type fructans induce specific changes in the human gut microbiota. *Gut, 66*(11), 1968–1974.

Velasquez, M. T., Ramezani, A., Manal, A., & Raj, D. S. (2016). Trimethylamine N-oxide: The good, the bad and the unknown. *Toxins, 8*(10), 326.

Vijayanand, S., & Wesely, E. G. (2010). Phytochemical studies of Murraya koeingi. *International Journal of Pharmaceutical Sciences Research, 2*(5), 1298–1302.

Walle, T. (2011). Bioavailability of resveratrol. *Annals of the New York Academy of Sciences, 1215*, 9–15.

Watanabe, M., Risi, R., Masi, D., Caputi, A., Balena, A., Rossini, G., Tuccinardi, D., Mariani, S., Wintergerst, E. S., Maggini, S., & Hornig, D. H. (2007). Contribution of selected vitamins and trace elements to immune function. *Annals of Nutrition & Metabolism, 51*(4), 301–323.

Wildman, R. E. C. (2007). Nutraceuticals and functional foods. In R. E. C. Wildman (Ed.), *Handbook of Nutraceuticals and Functional Foods* (1st ed., pp. 1–9). CRC Press.

Yankuzo, H., Ahmad, Q. U., Santosa, R. I., Akhtar, S. F., & Talib, N. A. (2011). Beneficial effect of the leaves of Murraya koenigii (Linn.) Spreng (Rutaceae) on diabetes-induced renal damage in vivo. *Journal of Ethnopharmacology, 135*(1), 88–94.

Yasukawa, Z., Inoue, R., Ozeki, M., Okubo, T., Takagi, T., Honda, A., & Naito, Y. (2019). Effect of repeated consumption of partially hydrolyzed guar gum on fecal characteristics and gut microbiota: A randomized, double-blind, placebo-controlled, and parallel-group clinical trial. *Nutrients, 11*(9), 2170.

Yuan, X. J., Long, Y., Ji, Z. H., Gao, J., Fu, T., Yan, M., Zhang, L., Su, H. X., Zhang, W. L., Wen, X. H., et al. (2018). Green tea liquid consumption alters the human intestinal and oral microbiome. *Molecular Nutrition & Food Research, 62*(18), 1800178.

CHAPTER 6

ROLE OF VITAMINS AND SUPPLEMENTS IN THE TREATMENT OF OBESITY

SHWETA VERMA and ALANKAR SHRIVASTAV

Faculty of Pharmacy, IFTM University, Moradabad, Uttar Pradesh, India

ABSTRACT

Obesity is a major health problem all over the world. It is increasing in both children and adults. Approximately one-third of the population is found to be obese. The healthcare costs of obesity are significant. This includes taking obesity treatment supplements, the cost of weight loss surgeries, prescription medications, as well as secondary effects like deaths and treatment of obesity-caused diseases. So, it is important to understand other significant ways to control obesity without harming the body much. Through much research, it is found that many vitamins and different supplements have the ability to control obesity. This chapter helps to understand the possible role of dietary vitamins and supplements in body weight regulation and obesity.

6.1 INTRODUCTION

According to epidemiological research, a body mass index (BMI) rise of 5 kg/m^2 raises the risk of mortality overall by 29%, the risk of death from cardiovascular disease by 41%, and the risk of death from diabetes by as much as 210% (Kamycheva et al., 2003). A total of 1.9 billion adults worldwide—or around 39% of the population over 20 years old—were obese in

Nutraceuticals in Obesity Management and Control. Raj K. Keservani & Alka Lohani (Eds.)

2016. By age 40, men make up the majority of obese patients, but this trend later in life reverses itself, maybe as a result of menopause, which is linked to a higher incidence of obesity in women. The prevalence of obesity has increased by 80% during the previous 35 years, while the number of obese persons has doubled. North America and Europe are the continents with the largest proportions of obese persons worldwide (Dos Santos et al., 2008). Obesity increases the likelihood of developing a variety of illnesses, such as type 2 diabetes, dyslipidemia, and cardiovascular conditions. On the other hand, insufficient eating habits and low levels of physical activity are the main risk factors for obesity. It may turn out that changing one's eating habits is not enough to treat obesity. Pharmacotherapy may therefore be used in the treatment of obesity in obese patients. Orlistat is one medication that helps in the treatment of obesity and has been authorized for use in Europe. This medication decreases the absorption of lipids from the digestive system. Bariatric surgery is becoming a more popular therapeutic option for people with morbid obesity as medication, better eating habits, and increased physical activity may not have the desired effects on reducing excess body weight (Harkness et al., 2005). Dietary supplements can help with weight loss in addition to boosting physical activity and making dietary improvements. These contain a wide range of chemicals that aid in weight loss. The properties of the most popular dietary supplements used to treat obesity as well as the mechanisms underlying their effect are presented in this review.

Obesity is a complex condition that affects more than 1 billion people worldwide. It is characterized by excess body fat, which may be caused by heredity, nutrition, age, and physical inactivity or by certain over-the-counter or prescription medications. Obesity is also a known risk factor for heart disease, stroke, high blood pressure, high cholesterol, diabetes, sleep apnea, gallbladder disease, osteoarthritis, and certain types of cancer (Berkey et al., 2005).

When we talk about obesity, we usually mean the presence of too much body fat, which can put you at risk for serious medical problems. People with obesity may have a hard time losing weight, even when they try hard to do so.

6.2 CAUSES OF OBESITY

Obesity has a variety of complex factors that differ from individual to person. Because their bodies are more likely to accumulate fat, some people are genetically predisposed to obesity. In general, an imbalance between calories consumed and burned results in obesity (Troiano et al., 1990). The majority of obese persons experience excess body fat. The overconsumption of calories and a lack of exercise are other variables that contribute to weight gain.

In the United States, obesity is a major contributor to avoidable death and disability. The prevalence of obesity is increasing globally and is predicted to keep increasing in the coming years (WHO, 2015).

6.3 OBESITY RISK FACTORS

As varied as the persons who are obese are the dangers of becoming obese and the effects of being obese. Regardless of the overall obesity prevalence, there are risk factors for obesity in practically every community. To assist people in preventing and managing overweight and obesity, it is crucial to fully comprehend these risk factors. Age, gender, and heredity are three of the most prevalent risk factors for obesity. Major risk factors for obesity include older age, gender, heredity, and higher BMI. Males are less likely to be obese than females. Compared to white people, black and Hispanic people are less likely to be obese (Pereira et al., 2002).

6.4 OBESITY TREATMENT OPTIONS

We should be aware that treating obesity requires a multi-step process that includes education, behavior modification, and physical activity. The majority of those who successfully reduce weight maintain it. Treatments for obesity can aid in weight loss and maintenance. "There are several ways to lose weight, including vitamins for treating obesity, prescription drugs, and surgery." Diet and exercise are the two main types of treatment for obesity. Other methods of treating obesity include diet pills, bariatric surgery, and gastric bypass (Teegarden et al., 2003).

6.4.1 WEIGHT LOSS SURGERY

For those who have tried and failed to lose weight with diet and exercise or who have a body mass index (BMI) of 50 or more, weight management surgery is an additional alternative. One of the most popular and risky methods of treating obesity is surgery. Laparoscopic gastric bypass is one of the most popular procedures, with about 135,000 procedures carried out in the United States in 2014 (Kull et al., 2009). A surgical weight loss surgery called gastric bypass can change a person's digestive system and speed up weight loss. Liposuction is another prevalent weight-loss procedure. This is a surgical treatment where extra fat is removed by inserting a tiny tube through skin incisions. Liposuction procedures frequently include general anesthesia and necessitate an overnight hospital stay for the patients. Thin layers of fat are removed from various parts of your body during this treatment. The thighs, back, arms, and belly are the areas that get liposuction the most frequently. There are numerous varieties of liposuction. Based on a variety of factors, including your preferences, your health, and how much fat you want to remove, your surgeon will choose which is ideal for you (Phillips et al., 2003).

6.4.2 PRESCRIPTION WEIGHT LOSS MEDICATIONS

For some obese persons who have failed to lose a considerable amount of weight with diet and exercise, prescription weight loss medication is also a possibility. "The majority of weight loss drugs are viewed as a supplement to diet and exercise." A healthy diet and moderate exercise are frequently combined with prescription weight loss medication (Garcia et al., 2009).

6.4.3 FAT BURNERS

An additional choice for certain obese individuals is a fat burner. Fat burners are a type of over-the-counter dietary supplement that aims to help with weight loss by converting excess body fat into energy. Some fat burners contain active ingredients that have been shown to assist in weight loss by increasing the calories burned during exercise. It is not recommended to rely on fat burners as a long-term solution for weight loss (Rajakumar et al., 2011).

6.4.4 APPETITE SUPPRESSANTS

An appetite suppressant is a medication or dietary supplement that reduces or suppresses hunger. By decreasing the urge to eat, appetite suppressants help individuals consume fewer calories overall. "Individuals who use appetite suppressants typically experience weight loss." It is important to note that appetite suppressants are effective only when combined with a healthy diet and exercise regimen. They are not a substitute for making healthy lifestyle choices (Bischoff-Ferrari et al., 2009).

6.4.5 *METABOLISM BOOSTERS*

Another option for some obese individuals is a metabolism booster. Metabolism boosters are dietary supplements designed to increase the body's basal metabolic rate (the number of calories the body burns at rest). "Using a metabolism booster should not replace leading a healthy lifestyle." It is important to be aware that using a metabolism booster may increase the risk of unpleasant side effects (Mansbach et al., 2009).

6.4.6 *FIBER SUPPLEMENTS*

Dietary fiber-based supplements are those that have this component. Fiber is a form of carbohydrate that the small intestine cannot completely break down. It is more difficult to eat as much when you are full and regular, which can help you avoid overeating and lose weight (Kulie et al., 2009).

6.5 ROLE OF VITAMINS IN THE MANAGEMENT OF OBESITY

According to the Global Health Observatory (GHO), the prevalence of obesity among people (18 and older) between 1975 and 2016 was 27.8% in the UK and 31.7% in the United Arab Emirates (UAE) (Wagner et al., 2008). According to the National Health Survey, adult obesity in the UAE was at 27.8% in 2019. The imbalance between calories consumed and expended as a result of dietary and physical activity changes is one of the factors causing obesity. The prevalence of obesity was found to be influenced by a variety of factors, most notably modifications in lifestyle choices in addition to genetic contribution and other factors, and this suggests that specific healthcare awareness initiatives and specific interventions can help and contribute to overcoming this issue (Wortsman et al., 2000). The maintenance of bone tissues, the balance of calcium and phosphorus, as well as other cell activities, depend on vitamin D, a critical nutrient. When exposed to sunlight, ultraviolet

B photons penetrate the skin, and heat from the body causes pre-vitamin D3 to be isomerized into vitamin D3. Despite many current debates that maintain vitamin D is unrelated to any health concerns and is only a measure of general good health, the association between vitamin D level and cancers as well as mental health, bone health, and other health issues is also strongly supported by studies (Sun et al., 2008). Since it aids in the body's ability to absorb calcium and phosphorus through the digestive system, vitamin D is crucial for sustaining good health. As a result, it can be used to treat and prevent osteoporosis, chronic fatigue, tooth and dental problems, and aches in the muscles and bones. Vitamin D insufficiency aggravates a variety of chronic metabolic and endocrine diseases (Keservani et al., 2017, 2020). Growth retardation, rickets, and adult fractures are all made more likely by vitamin D deficiency. Obesity, particularly abdominal obesity, was found to be significantly linked with low calcium serum levels. It is associated with a number of additional issues, such as an increased risk of contracting common cancers, infectious diseases, cardiovascular ailments, and other illnesses (Schrager et al., 2005). A 2018 study found that vitamin D supplements only increase bone density in people with 25-hydroxyvitamin D levels under 30 nmol/L. The study also suggested taking supplements. Although the precise mechanism is yet unknown, vitamin D deficiency is also associated with increased myocardial disease and cardiovascular risk. According to a recent study published in 2018, there is a significant link between the prevalence of hypertension and low plasma vitamin D levels. Vitamin D deficiency and acute coronary syndrome were statistically substantially associated (Harkness et al., 2005). However, research found that adding calcium to vitamin D supplements had no effect on the prevalence of hypertension and did not lower the risk of developing chronic heart disease or stroke. Because their bone chemistry tests fall within reference ranges, many people with low vitamin D levels go undetected without causing clinical concern. Clinical suspicion based on prior experiences and awareness of risk factors ought to continue to be the gold standard for requesting vitamin D testing (Keller et al., 2009).

6.6 SUGGESTED MECHANISM OF ACTION

Energy from ingested food is needed to maintain basic bodily activities and can also be stored in adipose tissue, which can measure the body's energy levels. When the body creates more energy than is required, triglycerides in lipid droplets start to form in adipose tissue (Jennings et al., 2006). Catecholamines increase the lipolysis process, which breaks down triglycerides into free fatty acids, by activating the protein kinase A pathway, which in turn causes the cAMP signaling pathway to become active. The hormone-sensitive lipase enzyme (HSL), which facilitates the translocation of lipid droplets to open up access to triglyceride stores, is phosphorylated by protein kinase A (Kumar et al., 2009). After the proteins are produced, their activity can be changed by a procedure called phosphorylation. By introducing a phosphate group that is provided by ATP, kinase enzymes alter proteins. The body breaks down fat when it needs energy. The adipose triglyceride lipase (ATGL) enzyme initiates the hydrolysis of the triglycerides into diacylglycerides. The diacylglyceride is subsequently transformed into a monoglyceride by the enzyme hormone-sensitive lipase (HSL), and the ester bond in the monoglyceride is then broken to release glycerol (Kumar et al., 2009). As a defense against the body's natural lipases like hormone-sensitive lipase (HSL), which breaks down triglycerides into glycerol and free fatty acids for use in metabolism during lipolysis, perilipin, a protein, covers the lipid droplets in the fat-storing cells of adipose tissue. The phosphorylation of perilipin is necessary for the mobilization of fats in adipose tissue, which is essential for the regulation of lipid storage. Insulin inhibits the enzymes hormone-sensitive lipase (HSL) and adipose triglyceride lipase in addition to increasing the quantity of perilipin around lipid droplets to prevent their access to triglycerides (ATGL). Poor sun exposure caused by reduced mobility brought on by obesity is one of the alleged causes of vitamin D insufficiency. It is well recognized that vitamin D insufficiency can occur for a variety of reasons and through a variety of means. Vitamin D is absorbed from a variety of sources by the adipose tissue, which is encouraged to store this vitamin for times when production is reduced. The amount of this vitamin is negatively correlated with adipose tissue levels (Yang et al., 2010). There are many ideas tying vitamin D deficiency to obesity, but few of them link the two to inadequate sun exposure or insufficient physical exercise. Obesity is associated with an increased frequency of deficiencies, according to an observational study, and there is evidence that vitamin D metabolism, action, and storage have an impact on adiposity, albeit the exact processes are unclear (Wise et al., 2002). The 1,25-dihydroxy vitamin D hormone is the hormonal version of vitamin D, and in addition to its well-known function in controlling calcium levels, it also controls adipocytes. Another suggestion is that the amount of the vitamin D-stimulating enzyme 1-hydroxylase in fat cells may be able to account for the greater local 25(OH)D use. Doctors examine the levels of this metabolite to assess a patient's vitamin D status. The liver's cholecalciferol 25-hydroxylase produces the prehormone 25-hydroxyvitamin D, also known as calcifediol, by hydroxylating vitamin D3 (cholecalciferol). It takes around 7 days for vitamin D3 to change into calcifediol, which is then changed in the kidneys by the enzyme 25(OH)D-1-hydroxylase into calcitriol (1,25-(OH)2D3), a secosteroid hormone that is the active form of vitamin D. According to this theory, fluctuations in vitamin D and blood 25(OH)D reserves are closely correlated with variations in subcutaneous body fat (Burrows et al., 2010). A cohort analysis revealed that this theory was insufficient to account for the association between vitamin D deficiency and obesity. The 1,25-dihydroxyvitamin D, which is the active form of vitamin D, can influence the mobilization of free fatty acids from adipose tissue. According to animal research, high vitamin D dosages can increase energy expenditure via decoupling oxidative phosphorylation in adipose tissues.

It has also been suggested that the weather may play a role since obesity can be generated by a winter adaptation and because the availability of vitamin D from the sun decreases in the winter, which may affect the potential for fat mass to increase in cold weather. Since vitamin D is stored in adipose tissue, another theory explaining the connection between vitamin D levels and obesity is that the more space an individual has for this vitamin's storage, the lower their blood levels of (25(OH)D) are at any given time. A second suggested connection was made between the interesting outcome and genetic variations that resemble the effects of variable environmental exposure. A genetic variation connected to decreased 25(OH)D concentrations should be linked with BMI if reduced vitamin consumption is causally related to obesity. The genetic links are believed to be less sensitive to confounding variables, socioeconomic factors, and lifestyle factors since genotypes remain stable. Given that different types of human cells include vitamin D receptors (VDR), which can affect a variety of cell functions and regulation, numerous studies on vitamin D have been carried out (Novotny et al., 2004). It was noted that multiple body parts were affected when these receptors were inhibited in some animal trials, making it difficult to interpret the data and draw a definite relationship. Prior research clarified the role of the vitamin D receptor (VDR) in the control of body energy *in vivo*. According to certain studies, vitamin D-dependent receptors regulate 1.25(OH)D's ability to suppress adipogenesis; as a result, a drop in vitamin D levels may cause an excessive amount of pre-adipocytes to differentiate into adipocytes. In certain studies, it was found that obese people responded less to a dosage of ultraviolet (UV-B) radiation than normal-weight subjects (Goldberg et al., 2009). It was implied by the previous process, even though it was not mentioned directly, that vitamin D is rather securely bound in tissue depots and is not released in a way that keeps the blood's serum vitamin level stable. However, this method stopped short of describing how this vitamin might be stored in fat. Variable sun exposure cannot account for the link between obesity and vitamin D insufficiency discovered in some studies. As an alternative, it was suggested that extra fat accumulates vitamin D metabolites and partially sequesters cholecalciferol before it is transported to the liver for first hydroxylation (Sun et al., 2008). Obese participants had serum vitamin D levels that were (53%) lower, according to a study. According to some research, vitamin D insufficiency can cause parathyroid hormone levels to rise and more calcium to enter adipocytes, which will accelerate lipogenesis and speed up the conversion of acetyl-CoA to triglycerides for fat storage and packaging in lipid droplets (Carafoli et al., 2001). It is important to recognize and understand the process beyond low vitamin D status in obesity for determining the appropriate vitamin D replacement doses for obese persons.

6.7 ROLE OF CALCIUM

According to estimates, calcium supplements are consumed by 43% of US citizens. Calcium carbonate and calcium citrate are the two main calcium supplements (Blair et al., 2007). Both forms are equally well absorbed, but citrate may be more effectively taken by persons with more acidic stomachs. While calcium carbonate is better absorbed with meals, calcium citrate can be absorbed equally well with or without food. The amount of calcium absorbed is influenced by a number of variables, such as what the calcium was taken with (foods and medications that bind calcium), how much elemental calcium is consumed at once (a higher intake at once reduces absorption), and the individual's current calcium status (Sergeev et al., 2005).

6.7.1 MECHANISMS

Through potential impacts on hunger and food intake, calcium intake has been hypothesized to aid in weight loss and maintenance. In the prehistoric environment, calcium might have served as a sign of the presence of food. Fat accumulation slows down when food is abundant (high calcium intake), and it speeds up when food is limited (low calcium intake) (Sargeev et al., 1995). The capacity of dietary calcium to inhibit calcitriol, the active form of vitamin D, which has both genomic and nongenomic effects on adipocyte metabolism, is one way that higher calcium consumption may affect fat loss. Genes that enhance adipocyte proliferation, and inflammatory factors, and block adipocyte death are upregulated when calcitriol levels are elevated. Although a substantial body of research suggests vitamin D status is inversely associated with weight status and BMI, a definitive association (as well as underlying mechanisms) has not been identified. Conclusions from the few research studies that have looked at calcium and vitamin D separately have been conflicting, and there have been few clinical trials. Meanwhile, both adults and children get more than 50% of their daily calcium needs from dairy (Wright et al., 2003). Drawing inferences from dairy consumption, however, is complicated by the fact that milk has strong satiety qualities irrespective of its calcium and vitamin D concentration. Casein macropeptides (CMP), one of the components of dairy, may assist in controlling body weight, body composition, and food consumption. Additionally, cholecystokinin (CCK), ghrelin, and glucagon-like peptide-1, three gut hormones that control satiety, food intake, and stomach emptying, may respond differently to calcium and dairy (GLP-1). To draw conclusions, more research is required because the current body of knowledge is limited.

6.8 ROLE OF OTHER SUPPLEMENTS

6.8.1 CAPSAICIN

The alkaloid in chili peppers called capsaicin (8-methyl-N-vanillyl-6-nonenamide) is what gives them their hot, spiciness. For thousands of years, people have used chili peppers in food and medicine. It is utilized as a natural preservative as well as a flavor-enhancing spice in many tribes and cultures (Spadari et al., 2013). Studies in both experimental and clinical settings have demonstrated the multiple ways that capsaicin affects the body. Preclinical and clinical studies have demonstrated that the regulation of the nervous system in the hypothalamus and modulation of the functions of the digestive system and intestinal microbiome are the potential mechanisms of capsaicin's anti-obesity action. These mechanisms include inhibition of adipogenesis, activation of brown adipose tissue (BAT), stimulation of thermogenesis, increased lipolysis, decreased appetite, and increased satiety (Zhang et al., 2015).

The activation of TRPV1 is the major mechanism by which capsaicin affects metabolism (transient receptor potential vanilloid subfamily 1). Given their crucial roles in the control of body weight, glucose, lipid metabolism, and the cardiovascular system, these receptors could be viable targets in the fight against obesity. Through the inhibition of NF-κB (nuclear factor kappa-light-chain-enhancer of activated B cells) and activation of the PPARγ receptor, it has been demonstrated that capsaicin can control how adipocytes operate. Randomized clinical trials have demonstrated a relationship between dietary intake of capsaicin and a reduction in hunger, as well as an increase in resting energy expenditure, fat oxidation, BAT activity, and thermogenesis (Ríos-Hoyo et al., 2016). Increased consumption of capsaicin was linked to improved lipid profiles, lower blood sugar levels, and reduced tissue insulin resistance in obese people. Numerous research findings point to the possibility of using capsaicin to treat and prevent obesity. Additionally, it has been discovered that using inpatients with normal and low body weight is safe. It should be noted, nevertheless, that not all research has supported capsaicin's favorable effects on helping obese persons lose weight.

6.8.2 CHITOSAN

A chain polysaccharide produced from chitin is chitosan. Shells from crustaceans are its main source. It is one of numerous dietary supplements offered on the Polish market with the goal of assisting in the management of hypertension, hypercholesterolemia, and obesity.

Chitosan's primary mode of action in the body is to lessen the absorption of fat and cholesterol. Chitosan lowers tissue resistance to leptin and suppresses adipogenesis, as demonstrated in studies on obese mice using the leptin signaling pathway (JAK2-STAT3) (Pan et al., 2018). In other research, obese rats fed a diet supplemented with chitosan showed an increase in BAT and an increase in thermogenesis. Meta-analyzes have shown that taking chitosan supplements causes obese persons to lose weight, although the weight reduction in the assessed studies was not statistically significant. Humans were examined at various doses for both a short and a reasonably long length of time to determine the effectiveness of chitosan in lowering extra body weight, and similar results were obtained. The effects of orlistat and chitosan were compared, and it was found that orlistat considerably increased the excretion of fat in the stools whereas chitosan did not. However, it has been shown that its use decreases blood pressure and improves lipid profiles in obese individuals (Stohs et al., 2017). Based on the results of many clinical studies, it can be concluded that chitosan only has a slight effect on body weight but may reduce cardiometabolic risk in obese people.

6.8.3 BITTER ORANGE

Citrus aurantium L., a plant, produces an extract that is used to cure a variety of afflictions and illnesses. While *C. aurantium* extract is used to treat epilepsy, anxiety, and sleeplessness in South America, bitter orange is traditionally used in Chinese medicine to prevent indigestion, diarrhea, and constipation. Due to its ability to aid in weight loss, including hunger control and energy conversion, bitter orange extract is used in weight loss supplements. P-synephrine, a phenylethylamine derivative chemically related to ephedrine (a substance whose usage in supplements was outlawed in 2004 due to the development of harmful cardiovascular symptoms), makes up more than 90% of the protoalkaloids found in bitter orange (Schwiertz et al., 2010).

The physiological characteristics, pharmacokinetics, and binding to adrenergic receptors of p-synephrine set it apart from ephedrine. Therefore, one need not be concerned about p-synephrine-containing supplement side effects resembling those of ephedrine. In tests on animals, adding bitter orange to the diet resulted in a small rise in blood pressure and heart rate; these modifications became worse when caffeine was also consumed (Gorji et al., 2019). Pure p-synephrine or bitter orange taken for 6 to 12 weeks together with caffeine boosts energy expenditure and resting metabolism, leading to weight loss, according to clinical trials. An experiment using a double-blind placebo proved the bitter orange's safety. No changes in blood pressure or substantial changes in blood morphological and biochemical markers were seen after using p-synephrine for 60 days at a dose of 98 mg per day. Bitter orange extract has a variety of health benefits in addition to helping with weight loss. Antitumor, cytotoxic, sedative, antidiabetic, antioxidant, and anti-ulcer activities are all present in *C. aurantium.*

6.8.4 GREEN COFFEE

One of the bioactive components of green coffee is chlorogenic acid, a polyphenol from the phenolic acid subfamily that has been shown to have positive impacts on the body's ability to burn fat. It has been noted that green coffee extract influences the release of fatty acids from human adipocytes. Both short-term (2 h) and long-term (192 h) therapy have shown this effect. Short-term consumption of green coffee is thought to have a higher lipolytic effect on the body than long-term consumption, which clearly shows how chlorogenic acid affects the release of fatty acids (Skrypnik et al., 2018). Due to the reduction of the expression of genes linked to adipogenesis and inflammation in the perioral adipose tissue, decaffeinated green coffee decreases the formation of fat and lowers insulin resistance.

Clinical studies have demonstrated that green coffee supplementation along with a low-calorie diet can help obese persons lose weight. A larger decrease in body weight, fatty tissue content, and waist-hip ratio was seen in the intervention group (WHR). Leptin levels were not substantially different between green coffee users and the placebo group, but adiponectin levels were. By reducing both the concentration of total cholesterol and the LDL fraction as well as the level of free fatty acids, green coffee extract also enhanced the lipid profile. It should be noted that green coffee had no effects on body weight in individuals who were at a healthy weight (Song et al., 2014). The experiments also showed that chlorogenic acid has an impact on how a high-fat diet-induced repair of the gut microbiota occurs. Because of this, using supplements containing green coffee extract is advised in order to aid in weight loss and restore microbial equilibrium.

6.8.5 BERBERINE

Barberry (*Berberis vulgaris* L.) contains the alkaloid berberine in its stem, rhizome, roots, and bark. This chemical has numerous known therapeutic benefits, including anti-cancer qualities, and it also safeguards the central nervous system and digestive system. As berberine affects the mechanisms of weight reduction, numerous studies have demonstrated the benefits of utilizing it in the weight loss process. Berberine use improves metabolic performance by raising energy expenditure and glucose tolerance while decreasing the expression of pro-inflammatory cytokines in white adipose tissue (Wawrzyniak et al., 2022). Adipose tissue is classified as either white or brown; beige adipose tissue is white adipose tissue that turns brown when subjected to environmental stressors. The activation of BAT results in weight reduction and is a method to avoid obesity because white adipose tissue stores triglycerides for energy whereas BAT regulates body temperature by burning energy from the oxidation of blood lipids (Haywood et al., 2018). In a study on mice, browning, or the change from white to beige adipose tissue, as well as BAT activation during a 4-week administration of 5 mg/kg of berberine per day, which boosted thermogenesis and energy burning, were observed. The production of UCP1 (uncoupling protein) and PGC1 (PPAR coactivator-1), as well as enhanced MPK (adenosine 5′-monophosphate-activated protein kinase) phosphorylation, are the mechanisms behind these activities. A 1.5 g dosage of berberine, also given for a month, stimulated brown adipose tissue in human research by activating the AMPK-PRDM16 (PR domain-containing 16) pathway. The expression of genes necessary for adipocyte proliferation and differentiation has been seen to be inhibited by berberine (Barengolts et al., 2016). In overweight and obese people, *Berberis vulgaris* L. extract also decreases leptin levels, resulting in weight loss. The waist-to-hip ratio (WHR) was dramatically decreased by berberine, although there was no discernible impact on BMI. Similar research on waist circumference has produced contradictory findings. After giving obese persons 500 mg of berberine three times a day for 12 weeks, minor weight reduction was seen, and the lipid profile dramatically improved (12.2% lower total cholesterol and 23% lower triglycerides). The approximately 60% increase in blood calcitriol concentration was an additional benefit (Abenavoli et al., 2019). Berberine reduces LDL cholesterol and total cholesterol when combined with other nutrients that are good for you, such as red yeast rice. Berberine lowers insulin resistance, which leads to lowering blood glucose levels as well as weight loss by modifying the gut microbiota. Because type 2 diabetes mellitus is one of the risk factors for obesity, it is crucial to understand how berberine affects blood glucose levels therapeutically. Berberine, like metformin, has the capacity to raise the quantity of SCFA-producing bacteria in the gut and to make up for structural modifications to the microbiota brought on by a high-fat diet (Caraj et al., 2011). Diabetes patients who consumed 1 g of berberine daily for three months saw a reduction in their fasting blood glucose levels, even after meals. Blood sugar and hemoglobin A1c levels were dramatically lowered even after a weekly intake of 0.5 g of berberine per day (Pan et al., 2017). Additionally, berberine affects the genes for glucose-6-phosphatase and phosphoenolpyruvate carboxykinase (PEPCK), which inhibits the production of glucose from scratch. Pharmacokinetic studies (Osman et al., 2008) have shown that berberine is a safe and effective supplement and pharmaceutical constituent, but that it has poor systemic oral bioavailability. Although studies have shown that berberine has beneficial effects on mechanisms relating to weight reduction, oral slimming products containing *Berberis vulgaris* L. extract may not work as well as they could because of their low bioavailability.

6.9 CONCLUSION

Capsaicin, bitter orange, white bean seeds, green coffee, berberine, and single and multi-strain probiotics are dietary supplements with documented effects that help people lose excess body weight. Some of these supplements also offer added health advantages. Antioxidant and anti-ulcer effects are present in bitter orange. Blood glucose levels are decreased, and fat metabolism is improved with berberine. In the therapy of neurodegenerative illnesses, capsaicin has found use. Chitosan and vitamin D supplements do not considerably reduce body weight. While vitamin D increases the sensitivity of tissues to insulin, chitosan lowers blood pressure.

KEYWORDS

- **chitosan**
- **dietary supplements**
- **glucose**
- **metabolism**
- **nutraceuticals**
- **obesity**
- **supplements**
- **vitamins**
- **weight regulation**

REFERENCES

Abenavoli, L., Scarpellini, E., Colica, C., Boccuto, L., Salehi, B., Sharifi-Rad, J., Aiello, V., Romano, B., De Lorenzo, A., Izzo, A. A., & Capasso, R. (2019). Gut microbiota and obesity: A role for probiotics. *Nutrients, 11*(11), 2690.

Barengolts, E. (2016). Gut microbiota, prebiotics, probiotics, and synbiotics in management of obesity and prediabetes: Review of randomized controlled trials. *Endocrine Practice, 22*(10), 1224–1234.

Berkey, C. S., Rockett, H. R., Willett, W. C., & Colditz, G. A. (2005). Milk, dairy fat, dietary calcium, and weight gain: A longitudinal study of adolescents. *Archives of Pediatrics & Adolescent Medicine, 159*(6), 543–550.

Bischoff-Ferrari, H. (2009). Vitamin D: What is an adequate vitamin D level and how much supplementation is necessary? *Best Practice & Research Clinical Rheumatology, 23*(6), 789–795.

Blair, H. C., Schlesinger, P. H., Huang, C. H., & Zaidi, M. (2007). Calcium signaling and calcium transport in bone disease. In H. M. S. Calcium Signaling and Disease (pp. 539–562).

Burrows, T. L., Martin, R. J., & Collins, C. E. (2010). A systematic review of the validity of dietary assessment methods in children when compared with the method of doubly labeled water. *Journal of the American Dietetic Association, 110*(10), 1501–1510.

Carafoli, E., Santella, L., Branca, D., & Brini, M. (2001). Generation, control, and processing of cellular calcium signals. *Critical Reviews in Biochemistry and Molecular Biology, 36*(2), 107–260.

Carai, M. A., Fantini, N., Loi, B., Colombo, G., Gessa, G. L., Riva, A., Bombardelli, E., & Morazzoni, P. (2011). Multiple cycles of repeated treatments with a Phaseolus vulgaris dry extract reduce food intake and body weight in obese rats. *British Journal of Nutrition, 106*(5), 762–768.

Dos Santos, L. C., de Padua Cintra, I., Fisberg, M., & Martini, L. A. (2008). Calcium intake and its relationship with adiposity and insulin resistance in post-pubertal adolescents. *Journal of Human Nutrition and Dietetics, 21*(2), 109–116.

García, O. P., Long, K. Z., & Rosado, J. L. (2009). Impact of micronutrient deficiencies on obesity. *Nutrition Reviews, 67*(10), 559–572.

Goldberg, B. L. T., Cristiane, S. C., Natal, L. P. L., Nogueira, B. M., Braz, H. M., et al. (2009). Calcium intake and its relationship with risk of overweight and obesity in adolescents. *Archivos Latinoamericanos de Nutrición, 59*(1), 14–21.

Gorji, Z., Varkaneh, H. K., Nazary-Vannani, A., Clark, C. C., Fatahi, S., Rahmani, J., Salamat, S., & Zhang, Y. (2019). The effect of green-coffee extract supplementation on obesity: A systematic review and dose-response meta-analysis of randomized controlled trials. *Phytotherapy Research, 63*, 153018.

Harkness, L. S., & Bonny, A. E. (2005). Calcium and vitamin D status in the adolescent: Key roles for bone, body weight, glucose tolerance, and estrogen biosynthesis. *Journal of Pediatric and Adolescent Gynecology, 18*(5), 305–311.

Haywood, C. J., Prendergast, L. A., Purcell, K., Le-Fevre, L., Lim, W. K., Galea, M., & Proietto, J. (2018). Very low-calorie diets for weight loss in obese older adults—A randomized trial. *The Journals of Gerontology Series A: Biological Sciences and Medical Sciences, 73*(1), 59–65.

Jennings, A., Costarelli, V., Davies, G. J., & Dettmar, P. W. (2006). Habitual dietary calcium intake and body weight in 7–10-year-old children. *Nutrition & Food Science, 36*(1), 34–38.

Kamycheva, E., Joakimsen, R. M., & Jorde, R. (2003). Intakes of calcium and vitamin D predict body mass index in the population of Northern Norway. *The Journal of Nutrition, 133*(1), 102–106.

Keller, K. L., Kirzner, J., Pietrobelli, A., St-Onge, M. P., & Faith, M. S. (2009). Increased sweetened beverage intake is associated with reduced milk and calcium intake in 3-to 7-year-old children at multi-item laboratory lunches. *Journal of the American Dietetic Association, 109*(3), 497–501.

Keservani, R. K., Sharma, A. K., & Kesharwani, R. K. (2017). An overview and therapeutic applications of nutraceutical and functional foods. In Recent Advances in Drug Delivery Technology (pp. 160–201). ISBN: 9781522507543.

Keservani, R. K., Sharma, A. K., & Kesharwani, R. K. (Eds.). (2020). *Nutraceuticals and Dietary Supplements: Applications in Health Improvement and Disease Management*. pp. 1–344. CRC Press. ISBN: 9781771888738.

Kulie, T., Groff, A., Redmer, J., Hounshell, J., & Schrager, S. (2009). Vitamin D: An evidence-based review. *Journal of the American Board of Family Medicine, 22*(6), 698–706.

Kull, M., Kallikorm, R., & Lember, M. (2009). Body mass index determines sunbathing habits: Implications on vitamin D levels. *Internal Medicine Journal, 39*(4), 256–258.

Kumar, J., Muntner, P., Kaskel, F. J., Hailpern, S. M., & Melamed, M. L. (2009). Prevalence and associations of 25-hydroxyvitamin D deficiency in US children: NHANES 2001–2004. *Pediatrics, 124*(3), 362–370.

Mansbach, J. M., Ginde, A. A., & Camargo, C. A. (2009). Serum 25-hydroxyvitamin D levels among US children aged 1 to 11 years: Do children need more vitamin D? *Pediatrics, 124*(5), 1404–1410.

Novotny, R., Daida, Y. G., Acharya, S., Grove, J. S., & Vogt, T. M. (2004). Dairy intake is associated with lower body fat and soda intake with greater weight in adolescent girls. *The Journal of Nutrition, 134*(8), 1905–1909.

Osman, N., Adawi, D., Ahrné, S., Jeppsson, B., & Molin, G. (2008). Probiotics and blueberry attenuate the severity of dextran sulfate sodium (DSS)-induced colitis. *Digestive Diseases and Sciences, 53*(9), 2464–2473.

Pan, C. W., Qian, D. J., & Saw, S. M. (2017). Time outdoors, blood vitamin D status and myopia: A review. *Photochemical & Photobiological Sciences, 16*(3), 426–432.

Pan, H., Fu, C., Huang, L., Jiang, Y., Deng, X., Guo, J., & Su, Z. (2018). Anti-obesity effect of chitosan oligosaccharide capsules (COSCs) in obese rats by ameliorating leptin resistance and adipogenesis. *Marine Drugs, 16*(6), 198.

Pereira, M. A., Jacobs, Jr., D. R., Van Horn, L., Slattery, M. L., Kartashov, A. I., & Ludwig, D. S. (2002). Dairy consumption, obesity, and the insulin resistance syndrome in young adults: The CARDIA Study. *JAMA, 287*(16), 2081–2089.

Phillips, S. M., Bandini, L. G., Cyr, H., Colclough-Douglas, S., Naumova, E., & Must, A. (2003). Dairy food consumption and body weight and fatness studied longitudinally over the adolescent period. *International Journal of Obesity, 27*(9), 1106–1113.

Rajakumar, K., Holick, M. F., Jeong, K., Moore, C. G., Chen, T. C., Olabopo, F., Haralam, M. A., Nucci, A., Thomas, S. B., & Greenspan, S. L. (2011). Impact of season and diet on vitamin D status of African American and Caucasian children. *Clinical Pediatrics, 50*(6), 493–502.

Ríos-Hoyo, A., & Gutiérrez-Salmeán, G. (2016). New dietary supplements for obesity: What we currently know. *Current Obesity Reports, 5*(2), 262–270.

Schrager, S. (2005). Dietary calcium intake and obesity. *Journal of the American Board of Family Practice, 18*(3), 205–210.

Schwiertz, A., Taras, D., Schafer, K., Beijer, S., Bos, N. A., Donus, C., & Hardt, P. D. (2010). Microbiota and SCFA in lean and overweight healthy subjects. *Journal of Obesity, 18*(1), 190–195.

Sergeev, I. N. (2005). Calcium signaling in cancer and vitamin D. *Journal of Steroid Biochemistry and Molecular Biology, 97*(1–2), 145–151.

Sergeev, I. N., & Rhoten, W. B. (1995). 1, 25-Dihydroxyvitamin D3 evokes oscillations of intracellular calcium in a pancreatic beta-cell line. *Endocrinology, 136*(7), 2852–2861.

Skrypnik, K., Bogdański, P., Łoniewski, I., Reguła, J., & Suliburska, J. (2018). Effect of probiotic supplementation on liver function and lipid status in rats. *Acta Scientiarum Polonorum Technologia Alimentaria, 17*(2), 185–192.

Song, S. J., Choi, S., & Park, T. (2014). Decaffeinated green coffee bean extract attenuates diet-induced obesity and insulin resistance in mice. *Evidence-Based Complementary and Alternative Medicine, 2014*, Article 208567.

Spadari, A., Romagnoli, N., Predieri, P. G., Borghetti, P., Cantoni, A. M., & Corradi, A. (2013). Effects of intraarticular treatment with stanozolol on synovial membrane and cartilage in an ovine model of osteoarthritis. *Research in Veterinary Science, 94*(3), 379–387.

Stohs, S. J. (2017). Safety, efficacy, and mechanistic studies regarding Citrus aurantium (bitter orange) extract and p-synephrine. *Phytotherapy Research, 31*(10), 1463–1474.

Sun, X., & Zemel, M. B. (2008). 1α, 25-Dihydroxyvitamin D and corticosteroid regulate adipocyte nuclear vitamin D receptor. *International Journal of Obesity, 32*(8), 1305–1311.

Sun, X., Morris, K. L., & Zemel, M. B. (2008). Role of calcitriol and cortisol on human adipocyte proliferation and oxidative and inflammatory stress: A microarray study. *Lifestyle Genomics, 1*(1–2), 30–48.

Teegarden, D., & Zemel, M. B. (2003). Dairy product components and weight regulation: symposium overview. *The Journal of Nutrition, 133*(1), 243S–244S.

Troiano, R. P., & Flegal, K. M. (1998). Overweight children and adolescents: description, epidemiology, and demographics. *Pediatrics, 101*(2), 497–504.

Wagner, C. L., & Greer, F. R., Section on Breastfeeding and Committee on Nutrition. (2008). Prevention of rickets and vitamin D deficiency in infants, children, and adolescents. *Pediatrics, 122*(5), 1142–1152.

Wawrzyniak, N., Skrypnik, K., & Suliburska, J. (2022). Dietary supplements in therapy to support weight reduction in obese patients. *Acta Scientiarum Polonorum Technologia Alimentaria, 21*(1), 67–80.

Wise, A., & Birrell, N. M. (2002). Design and analysis of food frequency questionnaires—review and novel method. *International Journal of Food Sciences and Nutrition, 53*(3), 273–279.

Wortsman, J., Matsuoka, L. Y., Chen, T. C., Lu, Z., & Holick, M. F. (2000). Decreased bioavailability of vitamin D in obesity. *American Journal of Clinical Nutrition, 72*(3), 690–693.

Wright, J. D. (2003). Dietary intake of ten key nutrients for public health, United States, 1999-2000. US Department of Health and Human Services, Centers for Disease Control and Prevention, National Center for Health Statistics.

Yang, Y. J., Kim, M. K., Hwang, S. H., Ahn, Y., Shim, J. E., & Kim, D. H. (2010). Relative validities of 3-day food records and the food frequency questionnaire. *Nutrition Research and Practice, 4*(2), 142–148.

Zhang, X., Zhao, Y., Xu, J., Xue, Z., Zhang, M., Pang, X., Zhang, X., & Zhao, L. (2015). Modulation of gut microbiota by berberine and metformin during the treatment of high-fat diet-induced obesity in rats. *Scientific Reports, 5*(1), 1–10.

CHAPTER 7

THE ROLE OF GREEN TEA IN THE MANAGEMENT OF OBESITY

NIHARIKA, SAKSHI MINOCHA, RASHMI SINGH, and PRAVEEN KUMAR GAUR

Department of Pharmacy, Metro College of Health Sciences and Research, Greater Noida, Uttar Pradesh, India

ABSTRACT

Obesity is the most common health concern, affecting people of all ages and leading to many consequences such as chronic heart disease, Type 2 diabetes, and stroke. According to a literature review, it is linked to at least 18 co-morbidities that are associated with being overweight or obese. Obese people are also more likely to have substantial joint pains and hormonal disorders, as well as social and psychological problems. Green tea catechins (GTC) are polyphenolic chemicals found in the unfermented dried leaves of the plant Camellia sinensis. Ingestion of GTC (270 mg to 1,200 mg/day) has been shown to lower body weight and fat in various randomized, controlled intervention trials. GTC is believed to affect body weight and composition through several processes. The most popular theory is that GTC increases energy expenditure and promotes fat oxidation by influencing sympathetic nervous system (SNS) activity. Caffeine, naturally found in green tea, affects SNS activity and may work synergistically with GTC to enhance energy expenditure and fat burning. Changes in appetite, up-regulation of enzymes involved in hepatic fat oxidation, and reduced nutritional absorption are all possible explanations. This chapter explores the potential of green tea as a vital nutraceutical for managing obesity. Additionally, we reviewed the

Nutraceuticals in Obesity Management and Control. Raj K. Keservani & Alka Lohani (Eds.)

evidence for each of these proposed mechanisms, with a focus on human studies.

7.1 INTRODUCTION

A growing global public health concern is obesity. Patients with obesity are significantly more likely to develop a variety of comorbid conditions, such as cardiovascular disease (CVD), gastrointestinal disorders, type 2 diabetes, joint and muscular disorders, respiratory issues, and psychological problems (Amagase, 2011). These conditions may have a significant impact on patient's daily lives and increase their mortality risk. It has been found that even minor weight loss may help patients lower their risk for CVD, diabetes, Obstructive sleep apnea (OSA), and Hypertension, among many other comorbidities, which are directly or indirectly related to obesity (Cabrera et al., 2006).

Almost half of adults today are too busy to exercise. The overall prevalence of obesity is projected to increase from about 12% in 1992 to 41% in men and 21% to 78% in women by 2022. The predicted prevalence in women was much higher than in men, especially in the 35–44, 45–54, and 55–64 age groups (Barnes et al., 2004; Basu et al., 2007). Tea is one of the most commonly consumed beverages worldwide and comes in many forms. Next to water, it is the cheapest drink most people consume. Since ancient times, tea made from the Camellia family has been the most commonly consumed. According to the manufacturing method, tea is classified into green tea (unfermented), black tea (fully fermented), oolong tea (semi-fermented), and Pu-erh tea (post-fermented). The most commonly consumed type of tea in Asian countries is green tea, one of the most popular types, accounting for 23% of all tea products (Eikelis & Esler, 2005). Green tea contains various elements with potential health benefits, including catechins and polyphenols that may help prevent cancer, cardiovascular disease, obesity, and type 2 diabetes.

Phytochemicals included in green tea are recognized to support the central nervous system and maintain overall human health. A growing body of research indicates that green tea may also be used as a potential agent to mediate skin aging and neurological disorders like Alzheimer's. Furthermore, many studies examine the evidence that green tea can help in increasing fat burning and be beneficial for weight loss (Cooper et al., 2005). The current chapter provides an overview of the significance of the role of green tea in weight loss. There are many controversies about the role of green tea and its effects on health and diseases. With this in mind, this chapter examines the beneficial effects of green tea and green tea catechins in healthy obese individuals (Di Pierro et al., 2009).

In general, green tea is an infusion made from the roasted leaves of the plant *Camellia sinensis* (formerly known as *Theasinensis*), and the beverage has a long tradition in China (lǜchá), Japan (ryokucha), Korea (nokcha), Vietnam (chèxanh), and elsewhere in the Orient. The tea plant is native to southwestern China; however, its cultivation has spread to many other regions of the world in line with the spread of tea drinking (Han et al., 2005; Abdollahi & Afshar-Imani, 2003).

Throughout the course of recent years, green tea has detonated into an incredibly famous refreshment decision for tea consumers around the world. It has been consumed for quite a long time in Asian nations like China, Japan, and India (Chacko et al., 2010).

7.2 ERA OF TEA CULTURE

Tea was first recorded in ancient China about 5,000 years ago. Legend has it that in 2732 BC Emperor Shennong discovered tea when leaves from a wild tree were blown into a pot of boiling water. He was immediately intrigued by the pleasant aroma of the finished tea and took a sip of it. Shennong called the tea the Chinese character "ch'a," which means "investigate" or "investigation." The popularity of tea in China continued to grow rapidly from the 4th century to the 8th century (Kurogi et al., 2012). Tea was valued not only for its therapeutic benefits but also for daily enjoyment and refreshment. Tea merchants became wealthy, tea plantations spread across China, and expensive and elegant teaware symbolized the wealth and status of their owners. Harvest, cultivation, and preparation were strictly controlled by the Chinese Empire. Specifically, only young women were allowed to handle the tea leaves, ostensibly because of their purity. These young female handlers were forbidden from consuming strong spices, garlic, or onions for fear that the smell from their fingertips would contaminate the precious tea leaves (Tian et al., 2004).

Until the mid-17th century, all Chinese tea was green tea. However, as international trade expanded, Chinese growers learned that a unique fermentation process could be used to preserve the tea leaves. The resulting black tea was better prepared for export trips to other nations and retained its flavor and scent longer than the more delicate green teas. Tea has been an essential component of Chinese culture (Swinburn et al., 2004).

It was well-liked before the Egyptians constructed the great pyramids, and it was traded with other Asian nations long before Europe emerged from the Dark Ages. Even today, tea is significant and well-liked in China and has come to represent its history, culture, and religion. In India, green tea was introduced by British cultivators. Around 1774, Warren Hastings sent a selection of Chinese seeds to plant to George His Bogle, a British envoy stationed in Bhutan at the time. However, nothing seems to come out of this experiment. In 1776, Sir Joseph Banks, the great English botanist, was commissioned to compose a series of notes. It was his recommendation to start growing tea in India. In 1780, Robert Kyd attempted to grow tea in India using a cargo of seeds allegedly arriving from China. In 1788, the Royal Society of Arts began considering the idea of transplanting saplings from China. Decades later, Robert Bruce found wild tea plants in the upper Brahmaputra Valley (Nammi et al., 2004).

Around this time, carpenters and shoemakers were sent to Darjeeling and Assam from the Chinese settlement in Calcutta, according to a 19th-century lecture to the Royal Society. Many of them had never seen a tea tree. Boxes of tea made from native Assamese leaves were sent to London and sold at auction there, resulting in the formation of the Bengal Tea Society in Calcutta. The Assam Company, the first tea joint-stock company in London, was established. After the success, other companies were established to start growing tea (Wu & Wei, 2002; Wu et al., 2007). Jorehaut Tea Company and George Williamson are two of the other pioneering companies. After developing a profitable industry in the Brahmaputra valley of Assam, researchers studied the profitability of tea cultivation throughout the Himalayan foothills and other parts of India. Around 78 plantations were established in the Garhwal, Kangra Valley, and Kullu areas (Pinnell, 2007).

After the transfer of the present-day Darjeeling area to the East India Company in 1835 and the first attempts in the 1840s, commercial plantations were established in Darjeeling in the 1850s and by 1874 had grown to 18,888 acres of tea. A total of 113 gardens were opened and production was recorded at £3.9 million (Rehman et al., 2011). The Indian Tea Association and the United Planters Association of South India (UPASI) were established in 1881 and 1895, respectively to address labor, legal and regulatory issues, communications, the need for market expansion, and the industry related to tea packaging. India is currently one of the world's leading producers of tea (Swinburn et al., 2004; Pal et al., 2011).

7.3 COMPOSITION OF GREEN TEA

Polyphenols make up the majority of green tea (90%), followed by amino acids (7%), theanine, proanthocyanidins, and caffeine (3%). Catechins and flavonols (myricetin, kaempferol, quercetin, chlorogenic acid, coumarylquinic acid, and theogallin) make up the majority of the various polyphenols. The main catechins found in green tea are catechin (C), epicatechin (EC), gallocatechin (GC), epigallocatechin (EGC), epicatechin gallate (ECG), epigallocatechin gallate (EGCG), and gallocatechin gallate (GCG). Of these, EGCG, ECG, and EGC make up 80% of all catechins (Boon, 2008; Chacko, 2010). The harvesting season and leaf age have a significant impact on the quality of green tea. Later harvests have lower concentrations of theanine, theobromine, caffeine, catechin, and GCG. However, under the same circumstances, EC, EGCG, and EGC concentrations rose. Similar findings showed that young leaves (up to the seventh leaf) had higher concentrations of caffeine, EGCG, ECG, and other catechins than older leaves (Sueoka et al., 2001). This is supposed to happen as a result of withering. The majority of the catechins in green tea, about 50%–80% of them, are found in EGCG. It is also regarded as the primary cause of the numerous health advantages of green tea (Cooper, 2005; Chu et al., 2011).

An average fresh tea leaf contains 30% catechins by dry weight, which belong to the flavonol family of polyphenols. In addition, tea has theogallin (3-galloylquinic acid), theanine (5-N-ethyl glutamine), chlorogenic acid, and coumarylquinic acid, which are all specific to tea. Tea contains caffeine as well as small levels of theophylline, theobromine, and other common methylxanthines. Tea can also store manganese and aluminum (Forester, 2012; Hasani-Ranjbar et al., 2009). The leaf structure is initially broken down during the production of black tea, allowing the aerobic oxidation of catechins. Polyphenol oxidase, one of several enzymes found in tea leaves, mediates this (Hara et al., 2012). The condensation of different quinones results in the production of a number of substances, including bisflavanols, theaflavins, epitheaflavic acids, and thearubigens. These are renowned for delivering black tea's distinctive flavor and color. The composition of effective components present in green tea is mentioned in Table 7.1.

TABLE 7.1 Composition of Green Tea Phytoconstituents

Components	Amount mg/100 g (100 ml)
Epigallocatechin 3-gallate	77.8 ± 7.0
Epicatechin 3-gallate	19.7 ± 2.8
Epigallocatechin	16.7 ± 1.4
Epicatechin	8.3 ± 0.5
Quercetin	2.7 ± 0.3
Catechin	2.6 ± 1.5
Gallocatechin	1.5 ± 0.0
Thiarubigins	1.1 ± 1.1

7.3.1 CATECHINS

Several studies support the high antioxidant properties of tea beverages, suggesting that this is due to the high content of catechins (Higdon, 2003). It is a kind of phenolic compound that has a positive effect on human health. Green tea contains four main catechins, namely epicatechin (EC), epicatechin-3-gallate (ECG), epigallocatechin (EGC), and epigallocatechin-3-gallate (EGCG), the last of which is the most active. Catechin derivatives exhibit dominant antioxidant activity as they can neutralize free radicals and enhance the detoxification activity of enzymes including glutathione peroxidase, catalase, and glutathione reductase (Subramani & Natesh, 2013; Koh et al., 2010).

Grzesik et al. reported that catechins have a higher antioxidant capacity than glutathione, vitamin C, and flavonoids, confirming their central role in maintaining cellular redox homeostasis (Grzesik et al., 2018). Koláčková et al., according to the study conducted, the total polyphenol content of matcha tea is 1,69,273 mg GAE/g (Koláčková et al., 2020). However, Nishitani & Sagesaka saw low levels of polyphenols in matcha compared to other green teas. Therefore, it was suggested that this difference in results may be due to the shade of the teas, which limits the synthesis of polyphenols. However, the amount of catechin in green tea is much higher than in black tea at 5,467.44 mg/g compared to 0.47 mg/g in black tea (Nishitani & Sagesaka, 2014).

7.3.2 CAFFEINE

Caffeine is an integral component of tea beverages and is responsible for their remarkable and desirable taste. The caffeine content can be related to the time of harvest and the age of the leaves. The older the leaves, the lower the caffeine content. Caffeine content can also depend on tea type, vegetation, weather conditions, and brewing method (Wang et al., 2006). The effects of caffeine are related to its antioxidant potential, neutralizing free oxygen species, and improving the activity of antioxidant enzymes and total glutathione levels. In normal doses, caffeine can reduce persistent oxidative stress and reduce the incidence of free radical-induced diseases. In addition, caffeine can limit the secretion of pro-inflammatory cytokines that have anti-inflammatory effects (Westerterp-Plantenga et al., 2006). Matcha (finely ground powder from specially grown and processed green tea leaves) has a relatively high caffeine content compared to other green teas, giving it a unique aroma and taste. The caffeine content of green tea ranges from 11.324.67 mg/g, while matcha ranges from 18.9 to 44.4 mg/g. Compared to green tea, most coffee beans contain 10,012.0 mg caffeine/g.

7.3.3 PHENOLIC ACIDS

Phenolic acids are minor plant metabolites with high antioxidant and anti-inflammatory effects, as well as neuroprotective and hypoglycemic effects. It has also been reported to inhibit cancer cell growth and prevent metastasis. Few phenolic acids support the regulation of metabolic disorders by modulating lipid and glucose metabolism.

Kolackova et al. conducted research and found that the total amount of phenol in alcoholic extracts can reach up to 273 mg GAE/g. Detailed analysis revealed that the highest concentrations of phenolic acids in matcha tea samples, which differ in several criteria, are: gallic acid 423 μg/g, p-hydroxybenzoic acid 243 μg/g, chlorogenic acid 4,800 μg/g, caffeic acid 223 μg/g, ferulic acid 289 μg/g, and ellagic acid 371 μg/g (Kolácková et al., 2020).

7.3.4 RUTIN

Rutin is a polyphenolic compound (Keservani & Sharma, 2014), a powerful antioxidant. Synergistic interaction with ascorbic acid enhances the protective effect of both substances on the cardiovascular system and strengthens blood vessels. It also has anti-diabetic and anti-inflammatory effects, thus preventing diabetes-related pathologies. Its antioxidant and anti-inflammatory effects offer the potential to prevent free radicals or inflammatory diseases, including neurodegenerative disorders.

According to Jakubczyk et al., matcha green tea contains an extraordinary amount of rutin compared to other teas on the market. The authors point out that the rutin content of matcha (1968.8 mg/l) and buckwheat (62.30 mg/100 g), the latter considered one of the richest sources of rutin in the human diet, and confirmed that matcha tea is a better source of the compound than other foods (Jakubczyk et al., 2020). Jakubczyk et al.'s findings are consistent with those of Kolácková et al. (2020).

7.3.5 QUERCETIN

Quercetin is a phytochemical with antioxidant and neuroprotective activity. It also normalizes carbohydrate metabolism, as it inhibits the absorption of glucose from the digestive tract, regulates insulin secretion, and develops tissue sensitivity to insulin. The combination of quercetin and epigallocatechin gallate (EGCG) enhances the anticancer effect. Schröder et al. measured the amount of quercetin in an aqueous matcha extract to be 1.2 mg/ml, which is slightly higher than that found in traditional green tea (1.1 mg/ml). In contrast, Koláčková et al. found the content of quercetin in alcoholic extracts to be 17.2 µg/g (Koláčková et al., 2020).

7.3.6 VITAMIN C

Vitamin C is a powerful antioxidant that strengthens the immune system, as it is an essential trace element in human nutrition. Jakubczyk et al. concluded that matcha green tea infusions contained between 32.12 and 44.8 mg/L of vitamin C, the range depending on the temperature of the water used to prepare the infusion and the type of tea (Jakubczyk et al., 2020). Koláčková et al., in a study conducted, found that matcha has more than twice the vitamin C content of other green teas. The amount was found to be 1,633.98 mg/g depending on the type of product and its origin (Koláčková et al., 2020).

7.3.7 CHLOROPHYLL

Matcha tea has an increased amount of chlorophyll due to the growth of the shade, which leads to a distinctive bright color. Chlorophyll and its derivatives have strong antioxidant and anti-inflammatory effects. Ku and others note the number of bioactive compounds, including chlorophyll, in the Tencha-type tea leaves used specifically for matcha. Tencha leaves contain higher levels of chlorophyll than traditional green tea at 5.65 mg/g and 4.33 mg/g, respectively (Ku et al., 2010).

7.3.8 THEANINE

Theanine is an amino acid found in the Camellia sinensis tea plant. For the production of matcha, the plants are grown in the shade so that the theanine does not break down. As a result, Tencha leaves contain higher amounts than other teas. The high amount of theanine in matcha tea results in a unique, unbitter taste, and together with caffeine, it gives this tea its characteristic taste, feel, and umami. The combination of theanine and caffeine improves concentration, alertness, and efficiency more than others, as well as reducing stress. According to Kaneko et al., the theanine content of matcha tea infusions is 6.1 mg/L, while Unno et al. found up to 44.65 mg/g of that compound in matcha tea samples (Kaneko et al., 2006; Unno et al., 2019).

7.4 OBESITY

Worldwide, the sudden increase in overweight and obesity is of great concern. Globally, it is estimated to cause more than 3.4 million deaths, 4% of life-years lost (YLL), and at least 4% of disability-adjusted life-years (DALY). Health problems due to the attractive appearance of thin bodies and poor health outcomes due to overweight and obesity (Kritchevsky et al., 2015). Obese people tend to be in worse health than people of normal weight, and their life expectancy is on average two years shorter. Cancer, type 2 diabetes, high blood pressure, stroke, coronary heart disease, congestive heart failure, asthma, chronic back pain, osteoarthritis, pulmonary embolism, gallbladder disease, as well as an increased risk of disability. All this leads to more than 3 million deaths per year worldwide. There is no doubt that obesity is the result of an imbalance between energy intake and energy expenditure. A growing body of evidence and knowledge demonstrates the complexity of the problem (DPP Research Group, 2009, 2015). Based on the evidence from these studies, the purpose of this comprehensive review is to provide a detailed analysis of the various factors contributing to the development of the obesity epidemic. A detailed breakdown of the causes of obesity is discussed in subsections.

7.4.1 CAUSES

7.4.1.1 DIET CULTURE

Obesity does not happen overnight. It develops gradually over time due to poor eating habits and lifestyle choices. Nutritional analysis shows that fast food is high in fat, saturated fat, energy density, fructose, and glycemic index, but low in fiber, vitamins A and C, and calcium. A typical fast-food meal contains 1,400 kcal, 85% of the recommended daily fat intake, and 73% of the recommended saturated fat, but only 40% of the recommended fiber and 30% of the recommended calcium (Pulgaron, 2013). Cross-sectional observational studies have repeatedly linked fast food with obesity and insulin resistance. Adults who report eating fast food have a higher mean BMI than those who do not, even after controlling for demographic variables. In the same study, people who ate fast food more than twice a week gained 4.5 kg over 15 years and were more insulin-resistant. In a second prospective study, increasing the frequency of fast-food consumption to 1 meal per week was associated with a 1.6-pound weight gain, compared with an average weight gain of 3.7 pounds over 2 weeks. A 3-year study. A second epidemiological link between fast food and obesity can be found by examining studies of sugary drink consumption. As mentioned, soft drinks are often added to fast food meals (Emery et al., 2015). Consumption of sugar-sweetened beverages increases the risk of obesity in preschool children and older children and increases the risk of obesity and type 2 diabetes in adults. In one study of 6th and 7th graders, each daily serving of sugary drinks increased the relative risk of obesity by 60%. The reverse also appears to be true, as studies aimed at reducing sugary drink consumption in school-aged children have been shown to be effective in reducing the prevalence of obesity (Haufe et al., 2013; Li et al., 2008).

7.4.1.2 HEREDITARY

Obesity is a complex heritable trait influenced by genetics, epigenetics, metagenomics, and the environment. A large number of genes influencing the phenotype have been discovered as a result of improved access to highly accurate diagnostic methods of genetic testing, especially in early-onset severe obesity (Farooqi & Rahilly, 2006). The idea of an innate (endogenous) biological cause of obesity was first proposed by Von Noorden in 1907. Silventoinen et al. found that the heritability of weight varies over time with a total influence of 45%–90% (Silventoinen, 2010). However, there are individual differences in body weight and fat mass within a given environment, implying that adiposity is regulated by a complex interplay of genetic, developmental, behavioral, and environmental factors (Ogden, 2010). Obesity is caused by a variety of genetic factors, which can be divided into three categories:

1. **Monogenic Causes:** These are caused by a single gene mutation, usually in the leptin-melanocortin pathway:
2. **Syndromic Obesity:** It is associated with additional features such as neurodevelopmental disorders and organ/system malformations.
3. **Polygenic Obesity:** This is caused by the combined effect of many genes, which are amplified in an environment that "promotes weight gain."

Through the brain-gut axis, the central nervous system regulates food intake, and the hypothalamic leptin-melanocortin pathway is a key regulator of energy balance (Huang & Tao, 2014). The leptin-melanocortin pathway has been implicated in the genetic origin of monogenic obesity. This pathway is critical for energy balance and food intake; severe obesity will occur upon discontinuation. Some of the genes associated with monogenetic severe obesity are leptin (LEP), leptin receptor (LEPR), proopiomelanocortin (POMC), MC4R, proconvertase 1 (PCSK1), single-minded 1 (SIM1), brain-derived neurotrophic factor (BDNF), and the tropomyosin receptor kinase B (TrkB). Leptin activates POMC-expressing neurons, causing them to produce melanocortin peptides that bind to MC4R, which regulates energy balance. Hyperphagia is caused by mutations in the POMC and MC4R genes, leading to extreme obesity. MC4R mutations are common in monogenetic obesity, accounting for more than 5% of all pediatric cases (Ibrahim et al., 2003; Koo & Noh, 2007). PCSK1 mutations lead to inappropriate processing of melanocortin peptides, resulting in obesity and impaired glucose homeostasis and adrenal function. The transcription factor SIM1 causes severe obesity by downregulating the hypothalamic paraventricular nucleus (PVN) and causing hyperphagia. BDNF is also expressed in the hypothalamus and promotes anorexia signaling and locomotor activity through MC4R signaling.

Obesity and hyperphagia have been linked to BDNF and its receptor TrkB in both humans and animals (Kopelman, 2007). Obesity associated with multiple comorbidities such as craniofacial dysmorphism, cognitive impairment, and other forms of congenital abnormalities is called syndromic obesity. Neurodevelopmental disorders can cause severe cognitive impairment and may be associated with adaptive behavior that occurs in childhood or adolescence. Chromosomal abnormalities (e.g., aneuploidies, microdeletions, and duplications) and monogenic mutations can cause syndromic obesity (Azadbakht et al., 2007; Genta et al., 2009). Comorbidities of syndromic obesity associated with monogenic and/or polygenic disorders include behavioral problems, neurodevelopmental delays, dysmorphic features, and organ-specific developmental malformations (Granell et al., 2012). Breakthroughs in laboratory genetic tools continue to expand the list of syndromic conditions associated with increased obesity risk and developmental delay, highlighting the need for targeted approaches to the management of syndromic obesity.

Polygenetic obesity is defined as a condition in which many different gene variations or polymorphisms are linked. These polymorphisms, called single nucleotide variants (SNVs), are common in the population and involve single nucleotide changes in the DNA sequence. GWAS (genome-wide association studies) have been developed by studying thousands or millions of variants (covering more than 75% of the human genome) in thousands of people at a time (case-control groups). FTO was the first obesity-related gene discovered in 2007 using the GWAS method. The first three obesity GWAS were published in 2009 and revealed 16 loci associated with obesity (Gout et al., 2010; Hasani-Ranjbar et al., 2010). Since then, a number of meta-analyses have shown clear differences in obesity in different populations or obesity-related traits such as body fat distribution over 300,000 or 700,000 people. There are now 941 nearly independent variants associated with BMI and 346 loci associated with body fat distribution. Some obesity-related genes discovered by the GWAS approach include MC4R, POMC, FTO, NRXN3, NPC1, NEGR1, GNPDA2, MTCH2, ETV5 (Hatzikotoulas et al., 2014). Some of these are involved in synaptic function and neurotransmitter signaling (NEGR1, NRXN3, CADM2, GRID1, ELAVL4, and SCG3) and energy homeostasis (POMC, MC4R, BDNF, ETV5, HNF4G, and TLR4). Polymorphic changes have little effect. Therefore, the GRS (Genetic Risk Score) was developed to show the "genome-wide number of risk variations," and the higher the GRS, the higher the risk of obesity (Visscher et al., 2017). Over the past 15 years of the genomic era, hundreds of variants have been associated with obesity. Finally, genetic risk prediction for obesity can be used to determine an individual's genetic predisposition to the condition.

7.4.1.3 PSYCHOLOGICAL

Although the evidence for a biological link between overweight, obesity, and depression is complex and inconclusive, it is important to highlight newer arguments about the possibility of a biological pathway. We first discuss the effect of obesity on depressive outcomes (Finucane et al., 2011). Obesity can be viewed as an inflammatory condition, as weight gain has been shown to activate inflammatory pathways that have been associated with depression, which was measured using the depression symptom ratio in this study. As inflammation affects both obesity and depression, it is possible that inflammation is a link between the two (IIPS and Macro-International, 2007). In addition, the hypothalamic-pituitary-adrenal (HPA) axis may play an important role, as obesity has been associated with dysregulation of the HPA axis, which has been linked to depression. Obesity may contribute to the development of depression by disrupting the HPA axis. Finally, obesity increases the risk of diabetes and insulin resistance, both of which can cause changes in the brain and increase the risk of depression. In addition to biological mechanisms, psychological pathways should be mentioned (Kreier et al., 2003; Dansinger & Schaefer, 2006). Obesity, like the perception of obesity, causes psychological experiences. Obesity can lead to body dissatisfaction and low self-esteem, risk factors for depression in both the United States and Europe, where thinness is considered the ideal of beauty. This is partly due to social recognition and sociocultural influence. Disordered eating patterns and eating disorders, as well as physical pain directly caused by obesity, were associated with an increased risk of depression. The fact that depression eventually leads to weight gain may be due to neuroendocrine disturbances (Puhl & Heuer, 2009). Depression, according to Björntorp, causes (abdominal) obesity by activating the HPA axis over time (Bjorntorp & Rosmond, 2000). Cortisol inhibits lipid-mobilizing enzymes in the presence of insulin, a mechanism mediated by glucocorticoid receptors in fat stores, particularly intra-abdominal visceral fat. Another important factor is a poor lifestyle, which can contribute to obesity if it is accompanied by insufficient movement and unhealthy eating habits. Finally, antidepressant use is known to cause weight gain, but many of the included studies were community-based studies in which participants with depression were often not treated with medication. Furthermore, studies using a clinical diagnosis of depression in which subjects were more frequently treated with antidepressants did not differ from studies of depressive symptoms (Chrousos & Gold, 1992). The social consequences of obesity can contribute to ongoing problems with weight management. Environmental factors, lifestyle choices, and the cultural milieu all contribute to the global obesity crisis. According to a recent study, most studies show a possible relationship between eating disorders and depression (Dallman et al., 2004). But this relationship is not a one-way street; depression can be both a cause and a consequence of obesity. In addition, obese adolescents in a clinical sample had a higher prevalence of anxiety disorders than nonobese controls. Despite this, some studies show no link between an increase in BMI and more anxiety symptoms. Therefore, the relationship between obesity and anxiety may not be unidirectional and less conclusive (Vogelzangs et al., 2007). Psychological Imbalance: Obesity is associated with various health problems. Fatty liver, sleep apnea, type 2 diabetes, asthma, cardiovascular disease, high cholesterol, gallstones, glucose intolerance and insulin resistance, skin disorders, menstrual disorders, balance, and orthopedic problems. Some of these health problems can even lead to death in the worst cases (Hach et al., 2006; Hallstrom & Noppa, 1981). Obesity affects a person's social and emotional health and is not only associated with various medical problems. Obesity, according to experts, is "one of the most stigmatizing and socially least acceptable childhood conditions." They also face many other difficulties, including negative stereotypes, discrimination, and social exclusion (Bornstein et al., 2006). The causes and possible remedies for obesity are mentioned in Figure 7.1.

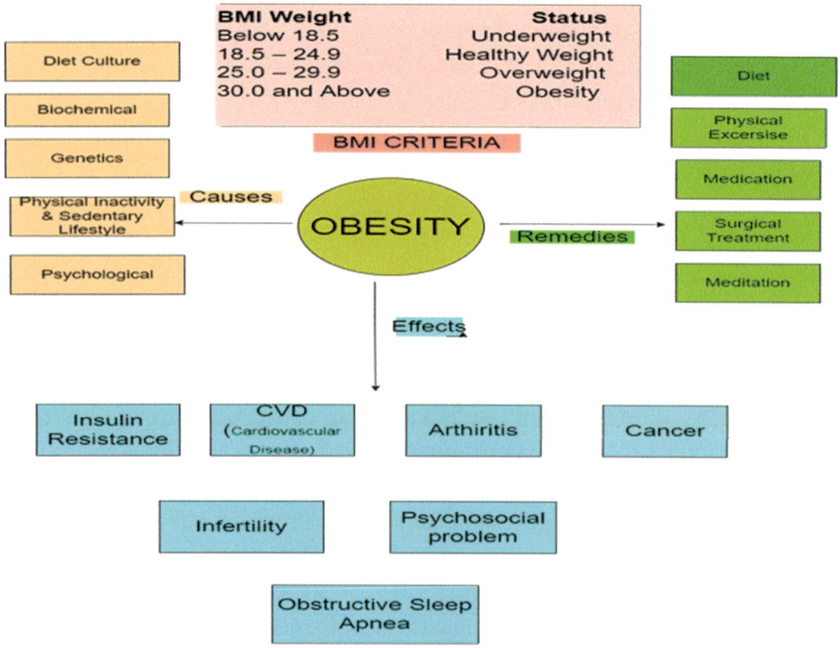

FIGURE 7.1 Schematic pictorial depiction of possible parameters associated with obesity.

7.4.2 REMEDY

Excess body fat management is one of the most pressing healthcare issues of our time. Losing weight through healthy eating, increasing physical activity, and making other lifestyle changes are all common remedies for overweight and obesity. Some measures that can be adopted for weight management are discussed in succeeding sections.

7.4.3 DIET

Popular weight-loss diets have attracted considerable attention and prompted a lot of debate. While energy balance (i.e., calories still count) remains the cornerstone of weight management, new diets and books promising weight loss by restricting certain foods or macronutrients rather than calories are continually emerging. One example of a low-fat (LF) dietary plan is provided by the Dietary Guidelines for Americans (Santesso et al., 2012).

The Dietary Guidelines are based on evidence indicating a low-fat (20–35% fat) diet can help people lose weight, improve their health, and lower their risk of chronic disease (Saad et al., 2021).

To maximize the nutrient content and health-enhancing potential of the diet, the guidelines recommend "foods to reduce" (i.e., saturated and trans-fat, cholesterol, sodium, added sugars, refined grains, alcohol) and "foods to increase" (i.e., fruits, vegetables, whole grains, low-fat dairy and protein foods, oils). The DASH diet, as well as those proposed by the American Diabetes Association, the American Heart Association, the American Cancer Society, and the commercial program Weight Watchers, are examples of LF diets (Bantle et al., 2008; Luke & Cooper, 2006). Low-fat diets are the most thoroughly researched of all weight-loss programs. One of the most significant obstacles to weight reduction success appears to be sticking to a calorie-controlled diet. Long-term adherence is not immune to LF eating.

Researchers have looked at a variety of interventions to promote long-term adherence to the diet, from altering the amount of fat in the diet to tailoring the diet to suit dietary preferences. A study comparing weight loss and cardiovascular risk factors in people eating calorie-restricted diets containing 10% or 30% fat found that both diets resulted in similar weight loss at 7 months, but that weight loss and heart rate decreased. Vascular risk factors were shown to be better maintained thereafter. This indicates that the 20% fat diet group has a more restricted intake, is more difficult to adhere to in the long term, and leads to more weight gain (Guh et al., 2009; Hu, 2013).

Some scientists investigated that a fat consumption of less than 20% of total calories is required for optimal health. Very low-fat diets are characterized as those that include 10% to 20% fat. Very low-fat diets include the Pritikin and Ornish diets. They are mostly plant-based diets (e.g., fruits, vegetables, whole grains, legumes, and soy), with some reduced-fat dairy, eggs, lean meats, and fish in limited amounts (Kobayashi et al., 2013). Unlike low-fat diets, which include all foods, very low-fat diets actively restrict the use of refined carbohydrate-rich meals. Given that low-fat (LF) diets can contain up to 30% fat, moderate-fat (MF) diets comprise between 35 and 45% fat. Many people mistakenly associate MF diets with Mediterranean diets, yet Mediterranean diet fat content varies greatly. Some have recorded fat concentrations as high as 47%, while others have reported fat contents as low as 25%; consequently, while some Mediterranean diets can be considered moderate in fat, this cannot be assumed for everyone.

Previous studies have found that people who followed an MF diet maintained their weight loss better over time, suggesting that MF diets may be easier to stick to in the long run than LF diets (Boone et al., 2007). Recent research assessing MF (35%–46% fat) and LF (25%–30% fat) diets found that MF diets resulted in similar to slightly better weight reduction. These diets are high in monounsaturated fatty acids (MUFAs), primarily from MUFA-rich oils, and high in plant-based foods (fruits, vegetables, whole grains, legumes, etc.), resembling a Mediterranean diet. They also include nuts dietary fiber and small amounts of saturated fat from animal foods (Koh et al., 2012).

One study evaluated the effectiveness of MF diets in terms of weight maintenance. Participants in this study were randomized to one of three ad libitum diets for 6 months after losing at least 8% of their baseline body weight on an 8-week low-energy diet: (i) Mediterranean-style diet (35–45% fat with > 20% MUFA); (ii) low-fat (20–30% fat); or (iii) control (35% fat with > 15% saturated fat). All subjects regained weight after 6 months, with no notable variations between groups (MF, 2.5 kg; LF, 2.2 kg; control, 3.8 kg). However, the MF and LF groups had reduced body fat regain. The MF diet had a positive impact on diabetes risk indicators (i.e., fasting insulin levels were lower, and the homeostasis model assessment of insulin resistance improved) (Aitsi-Selmi et al., 2014).

The degree to which carbohydrates elevate blood glucose and insulin levels varies. The term "glycemic index" (GI) refers to a characteristic of carbohydrate-containing foods that affects blood glucose levels after consumption. Carbohydrate-rich foods are typically compared to glucose or white bread, both of which have a GI of 100 (Durand et al., 2011). Foods with a GI of 0 to 55 are classified as low GI, those with a GI of 70 or higher are classified as high GI, and those in between are classified as intermediate GI. The GI is influenced by various factors, including the type of carbohydrate, amount and type of fiber, level of processing, cooking method, storage, acidity, dietary structure, and macronutrient content (Clarke et al., 2012).

Glycemic load (GL) is a related term that takes into account both the type and quantity of carbohydrates consumed. A low GI or GL diet combines principles of low fat and low carbohydrate intake. The dietary recommendations of this approach are not solely based on the GI values of foods but also the overall nutritional composition of the diet. The main objective of consuming low-GI foods is to obtain sufficient energy and nutrients while avoiding significant spikes in insulin and blood glucose levels (Garvey et al., 2012).

There has been considerable debate regarding whether clinicians should recommend low-GI diets to overweight and obese patients. Results from adult trials discussed in our previous assessment indicated that altering the GI without changing the energy and macronutrient composition did not lead to weight loss benefits. However, low GI diets may play a crucial role in the prevention and management of metabolic and cardiovascular diseases, as suggested by the findings.

Of course, all of these diets have their benefits, but they only work if you stick to them. Long-term poor adherence and weight gain are recurring themes in research. Dansinger et al. studied finding a clear link between dietary adherence and clinically meaningful weight loss. The key to successful weight management is 'consistent dietary adherence' rather than 'adherence to a specific type of diet' (Shen et al., 2013).

7.4.4 PHYSICAL EXERCISE

The increasing energy expenditure can aid in lowering obesity and extra adipose tissue. Recent recommendations from the American College of Sports Medicine (ACSM) call for both aerobic and anaerobic exercise. Running, cycling, rowing, and other forms of aerobic exercise deplete the oxygen in your muscles, but your oxygen consumption is sufficient to meet your muscles' energy needs without needing to obtain energy from another source (Blair, 2013). Contrarily, anaerobic exercise (also known as resistance training or weightlifting) involves oxygen consumption that is insufficient to meet the energy demands placed on the muscles. As a result, the muscles must break down additional energy sources, such as carbohydrates, to produce energy and lactic acid. Exercise includes physical activity (PA), albeit PA is not always associated with planned exercise plans or sessions (Borodulin et al., 2015). Exercise is measured in "metabolic equivalent tasks" (METs), which roughly correspond to the effort and energy required for an individual to sit quietly. The requirement for consistent quantities of physical exercise throughout the day is emphasized by the frequent integration of physical activity into various lifestyle treatments. Goal setting, problem-solving, leisure-time physical activity, and exercise used for transportation are all examples of physical activity in a general lifestyle (Finkelstein et al., 2012). Cardiorespiratory fitness, body composition, and muscular fitness are some of the outcomes of interest. Numerous studies have recently demonstrated the benefits of exercise for people of all ages in terms of their physical, mental, and emotional health.

The same exercise regimens that are recommended for those who are normal weight are also appropriate for overweight and obese people. However, one should consider certain factors such as current comorbidities like orthopedic risks (such as arthritis), and pulmonary and/or cardiac comorbidities that may be associated with obesity (Blair et al., 2013). Exercise is essential to overall health and should not discourage individuals from enrolling in exercise programs.

The American College of Sports Medicine (ACSM), the Obesity Medical Association (OMA), and the Obesity Society (TOS) are all clinically available to help individuals prescribe exercise and are currently assisting people living with obesity.

To prevent weight gain, accelerate weight loss, and enhance fitness, one must engage in at least 150 to 300 minutes of weekly moderate exercise or 75 to 150 minutes of weekly intense exercise. To assist long-term weight loss, it is advised that those who want to lose weight engage in at least 200 to 300 minutes of moderate to strenuous physical activity per week (Ng & Popkin, 2012).

7.4.5 MEDICATION

Drug therapies that aid in weight loss are becoming more popular since they can lower the prevalence of obesity and its comorbidities. Intensive lifestyle changes for obese patients have been shown to significantly improve weight, among other characteristics. A 5% decrease in body weight was linked to long-lasting reductions in significant cardiovascular risk factors like blood pressure and lipid profile, according to the Look AHEAD trial (Garvey et al., 2012; Kastin, 2002). In order to assess whether a medicine causes significant weight loss, several regulatory authorities utilize a 5% overall weight loss. While the European Medicines Agency (EMA) has only approved three drug therapies— orlistat, bupropion/naltrexone, and liraglutide— to treat obesity, the US Food and Drug Administration (FDA) has approved five— orlistat, phentermine/topiramate, lorcaserin, naltrexone/bupropion, and liraglutide to date (Bhat & Sharma, 2017). Bariatric surgery is a last resort for some people if medical treatments are ineffective in helping them lose enough weight. These treatments typically promote weight reduction by either improving satiety, decreasing hunger, or boosting catabolism. But as our knowledge of the pathophysiology underlying obesity grows, more drug targets are being found, and it is anticipated that more drugs will be approved by regulatory bodies like the FDA and EMA to combat the obesity epidemic (Courcoulas et al., 2013; Mingrone et al., 2015).

Several medications have been created specifically to help people lose weight; some of these have been approved for sale in the past five years, while others are still in the research and development stage. In addition, weight loss is a significant side effect of numerous prescribed drugs. Topiramate, an antiepileptic medication also used for migraine prevention, Roflumilast in the treatment of chronic obstructive pulmonary disease (COPD), and Bupropion and Fluoxetine in the management of depression are a few well-known examples (Shank & Maryanoff, 2008). Although weight loss is not the primary indication for treatment for some other medications, the weight-reducing impact is nevertheless desirable and likely accounts for some of their success. When used to treat type 2 diabetes mellitus, important examples are sodium-glucose transport protein 2 (SGLT2) inhibitors and glucagon-like peptide-1 receptor (GLP1) agonists. Topiramate, for instance, appears to be an effective therapeutic choice for obese migraine patients. In some conditions where a variety of medications are available, a single medication may be chosen because of its known weight-lowering side effect. However, the effects of some medications on weight loss may also encourage off-label use, and it is possible that some of these medications, like methylphenidate, could be abused (Pineyro-Lopez et al., 2009).

Not every obese patient requires medication to help them lose weight. The cornerstones of any anti-obesity treatment should always be behavior modification, food, and exercise (Yanovski & Yanovski, 2014). With that strategy, however, many affected people fail to lose weight or fail to keep it off. There is agreement that those with a body mass index (BMI) of >30 kg/m^2 or a BMI of >27 kg/m^2 with weight-related comorbidities may be candidates for anti-obesity medication therapy if they continue to show no improvement after six months of treatment (Barrera et al., 2011). However, the primary objective of treatment shouldn't be weight loss in and of itself. At least equally important is addressing obesity-related comorbidities such as hyperglycemia, hyperlipidemia, and hypertension. However, expectations for effective weight loss are frequently highly irrational. Patients and healthcare professionals should be aware that the effectiveness of currently available anti-obesity medications is frequently restricted to a decrease of 5–10% in body weight over the course of a year (Astrup et al., 2012). Drug-induced weight loss often takes longer than 6–8 months to manifest. Since obesity is a chronic condition, long-term care is necessary. Still, many individuals and healthcare professionals do not behave in accordance with this concept.

When hemoglobin A1c (HbA1c) improves after a new medicine is started, no one would advise stopping anti-diabetic medication. When it comes to obesity, there is much debate concerning weight gained after anti-obesity medication is stopped, which underscores the necessity for efficient weight control techniques (U.S. Food and Drug Administration, 2020). Anti-obesity medicine should be seen, like with other chronic conditions, as a possible next step in treatment after maintaining a healthy lifestyle regimen that includes regular exercise and calorie restriction. Drug therapy should never be used as a stand-alone treatment for obesity or even as a general cure. To maintain weight and avoid weight regain after bariatric surgery, pharmacotherapy might be thought of as an adjuvant. In some situations, these individuals' continued weight loss may be aided by further medication therapy (Peterli et al., 2008).

7.4.6 SURGICAL TREATMENT

Due to hardwired survival mechanisms that link stress and appetite and have grown egregiously maladaptive in the industrial period, the majority of therapies fail. An apparently drastic, effective treatment for this serious disease of excess energy is bariatric (anti-obesity) surgery (Cavin et al., 2017). Its safety has significantly increased because of technological advancement during the past 20 years. Although methods of action have been clarified concurrently with advancements in knowledge of the molecular biology of energy balance and appetite regulation, the surgical concepts of gastric restriction and/or gastrointestinal diversion have remained unchanged over the past 40 years (Ikramuddin et al., 2013).

A large case series of patients who underwent bariatric surgery and were followed up for at least 10 years afterward demonstrated consistent improvements in the symptoms of insulin-resistant metabolic syndrome and other comorbidities, significantly enhancing the quality of life of the patients (Risstad et al., 2015). Additionally, it has been conclusively demonstrated that bariatric surgery reduces mortality when compared to nonoperative methods. This procedure requires thorough preoperative and postoperative evaluation, as well as monitoring and education, to produce the greatest results. In the absence of effective societal changes to reestablish a healthy energy balance, bariatric surgery is a critical treatment option for a very serious disease.

Around the world, bariatric surgery is becoming more and more common (Nuttall et al., 2015). The variety of bariatric surgeries performed, along with other procedures, is also increasing. There are various innovative types of endoscopic procedures in preclinical or clinical testing, aside from evolving experimental operations (such as one-anastomosis/single-anastomosis gastric bypass and gastric plication) (e.g., gastric balloons and duodenal mucosal resurfacing). Given the variety of newly developed gadgets, we are here concentrating solely on the most widespread procedures for treating obesity, which is an active area of study. Despite this, experimental techniques and equipment do not currently account for a sizable portion of surgeries performed around the world, but these developing instruments might do so in the future as the need to manage obesity rises (Hedberg et al., 2014).

7.5 NUTRACEUTICAL

The words "nutrition" and "pharmaceutics" are the roots of the term "nutraceutical." The word is used to describe goods that are isolated from herbal products, dietary supplements (nutrients), certain diets, and processed meals like cereals, soups, and drinks that are also utilized as medicine in addition to providing nutrition (Keservani et al., 2010a, b; Institute of Medicine, 2000; Kanteev et al., 2015). As the term "nutraceutical" products are regulated as drugs, food ingredients, and dietary supplements. Although the definition of the term varies from country to country, it is typically understood to define a product that has been separated from foods and is typically sold in medical forms unrelated to food. A substance that has physiological benefits or offers protection from chronic diseases might be described as a nutraceutical product (Wu et al., 2017).

Nutraceuticals can be used to boost well-being, slow down aging, stop chronic diseases from occurring, increase life expectancy, or support the body's structure or functions.

Contrary to medications, nutritional supplements typically lack patent protection. Although both pharmaceutical and nutraceutical substances may be used to treat or prevent disease, only pharmaceutical substances are approved by the government. A product is considered to be a dietary supplement if it bears or contains one or more of the dietary components listed below: a concentration, metabolite, constituent, extract, or mixture of these ingredients; a mineral, vitamin, amino acid, medicinal plant or other botanical; nutritional supplement used by humans to boost daily intake (Wintergerst et al., 2007). The nutritional supplements known as nutraceuticals are utilized for medical conditions other than nutrition. Ginseng, Echinacea, green tea, glucosamine, omega-3, lutein, folic acid, and cod liver oil are a few well-known nutraceuticals (Keservani et al., 2017, 2020). The majority of nutritional supplements have several therapeutic benefits (Pinnell, 2003).

Due to their potential for providing nutrition, safety, and therapeutic benefits, nutraceuticals are receiving a lot of attention nowadays. A recent industry study predicted that the global market for nutraceuticals is growing and will reach US $250 billion by 2018.

A number of clinical consequences, including diabetes, atherosclerosis, cardiovascular diseases (CVDs), cancer, and neurological illnesses, have demonstrated encouraging results for these substances in recent research. These conditions bring about a variety of modifications, including redox state changes. The majority of dietary supplements have antioxidant activity that can help to prevent these conditions. As a result, they are regarded as beneficial sources for promoting health, particularly in terms of preventing fatal diseases like diabetes, infections, renal, and gastrointestinal disorders. Obesity and overweight are linked pathological diseases that have serious effects on the cardiovascular, metabolic, musculoskeletal, and oncological systems (Institute of Medicine, 2000). They pose a serious threat to worldwide public health. In addition to the use of food supplements, the traditionally recommended therapeutic approaches have effects on pharmacological, psychological, lifestyle (eliminating sedentary behavior and encouraging physical activity), nutritional, and lifestyle levels. Recent research by Watanabe et al. identified and evaluated 33 food supplements that are most commonly used for weight loss, classifying them according to their key effects on nutrient absorption, hunger control, energy expenditure modulation, and fat and carbohydrate metabolism (Watanabe et al., 2020).

Obesity and overweight are linked pathological diseases that have serious effects on the cardiovascular, metabolic, musculoskeletal, and oncological systems. We discovered reliable information regarding the following in-depth: (i) dietary supplements that are primarily intended to increase nutritional absorption (inulin, chitosan, psyllium, guar gum, green tea, and ginseng); (ii) dietary supplements with whey proteins and chlorogenic acid as their primary ingredients; (iii) dietary supplements with curcumin and L-carnitine as their primary ingredients; and (iv) dietary supplements with a primary focus on fat metabolism (resveratrol and flaxseed). Additionally, we included information on how each medication affected weight loss by altering the microbiome in animal models, keeping in mind that results in animal models do not always correspond to observations in humans (Watanabe et al., 2020).

7.6 GREEN TEA REVOLUTION

Green, black, or oolong tea made from the Camellia sinensis plant is drunk in various parts of the world. However, drinking green tea (Kesharwani et al., 2016) has been found to have the greatest impact on human health. In the 17th century, India shipped the first green tea to Japan. Produced mainly in Asia, parts of North Africa, the United States, and Europe, green tea accounts for over 20% of the estimated 2.5 million tons of tea leaves produced annually worldwide. The health benefits of drinking tea, especially green tea, have long been recognized (Chen et al., 2003). Black tea and green tea have different manufacturing processes. The freshly picked leaves are steamed as soon as possible to prevent fermentation and result in a dry and reliable green tea. Subsequent rolling and drying preserve the green color of the tea because steaming kills the enzymes that break down the pigments in the tea leaves. In terms of health-promoting properties, these processes retain the natural polyphenols (Zheng et al., 2011). Polyphenolic chemicals (catechins) in green tea dimerize to produce different theaflavins when fermented into oolong and black teas, so these teas may have different biological functions.

The ancient Chinese medical system has made considerable use of the herbal preparations of green tea (Camellia sinensis Kuntze). Due to polyphenols, which are its main bioactive constituents and have exhibited numerous capabilities, including antioxidant, anti-aging, and anti-inflammatory action, it has a number of beneficial health impacts (Chikara et al., 2018). Green tea use was observed to increase the relative abundance of Firmicutes and Actinobacteria in humans and reduce the concentration of the phylum Bacteroidetes using 16S rRNA sequencing (Kajimura & Saito, 2014). Additionally, green tea raised some species of the genus Prevotella while decreasing others, including those that produce short-chain fatty acids (SCFAs), including *Roseburia* spp., *Faecalibacterium* spp., *Eubacterium rectale group, Blautia* spp., *Coprococcus* spp., and *Bifidobacterium longum*. Barcena et al. observed that green tea polyphenols were able to increase the concentration of *Faecalibacterium prausnitzii* in a mouse model (Virtanen et al., 2009; van Marken Lichtenbelt et al., 2009). In mice fed a high-fat diet (HFD), the manipulation of this gut microbiota species appears to be related to the reduction of weight gain and the intestinal and liver inflammatory response (Yoneshiro et al., 2013; van der Lans et al., 2013). Green tea extract supplementation led to an increase in the *Bacteroidetes* and *Oscillospira* spp. families and a decrease in the Peptostreptococcaceae concentration in mice on an HFD diet. Additionally, green tea polyphenols lowered the *Firmicutes/Bacteroidetes* ratio and positively regulated *Akkermansia muciniphila* (Lee et al., 2014; Cypess et al., 2015). Numerous *in vitro* studies have looked into the possible prebiotic function of green tea; in particular, the polyphenols in green tea have been shown to be able to regulate the gut microbiota. Considering the evidence, green tea may have a potential anti-obesity activity by modulating gut microbiota.

7.7 ANTI-OBESITY EFFECTS OF GREEN TEA *IN VITRO*

7.7.1 *EFFECTS ON ADIPOCYTE DIFFERENTIATION*

Green tea catechins significantly reduce adipocyte development in cultured adipocyte models. In C3H10T1/2 cells, it was recently discovered that EGCG (TEAVIGOTM, DSM Nutritional Products) suppressed adipogenesis caused by the standard adipogenic combination of insulin, dexamethasone, and 3-isobutyl-1-methylxanthine (IBMX) dose-dependently (Mori & Hasegawa, 2003). Furuyashiki et al. discovered catechin in 3T3-L1 cells, in another adipocyte model. CG, EGC, ECG, and EGCG at 5 μM inhibited lipid accumulation generated by the same combination. In a time-course experiment,

CG and EGC inhibited lipid accumulation starting on day 3 and reduced the amount of lipid by 50% by day 8, indicating that catechins inhibit both early-stage and late-stage differentiation processes (Furuyashiki et al., 2004). Green tea catechins also suppressed the proliferation of 3T3-L1 preadipocytes, according to Hung et al. (2005). These inhibitory effects require the involvement of two cell cycle regulatory kinases, ERK and cyclin-dependent kinase 2 (Cdk2). EGCG had no effect on total levels of ERK1 (extracellular signal-regulated kinase 1) and ERK2 (extracellular signal-regulated kinase 2), but it did considerably reduce phospho-ERK1 and phospho-ERK2, the active forms of ERK, at 50 μM. Cdk2, another important cell cycle regulator, was lowered by EGCG at both the protein and activity levels after 4, 24, and 48 hours of administration. EGCG outperformed EC, ECG, and EGC in terms of antimitogenic characteristics, arresting preadipocytes in the G0/G1 phase (Hung et al., 2005).

Obesity is caused by an increase in adipocyte size (hypertrophy) as well as an increase in adipocyte number (hyperplasia) (Kajimura et al., 2014). According to the research, green tea catechins suppress adipocyte differentiation as well as proliferation, two factors that contribute to increasing adipose mass. CCAAT/enhancer binding protein beta (C/EBPb), CCAAT/enhancer binding protein delta (C/EBPd), peroxisome proliferator-activated receptor gamma 2 (PPARc2), and CCAAT/enhancer binding protein alpha (C/EBPa) are all transcription factors that govern adipocyte development (Saito et al., 2009). C/EBPb and C/EBPd, which can be stimulated by IBMX and dexamethasone, respectively, are responsible for its induction. C/EBPb and C/EBPd work cooperatively to activate PPARc2, a major adipogenesis regulator, and C/EBPa (Virtanen et al., 2009; Yoneshiro et al., 2011). C/EBPa and PPARc work together to promote adipocyte differentiation by activating the production of adipocyte-specific genes, and they're also required for each other's expression to stay high. Thus, the antiadipogenic actions of green tea catechins are mediated, at least partially, by PPARc2 and C/EBPa suppression. The direct molecular targets of action, on the other hand, have yet to be identified (Yoneshiro et al., 2013).

In 2004, Tachibana et al. cloned a 67 kDa laminin receptor from a cancer cell line that binds EGCG with a very low Kd value. It is unknown whether this receptor is expressed in adipocytes or if it is involved in EGCG-induced signaling. Thus, the most abundant green tea catechin, EGCG, suppresses adipocyte proliferation and differentiation, which is at least partially mediated through inhibition of phospho-ERK1, phospho-ERK2, Cdk2, PPARγ2, and C/EBPα (Tachibana et al., 2004).

7.7.2 EFFECTS ON BROWN ADIPOSE TISSUE (BAT) THERMOGENESIS

Brown adipose tissue (BAT) is an attractive target for treating obesity and associated metabolic diseases since it is specialized for non-shivering metabolic thermogenesis. Cold exposure has long-term consequences, such as increased BAT activity and thermogenic uncoupling protein 1 expression, which are linked to higher energy expenditure (EE), lower adiposity, and improved insulin sensitivity (Park et al., 2011). BAT thermogenesis is acutely stimulated by cold exposure. Bile acids and a β3-adrenergic receptor agonist can both activate human BAT; however, due to unfavorable side effects, neither the cold regimen nor these pharmacologic treatments would be suitable for long-term interventions.

By ingesting natural dietary ingredients, it is possible to stimulate the sympathetic nervous system and temperature-sensitive transient receptor potential (TRP) channel activation of BAT that is brought on by cold. As an illustration, capsaicin analogs, or capsinoids, which have agonistic actions at TRPV1 and TRPA1, boost efferent discharges of sympathetic neurons connected to BAT, thus inducing thermogenesis (Sugiura et al., 2012; Zheng et al., 2004).

Green tea extract (GTE) promotes BAT thermogenesis to a significantly greater extent than an equal amount of caffeine alone, according to Dulloo et al. According to the findings, the strong effect of GTE on BAT thermogenesis is due to the interplay of catechins and caffeine, as well as sympathetically generated noradrenaline (NA) (Dulloo et al., 2004). A synergistic increase of thermogenesis was reported when EGCG was given with a mixture of caffeine and ephedrine. The authors theorized that the synergistic effects seen could be mediated by catechins and caffeine acting at separate control points of the NA-cyclic adenosine monophosphate (cAMP) axis. EGCG inhibits COMT (catechol-O-methyltransferase), an enzyme that destroys NA, allowing sympathetically produced NA to last longer. Caffeine blocks the enzyme phosphodiesterase, which breaks down cAMP, a second messenger generated in response to NA. Thus, EGCG and caffeine may enhance intracellular cAMP levels in a synergistic manner, mediating the thermogenic impact of GTE.

Even though catechin has a strong thermogenic impact, there is still a lack of knowledge regarding how exactly its active ingredient works. Although catechin is thought to encourage fatty acid breakdown in the liver and adipose tissue, there is still debate regarding how this food element produces heat (Ipsen et al., 2018). One of the primary catechins in green tea, epigallocatechin gallate (EGCG), was revealed to have agonistic effects on the cold-sensitive TRPA1 by Kurogi et al. Additionally, green tea and exercise cause the production of brown-like (beige) adipocytes in mice. It is likely that the thermogenic impact of catechin is mediated through the activation of BAT given that adult humans' BAT primarily contains beige adipocytes. We examined the acute and long-term effects of oral catechin and caffeine administration on whole-body EE in the current investigation to test this, paying particular attention to BAT activity in healthy adults (Kurogi et al., 2012).

7.7.3 EFFECTS ON LIPOLYSIS

The development of type 2 diabetes is known to be influenced by lipid accumulation, which is one of the obvious factors contributing to overweight and obesity. Insulin resistance in the muscle and liver is also related to lipid accumulation (Koo & Noh, 2007). Lipid buildup results from either increased lipogenesis, intake of fatty acids, or decreased fatty acid oxidation (Ngondi et al., 2009).

Recently, the modification of serum lipid homeostasis has been studied in relation to green tea catechins. After 24 hours of incubation with 10 mM green tea catechins, Mak-Soon Lee et al. noticed that lipid droplets in 3T3-L1 adipocytes were repressed without having any negative impacts on the viability of the cells during differentiation. CG and ECG reduced the number of lipid droplets from day 3 and a 50% reduction on day 8 implies that green tea has impacts in the early and late stages of the differentiation process (Mak-Soon Lee et al., 2016). Furuyashiki et al. also discovered that green tea components reduced the accumulation of lipids in 3T3-L1 (Furuyashiki et al., 2004).

In both the mouse experiments and the human trials, similar outcomes following green tea therapy were seen. It was evident that after giving HDF mice 3.2 g of EGCG/kg over the course of 16 weeks, hepatocyte lipid buildup decreased. Human body weight and abdominal fat were significantly lower in the experimental group than in the control group (lower green tea catechin diet). Caffeine and green tea catechins both control lipid buildup. EGCG, green tea extract, or caffeine alone do not have the same anti-obesity effects as a combination of high catechin, EGCG, or caffeine, which can reduce body weight and lipid buildup. By preventing the synthesis of new lipids and increasing the β-oxidation of existing lipids in the mouse liver, green tea catechins and caffeine limit the buildup of lipids (Moon et al., 2007; Basu et al., 2011). Catechins significantly decreased the expression of genes involved in lipogenesis such as acyl-CoA oxidase and dehydrogenase, sterol regulatory element-binding protein-1c (SREBP-1c), and FAS, but they increased the expression of genes involved in oxidative processes such as peroxisome proliferator-activated receptor γ2 (PPARγ2), C/EBP, carnitine palmitoyltransferase-I. In another adipocyte model, 3T3-L1 cells, Furuyashiki et al. showed that catechin, CG, EGC, ECG, and EGCG at 5 μM inhibited lipid accumulation generated by the same combination. According to a time-course experiment, catechins (CG and EGC) block both early-stage and late-stage differentiation programs because they slow down lipid accumulation starting on day 3 and lower it to 50% less than the control by day 8. In another adipocyte model, 3T3-L1 cells, Furuyashiki et al. showed that catechin, CG, EGC, ECG, and EGCG at 5 μM inhibited lipid accumulation generated by the same combination (Furuyashiki et al., 2004).

In a time-course experiment, catechins (CG and EGC) reduced the amount of fat by 50% by day 8 compared to day 3 of the control, indicating that they can inhibit both early-stage and late-stage differentiation processes. The ingestion of a green tea water extract for two weeks reduced the buildup of body fat in Sprague-Dawley rats fed a high-fat diet. While food intake was unaffected, it appeared that this impact was mediated by increased energy expenditure and a modest but statistically significant impairment in food digestibility.

7.7.4 EFFECTS ON NUTRIENT ABSORPTION

The health advantages of drinking green tea, such as green tea and isolated green tea constituents, have been shown to have anti-inflammatory, anti-arthritic, antibacterial, anti-angiogenic, antioxidative, antiviral, neuroprotective, and cholesterol-lowering properties. Currently being studied. However, consuming more green tea could have a negative impact on your health in other ways (Watanabe et al., 2020).

Green tea's polyphenol content, especially flavanols and flavonols which make up 30% of the dry weight of fresh leaves, is primarily responsible for its health-promoting properties. Recently, the majority of the positive effects of green tea stated above were linked to its most prevalent catechin, (–)-epigallocatechin-3-gallate (EGCG).

Ten weeks of oolong tea consumption in rats with diet-induced obesity reduced obesity and fatty liver. These effects could be caused by both decreased nutrition absorption and higher energy expenditure (Hursel et al., 2009). More than could be explained by caffeine alone, green tea extracts increased brown adipose tissue thermogenesis in rats. When compared to placebo and caffeine treatments, healthy young men who consumed green tea extract with each meal had significantly higher 24-hour energy expenditure and significantly lower 24-hour respiratory quotients. According to these authors, caffeine and tea polyphenols work together to prolong sympathetic activation of thermogenesis by inhibiting catechol-O-methyltransferase activity (Takase et al., 2008).

Tea polyphenols may have an impact on nutritional status because of their significant affinity for minerals and proteins. Through hydrophobic interactions and hydrogen bonds, the different phenolic groups in tea can bind to several locations on a protein. Proteins having a high proline content, such as milk caseins, gelatin, and salivary proline-rich proteins, have a great affinity for polyphenols. It is yet unknown if drinking tea affects how well humans absorb protein. The effects of tea on the absorption of these nutrients are crucial because of the tea polyphenols' high affinity for binding metal ions (Basu et al., 2010).

Tea consumption has been linked to decreased iron absorption. It appears that nonheme iron is the main target of this effect, particularly when tea and iron are both eaten. Tea drinking had no impact on the absorption of heme iron from cooked meats. Tea consumption has been linked to neonatal microcytic anemia (Ichinose et al., 2011). The National Health and Nutrition Examination Survey II study, which included 11,684 people, found no link between anemia and tea or coffee use. Rats administered a methanol extract of black tea had poorer apparent calcium absorption than control rats between days 11 to 18, but by week four there was no difference; the treatment had no effect on apparent protein or magnesium absorption (Ferreira et al., 2016).

Consuming tea was linked to higher bone mineral density measures in women between the ages of 65 and 76, which is in line with other studies that suggested tea may prevent hip fractures. These results indicated that elements other than polyphenols, such as fluoride or phytoestrogens, might affect bone mineral density. The glucosyltransferase activity of oral streptococci and the onset of dental caries in rats were both found to be inhibited by tea. Fluoride, which is present in tea, may help to promote dental health by fortifying tooth enamel.

Green tea polyphenols significantly decreased the incidence and severity of arthritis in a mouse model of arthritis caused by collagen. When mice were administered green tea polyphenols, the expression of inflammatory mediators such as cyclooxygenase-2, interferon, and TNF was dramatically reduced in the arthritic joints. Increased tea drinking may help prevent cataracts, which happen when proteins precipitate in the eye's lens (Kim et al., 2009).

ECG has been shown to limit glucose uptake in Caco-2 cells. ECG inhibited sodium/glucose cotransporter 1 (SGLT1) in brush border membrane vesicles in a competitive way. Green tea catechins inhibited the activities of α-amylase and sucrase in the rat gut. More research into this phenomenon demonstrated that EGCG has just a moderate inhibitory effect on sucrase activity, whereas theaflavins, which are contained in black tea to a greater level, are significantly more effective (Kurogi et al., 2012; Bose et al., 2008). EGCG blocked the sodium-dependent glucose transporter and lowered glucose uptake in the rat gut, but it was less effective than ECG. Green tea extract (GTE) was discovered to suppress stomach and pancreatic lipase activities, leading to reduced fat digestion in humans and contributing to green tea's anti-obesity benefit. Green tea may thereby lower glucose and fat absorption by blocking gastrointestinal enzymes involved in nutrition breakdown, according to currently known *in vitro* research. The exact contribution of these actions to the documented anti-obesity effects of green tea, green tea catechins, and EGCG *in vivo* is still unknown (Lee et al., 2009).

7.7.5 THE ANTI-OBESITY EFFECTS OF GREEN TEA ON HUMAN TRIALS ASSESSING UNDERLYING MECHANISMS

Adipose tissue in excess is the definition of obesity. Body mass index (BMI; weight in kg/height in m^2), which has a good connection with the percentage of body fat, is frequently used as a screening indicator for obesity. Adult obesity is defined by the World Health Organization (WHO) as a BMI of 30 kg/m^2 or greater. The prevalence of obesity has dramatically increased over the past 40 years, rising from 3% in 1975 to 11% in 2016 for men and from 6% to 15% in the same time frame for women (Sugiura et al., 2012).

The main source of green tea's health-promoting properties is thought to be its high polyphenol content, which accounts for about 30% of the fresh leaf's dry weight. Its catechin content, specifically EGCG, the most active catechin in green tea, is best correlated with its well-known antioxidant and anti-inflammatory properties, leading to its evaluation in a number of diseases like cancer, cardiovascular and neurodegenerative diseases, as well as obesity and metabolic syndrome (MetS), because these illnesses are linked when its complex physiopathology is taken into account. Therefore, the aim of this review was to evaluate the effect of the consumption of green tea on the treatment of obesity (Zheng et al., 2012).

The anti-obesity effects of green tea, GTE, and EGCG are exerted via a number of mechanisms and target tissues. However, the effect of green tea catechins on thermogenesis and substrate oxidation has been the only mechanism of action evaluated in human trials so far. Dulloo et al. and Rumpler et al. measured energy expenditure and substrate oxidation in their study subjects over 24-hour periods using a metabolic chamber. Although the two trials had similar goals, they used distinct methods of administration, such as capsules or beverages, respectively (Dulloo et al., 2000; Rumpler et al., 2001). The study by Komatsu et al. appears to have methodological flaws, such as the test time, which may have been too short, and the use of Douglas bags for gas measurements, which is less reliable than more current technologies. All three studies found significant increases in energy expenditure; two of the studies, which used cutting-edge techniques and proper research designs, found increases in energy expenditure of 2.9 and 4, respectively, and fat oxidation of 12 and 35%, respectively (Komatsu et al., 2003).

7.8 MARKETED PRODUCTS

Growing consumer attention on living a healthy lifestyle and increasing knowledge of the health benefits are two important aspects that are anticipated to support market expansion over the course of the projected period. Additionally, it is predicted that the global demand for green tea will increase because of the sharp rise in obesity and cardiovascular disease incidences. The global green tea market is expected to produce $34,044.28 million in sales by 2028, up from $13,850.94 million in 2020, at a significant CAGR of 11.9%.

Increased consumer demand for healthy drinks as a result of the increased prevalence of lifestyle-related health issues such as obesity and high blood pressure is expected to boost the green tea market in the anticipated time period.

The Asia-Pacific green tea market is expected to grow at an 11.30% CAGR during the study period, creating a value of $21,754.29 million.

7.8.1 MARKET INSIGHTS

Green tea market growth in India is being fueled by merger and acquisition activity as well as product launches. The green tea industry is seeing expansion due to consumer desire for green tea blends with distinctive flavors, rich aromas, and tantalizing tastes. Large companies like Unilever and Tata Global Beverages dominate the market. These leading companies never stop putting their R&D efforts into strengthening their product portfolios. Additionally, they are attempting to acquire as many customers as possible in India by engaging in merger and acquisition activities with rival businesses that have bright futures in the region.

India green tea market – type (Tables 7.2 and 7.3):

- Green tea bags;
- Green tea instant mixes;
- Iced green tea;
- Loose leaf;
- Others.

India green tea market – by flavor:

- Lemon;
- Aloe vera;
- Cinnamon.

TABLE 7.2 A List of Key Market Segments of Green Tea

Segments	Sub-Segment
By type	1. Flavored green tea: • Lemon; • Aloe vera; • Cinnamon; • Wildberry; • Jasmine; • Basil; • Others. 2. Unflavored green tea

Segments	Sub-Segment
By form	• Green tea bags; • Green tea instant mixes; • Iced green tea; • Loose leaf; • Capsules; • Tablets.
Key market players (green tea sachets)	• Tetley GB Ltd. • Tata Global Beverages • AMORE Pacific Corp. • Associated British Foods LLC. • Nestle S.A. • Celestial Seasonings • Cape Natural Tea Products • Finlay Beverages Ltd. • Hambleden Herbs • Hankook Tea

TABLE 7.3 A List of Marketed Products of Green Tea

Dose Type	Dosage	Brand
Green tea extract capsule	500 mg	InLife
Green tea extract capsule	400 mg	Now foods
Green tea capsules	500 mg	BioAyurveda
Green tea leaf extract capsule	500 mg	HealthyHey Nutrition
Green tea fat burner liquid soft gels	400 mg	Applied nutrition
Green tea fat mobilizer liquid soft gel	400 mg	Irwin naturals
Green tea tablets	18 mg extract equivalent to 6.3 g green tea	Vita biotics
Green tea effervescent tablets	500 mg	Suprfit
Green tea with EGCG tablets	500 mg	GoYNFSx
Green tea tablets	200 mg	Doctor's nutrition
Matcha green tea gummies	200 mg	Plix
Matcha green tea gummies	200 mg	Novomins
Green tea extract	500 mg	Carmine county
Liquid		
Green tea extract mouth-dissolving strip	200 mg	BonAyu

KEYWORDS

- **blood pressure**
- **catechins**
- **fat oxidation**
- **green tea**
- **metabolic chamber**
- **nutraceuticals**
- **obesity**
- **polyphenol content**

REFERENCES

Abdollahi, M., & Afshar-Imani, B. (2003). A review on obesity and weight loss measures. *Middle East Pharmacy, 11*, 6–10.

Aitsi-Selmi, A., Bell, R., Shipley, M. J., & Marmot, M. G. (2014). Education modifies the association of wealth with obesity in women in middle-income but not low-income countries: An interaction study using seven national datasets, 2005–2010. *PloS One, 9*(3), e90403.

Amagase, H., & Nance, D. M. (2011). Lycium barbarum increases caloric expenditure and decreases waist circumference in healthy overweight men and women: Pilot study. *Journal of the American College of Nutrition, 30*, 304–309.

American Diabetes Association, Bantle, J. P., Wylie-Rosett, J., Albright, A. L., Apovian, C. M., Clark, N. G., Franz, M. J., Hoogwerf, B. J., Lichtenstein, A. H., Mayer-Davis, E., Mooradian, A. D., & Wheeler, M. L. (2008). Nutrition recommendations and interventions for diabetes: A position statement of the American Diabetes Association. *Diabetes Care, 31*(Suppl 1), S61–S78.

Azadbakht, L., Mirmiran, P., Esmaillzadeh, A., & Azizi, F. (2007). Better dietary adherence and weight maintenance achieved by a long-term moderate-fat diet. *British Journal of Nutrition, 97*, 399–404.

Barnes, P. M., Powell-Griner, E., McFann, K., & Nahin, R. L. (2004). Complementary and alternative medicine use among adults: United States, 2002. *Advance Data, 343*, 1–19.

Basu, A., & Lucas, E. A. (2007). Mechanisms and effects of green tea on cardiovascular health. *Nutrition Reviews, 65*, 361–375.

Basu, A., Du, M., Sanchez, K., Leyva, M. J., Betts, N. M., Blevins, S., Wu, M., Aston, C. E., & Lyons, T. J. (2011). Green tea minimally affects biomarkers of inflammation in obese subjects with metabolic syndrome. *Nutrition, 27*, 206–213.

Björntorp, P., & Rosmond, R. (2000). Neuroendocrine abnormalities in visceral obesity. *International Journal of Obesity and Related Metabolic Disorders, 24*(Suppl 2), S80–S85.

Blair, S. N., Archer, E., & Hand, G. A. (2013). Commentary: Luke and Cooper are wrong: Physical activity has a crucial role in weight management and determinants of obesity. *International Journal of Epidemiology, 42*(6), 1836–1838.

Boon, N. (2008). Health potential for functional green teas? *International Journal for Vitamin and Nutrition Research, 78*, 275–281.

Boone, J. E., Gordon-Larsen, P., Adair, L. S., & Popkin, B. M. (2007). Screen time and physical activity during adolescence: Longitudinal effects on obesity in young adulthood. *International Journal of Behavioral Nutrition and Physical Activity, 4*(1), 26.

Bornstein, M. H., & Cheah, C. S. L. (2006). The place of "Culture and Parenting" in the ecological contextual perspective on developmental science. In K. H. Rubin & O. B. Chung (Eds.), *Parenting Beliefs, Behaviors, and Parent-Child Relations: A Cross-Cultural Perspective* (pp. 3–33). Psychology Press.

Bose, M., Lambert, J. D., Ju, J., Reuhl, K. R., Shapses, S. A., & Yang, C. S. (2008). The major green tea polyphenol, (–)-epigallocatechin-3-gallate, inhibits obesity, metabolic syndrome, and fatty liver disease in high-fat-fed mice. *The Journal of Nutrition, 138*, 1677–1683.

Chacko, S. M., Thambi, P. T., Kuttan, R., & Nishigaki, I. (2010). Beneficial effects of green tea: A literature review. *Chinese Medicine, 5*(13), 1–9.

Chantre, P., & Lairon, D. (2002). Recent findings of green tea extract AR25 (Exolise) and its activity for the treatment of obesity. *Phytomedicine, 9*, 3–8.

Chrousos, G. P., & Gold, P. W. (1992). The concepts of stress and stress system disorders: Overview of physical and behavioral homeostasis. *JAMA, 267*(9), 1244–1252.

Chu, S. L., Fu, H., Yang, J. X., Liu, G. X., Dou, P., Zhang, L., Tu, P. F., & Wang, X. M. (2011). A randomized double-blind placebo-controlled study of Pu'er tea extract on the regulation of metabolic syndrome. *Chinese Journal of Integrative Medicine, 17*, 492–498.

Clarke, S. F., Murphy, E. F., Nilaweera, K., Ross, P. R., Shanahan, F., & O'Toole, P. W. et al. (2012). The gut microbiota and its relationship to diet and obesity: new insights. *Gut Microbes, 3*(3), 186–202.

Cooper, R., Morré, D. J., & Morré, D. M. (2005). Medicinal benefits of green tea: Part I. Review of noncancer health benefits. *Journal of Alternative and Complementary Medicine, 11*, 521–528.

Dallman, M. F., Warne, J. P., Foster, M. T., & Pecoraro, N. C. (2007). Glucocorticoids and insulin both modulate caloric intake through actions on the brain. *Journal of Physiology, 583*(Pt 2), 431–436.

Dansinger, M. L., & Schaefer, E. J. (2006). Low-fat diets and weight change. *JAMA, 295*, 94–95.

Di Pierro, F., Menghi, A. B., Barreca, A., Lucarelli, M., & Calandrelli, A. (2009). Green select phytosome as an adjunct to a low-calorie diet for treatment of obesity: A clinical trial. *Alternative Medicine Review, 14*, 154–160.

Diabetes Prevention Program (DPP) Research Group, Knowler, W. C., Fowler, S. E., Hamman, R. F., Christophi, C. A., Hoffman, H. J., & Nathan, D. M. (2009). 10-year follow-up of diabetes incidence and weight loss in the Diabetes Prevention Program Outcomes Study. *Lancet, 374*(9702), 1677–1686.

Diabetes Prevention Program (DPP) Research Group. (2015). Long-term effects of lifestyle intervention or metformin on diabetes development and microvascular complications over 15-year follow-up: The Diabetes Prevention Program Outcomes Study. *Lancet Diabetes & Endocrinology, 3*(11), 866–875.

Dulloo, A. G., Seydoux, J., Girardier, L., Chantre, P., & Vandermander, J. (2000). Green tea and thermogenesis: interactions between catechin-polyphenols, caffeine and sympathetic activity. *International Journal of Obesity and Related Metabolic Disorders, 24*(2), 252–258.

Durand, C. P., Andalib, M., Dunton, G. F., Wolch, J., & Pentz, M. A. (2011). A systematic review of built environment factors related to physical activity and obesity risk: implications for smart growth urban planning. *Obesity Reviews: An Official Journal of the International Association for the Study of Obesity, 12*(5), e173–e182.

Eikelis, N., & Esler, M. (2005). The neurobiology of human obesity. *Experimental Physiology, 90*, 673–682.

Emery, C. F., Olson, K. L., Lee, V. S., Habash, D. L., Nasar, J. L., & Bodine, A. (2015). Home environment and psychosocial predictors of obesity status among community-residing men and women. *International Journal of Obesity, 39*(9), 1401–1407.

Farooqi, S., & O'Rahilly, S. (2006). Genetics of obesity in humans. *Endocrine Reviews, 27*, 710–718.

Ferreira, M. A., Silva, D. M., de Morais, A. C. Jr., Mota, J. F., & Botelho, P. B. (2016). Therapeutic potential of green tea on risk factors for type 2 diabetes in obese adults: a review. *Obesity Reviews, 17*, 1316–1328.

Finucane, M. M., Stevens, G. A., Cowan, M. J., Danaei, G., Lin, J. K., Paciorek, C. J., Singh, G. M., Gutierrez, H. R., Lu, Y., Bahalim, A. N., Farzadfar, F., Riley, L. M., & Ezzati, M.; Global Burden of Metabolic Risk Factors of Chronic Diseases Collaborating Group (Body Mass Index). (2011). National, regional, and global trends in body-mass index since 1980: systematic analysis of health examination surveys and epidemiological studies with 960 country-years and 9.1 million participants. *Lancet, 377*(9765), 557–567.

Forester, S. C., Gu, Y., & Lambert, J. D. (2012). Inhibition of starch digestion by the green tea polyphenol, (–)-epigallocatechin-3-gallate. *Molecular Nutrition & Food Research, 56*, 1647–1654.

Garvey, W. T., Ryan, D. H., Look, M., Gadde, K. M., Allison, D. B., Peterson, C. A., Schwiers, M., Day, W. W., & Bowden, C. H. (2012). Two-year sustained weight loss and metabolic benefits with controlled-release phentermine/topiramate in obese and overweight adults (SEQUEL): A randomized, placebo-controlled, phase 3 extension study. *American Journal of Clinical Nutrition, 95*, 297–308.

Genta, S., Cabrera, W., Habib, N., Pons, J., Carillo, I. M., Grau, A., & Sánchez, S. (2009). Yacon syrup: beneficial effects on obesity and insulin resistance in humans. *Clinical Nutrition, 28*, 182–187.

Goldfein, J. A., Walsh, B. T., LaChaussée, J. L., Kissileff, H. R., & Devlin, M. J. (1993). Eating behavior in binge eating disorder. *International Journal of Eating Disorders, 14*, 427–431.

Gout, B., Bourges, C., & Paineau-Dubreuil, S. (2010). Satiereal, a crocus sativus L-extract, reduces snacking and increases satiety in a randomized placebo-controlled study of mildly overweight, healthy women. *Nutrition Research, 30*, 305–313.

Granelljose, J., Garrido, L., Millas, T., & Gutierrez-Fonseca, R. (2012). Management of Oropharyngeal Dysphagia in Laryngeal and Hypopharyngeal Cancer. *International Journal of Otolaryngology*, 2012, Article ID 157630, 9 pages.

Grzesik, M., Naparło, K., Bartosz, G., & Sadowska-Bartosz, I. (2018). Antioxidant properties of catechins: comparison with other antioxidants. *Food Chemistry, 241*, 480–492.

Guh, D. P., Zhang, W., Bansback, N., Amarsi, Z., Birmingham, C. L., & Anis, A. H. (2009). The incidence of co-morbidities related to obesity and overweight: a systematic review and meta-analysis. *BMC Public Health, 9*, 88.

Hach, I., Ruhl, U. E., Klose, M., Klotsche, J., Kirch, W., & Jacobi, F. (2007). Obesity and the risk for mental disorders in a representative German adult sample. *European Journal of Public Health, 17*, 297–305.

Hallstrom, T., & Noppa, H. (1981). Obesity in women in relation to mental illness, social factors and personality traits. *Journal of Psychosomatic Research, 25*, 75–82.

Han, L., Kimura, Y., & Okuda, H. (2005). Anti-obesity effects of natural products. *Studies in Natural Products Chemistry, 30*, 79–110.

Hara, K., Ohara, M., Hayashi, I., Hino, T., Nishimura, R., Iwasaki, Y., & Nakamura, H. (2012). The green tea polyphenol (–)-epigallocatechin gallate precipitates salivary proteins including alpha-amylase: biochemical implications for oral health. *European Journal of Oral Sciences, 120*, 132–139.

Hasani-Ranjbar, S., Larijani, B., & Abdollahi, M. (2009). A systematic review of the potential herbal sources of future drugs effective in oxidant-related diseases. *Inflammation & Allergy-Drug Targets, 8*, 2–10.

Hasani-Ranjbar, S., Nayebi, N., Moradi, L., Mehri, A., Larijani, B., & Abdollahi, M. (2010). The efficacy and safety of herbal medicines used in the treatment of hyperlipidemia: A systematic review. *Current Pharmaceutical Design, 16*, 2935–2947.

Haufe, S., Haas, V., Utz, W., Birkenfeld, A. L., Jeran, S., Bohnke, J., & Engeli, S. (2013). Long-lasting improvements in liver fat and metabolism despite body weight regain after dietary weight loss. *Diabetes Care, 36*(11), 3786–3792.

Higdon, J. V., & Frei, B. (2003). Tea catechins and polyphenols: Health effects, metabolism, and antioxidant functions. *Critical Reviews in Food Science and Nutrition, 43*, 89–143.

Hu, F. B. (2013). Resolved: There is sufficient scientific evidence that decreasing sugar-sweetened beverage consumption will reduce the prevalence of obesity and obesity-related diseases. *Obesity Reviews, 14*(8), 606–619.

Huang, T., Qi, Q., Li, Y., Hu, F. B., Bray, G. A., Sacks, F. M., Williamson, D. A., & Qi, L. (2014). FTO genotype, dietary protein, and change in appetite: The Preventing Overweight Using Novel Dietary Strategies trial. *American Journal of Clinical Nutrition, 99*(5), 1126–1130.

Hursel, R., Viechtbauer, W., & Westerterp-Plantenga, M. S. (2009). The effects of green tea on weight loss and weight maintenance: A meta-analysis. *International Journal of Obesity (London), 33*(9), 956–961.

Ibrahim, A., Dahham, S., Al-Muffti, S., & Al-Rawi, S. (2018). Obesity study among secondary school students at Duhok city. *IOP Conference Series: Materials Science and Engineering*, 454, p. 012165.

Ichinose, T., Nomura, S., Someya, Y., Akimoto, S., Tachiyashiki, K., & Imaizumi, K. (2011). Effect of endurance training supplemented with green tea extract on substrate metabolism during exercise in humans. *Scandinavian Journal of Medicine & Science in Sports, 21*, 598–605.

International Institute for Population Sciences (IIPS) & Macro International. (2007). *National Family Health Survey India, 2005–2006 NFHS-3*. International Institute for Population Sciences, Mumbai.

Jakubczyk, K., Kochman, J., Kwiatkowska, A., Kałduńska, J., Dec, K., Kawczuga, D., & Janda, K. (2020). Antioxidant properties and nutritional composition of matcha green tea. *Foods, 9*, 483.

Kaneko, S., Kumazawa, K., Masuda, H., Henze, A., & Hofmann, T. (2006). Molecular and sensory studies on the umami taste of Japanese green tea. *Journal of Agricultural and Food Chemistry, 54*, 2688–2694.

Keservani, R. K., & Sharma, A. K. (2014). Flavonoids: Emerging trends and potential health benefits. *Journal of Chinese Pharmaceutical Sciences, 23*(12), 815.

Keservani, R. K., Kesharwani, R. K., Sharma, A. K., Vyas, N., & Chadoker, A. (2010b). Nutritional supplements: An overview. *International Journal of Current Pharmaceutical Review and Research, 1*(1), 59–75.

Keservani, R. K., Kesharwani, R. K., Vyas, N., Jain, S., Raghuvanshi, R., & Sharma, A. K. (2010a). Nutraceutical and functional food as future food: A review. *Der Pharmacia Lettre, 2*(1), 106–116.

Keservani, R. K., Sharma, A. K., & Kesharwani, R. K. (2017). An overview and therapeutic applications of nutraceutical and functional foods. In *Recent Advances in Drug Delivery Technology* (pp. 160–201). ISBN: 9781522507543.

Keservani, R. K., Sharma, A. K., & Kesharwani, R. K. (Eds.). (2020). *Nutraceuticals and Dietary Supplements: Applications in Health Improvement and Disease Management*. CRC Press. ISBN: 9781771888738.

Kesharwani, R. K., Singh, P., & Keservani, R. K. (2016). Green coffee bean extract and chlorogenic acids: Chemistry and novel antioxidant benefits. In D. Bagchi, H. Moriyama, & A. Swaroop (Eds.), *Green Coffee Bean Extract in Human Health* (pp. 1–17). Boca Raton: Taylor and Francis. ISBN: 9781498716376.

Kobayashi, D., Takahashi, O., Deshpande, G. A., Shimbo, T., & Fukui, T. (2012). Association between weight gain, obesity, and sleep duration: A large-scale 3-year cohort study. *Sleep and Breathing, 16*(3), 829–833.

Koh, K. A., Hoy, J. S., O'Connell, J. J., & Montgomery, P. (2012). The hunger-obesity paradox: Obesity in the homeless. *Journal of Urban Health: Bulletin of the New York Academy of Medicine, 89*(6), 952–964.

Koh, L. W., Wong, L. L., Loo, Y. Y., Kasapis, S., & Huang, D. (2010). Evaluation of different teas against starch digestibility by mammalian glycosidases. *Journal of Agricultural and Food Chemistry, 58*, 148–154.

Kolákucková, T., Kolofiková, K., Sytarová, I., Snopek, L., Sumczynski, D., & Orsavová, J. (2020). Matcha tea: Analysis of nutritional composition, phenolics and antioxidant activity. *Plant Foods for Human Nutrition, 75*, 48–53.

Komatsu, T., Nakamori, M., Komatsu, K., Hosoda, K., & et al. (2003). *Journal of Medical Investigation, 50*, 170–175.

Koo, S. I., & Noh, S. K. (2007). Green tea as inhibitor of the intestinal absorption of lipids: Potential mechanism for its lipid-lowering effect. *Journal of Nutritional Biochemistry, 18*, 179–183.

Kopelman, P. G. (2000). Obesity as a medical problem. *Nature, 404*, 635–643.

Kreier, F., Yilmaz, A., Kalsbeek, A., Romijn, J. A., Sauerwein, H. P., & Fliers, E. (2003). Hypothesis: Shifting the equilibrium from activity to food leads to autonomic unbalance and the metabolic syndrome. *Diabetes, 52*, 2652–2656.

Kritchevsky, S. B., Beavers, K. M., Miller, M. E., Shea, M. K., Houston, D. K., Kitzman, D. W., & Nicklas, B. J. (2015). Intentional weight loss and all-cause mortality: A meta-analysis of randomized clinical trials. *PLoS One, 10*(3), e0121993.

Ku, K. M., Choi, J. N., Kim, J., Kim, J. K., Yoo, L. G., Lee, S. J., Hong, Y. S., & Lee, C. H. (2010). Metabolomics analysis reveals the compositional differences of shade grown tea (Camellia sinensis L.). *Journal of Agricultural and Food Chemistry, 58*(1), 418–426.

Kubota, K., Sumi, S., Tojo, H., & Sumi-Inoue, Y. (2011). Improvements of mean body mass index and body weight in preobese and overweight Japanese adults with black Chinese tea (Pu-Erh) water extract. *Nutrition Research, 31*(6), 421–428.

Kurogi, M., Miyashita, M., Emoto, Y., Kubo, Y., & Saitoh, O. (2012). Green tea polyphenol epigallocatechin gallate activates TRPA1 in an intestinal enteroendocrine cell line, STC-1. *Chemical Senses, 37*(2), 167–177.

Lee, M. S., Kim, C. T., Kim, I. H., & Kim, Y. (2009). Inhibitory effects of green tea catechin on the lipid accumulation in 3T3-L1 adipocytes. *Phytotherapy Research, 23*(8), 1088–1091.

Li, G., Zhang, P., Wang, J., Gregg, E. W., Yang, W., Gong, Q., & Bennett, P. H. (2008). The long-term effect of lifestyle interventions to prevent diabetes in the China Da Qing Diabetes Prevention Study: A 20-year follow-up study. *The Lancet, 371*(9626), 1783–1789.

Luke, A., & Cooper, R. S. (2013). Physical activity does not influence obesity risk: Time to clarify the public health message. *International Journal of Epidemiology, 42*(6), 1831–1836.

Mak-Soon, L., Seohyun, L., Miae, D., & Yangha, K. (2016). Green tea (–)-Epigallocatechin-3-Gallate induces PGC-1α gene expression in HepG2 cells and 3T3-L1 adipocytes. *Preventive Nutrition and Food Science, 21*(1), 62–67.

Moon, H. S., Chung, C. S., Lee, H. G., Kim, T. G., Choi, Y. J., & Cho, C. S. (2007). Inhibitory effect of (–)-epigallocatechin-3-gallate on lipid accumulation of 3T3-L1 cells. *Obesity, 15*(11), 2571–2582.

Nammi, S., Koka, S., Chinnala, K. M., & Boini, K. M. (2004). Obesity: An overview on its current perspectives and treatment options. *Nutrition Journal, 3*(1), 3.

Nishitani, E., & Sagesaka, Y. M. (2004). Simultaneous determination of catechins, caffeine and other phenolic compounds in tea using new HPLC method. *Journal of Food Composition and Analysis, 17*(5), 675–685.

Ogden, J. (2010). The psychology of eating: From healthy to disordered behavior (2nd edn.). Wiley-Blackwell.

Pal, S., Khossousi, A., Binns, C., Dhaliwal, S., & Ellis, V. (2011). The effect of a fibre supplement compared to a healthy diet on body composition, lipids, glucose, insulin and other metabolic syndrome risk factors in overweight and obese individuals. *British Journal of Nutrition, 105*(1), 90–100.

Pinnell, S. R. (2003). Cutaneous photodamage, oxidative stress, and topical antioxidant protection. *Journal of the American Academy of Dermatology, 48*(1), 1–19.

Puhl, R. M., & Heuer, C. A. (2009). The stigma of obesity: A review and update. *Obesity, 17*(5), 941–964.

Pulgaron, E. R. (2013). Childhood obesity: A review of increased risk for physical and psychological comorbidities. *Clinical Therapeutics, 35*(1), A18–A32.

Rehman, R. U., Usmanghani, K., Nazar, H., Uddin, S., Akram, M., & Asif, H. M. (2011). Clinical study on the management of obesity with certain natural medicine. *Journal of Medicinal Plants Research, 5*(18), 4094–4098.

Rumpler, W., Seale, J., Clevidence, B., Judd, J., et al. (2001). *Journal of Nutrition, 131*, 2848–2852.

Saad, B., Ghareeb, B., & Kmail, A. (2021). Metabolic and epigenetics action mechanisms of antiobesity medicinal plants and phytochemicals. *Evidence-Based Complementary and Alternative Medicine, 2021*, 9995903.

Santesso, N., Akl, E. A., Bianchi, M., Mente, A., Mustafa, R., Heels-Ansdell, D., & Schünemann, H. J. (2012). Effects of higher- versus lower-protein diets on health outcomes: A systematic review and meta-analysis. *European Journal of Clinical Nutrition, 66*(7), 780–788.

Shen, J., Obin, M. S., & Zhao, L. (2013). The gut microbiota, obesity and insulin resistance. *Obesity, 34*(1), 39–58.

Silventoinen, K., Rokholm, B., Kaprio, J., & Sørensen, T. I. (2010). The genetic and environmental influences on childhood obesity: A systematic review of twin and adoption studies. *International Journal of Obesity, 34*(1), 29–40.

Subramani, C., & Natesh, R. K. (2013). Molecular mechanisms and biological implications of green tea polyphenol, (–)-epigallocatechin-3-gallate. *International Journal of Pharmacy & Bio Sciences, 1*(1), 54–63.

Sueoka, N., Suganuma, M., Sueoka, E., Okabe, S., Matsuyama, S., Imai, K., Nakachi, K., & Fujiki, H. (2001). A new function of green tea: Prevention of lifestyle-related diseases. *Annals of the New York Academy of Sciences, 928*, 274–280.

Sugiura, C., Nishimatsu, S., Moriyama, T., Ozasa, S., Kawada, T., & Sayama, K. (2012). Catechins and caffeine inhibit fat accumulation in mice through the improvement of hepatic lipid metabolism. *Journal of Obesity, 2012*, 2012.

Swinburn, B. A., Caterson, I., Seidell, J. C., & James, W. P. (2004). Diet, nutrition and the prevention of excess weight gain and obesity. *Public Health Nutrition, 7*(1a), 123–146.

Tachibana, H., Koga, K., Fujimura, Y., & Yamada, K. (2004). A receptor for green tea polyphenol EGCG. *Nature Structural & Molecular Biology, 11*(4), 380–381.

Takase, H., Nagao, T., Otsuka, K., Kozuma, K., Kataoka, K., Meguro, S., Komikado, M., & Tokimitsu, I. (2008). Effects of long-term ingestion of tea catechins on visceral fat accumulation and metabolic syndrome: Pooling-analysis of 7 randomized controlled trials. *Japanese Pharmacology & Therapeutics, 36*, 509–514.

Tian, W. X., Li, L. C., Wu, X. D., & Chen, C. C. (2004). Weight reduction by Chinese medicinal herbs may be related to inhibition of fatty acid synthase. *Life Sciences, 74*(19), 2389–2399.

Unno, K., Furushima, D., Hamamoto, S., Iguchi, K., Yamada, H., Morita, A., Pervin, M., & Nakamura, Y. (2019). Stress-reducing effect of cookies containing matcha green tea: Essential ratio among theanine, arginine, caffeine and epigallocatechin gallate. *Heliyon, 5*(1), e02236.

Visscher, P. M., Wray, N. R., Zhang, Q., Sklar, P., McCarthy, M. I., Brown, M. A., & Yang, J. (2017). 10 years of GWAS discovery: Biology, function, and translation. *American Journal of Human Genetics, 101*(1), 5–22.

Vogelzangs, N., & Penninx, B. W. (2007). Cortisol and insulin in depression and metabolic syndrome. *Psychoneuroendocrinology, 32*(7), 856–861.

Wang, S., Noh, S. K., & Koo, S. I. (2006). Epigallocatechin gallate and caffeine differentially inhibit the intestinal absorption of cholesterol and fat in ovariectomized rats. *Journal of Nutrition, 136*(11), 2791–2796.

Watanabe, M., Risi, R., Masi, D., Caputi, A., Balena, A., Rossini, G., Tuccinardi, D., Mariani, S., Basciani, S., Manfrini, S., Gnessi, L., & Lubrano, C. (2020). Current evidence to propose different food supplements for weight loss: A comprehensive review. *Nutrients, 12*(9), 2873.

Westerterp-Plantenga, M., Diepvens, K., Joosen, A. M., Bérubé-Parent, S., & Tremblay, A. (2006). Metabolic effects of spices, teas, and caffeine. *Physiology & Behavior, 89*(1), 85–91.

World Health Organization. (2013). Obesity and overweight. Retrieved from: https://www.who.int/news-room/fact-sheets/detail/obesity-and-overweight (accessed on 15 June 2024).

Wu, C. D., & Wei, G. X. (2002). Tea as a functional food for oral health. *Nutrition, 18*(5), 443–444.

Wu, X., Cheng, J., & Wang, X. (2017). Dietary antioxidants: Potential anticancer agents. *Nutrition and Cancer, 69*(4), 521–533.

Zheng, X. X., Xu, Y. L., Li, S. H., Liu, X. X., Hui, R., & Huang, X. H. (2011). Green tea intake lowers fasting serum total and LDL cholesterol in adults: A meta-analysis of 14 randomized controlled trials. *American Journal of Clinical Nutrition, 94*(2), 601–610.

PART III

SPICES AND CEREALS IN OBESITY

CHAPTER 8

POTENTIAL OF PSEUDOCEREALS IN THE MANAGEMENT OF OBESITY

HARPREET SINGH,[1] AMRITA MISHRA,[2] ARVIND KUMAR,[1] and ARUN KUMAR MISHRA[3]

[1]*School of Pharmaceutical Sciences, IFTM University, Moradabad, Uttar Pradesh, India*

[2]*Delhi Pharmaceutical Science and Research University, New Delhi, India*

[3]*Pharmacy Academy, IFTM University, Moradabad, Uttar Pradesh, India*

ABSTRACT

In modern times, there has been a rise in research related to pseudocereals all over the world. Pseudocereals are non-grass seeds or fruits that can be eaten in the same way that cereals are. Some of the most commonly used pseudocereals are amaranth, buckwheat, and quinoa, among others. Each of them has bioactive and nutritional compounds that are good for human health, including essential amino acids, essential fatty acids, phenolic acids, flavonoids, minerals, vitamins, dietary fibers, and healthy fats. The build-up of extra fat to the point where it begins to adversely affect a person's health or the ways in which the body works is known as obesity. Obesity is one of the common problems in present society, which is detrimental to people's health. Balanced pseudocereal consumption can reduce body weight and prevent obesity. The present chapter will delve in-depth into the different kinds of pseudocereals, the dietary value of pseudocereals, the health

Nutraceuticals in Obesity Management and Control. Raj K. Keservani & Alka Lohani (Eds.)

benefits of eating them, and the role and importance of pseudocereals in the fight against obesity.

8.1 INTRODUCTION

The terms "obesity" and "overweight" are used to indicate the levels of excess weight that are causative for more illness and even death too (Fruh, 2017). Being overweight is defined as having a body mass index greater than or equal to the 95th percentile for age and gender (Zhang et al., 2022). The risk of being overweight is defined as having a body mass index greater than or equal to the 85th percentile and less than the 95th percentile for age and gender (Wang & Beydoun, 2007). The risks related to overweight are increasing throughout the world, but they are most prevalent in the developed and near-developed worlds. There are innumerable biologically activated causes of obesity, but recent dietary (Keservani et al., 2017, 2020) and reduced physical activity appear to be the most significant contributing factors to increasing rates of obesity (Chaput et al., 2012). Consuming oily foods containing trans-fat and fast foods increases the weight of a person and makes him or her obese (Astrup et al., 2008).

The problem of obesity (Jarouliya & Keservani, 2019) can be improved by taking a low-fat diet, rich in fiber, vitamins, and proteins. Grain-based foods are essential for a fit and active lifestyle (Mozaffarian, 2016). The composition of each food is unique and contains a diverse range of macro- and micro-nutrients (Mazzeo et al., 2015). Nutritionally dense foods have a good mix of nutrients that are easily absorbed by the body (Demment & Van Soest, 1985). Pseudocereals are the fruits or seeds of non-grass species (Mosyakin & Schwartau, 2015). Supplementing traditional cereals with pseudocereals can be beneficial in reducing obesity (Coda et al., 2014). Pseudocereals such as amaranth, buckwheat, and quinoa provide better nutritional value than most major crops (Constantino & Garcia-Rojas, 2022). The pseudocereals have higher protein content and quality, and the protein quality of amaranth grain can be compared to milk (Alvarez-Jubete et al., 2010). In addition to having protein that doesn't come from gluten and being a great source of essential amino acids, pseudocereals are a great addition to a diet for someone who is overweight because they have both soluble and insoluble fiber (Brito et al., 2022). This chapter highlights various kinds of pseudocereals, the positive effects of consuming them on one's health, and the part that pseudocereals play and how important they are in order to reduce obesity.

8.2 EXAMPLES OF PSEUDOCEREALS

8.2.1 AMARANTH

There are more than 50 different species that belong to the genus Amaranthus, belonging to the family *Amaranthaceae* (Al-Tamimi et al., 2021). Some of these species are cultivated for their use as cereals, vegetables, and ornamentals, while others are considered to be weeds (Ruth et al., 2021). Grain-derived amaranth, which was a mainstay in the diet of the ancient Aztecs, is increasingly being used in the production of baked goods and breakfast cereals in almost all parts of the world (Colgrave et al., 2021). At the beginning of the 16th century, Mexico and other parts of Central America were major producers of Amaranth. Amaranth in the form of both grain and vegetable was grown in China, Southeast Asia, Southern India, West Africa, and the Caribbean basin before the recent resurgence in interest in the crop (Schnetzler, 1994). Amaranth grain is grown on a small scale by some farmers in the remote villages of Mexico, Guatemala, Peru, Northern India, and Nepal; whereas vegetable amaranth has been grown in northern India since ancient times. Amaranth grain has only recently been recognized as a potentially useful crop for human consumption as a result of its resilience in the face of adversity (such as drought, disease, salinity, alkalinity, acidic soil, or poor soil) as well as its high potential for producing biomass and grain yields (Shahzad et al., 2021). In some parts of Asia and Africa, as well as in some parts of Central and South America, it is cultivated as a supplementary crop.

Amaranth is a pseudocereal crop that produces grains that are similar to other cereals and contain high levels of nutritionally beneficial proteins (they have an amino acid composition that is close to that of the ideal protein, which is an unusual type of starch, and high-quality oil) (Mburu et al., 2011). Amaranth grows well in tropical and subtropical regions (Gerrano et al., 2017). It is classified as an important pseudocereal category because, despite having higher digestibility, its saccharide content (62.0%) is slightly lower than that of common cereals. This is one of the important reasons why it is considered an important pseudocereal. In addition, the consumption of amaranth has a positive effect on plasma lipid profiles which leads to a reduction in cholesterol levels, making it an appropriate food choice for patients who are gluten intolerant (Rinninella et al., 2021). An additional beneficial source of natural antioxidants is amaranth oil, which has a high proportion of unsaturated fatty acids and squalene in its composition (Baraniak & Kania-Dobrowolska, 2022). Squalene is a precursor that is used in the biosynthesis of all important steroids. Its IUPAC Name is 2,6,10,15,19,23-hexamethyl-2,6,10,14,18,22-tetracosahexaene and its chemical formula is $C_{30}H_{50}$ (Tarhan, 2021). In recent years, it has come to light that members of the genus *Amaranthus* possess antimalarial and antiviral properties (Moreno et al., 2008). Amaranth pectin, which is one of the important components that forms a gel, can also be used to bind toxic and radioactive metals aiming to remove them from the human body (Lara-Espinoza et al., 2018). Also, the plant parts of amaranth that are red have a lot of beta-cyanin pigments, which can be used as natural food dyes (Nowacka et al., 2021).

Although the demand for amaranth on the market has fluctuated over the past few decades, the crop has remained consistently utilized in the production of multigrain bread products, breakfast cereals, snack foods, etc. (Bvenura & Kambizi, 2022). Direct marketing, specialty and organic food stores, and grocery store health food sections are the most common distribution channels for amaranth products. Amaranth products can also be purchased online (Noort et al., 2022). Amaranth is one of the easiest plant species to grow because it can handle a wide range of tough environmental conditions (Sharma et al., 2021).

In addition, because it contains potentially health-enhancing compounds like rutin as well as peptides with anticarcinogenic and antihypertensive activities, amaranth is regarded as a "natural biopharmaceutical" plant that has the potential to improve human health. Because of these factors, amaranth has been gaining attention all over the world as a highly potential new crop that can be used in a variety of ways (Maldonado-Cervantes et al., 2010). The chemical structures of important constituents present in Amaranth are presented in Table 8.1.

8.2.2 BUCKWHEAT

Buckwheat is a crop that is typically grown for its triangular seeds that can be either black or gray in color (Yang et al., 2022). Additionally, it can be cultivated as a crop for the production of buckwheat honey, as a companion crop, as a cover crop, as a pharmaceutical plant that produces rutin, and as a green manure crop also (Singh & Verma, 2022). Buckwheat is a cereal that belongs to the grass family, like wheat, corn, and rice. However, the grain of buckwheat is a dry fruit, similar to other cereals (Shahbaz et al., 2022).

Buckwheat is thought to have originated in either central or northeastern Asia, and it was most likely first cultivated in China between the fifth and

TABLE 8.1 Chemical Structures of Important Constituents Present in Amaranth

Sl. No.	Name	Chemical Structure	IUPAC Name	References
1.	α-tocopherol	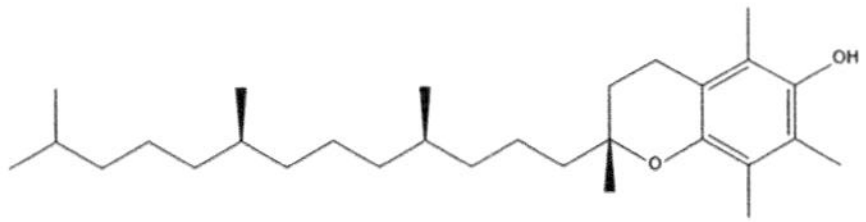	(2R)-2,5,7,8-Tetramethyl-2-[(4R,8R)-4,8,12-trimethyltridecyl]-3,4-dihydro-2H-1-benzopyran-6-ol	Kraujalis & Venskutonis (2013)
2.	β-Tocotrienol	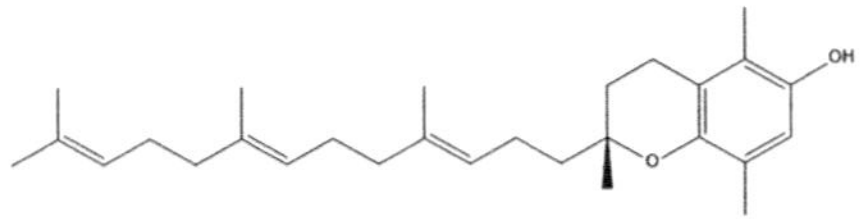	(2R)-2,5,8-trimethyl-2-[(3E,7E)-4,8,12-trimethyltrideca-3,7,11-trienyl]-3,4-dihydrochromen-6-ol	Kraujalis & Venskutonis (2013)
3.	ϒ-Tocotrienol	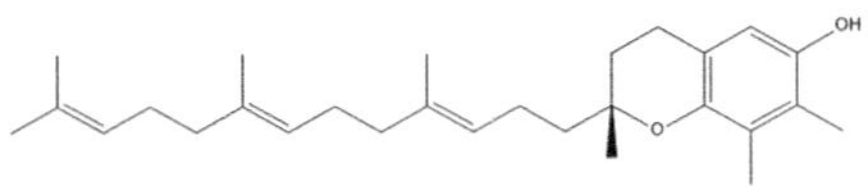	(2R)-2,7,8-trimethyl-2-[(3E,7E)-4,8,12-trimethyltrideca-3,7,11-trienyl]-3,4-dihydrochromen-6-ol	Kraujalis & Venskutonis (2013)
4.	β-tocopherol	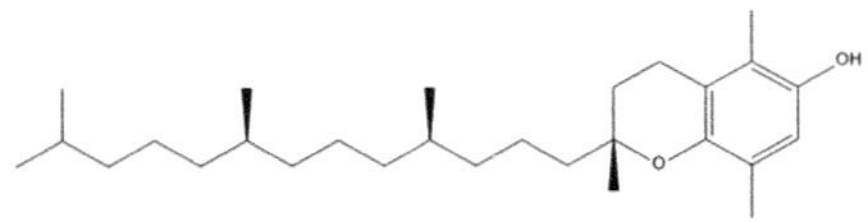	(2R)-2,5,8-trimethyl-2-[(4R,8R)-4,8,12-trimethyltridecyl]-3,4-dihydrochromen-6-ol	Kraujalis & Venskutonis (2013)
5.	Myricetin	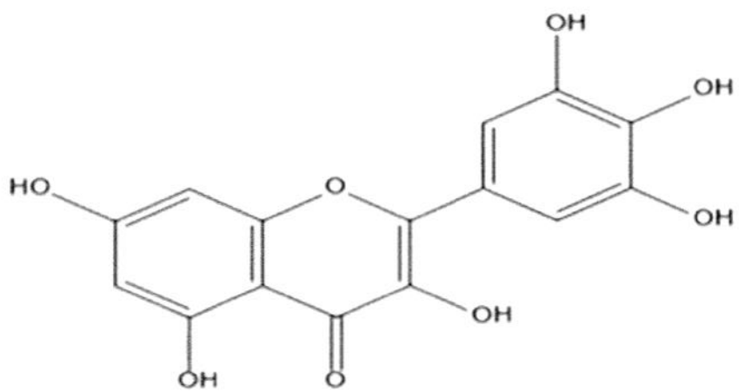	3,5,7-trihydroxy-2-(3,4,5-trihydroxyphenyl) chromen-4-one	Sarker & Oba (2020)

TABLE 8.1 *(Continued)*

Sl. No.	Name	Chemical Structure	IUPAC Name	References
6.	Catechin	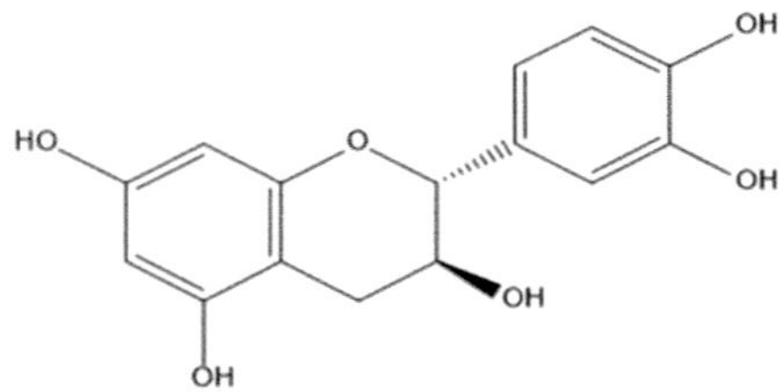	(2R,3S)-2-(3,4-Dihydroxyphenyl)-3,4-dihydro-2H-chromene-3,5,7-triol	Sarker & Oba (2020)
7.	Apigenin	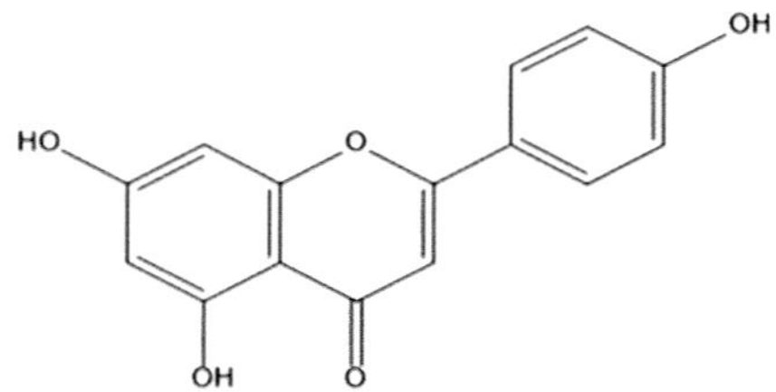	5,7-dihydroxy-2-(4-hydroxyphenyl) chromen-4-one	Sarker & Oba (2020)
8.	Naringenin	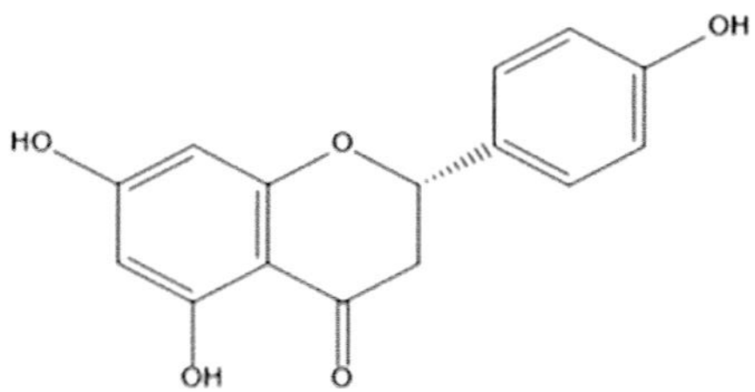	(2S)-5,7-dihydroxy-2-(4-hydroxyphenyl)-2,3-dihydrochromen-4-one	Sarker & Oba (2020)
9.	Squalene	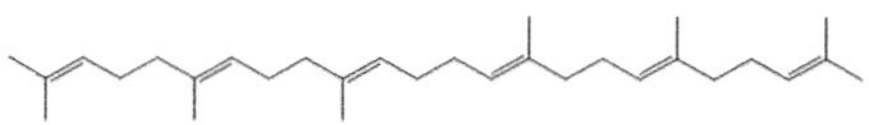	(6E,10E,14E,18E)-2,6,10,15,19,23-Hexamethyltetracosa-2,6,10,14,18,22-hexaene	Kraujalis & Venskutonis (2013)

sixth centuries (Xue et al., 2022). During the 14th and 15th centuries, Türkiye and Russia were the gateways to enter the market of Europe. In the 17th century, it arrived in North America. Buckwheat production around the world reached its zenith in the early 19th century. Countries like Brazil, Poland, the United States of America, Japan, Canada, France, Bhutan, and the Republic of Korea are also major producers of the same. South Africa is also one of them (Vanhaute, 2007).

Although the genus *Fagopyrum* contains at least 15 species of buckwheat, only two of those species are used as food or feed (Zhou et al., 2022). Wild buckwheat (*F. cymosum*), which is primarily found as a tetraploid, is occasionally used as a green vegetable or as forage for cattle (Suvorova, 2016). Buckwheat is classified into three main species: the common buckwheat (*Fagopyrum esculentum*), the Tartary buckwheat (*Fagopyrum tataricum*), and the perennial buckwheat (*Fagopyrum cymosum*) (Stojilkovski et al., 2013). Both tartary and common buckwheat come from perennial buckwheat and more specifically the diploid type (Gondola & Papp, 2010).

The Himalayan regions of India and China, the eastern provinces of Canada, and the mountainous regions of the eastern United States of America are the primary growing regions for Tartary buckwheat. Because it can withstand frost to some degree, it is typically cultivated at higher altitudes, where the potential for damage from frost is greater. The seeds and the products derived from seeds of buckwheat that can be made from them have a greenish color and a flavor that is somewhat bitter. It is most commonly utilized either as feed or as a combination of wheat and buckwheat flour. Additionally, it is frequently utilized as a source of rutin and given to needy patients to meet their nutritional requirements (Babu et al., 2018).

Buckwheat is found in several species. The most important of which is common buckwheat, which accounts for more than 90% of total global production (Mravlje et al., 2021). There are a great number of varieties and strains.

There are types that mature late and types that mature early; Japanese types and European types; summer types and fall types. There may be strains or varieties within a given type that have plants that are either tall or short, seeds that are either gray or black, and flowers that are either white or pink. In general, however, the common buckwheat varieties that can be found in various parts of the world can be separated into two primary categories. The first group consists of varieties that are tall, vigorous, mature late, and sensitive to the length of the photoperiod. They can be found in Japan, Korea, southern China, Nepal, and India. The second group isn't too much affected by the length of the sunlight. They are small and reach adulthood early. This type encompasses the different varieties that can be found in Europe and northern China (Li & Zhang, 2001).

Before the year 1950, farmers who grew buckwheat did so using unnamed strains of the grain that they either harvested from their fields or obtained from their neighbors or stores in the immediate area (Stoner & Gilman, 2008). In the 1950s, the first named varieties that had been developed through plant breeding were made available for crops. The Agriculture Canada Research Station in Ottawa issued a license for the Tokyo farmers in 1955, making it the oldest of the named cultivars that were brought into North America at the time. Tempest, Mancan, and Manor were three additional cultivars that were all developed at the Agriculture Canada Research Station in Morden, Manitoba, in 1965.

These cultivars are now licensed for production in Canada. Because of its large seeds, desirable flavor, color, and high yield of groats in the milling process, the Canadian cultivar Mancan is the one that is preferred in the Japanese market. Mancan has thick stems and large leaves, in addition to dark brown seeds that are quite large. Recently, newer cultivars like AC Manisoba, Koban, and Koto have been added to the mixture, supplementing the older cultivars that were previously available. The seeds from these newly developed cultivars are bigger and there are more of them.

Some cultivars are allowed to be grown in the United States. These include Pennquad, which was introduced to the public by the Pennsylvania Agricultural Experimental Station and the United States Department of Agriculture (USDA) in 1968, and Giant American, a Japanese-style cultivar that a farmer in Minnesota chose.

Among the cultivars that have been developed in what was formerly known as the Soviet Union (USSR) since the 1950s are Victoria, Galleya, Eneida, Podolyaka, Diadema, and Aestoria. Some cultivars that represent other parts of the world are Pulawska, Emka, Hruszowska, and Bednja from Poland, Bednja from Yugoslavia, Botan-Soba, Shinano No. 1, Kyushu Akisoba Shinshu, and Miyazaki Oosoba from Japan.

The buckwheat plant is tall, erect, and herbaceous, and can be grown to a height of 0.70–1.5 meters. The broad leaves of buckwheat take less than 90 days to reach full maturity despite having a main stem and several branches in addition to that. The stem, with the exception of the nodes, is typically grooved and hollow. The stem also contains succulent tissues. After reaching the highest level of maturity, the color of the stems and branches changes to a brownish hue, whereas before maturity, the color ranges from green to red.

The plant has a single, more extensive root called a taproot, which branches out into numerous lateral roots. It has a root system that is not as extensive as the one found in cereals, and it only accounts for 3% to 4% of the total dry weight of the plant (Luitel et al., 2017).

Buckwheat is characterized by a flowering pattern that is indeterminate. Buckwheat flowers are beautiful. Although they lack petals, the calyx is made up of five overlapping sepals that resemble petals and are typically white in color but can also be pink or red. Flowers are grouped in dense clusters at the ends of the branches or on short pedicels that grow from the sides of the leaves (Kasajima et al., 2019).

Buckwheat is a type of plant that can produce either one of two different kinds of flowers on its plants. The pin-type flower has long styles, which are known as the female parts of the flower, and short stamens, also known as the male parts of the flower. The thrum-type flower, on the other hand, has long styles but short pistils. The pistil consists of a superior ovary that only has one cell, a style that has three parts and stigmas that look like knobs, and it is surrounded by eight stamens. At the bottom of the ovary is where one will find the glands that produce nectar. Common buckwheat plants can't fertilize themselves because they aren't compatible with themselves. This means that the plants can't make fertile offspring on their own (Matsui & Yasui, 2020).

The buckwheat kernel is an achene that is triangular in shape and can range in length from 4 to 9 mm. It has a shell, called the pericarp, and three parts: the spermoderm, the endosperm, and the embryo (Karasch, 2000).

The sides of large seeds typically have a concave shape, while the sides of small seeds typically have a convex shape. The hull can have a glossy finish, and its color can range from gray to brown to black; it can also be solid or mottled. It may be smooth all the way across, or it may be rough with lateral furrows. The hulls make up between 17% and 26% of the weight of the kernel (or 30% and 35% in tartary buckwheat). In general, tetraploid varieties have a greater amount of hull than diploid varieties (Li et al., 2019).

In most cases, the production of seeds of buckwheat is dependent on the pin and thyme flowers being able to pollinate one another. Pollination becomes most successful when carried out by honeybees and leafcutter bees. They increase the number of seeds that are set and in turn yield per seed is also increased (Khalifa et al., 2021).

Rutin is one of the most important constituents present in high amounts of buckwheat. As a result of the high rutin content, common buckwheat, and the components that it contains are regarded as functional foods in Japan. It is a well-established and proven fact that rutin can improve the elasticity of blood vessels and, as a result, prevent the hardening of the arteries. In the traditional Chinese medicinal system, both the leaves and stem of Tartary buckwheat are considered to have medicinal properties. These properties include its ability to treat peptic ulcers, hemostasis, and hypertension (Kreft et al., 2003).

Stems and seeds of buckwheat may also improve vision and hearing, and they act as an adaptogen. It has been reported in contemporary research that eating tartary buckwheat can help treat stomach problems. The use of buckwheat in one's diet has been linked to both the prevention and treatment of hypercholesterolemia (Luthar et al., 2021).

This effect of common buckwheat is due to the fact that it contains a protein that possesses a stronger hypocholesterolemic activity than that of soy protein isolate and behaves in a manner that is comparable to that of dietary fiber. In recent years, it has been observed that the consumption of buckwheat protein extract slows the progression of mammary cancer in rats by reducing the amount of estradiol in the serum. Additionally, this extract reduces digestibility, which leads to a reduction in overall body fat. Buckwheat pollen contains bioactive peptides that have an immunostimulatory effect on lymphocytes. As a result, these peptides have the potential to act as immunomodulators, thereby increasing immunity and also acting as a cure for several kinds of cancer (Prakash & Yadav, 2016).

It has been suggested that the use of buckwheat flour in the treatment of hyperlipidemia, hyperglycemia, diabetes, and cardiovascular disease may have a positive impact on the physiological processes of the body system. In a clinical study involving 75 diabetic patients, Tartary buckwheat biscuits have exhibited encouraging results in reducing the amount of glucose in the blood. Buckwheat bran is known to contain fagopyritols, which are a group of phytochemicals that act as insulin mediators. These fagopyritols may have significant pharmacological use in the treatment of diabetes mellitus that is not dependent on insulin. When combined with vitamin C, the nutrient rutin obtained from buckwheat stops the oxidation of ascorbic acid and helps protect the endothelium. So, the combination of fagopyritols and rutin may have a significant effect on lowering the chance of getting diabetes (Qiu et al., 2016).

Patients with chronic venous insufficiency may benefit from drinking standardized buckwheat herbal tea containing 5% total flavonoids. This has been shown to reduce the risk of edema. It is believed that the capillary action of rutin is responsible for the formation of venous microcirculation, which contributes to the beneficial pharmacological effect. Due to the high rutin content, the leaves and flowers of buckwheat have been dehydrated and combined with other essential oils for packaging. This was done to provide protection for the vascular system. As buckwheat contains quercetin and rutin, Tartary buckwheat has been suggested as one of the possible treatments for periodontitis and bleeding gums (Ihme et al., 1996).

In Japan, green flour made by milling dried flowering buckwheat plants is already used as a natural food colorant in pasta, ice cream, and other food products as a source of dietary rutin. This green flour can be easily obtained by milling the dried flowering buckwheat plants (Huda et al., 2021). The chemical structures of important constituents present in buckwheat are presented in Table 8.2.

8.2.3 QUINOA

In the Chenopodiaceae family, Quinoa (*Chenopodium quinoa* Willd) is a pseudocereal that is native to the Andes region of South America. In Mexico, around Lake Titicaca in Bolivia and Peru, and in the Himalayan region, there are other chenopods that are closely related and act as pseudocereals (Goyat & Handa, 2018).

According to archaeological evidence, quinoa was grown some 7,000 years ago and 5,000 years ago in Peru and Chile, respectively. The Inca civilization relied heavily on quinoa as a source of protein and energy. War balls, a concoction of quinoa and fat, were apparently the Inca army's primary source of energy during long marches (Angeli et al., 2020).

Quinoa is known as chisiya mama in the Quechua language of the Incas, which translates to "mother grain." Quinoa is a Spanish word. Quinoa's ancient Inca ancestors revered it for its high nutritional content. In comparison to most cereals, it has a higher protein content and a better balance of amino acids. However, several saponins and plant glycosides are found in quinoa grain. When agitated, saponins produce a foam, which is why the Latin word "saponin" was coined (Murphy & Matanguihan, 2015).

Quinoa's saponins, which give the grain its bitter taste, also have important implications for grain processing and nutrition. Several South American food crops, such as Phaseolus beans, maize, and potatoes, have achieved global consumable status in part because of saponins including quinoa (El-Hazzam et al., 2020).

Quinoa is one of the few crops that can thrive at altitudes of up to 4,000 feet (Jancurová et al., 2009). It can be cultivated in areas with low rainfall

TABLE 8.2 Chemical Structures of Important Constituents Present in Buckwheat

Sl. No.	Name	Chemical Structure	IUPAC Name	References
1.	Rutin	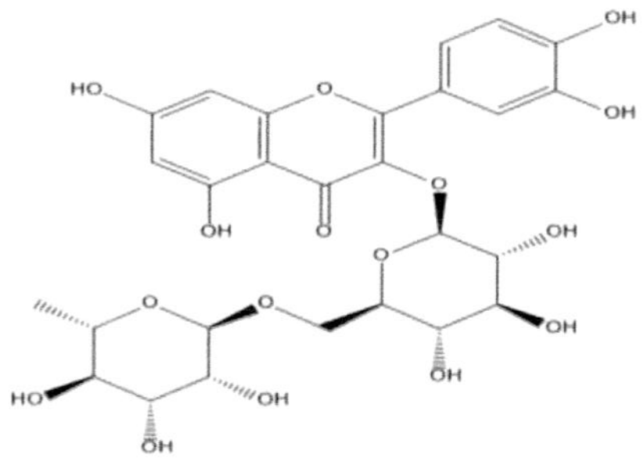	2-(3,4-dihydroxyphenyl)-5,7-dihydroxy-3-[(2S,3R,4S,5S,6R)-3,4,5-trihydroxy-6-[[(2R,3R,4R,5R,6S)-3,4,5-trihydroxy-6-methyloxan-2-yl]oxymethyl]oxan-2-yl]oxychromen-4-one	Huda et al. (2021)
2.	Quercetin	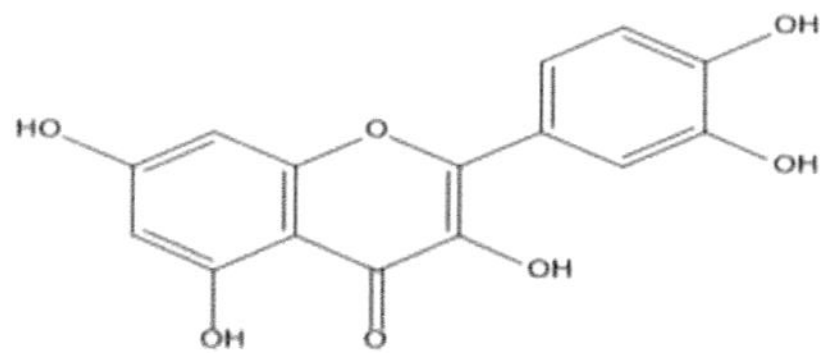	2-(3,4-dihydroxy phenyl)-3,5,7-trihydroxychromen-4-one	Huda et al. (2021)
3.	Orientin	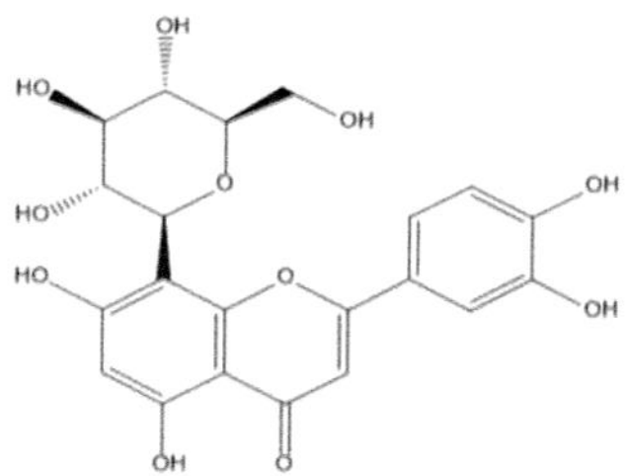	2-(3,4-dihydroxyphenyl)-5,7-dihydroxy-8-[(2S,3R,4R,5S,6R)-3,4,5-trihydroxy-6-(hydroxymethyl) oxan-2-yl]chromen-4-one	Huda et al. (2021)

TABLE 8.2 *(Continued)*

Sl. No.	Name	Chemical Structure	IUPAC Name	References
4.	Isoorientin	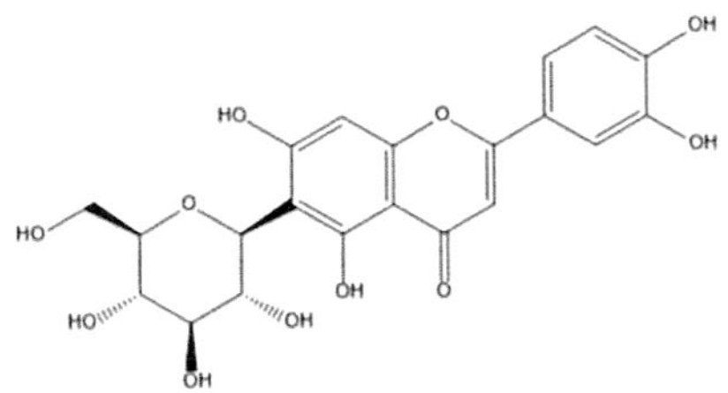	2-(3,4-dihydroxyphenyl)-5,7-dihydroxy-6-[(2S,3R,4R,5S,6R)-3,4,5-trihydroxy-6-(hydroxymethyl) oxan-2-yl] chromen-4-one	Huda et al. (2021)
5.	Vitexin	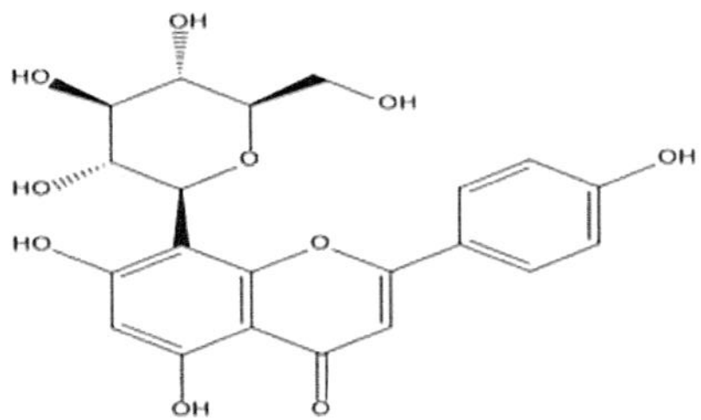	5,7-dihydroxy-2-(4-hydroxyphenyl)-8-[(2S,3R,4R,5S,6R)-3,4,5-trihydroxy-6-(hydroxymethyl) oxan-2-yl]chromen-4-one	Huda et al. (2021)
6.	Isovitexin	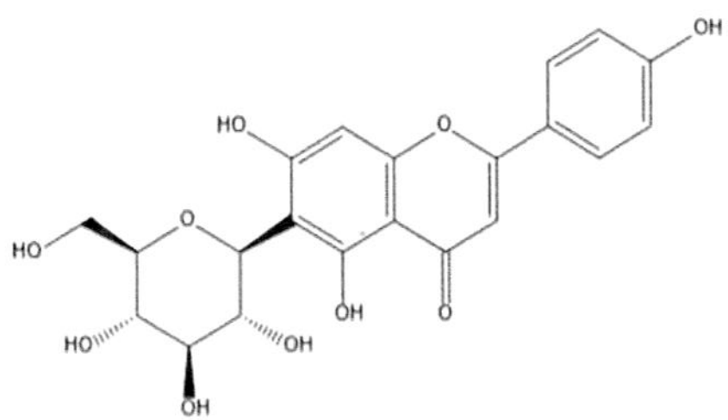	5,7-dihydroxy-2-(4-hydroxyphenyl)-6-[(2S,3R,4R,5S,6R)-3,4,5-trihydroxy-6-(hydroxymethyl) oxan-2-yl]chromen-4-one	Huda et al. (2021)

TABLE 8.2 *(Continued)*

Sl. No.	Name	Chemical Structure	IUPAC Name	References
7.	Kaempferol	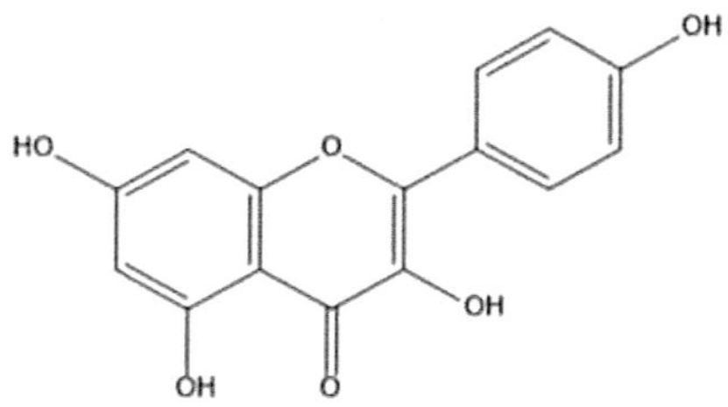	3,5,7-trihydroxy-2-(4-hydroxyphenyl) chromen-4-one	Huda et al. (2021)
8.	Isoquercetin	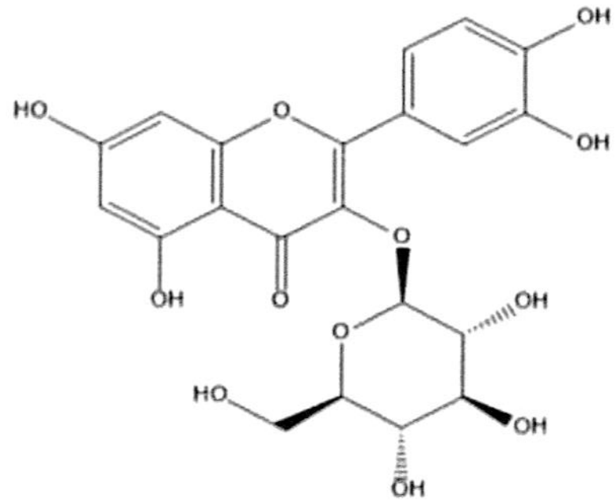	2-(3,4-dihydroxyphenyl)-5,7-dihydroxy-3-[(2S,3R,4S,5S,6R)-3,4,5-trihydroxy-6-(hydroxymethyl) oxan-2-yl] oxychromen-4-one	Huda et al. (2021)

(300–400 mm/yr) because it is frost-resistant. Quinoa is being grown more and more in South America and it is now being grown all over the world because of its useful qualities and high nutritional value (Vega-Gálvez et al., 2010).

Quinoa is a dioecious plant. Its height can range between 0.7 and 3.0 m, depending on the variety and environment. Root depth varies with plant height and can reach up to 30 cm. The erect stem can be branched or unbranched, and its leaves are alternate. The leaves and branches and the stem become angular. The leaves are alternate on all four sides (Kadam et al., 2018).

When the plants are young, the cortex of the stem is tough and soft, but as the plants mature, it becomes dry and spongy. Due to betacyanin pigments as in amaranth, the color of the stem changes from pale yellow to red in some varieties. Petioles and laminae of Quinoa are found on the leaves. Petioles are long, narrow, and channeled on one side. The petiole gives rise to three veins that run through the laminae. The leaves of a young plant are green, but as the plant grows older, they turn yellow or red (Berghofer & Schoenlechner, 2002).

Quinoa flowers are unremarkable because they lack petals. Quinoa has female and hermaphrodite flowers because it is gynomonoecious, and as a result, it is primarily an inbreeding species with only about 10% outcrossing. The hermaphrodite flowers are found at the distal end of a group, while the female flowers are found at the proximal end. The time from sowing to grain maturity varies between five and seven months, depending on variety and environment (Bhargava et al., 2007).

A crop can be harvested in three months under hydroponic conditions. The grains, like sorghum, are borne on an open panicle and, like sorghum, are vulnerable to bird predation. Quinoa saponins, like tannins in some sorghum varieties, are thought to be a defense mechanism against bird predation and fungal infection (Taylor & Parker, 2002). The chemical structures of important constituents present in Quinoa are presented in Table 8.3.

8.3 DIETARY VALUE OF PSEUDOCEREALS

Pseudocereals are absolutely full of nutrients that promote good health and enhance well-being. Amaranth, buckwheat, and quinoa are all good sources of carbohydrates (50–70%), which are primarily made up of starch and non-starch polysaccharides. Because their starch granules are smaller, their flour

TABLE 8.3 Chemical Structures of Important Constituents Present in Quinoa

Sl. No.	Name	Chemical Structure	IUPAC Name	References
1.	Betaine	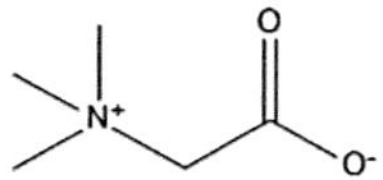	2-(trimethyl azaniumyl)acetate	Hernández-Ledesma (2019)
2.	Choline	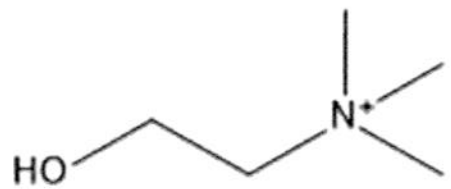	2-hydroxyethyl(trimethyl)azanium	Hernández-Ledesma (2019)
3.	α-tocopherol	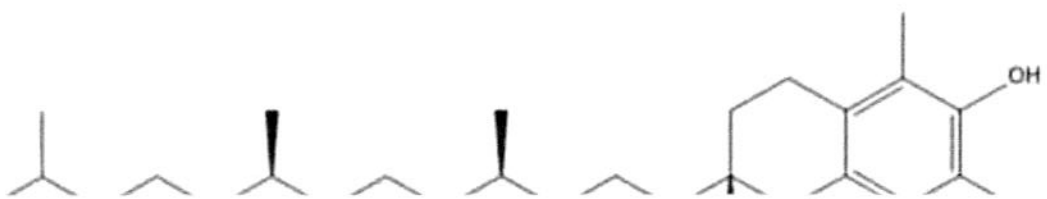	(2R)-2,5,7,8-Tetramethyl-2-[(4R,8R)-4,8,12-trimethyltridecyl]-3,4-dihydro-2H-1-benzopyran-6-ol	Hernández-Ledesma (2019)
4.	β-tocopherol	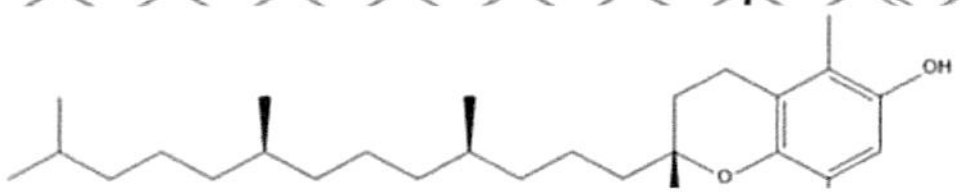	(2R)-2,5,8-trimethyl-2-[(4R,8R)-4,8,12-trimethyltridecyl]-3,4-dihydrochromen-6-ol	Hernández-Ledesma (2019)
5.	γ-tocopherol	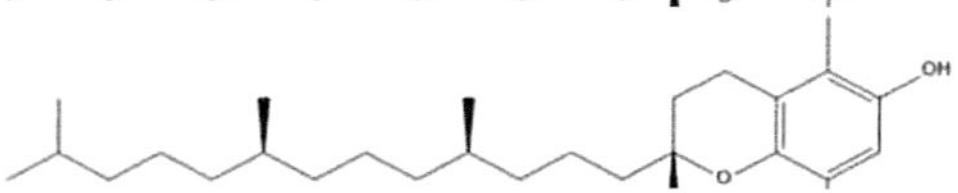	(2R)-2,7,8-trimethyl-2-[(4R,8R)-4,8,12-trimethyltridecyl]-3,4-dihydrochromen-6-ol	Hernández-Ledesma (2019)
6.	δ-tocopherol	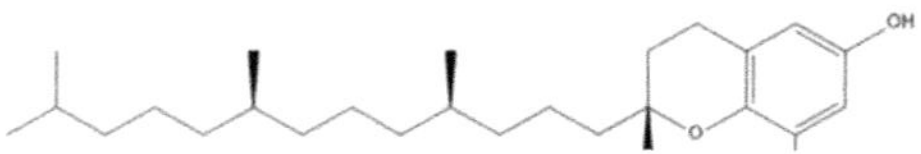	(2R)-2,8-dimethyl-2-[(4R,8R)-4,8,12-trimethyltridecyl]-3,4-dihydrochromen-6-ol	Hernández-Ledesma (2019)
7.	β-carotene	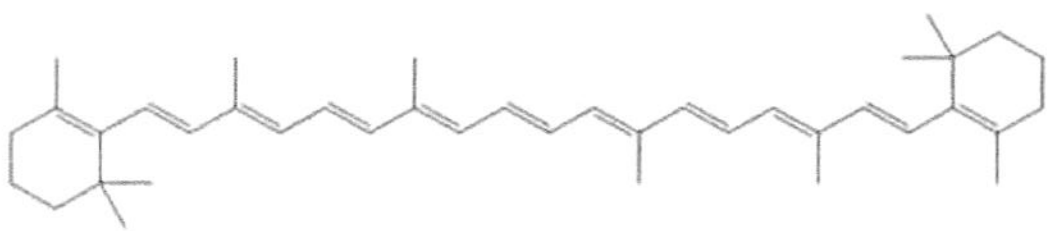	1,3,3-trimethyl-2-[(1E,3E,5E,7E,9E,11E,13E,15E,17E)-3,7,12,16-tetramethyl-18-(2,6,6-tri-methylcyclohexen-1-yl) octadeca-1,3,5,7,9,11,13,15,17-nonaenyl] cyclohexene	Hernández-Ledesma (2019)

TABLE 8.3 *(Continued)*

Sl. No.	Name	Chemical Structure	IUPAC Name	References
8.	Retinol	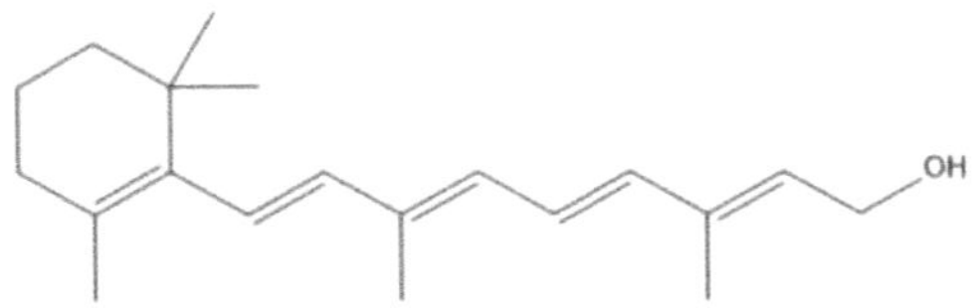	(2E,4E,6E,8E)-3,7-dimethyl-9-(2,6,6-trimethylcyclohexen-1-yl) nona-2,4,6,8-tetraen-1-ol	Hernández-Ledesma (2019)
9.	Lutein	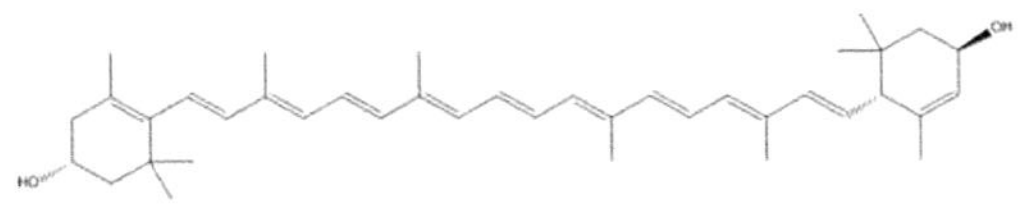	(1R)-4-[(1E,3E,5E,7E,9E,11E,13E,15E,17E)-18-[(1R,4R)-4-hydroxy-2,6,6-trimethylcyclohex-2-en-1-yl]-3,7,12,16-tetramethylocta-deca-1,3,5,7,9,11,13,15,17-nonaenyl]-3,5,5-trimethylcyclohex-3-en-1-ol	Hernández-Ledesma (2019)
10.	Zeaxanthin	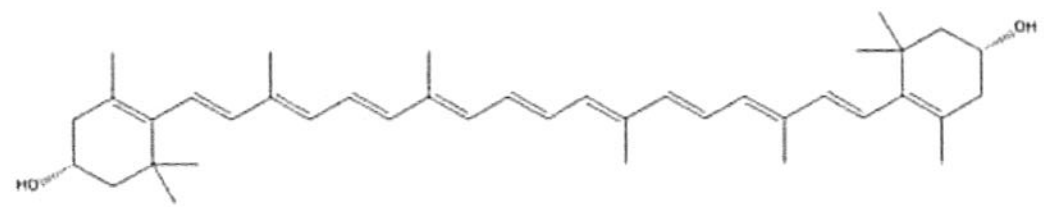	(1R)-4-[(1E,3E,5E,7E,9E,11E,13E,15E,17E)-18-[(4R)-4-hydroxy-2,6,6-trimethylcyclohexen-1-yl]-3,7,12,16-tetramethyloctadeca-1,3,5,7,9,11,13,15,17-nonaenyl]-3,5,5-trimethylcyclohex-3-en-1-ol	Hernández-Ledesma (2019)

has a smoother texture. Non-starchy polysaccharides contain 4–12% soluble and insoluble dietary fiber. The endosperm of all the pseudocereals contains a lot of cell wall matrix, therefore the enzymes have a hard time getting to the starch, which slows digestion. Amaranth, buckwheat, and quinoa are excellent sources of dietary fiber, and they impact the health system by reducing body weight (Martínez-Villaluenga et al., 2020).

Amaranth, buckwheat, and quinoa all have a protein content ranging from 7% to 16%. Their proteins are nutritionally superior to millet and major cereals in terms of essential amino acid profiles. Salt-soluble globulins and water-soluble albumins, both containing high levels of lysine, threonine, methionine, and other essential amino acids, are examples of pseudocereal storage proteins. Gluten-free and hypoallergenic proteins are also reported to be present in these pseudocereals, which are beneficial for human health (Mota et al., 2016).

Pseudocereals also provide a good source of dietary lipids (4–7%) and essential fatty acids. Quinoa is high in linoleate and linolenate, which are considered fatty acids. Amaranthus lipids are unique in that they contain a high proportion of squalene, which is an acyclic triterpene and is a precursor of cholesterol and other plant-derived sterols and triterpenoids (Alvarez-Jubete et al., 2010). Amaranth, buckwheat, and quinoa grains contain a variety of minerals, including Zn, Cu, Mn, K, Na, Ca, and Mg. Quinoa has a higher vitamin E content (2.44 g%) than rice (0.6 g%). Buckwheat seeds also have a lot of natural antioxidants like tocopherols, rutin, quercetin, flavonoids (Keservani & Sharma, 2014), and phenolic acids, as well as vitamins B1, B2, and B6 (De Bock et al., 2021).

This concludes that pseudocereals have very good dietary and nutritional value and therefore should be supplemented along with a normal diet (Vega-Gálvez et al., 2010).

8.4 HEALTH BENEFITS OF PSEUDOCEREALS WITH ESPECIAL EMPHASIS TO REDUCE OBESITY

The scientific evidence supporting health claims in *in vivo* models is still limited and restricted to a few animal studies and human trials, despite the composition and properties of pseudocereals (Comino et al., 2013). The consumption of pseudocereals or the bioactive components that make up these foods has primarily been linked to effects against obesity, prediabetes, and diabetes-related complications (Hernández-Ledesma, 2019). Therefore, diets that are based on amaranth protein have been found to reduce food intake and body weight as well. This is accomplished through the reduction of rat plasma ghrelin levels and the increase of postprandial leptin and cholecystokinin levels (Mlakar et al., 2009).

Furthermore, these diets have been found to modify the microbiota composition in a mouse model of diet-induced obesity (Etxeberria et al., 2015). Additionally, amaranth protein improved glucose tolerance and increased plasma insulin in a diabetes model induced by streptozotocin, while protein hydrolysates exerted significant anti-hypertensive activity in rats that were spontaneously hypertensive and antithrombotic effects in rats that were Wistar strains (Kehinde & Sharma, 2020). Researchers found that feeding mice a high-fat diet for six weeks caused the tartary buckwheat protein to exert hypocholesterolemic and anti-inflammatory activities in the mice (Gimenez-Bastida & Zielinski, 2015).

In addition, the protein was found to modulate the microbiota composition of the animals. Consumption of quinoa was found to protect Wistar rats and obese diabetic mice from developing hyperglycemia, as well as lower total cholesterol and LDL cholesterol levels. In the most recent study, it was discovered that quinoa can modulate inflammatory biomarkers and reduce the accumulation of hepatic steatosis and total cholesterol in the liver. These findings come from the use of a model. A diet-induced obesity mouse model was used to demonstrate the health benefits of quinoa phytoecdysteroid-enriched extracts (Noratto et al., 2019).

In this model, the extracts reduced adipose tissue decreased the expression of genes involved in lipid storage, and attenuated mRNA levels of inflammation and insulin resistance (Qin & Anderson, 2012). Additionally, the researchers observed that there was an increase in energy expenditure despite no change in the amount of food consumed or activity level, as well as an increase in glucose oxidation and fecal lipid excretion despite there being no change in the quantity of stool. At present, there have only been a limited number of studies done on humans to investigate the potential health advantages of consuming pseudocereals (Mir et al., 2018). The levels of insulin-like growth factor (IGF-1) in the plasma of boys aged 50–65 months who came from families in Ecuador with low incomes were significantly increased when quinoa was given to them twice a day in doses of 100 grams when compared to the levels in the control group (Ruales et al., 2002).

As a result, baby food containing quinoa was described as being able to provide sufficient protein in addition to other essential nutritional elements that could prevent malnutrition in children (Venlet et al., 2021). In addition, it has been demonstrated that adding quinoa to one's diet can modulate cardiovascular and metabolic parameters in a variety of individuals, including those who are healthy, overweight, and obese. In the same way, both short-term and long-term administration of buckwheat to diabetic subjects had effects on metabolic and cardiovascular markers (Soliman, 2019).

8.5 DEVELOPMENT OF GLUTEN-FREE DIET (GFD) TO COMBAT OBESITY

A gluten-free diet (GFD) is the need of the hour because obesity is creating problems for one-third of the entire population. Wheat is the cereal grain that is grown in the greatest number of locations across the globe, including in India and Pakistan, among other places (Zou et al., 2019). Due to the widespread adoption of diets, there has also been a rise in the demand for wheat intended for human consumption around the world (Henchion et al., 2021). This trend has been observed even in regions of the world where the climate is poorly suited to the cultivation of wheat (Fatima et al., 2020). Wheat has a fairly high concentration of micronutrients like minerals and vitamin B, and it provides up to 20% of the energy that the world's population needs (Galani et al., 2022).

Wheat, however, has the disadvantage of containing gluten, which research suggests may be the root cause of obesity (Xiong et al., 2019). The proliferation of wheat products has occurred concurrently with the expansion of people's waistlines (Popkin & Reardon, 2018). Wheat starch is different from the starch found in other carbohydrate-rich foods such as bananas, potatoes, and vegetables (Lal et al., 2021). Wheat starch can be broken down into smaller components (Cai et al., 1995). Because of the structure of amylopectin, it can be converted into glucose very effectively, which causes an increase in blood sugar (undesirably). Wheat is so addictive that it renders people unable to exercise self-control over their food consumption; conversely, eliminating wheat from the diet results in symptoms of withdrawal. "The glycemic index of whole-wheat bread is 72, which is higher than the glycemic index of sugar" (Glycemic Index of 59) (Radhika et al., 2010).

Therefore, the consumption of pseudocereals is required in order to counteract the negative effects of wheat (Cela et al., 2020). Because pseudocereals do not contain gluten, they are a potentially useful tool in the fight against obesity (Morales et al., 2021). Due to the high nutritional value of pseudocereals such as amaranth, buckwheat, and quinoa, these pseudocereals are increasingly being acknowledged as having relevance for a GFD (Alvarez-Jubete et al., 2010). Because pseudocereals are an excellent source of vitamins, minerals, and micro- and macro-nutrients in addition to being rich in starch and fiber, as well as high biological value proteins, they have been the subject of research as a potential alternative to broaden and improve the effectiveness of a GFD (Yilmaz et al., 2020).

Pseudocereals have a higher and superior protein bioavailability compared to common cereals, and their protein quality is comparable to that of animal protein (Rodríguez et al., 2020). This is important to consider when deciding whether or not to include pseudocereals in a GFD because eliminating certain cereals from the diet may result in a reduction in the number of protein sources (Vici et al., 2016). According to studies, both amaranth and quinoa contain protein that is easier to digest, more efficient, and has a more nutritionally balanced profile (De Bock et al., 2021). The analogy holds for fiber. The amount of fiber present in buckwheat, in particular, is significantly higher than that found in both traditional cereals and other pseudocereals (quinoa and amaranth) (Berti et al., 2005). Buckwheat, when included in a GFD, can help reduce the risk of fiber deficiency, which is extremely common in these patients (Di Nardo et al., 2019). The lipid content of pseudocereals is two to three times higher than that of common cereals like wheat, making this property of pseudocereals an additional important characteristic (Alvarez-Jubete et al., 2010). Overall, the majority of these lipids are unsaturated, which contributes to an increase in the nutritional value of the product. In terms of the vitamin B complex content, amaranth, quinoa, and buckwheat are all good sources of riboflavin; quinoa also contains thiamine and folic acid; and buckwheat also contains thiamine, riboflavin, and pyridoxine (Sindhu & Khatkar, 2019). These pseudocereals are an option that should be considered for inclusion in a GFD because patients with celiac disease frequently have insufficient levels of nutrients (Di Nardo et al., 2019).

Pseudocereals are not only sources of bioactive compounds that are not included in the definition of nutrients, but in addition, they are a beautiful source of vitamins, minerals, peptides, and fatty acids too which exhibit bioactive properties towards biological systems (Morales et al., 2021). Pseudocereals can be classified into two categories. Among these are saponins, polyphenols, phytosterols, phytosteroids, and betalains, the activities of which—anti-inflammatory, antioxidant, anticancer, and anti-diabetic, to name a few—are currently being investigated and are becoming more widely recognized as being significant (Martínez-Villaluenga et al., 2020).

Phenomenolic compounds are some of the most common and extensively researched phytochemicals that can be found in pseudocereals (Cotacallapa-Sucapuca et al., 2021). These compounds appear to be responsible (along with the nutritional density of pseudocereals) for the health benefits that are generally attributed to this food group (Fotschki et al., 2020). The metabolomic investigation of a number of gluten-free flours revealed the presence of a broad spectrum of phenolic compounds, the most representative of which were flavonoids (anthocyanins, flavones, flavanones, isoflavonoids, flavonols, and flavanols), phenolic acids (hydroxycinnamics, hydroxybenzoics, and hydroxyphenyl acetics), and tyrosol derivatives (Rocchetti et al., 2019). The lowest amount of total phenolics is found in amaranth (57.0 mg of gallic acid equivalents (GAE)/100 g), while buckwheat contains the highest amount [275.8 mg of gallic acid equivalents (GAE)/100 g], followed by quinoa (130.2 mg GAE/100 g), and then amaranth (Lin & Tang, 2007).

8.6 CONCLUSION

In modern times, there has been a rise in the number of people interested in researching pseudocereals all around the world.

The epidemic of obesity is a major cause for concern. Consuming an excessive quantity of unhealthy foods, such as junk food and fried foods, can lead to the development of a chronic condition known as obesity. Obesity has become an epidemic, which is a big reason for concern. It is possible to develop a long-term condition known as obesity if one consumes an excessive quantity of harmful foods, such as fast food and fried foods, such as junk food and other fried foods. One of the most prevalent factors that lead to obesity is having a caloric intake that is higher than the number of calories burned via movement and normal daily activities.

Obesity is defined as a body mass index of 25 or greater, at which point a person is regarded to be overweight. Excessive amounts of body fat are linked to an increased risk of significant health problems. Studies have connected the use of pseudocereals to health benefits such as a lower risk of heart disease, reduced obesity, improved blood sugar regulation, and enhanced digestion.

This chapter describes the nutritional benefits of various pseudocereals for living a healthy and active lifestyle. Amaranth, buckwheat, and quinoa are some of the best choices for pseudocereals because they are not only gluten-free but also rich in dietary fiber. Multiple studies have shown the use of amaranth, quinoa, and buckwheat in gluten-free consumables. The present chapter also covered the development of a Gluten-Free Diet (GFD) because the use of pseudocereals to combat obesity has been reported in several studies.

In a number of recent experiments, gluten-free cereal-based products including pseudocereals, such as bread, pasta, and confections, have been successfully manufactured. Examples of these products include Despite this, the availability of these things on the market is still somewhat restricted. Additional research is necessary in order to make full use of the seeds' potential as gluten-free ingredients in the production of palatable and nutritionally sound products so as to maximize their potential benefits.

Therefore, we can conclude that these pseudocereals, which have a high fiber content but no gluten, could be incorporated into the daily diet of an obese person to help them lose weight because of their high fiber content.

KEYWORDS

- **amaranth**
- **buckwheat**
- **gluten-free diet**
- **non-grass seeds**
- **pseudocereals**
- **quinoa**

REFERENCES

Al-Tamimi, A., Alfarhan, A., Al-Ansari, A., & Rajagopal, R. (2021). Antioxidant, enzyme inhibitory and apoptotic activities of alkaloid and flavonoid fractions of Amaranthus spinosus. *Physiological and Molecular Plant Pathology, 116*, 101728.

Alvarez-Jubete, L., Arendt, E. K., & Gallagher, E. (2010). Nutritive value of pseudocereals and their increasing use as functional gluten-free ingredients. *Trends in Food Science & Technology, 21*, 106–113.

Alvarez-Jubete, L., Auty, M., Arendt, E. K., & Gallagher, E. (2010). Baking properties and microstructure of pseudocereal flours in gluten-free bread formulations. *European Food Research and Technology, 230*, 437–445.

Angeli, V., Miguel Silva, P., Crispim Massuela, D., Khan, M. W., Hamar, A., Khajehei, F., Graeff-Hönninger, S., & Piatti, C. (2020). Quinoa (Chenopodium quinoa Willd.): An overview of the potentials of the "Golden Grain" and socio-economic and environmental aspects of its cultivation and marketization. *Foods, 9*, 1–31.

Astrup, A., Dyerberg, J., Selleck, M., & Stender, S. (2008). Nutrition transition and its relationship to the development of obesity and related chronic diseases. *Obesity Reviews, 9*, 48–52.

Babu, S., Yadav, G. S., Singh, R., Avasthe, R. K., Das, A., Mohapatra, K. P., Tahashildar, M., Kumar, K., Prabha, M., Devi, M. T., & Rana, D. S. (2018). Production technology and multifarious uses of buckwheat (Fagopyrum spp.): A review. *Indian Journal of Agricultural Sciences, 63*, 415–427.

Baraniak, J., & Kania-Dobrowolska, M. (2022). The dual nature of amaranth—Functional food and potential medicine. *Foods, 11*, 1–12.

Berghofer, E., & Schoenlechner, R. (2002). Grain amaranth. In Pseudocereals and Less Common Cereals (pp. 219–260). Springer, Berlin, Heidelberg.

Berti, C., Riso, P., Brusamolino, A., & Porrini, M. (2005). Effect on appetite control of minor cereal and pseudocereal products. *British Journal of Nutrition, 94*, 850–858.

Bhargava, A., Shukla, S., & Ohri, D. (2007). Gynomonoecy in Chenopodium quinoa (Chenopodiaceae): Variation in inflorescence and floral types in some accessions. *Biologia Plantarum, 62*, 19–23.

Brito, I. D. L., Chantelle, L., Magnani, M., & Cordeiro, A. M. T. D. M. (2022). Nutritional, therapeutic, and technological perspectives of quinoa (Chenopodium quinoa Willd.): A review. *Journal of Food Processing and Preservation, 46*, 1–12.

Bvenura, C., & Kambizi, L. (2022). Future grain crops. In Future Foods (pp. 81–105). Academic Press.

Cai, W., Diosady, L. L., & Rubin, L. J. (1995). Degradation of wheat starch in a twin-screw extruder. *Journal of Food Engineering, 26*, 289–300.

Cela, N., Condelli, N., Caruso, M. C., Perretti, G., Di Cairano, M., Tolve, R., & Galgano, F. (2020). Gluten-free brewing: Issues and perspectives. *Fermentation, 6*, 1–26.

Chaput, J. P., Doucet, E., & Tremblay, A. (2012). Obesity: a disease or a biological adaptation? An update. *Obesity Reviews, 13*, 681–691.

Coda, R., Di Cagno, R., Gobbetti, M., & Rizzello, C. G. (2014). Sourdough lactic acid bacteria: Exploration of non-wheat cereal-based fermentation. *Food Microbiology, 37*, 51–58.

Colgrave, M. L., Dominik, S., Tobin, A. B., Stockmann, R., Simon, C., Howitt, C. A., Belobrajdic, D. P., Paull, C., & Vanhercke, T. (2021). Perspectives on future protein production. *Journal of Agricultural and Food Chemistry, 69*, 15076–15083.

Comino, I., de Lourdes Moreno, M., Real, A., Rodríguez-Herrera, A., Barro, F., & Sousa, C. (2013). The gluten-free diet: testing alternative cereals tolerated by celiac patients. *Nutrients, 5*, 4250–4268.

Constantino, A. B. T., & Garcia-Rojas, E. E. (2022). Proteins from pseudocereal seeds: solubility, extraction, and modifications of the physicochemical and techno-functional properties. *Journal of the Science of Food and Agriculture, 102*, 2630–2639.

Cotacallapa-Sucapuca, M., Vega, E. N., Maieves, H. A., Berrios, J. D. J., Morales, P., Fernández-Ruiz, V., & Cámara, M. (2021). Extrusion process as an alternative to improve pulses products consumption. A review. *Foods, 10*, 1096.

De Bock, P., Daelemans, L., Selis, L., Raes, K., Vermeir, P., Eeckhout, M., & Van Bockstaele, F. (2021). Comparison of the chemical and technological characteristics of wholemeal flours obtained from amaranth (Amaranthus sp.), quinoa (Chenopodium quinoa) and buckwheat (Fagopyrum sp.) seeds. *Foods, 10*, 1–22.

Demment, M. W., & Van Soest, P. J. (1985). A nutritional explanation for body-size patterns of ruminant and nonruminant herbivores. *The American Naturalist, 125*, 641–672.

Di Nardo, G., Villa, M. P., Conti, L., Ranucci, G., Pacchiarotti, C., Principessa, L., Raucci, U., & Parisi, P. (2019). Nutritional deficiencies in children with celiac disease resulting from a gluten-free diet: A systematic review. *Nutrients, 11*, 1–12.

El Hazzam, K., Hafsa, J., Sobeh, M., Mhada, M., Taourirte, M., El Kacimi, K., & Yasri, A. (2020). An insight into saponins from Quinoa (Chenopodium quinoa Willd): A review. *Molecules, 25*, 1–22.

Etxeberria, U., Arias, N., Boqué, N., Macarulla, M. T., Portillo, M. P., Martínez, J. A., & Milagro, F. I. (2015). Reshaping faecal gut microbiota composition by the intake of trans-resveratrol and quercetin in high-fat sucrose diet-fed rats. *The Journal of Nutritional Biochemistry, 26*, 651–660.

Fatima, Z., Ahmed, M., Hussain, M., Abbas, G., Ul-Allah, S., Ahmad, S., Ahmed, N., Ali, M. A., Sarwar, G., Iqbal, P., & Hussain, S. (2020). The fingerprints of climate warming on cereal crops phenology and adaptation options. *Scientific Reports, 10*, 1–21.

Fotschki, B., Juśkiewicz, J., Jurgoński, A., Amarowicz, R., Opyd, P., Bez, J., Muranyi, I., Lykke Petersen, I., & Laparra Llopis, M. (2020). Protein-rich flours from quinoa and buckwheat favourably affect the growth parameters, intestinal microbial activity and plasma lipid profile of rats. *Nutrients, 12*, 1–12.

Fruh, S. M. (2017). Obesity: Risk factors, complications, and strategies for sustainable long-term weight management. *Journal of the American Association of Nurse Practitioners, 29*, S3–S14.

Galani, Y. J. H., Orfila, C., & Gong, Y. Y. (2022). A review of micronutrient deficiencies and analysis of maize contribution to nutrient requirements of women and children in Eastern and Southern Africa. *Critical Reviews in Food Science and Nutrition, 62*, 1568–1591.

Gerrano, A. S., Van Rensburg, W. J., Mavengahama, S., Bairu, M., Venter, S., & Adebola, P. O. (2017). Qualitative morphological diversity of Amaranthus species. *Journal of Tropical Agriculture, 55*, 12–20.

Gimenez-Bastida, J. A., & Zielinski, H. (2015). Buckwheat as a functional food and its effects on health. *Journal of Agricultural and Food Chemistry, 63*, 7896–7913.

Gondola, I., & Papp, P. P. (2010). Origin, geographical distribution and phylogenic relationships of common buckwheat (Fagopyrum esculentum Moench.). *The European Journal of Plant Science and Biotechnology, 4*, 17–32.

Goyat, J., & Handa, C. (2018). QUINOA (Chenopodium quinoa Willd.)–The forgotten golden grain. *International Journal of Food and Nutritional Sciences, 7*, 1–9.

Henchion, M., Moloney, A. P., Hyland, J., Zimmermann, J., & McCarthy, S. (2021). Trends for meat, milk and egg consumption for the next decades and the role played by livestock systems in the global production of proteins. *Animals, 15*, 100287.

Hernández-Ledesma, B. (2019). Quinoa (Chenopodium quinoa Willd.) as source of bioactive compounds: A review. *Bioactive Compounds in Health and Disease, 2*, 27–47.

Huda, M. N., Lu, S., Jahan, T., Ding, M., Jha, R., Zhang, K., Zhang, W., Georgiev, M. I., Park, S. U., & Zhou, M. (2021). Treasure from garden: Bioactive compounds of buckwheat. *Food Chemistry, 335*, 1–55.

Ihme, N., Kiesewetter, H., Jung, F. A., Hoffmann, K. H., Birk, A., Müller, A., & Grützner, K. I. (1996). Leg oedema protection from a buckwheat herb tea in patients with chronic venous insufficiency: a single-center, randomized, double-blind, placebo-controlled clinical trial. *European Journal of Clinical Pharmacology, 50*, 443–447.

Jancurová, M., Minarovičová, L., & Dandar, A. (2009). Quinoa–A review. *Czech Journal of Food Sciences, 27*, 71–79.

Jarouliya, U., & Keservani, Raj K. (2019). Pathways Leading to Child Obesity. In D. Bagchi (Ed.), *Global Perspectives on Childhood Obesity: Current Status, Consequences and Prevention, Second Edition* (pp. 137–146). Academic Press, Elsevier.

Kadam, V. P., Devi, K. S., Hussain, S. A., & Devi, M. U. (2018). Growth, yield attributes, yield and economics of quinoa (Chenopodium quinoa Willd.) as influenced by variable irrigation water supply through drip and surface methods. *International Journal of Current Microbiology and Applied Sciences, 7*, 3428–3438.

Karasch, M. (2000). May well become an important supplementary food crop in many developing countries in the future. *The Cambridge World History of Food, 1*, 81.

Kasajima, S., Yoshimaru, I., & Itoh, H. (2019). Differentiation and growth of a growing point until the stage of flower bud appearance in leading common buckwheat and Tartary buckwheat varieties in northern Japan. *Fagopyrum*, 36, 37–41.

Kehinde, B. A., & Sharma, P. (2020). Recently isolated antidiabetic hydrolysates and peptides from multiple food sources: A review. *Critical Reviews in Food Science and Nutrition, 60*(2), 322–340.

Keservani, R. K., & Sharma, A. K. (2014). Flavonoids: Emerging trends and potential health benefits. *Journal of Chinese Pharmaceutical Sciences, 23*(12), 815.

Keservani, R. K., Sharma, A. K., & Kesharwani, R. K. (Eds.). (2020). *Nutraceuticals and Dietary Supplements: Applications in Health Improvement and Disease Management*. CRC Press. ISBN: 9781771888738.

Khalifa, S. A., Elshafiey, E. H., Shetaia, A. A., El-Wahed, A. A. A., Algethami, A. F., Musharraf, S. G., & Halabi, M. F. (2021). Overview of bee pollination and its economic value for crop production. *Insects, 12*(1), 1–23.

Kraujalis, P., & Venskutonis, P. R. (2013). Supercritical carbon dioxide extraction of squalene and tocopherols from amaranth and assessment of extracts antioxidant activity. *The Journal of Supercritical Fluids, 80*, 78–85.

Kreft, I., Fabjan, N., & Germ, M. (2003). Rutin in buckwheat-protection of plants and its importance for the production of functional food. *Fagopyrum*, 20, 7–11.

Lal, M. K., Singh, B., Sharma, S., Singh, M. P., & Kumar, A. (2021). Glycemic index of starchy crops and factors affecting its digestibility: A review. *Trends in Food Science & Technology, 111*, 741–755.

Lara-Espinoza, C., Carvajal-Millán, E., Balandrán-Quintana, R., López-Franco, Y., & Rascón-Chu, A. (2018). Pectin and pectin-based composite materials: Beyond food texture. *Molecules, 23*(1), 1–35.

Li, C., Xie, Z., Wang, Y., Lu, W., Yin, G., Sun, D., & Wang, L. (2019). Correlation and genetic analysis of seed shell thickness and yield factors in Tartary buckwheat (*Fagopyrum tataricum* (L.) Gaertn.). *Breeding Science, 69*(5), 681–687.

Li, S. Q., & Zhang, Q. H. (2001). Advances in the development of functional foods from buckwheat. *Critical Reviews in Food Science and Nutrition, 41*(6), 451–464.

Lin, J. Y., & Tang, C. Y. (2007). Determination of total phenolic and flavonoid contents in selected fruits and vegetables, as well as their stimulatory effects on mouse splenocyte proliferation. *Food Chemistry, 101*(1), 140–147.

Luitel, D. R., Siwakoti, M., Jha, P. K., Jha, A. K., & Krakauer, N. (2017). An overview: distribution, production, and diversity of local landraces of buckwheat in Nepal. *Advances in Agriculture, Article ID 2738045*, 1–6.

Luthar, Z., Golob, A., Germ, M., Vombergar, B., & Kreft, I. (2021). Tartary buckwheat in human nutrition. *Plants, 10*(1), 1–14.

Maldonado-Cervantes, E., Jeong, H. J., León-Galván, F., Barrera-Pacheco, A., De León-Rodríguez, A., De Mejia, E. G., & De La Rosa, A. P. B. (2010). Amaranth lunasin-like peptide internalizes into the cell nucleus and inhibits chemical carcinogen-induced transformation of NIH-3T3 cells. *Peptides, 31*(9), 1635–1642.

Martínez-Villaluenga, C., Peñas, E., & Hernández-Ledesma, B. (2020). Pseudocereal grains: Nutritional value, health benefits and current applications for the development of gluten-free foods. *Food and Chemical Toxicology, 137*, 1–82.

Matsui, K., & Yasui, Y. (2020). Buckwheat heteromorphic self-incompatibility: genetics, genomics and application to breeding. *Breeding Science, 70*(1), 32–38.

Mattila, P. H., Pihlava, J. M., Hellström, J., Nurmi, M., Eurola, M., Mäkinen, S., & Pihlanto, A. (2018). Contents of phytochemicals and antinutritional factors in commercial protein-rich plant products. *Food Quality and Safety, 2*(4), 213–219.

Mazzeo, T., Cauzzi, S., Brighenti, F., & Pellegrini, N. (2015). The development of a composition database of gluten-free products. *Public Health Nutrition, 18*(8), 1353–1357.

Mburu, M. W., Gikonyo, N. K., Kenji, G. M., & Mwasaru, A. M. (2011). Properties of a complementary food based on amaranth grain (*Amaranthus cruentus*) grown in Kenya. *Journal of Agricultural and Food Technology, 1*, 153–178.

Mir, N. A., Riar, C. S., & Singh, S. (2018). Nutritional constituents of pseudocereals and their potential use in food systems: A review. *Trends in Food Science & Technology, 75*, 170–180.

Mlakar, S. G., Turinek, M., Jakop, M., Bavec, M., & Bavec, F. (2009). Nutrition value and use of grain amaranth: potential future application in bread making. *Agriculture, 6*, 43–53.

Morales, D., Miguel, M., & Garcés-Rimón, M. (2021). Pseudocereals: a novel source of biologically active peptides. *Critical Reviews in Food Science and Nutrition, 61*(10), 1537–1544.

Moreno, D. A., García-Viguera, C., Gil, J. I., & Gil-Izquierdo, A. (2008). Betalains in the era of global agri-food science, technology and nutritional health. *Phytochemical Reviews, 7*(2), 261–280.

Mosyakin, S., & Schwartau, V. (2015). Quinoa as a promising pseudocereal crop for Ukraine. *Agricultural Science and Practice, 2*, 3–11.

Mota, C., Santos, M., Mauro, R., Samman, N., Matos, A. S., Torres, D., & Castanheira, I. (2016). Protein content and amino acids profile of pseudocereals. *Food Chemistry, 193*, 55–61.

Mozaffarian, D. (2016). Dietary and policy priorities for cardiovascular disease, diabetes, and obesity: A comprehensive review. *Circulation, 133*(2), 187–225.

Mravlje, J., Regvar, M., Starič, P., Mozetič, M., & Vogel-Mikuš, K. (2021). Cold plasma affects germination and fungal community structure of buckwheat seeds. *Plants, 10*(1), Article 1.

Murphy, K. S., & Matanguihan, J. (Eds.). (2015). *Quinoa: Improvement and Sustainable Production*. John Wiley & Sons.

Noort, M. W., Renzetti, S., Linderhof, V., du Rand, G. E., Marx-Pienaar, N. J., de Kock, H. L., & Taylor, J. R. (2022). Towards sustainable shifts to healthy diets and food security in Sub-Saharan Africa with climate-resilient crops in bread-type products: A food system analysis. *Foods, 11*(1), Article 1.

Noratto, G. D., Murphy, K., & Chew, B. P. (2019). Quinoa intake reduces plasma and liver cholesterol, lessens obesity-associated inflammation, and helps to prevent hepatic steatosis in obese db/db mouse. *Food Chemistry, 287*, 107–114.

Nowacka, M., Dadan, M., Janowicz, M., Wiktor, A., Witrowa-Rajchert, D., Mandal, R., & Janiszewska-Turak, E. (2021). Effect of nonthermal treatments on selected natural food pigments and color changes in plant material. *Comprehensive Reviews in Food Science and Food Safety, 20*(8), 5097–5144.

Popkin, B. M., & Reardon, T. (2018). Obesity and the food system transformation in Latin America. *Obesity Reviews, 19*(8), 1028–1064.

Prakash, S., & Yadav, K. (2016). Buckwheat (*Fagopyrum esculentum*) as a functional food: A nutraceutical pseudocereal. *International Journal of Current Trends in Pharmacobiology and Medical Sciences, 1*(1), 1–15.

Qin, B., & Anderson, R. A. (2012). An extract of chokeberry attenuates weight gain and modulates insulin, adipogenic and inflammatory signaling pathways in epididymal adipose tissue of rats fed a fructose-rich diet. *British Journal of Nutrition, 108*(4), 581–587.

Qiu, J., Liu, Y., Yue, Y., Qin, Y., & Li, Z. (2016). Dietary tartary buckwheat intake attenuates insulin resistance and improves lipid profiles in patients with type 2 diabetes: A randomized controlled trial. *Nutrition Research, 36*(12), 1392–1401.

Radhika, G., Sumathi, C., Ganesan, A., Sudha, V., Henry, C. J. K., & Mohan, V. (2010). Glycaemic index of Indian flatbreads (rotis) prepared using whole wheat flour and 'atta mix'-added whole wheat flour. *British Journal of Nutrition, 103*(12), 1642–1647.

Rinninella, E., Cintoni, M., Raoul, P., Triarico, S., Dionisi, T., Gasbarrini, G. B., & Mele, M. C. (2021). The healthy gluten-free diet: Practical tips to prevent metabolic disorders and nutritional deficiencies in celiac patients. *Gastroenterology Insights, 12*(2), 166–182.

Rocchetti, G., Lucini, L., Rodriguez, J. M. L., Barba, F. J., & Giuberti, G. (2019). Gluten-free flours from cereals, pseudocereals and legumes: Phenolic fingerprints and in vitro antioxidant properties. *Food Chemistry, 271*, 157–164.

Rodríguez, J. P., Rahman, H., Thushar, S., & Singh, R. K. (2020). Healthy and resilient cereals and pseudo-cereals for marginal agriculture: Molecular advances for improving nutrient bioavailability. *Frontiers in Genetics, 11*, Article 1.

Ruales, J., Grijalva, Y. D., Lopez-Jaramillo, P., & Nair, B. M. (2002). The nutritional quality of an infant food from quinoa and its effect on the plasma level of insulin-like growth factor-1 (IGF-1) in undernourished children. *International Journal of Food Sciences and Nutrition, 53*(2), 143–154.

Ruth, O. N., Unathi, K., Nomali, N., & Chinsamy, M. (2021). Underutilization versus nutritional-nutraceutical potential of the Amaranthus food plant: A mini-review. *Applied Sciences, 11*(1), Article 1.

Sarker, U., & Oba, S. (2020). Nutraceuticals, phytochemicals, and radical quenching ability of selected drought-tolerant advance lines of vegetable amaranth. *BMC Plant Biology, 20*(1), Article 1.

Schnetzler, K. A. (1994). Food uses and amaranth product research: A comprehensive review. In *Amaranth Biology, Chemistry, and Technology* (1st ed., pp. 155–184). CRC Press.

Shahbaz, M., Raza, N., Islam, M., Imran, M., Ahmad, I., Meyyazhagan, A., & Gondal, T. A. (2022). The nutraceutical properties and health benefits of pseudocereals: A comprehensive treatise. *Critical Reviews in Food Science and Nutrition,* 63, *1–13.*

Shahzad, A., Ullah, S., Dar, A. A., Sardar, M. F., Mehmood, T., Tufail, M. A., & Haris, M. (2021). Nexus on climate change: Agriculture and possible solution to cope future climate change stresses. *Environmental Science and Pollution Research, 28*(26), 14211–14232.

Sharma, G., Barney, J. N., Westwood, J. H., & Haak, D. C. (2021). Into the weeds: New insights in plant stress. Trends in Plant Science, 26(11), 1050–1060.

Sindhu, R., & Khatkar, B. S. (2019). Pseudocereals: Nutritional composition, functional properties, and food applications. In R. K. Singh & D. Verma (Eds.), Food Bioactives (pp. 129–147). Apple Academic Press.

Singh, S., & Verma, D. (2022). Morphological and anatomical characterization of Fagopyrum esculentum Moench: A highly used medicinal plant in old and new world. Vegetos, 24, 1–10.

Soliman, G. A. (2019). Dietary fiber, atherosclerosis, and cardiovascular disease. Nutrients, 11(5), Article 1155.

Stojilkovski, K., Glavač, N. K., Kreft, S., & Kreft, I. (2013). Fagopyrin and flavonoid contents in common, tartary, and cymosum buckwheat. Journal of Food Composition and Analysis, 32(2), 126–130.

Stoner, K. A., & Gilman, S. (2008). Organic vegetable farms in New England-three case studies. Connecticut Agricultural Experiment Station.

Suvorova, G. (2016). Interspecific crosses in buckwheat breeding. In J. Zhou & M. Kreft (Eds.), Molecular Breeding and Nutritional Aspects of Buckwheat (pp. 87–97). Academic Press.

Tarhan, İ. (2021). A new and rapid analysis method for the most important herbal squalene source: Comparison of UV-visible, fluorescence, and FTIR techniques for the quantification of squalene in amaranth seed oil. Microchemical Journal, 168, Article 105142.

Taylor, J., & Parker, M. L. (2002). Quinoa. In J. Thomas & B. E. Marshall (Eds.), Pseudocereals and Less Common Cereals (pp. 93–122). Springer.

Vanhaute, E. (2007). 'So, worthy an example to Ireland.' The subsistence and industrial crisis of 1845–1850 in Flanders. In T. H. Courtin & P. D. Baten (Eds.), When the Potato Failed: Causes and Effects of the 'Last' European Subsistence Crisis, 1845–1850 (pp. 123–148). Brepols.

Vega-Gálvez, A., Miranda, M., Vergara, J., Uribe, E., Puente, L., & Martínez, E. A. (2010). Nutrition facts and functional potential of quinoa (Chenopodium quinoa Willd.), an ancient Andean grain: A review. Journal of the Science of Food and Agriculture, 90(14), 2541–2547.

Venlet, N. V., Hettinga, K. A., Schebesta, H., & Bernaz, N. (2021). Perspective: A legal and nutritional perspective on the introduction of quinoa-based infant and follow-on formula in the EU. Advances in Nutrition, 12(4), 1100–1107.

Vici, G., Belli, L., Biondi, M., & Polzonetti, V. (2016). Gluten-free diet and nutrient deficiencies: A review. Clinical Nutrition, 35(6), 1236–1241.

Wang, Y., & Beydoun, M. A. (2007). The obesity epidemic in the United States—Gender, age, socioeconomic, racial/ethnic, and geographic characteristics: A systematic review and meta-regression analysis. Epidemiologic Reviews, 29(1), 6–28.

Xiong, Y., Zhang, P., Warner, R. D., & Fang, Z. (2019). Sorghum grain: From genotype, nutrition, and phenolic profile to its health benefits and food applications. Comprehensive Reviews in Food Science and Food Safety, 18(6), 2025–2046.

Xue, Y., Dal Martello, R., Qin, L., Stevens, C. J., Min, R., & Fuller, D. Q. (2022). Post-Neolithic broadening of agriculture in Yunnan, China: Archaeobotanical evidence from Haimenkou. Archaeological Research in Asia, 30, Article 100364.

Yang, M., He, G., Hou, Q., Fan, Y., Duan, L., Li, K., & He, T. (2022). Systematic analysis and expression profiles of TCP gene family in Tartary buckwheat (Fagopyrum tataricum (L.) Gaertn.) revealed the potential function of FtTCP15 and FtTCP18 in response to abiotic stress. BMC Genomics, 23(1), Article 1.

Yilmaz, H. Ö., Ayhan, N. Y., & Meriç, Ç. S. (2020). Buckwheat: A useful food and its effects on human health. Current Nutrition & Food Science, 16(1), 29–34.

Zhang, X., Chen, H., Gu, K., & Jiang, X. (2022). Association of body mass index and abdominal obesity with the risk of airflow obstruction: National Health and Nutrition Examination Survey (NHANES) 2007–2012. COPD: Journal of Chronic Obstructive Pulmonary Disease, 19(2), 99–108.

Zhou, M., Huo, M., Wang, J., Shi, T., Li, F., & Liao, Z. (2022). Identification of Tartary buckwheat varieties suitable for forage via nutrient value analysis at different growth stages. International Journal of Plant Biology, 13(1), 31–43.

CHAPTER 9

FUNCTIONAL FOODS AND SPICES IN THE MANAGEMENT OF METABOLIC SYNDROME

SHRIYANSH SRIVASTAVA,[1] VISHAL KUMAR,[2] LAKSHAY KAPIL,[2] SONIMA PRASAD,[2] KRITIKA,[1] SHAHBAZ KHAN,[3] CHARAN SINGH,[4] and ARTI SINGH[2]

[1]*Department of Pharmacy, School of Medical and Allied Sciences, Galgotias University, Greater Noida, Uttar Pradesh, India*

[2]*Department of Pharmacology, ISF College of Pharmacy Affiliated to I.K. Gujral Punjab Technical University, Jalandhar, Punjab, India*

[3]*Pharmacy Academy, IFTM University, Lodhipur–Rajpoot, Moradabad, Uttar Pradesh, India*

[4]*Department of Pharmaceutics, ISF College of Pharmacy Affiliated to I.K. Gujral Punjab Technical University, Jalandhar, Punjab, India*

ABSTRACT

Syndrome X is also referred to as metabolic syndrome, characterized by the interconnected group of pathophysiological conditions such as obesity, cardiovascular diseases, coronary heart disease, atherosclerosis, hypertension, dyslipidemia, stroke, and diabetes. Apart from this, it is also associated with chronic kidney diseases, insomnia, depression, microglobulinuria, dementia, and cognitive decline. Herbs and spices such *as Curcuma longa, Trigonella foenum-graceum, Lagerstroemia speciosa, Emblica officinalis, Cinnamomum cassia, Vigna munga, Punica granatum, Murraya koenigii, Anacyclus pyrethrum,* and *Ficus religiosa* were widely used not only for the

Nutraceuticals in Obesity Management and Control. Raj K. Keservani & Alka Lohani (Eds.)

improvement of taste and food flavor but also for the prevention of several metabolic diseases from ancient times. Several studies have highlighted the molecular mechanism of active pharmaceutical ingredients present in herbs and spices. The available treatment therapy includes non-pharmacological approaches (functional foods, nutraceuticals, herbs, and spices) as well as pharmacological therapy such as statins, insulin, oral hypoglycemic agents, and beta-blockers, which have shown protective effects against metabolic syndrome. Nowadays, the demand for affordable, safe, and cost-effective alternative therapy has increased due to the high cost of synthetic drugs used to treat metabolic syndrome and associated complications. The current research scenario is focusing on evaluating the dosing schedule, long-term safety, and efficacy of herbal remedies, functional foods, antioxidants, nutraceuticals, and anti-inflammatory phototherapies to prevent disease progression. Several *in-vitro* and *in-vivo* studies reported the protective effect of several herbal remedies such as *Phaseolus vulgaris, Garcinia cambogia, Irvingia gabonensis, Berberine, and Tribulus terrestris a*gainst obesity, diabetes, and atherosclerosis caused by inflammatory cytokines and oxidative stress. We suggest that functional foods, spices, and herbal remedies could be novel treatment strategies against several metabolic disorders. Therefore, this chapter highlighted the protective effects of several herbal remedies, spices, and functional foods against various metabolic diseases with evidence from preclinical as well as clinical trials conducted with functional foods and spices against different metabolic diseases.

9.1 INTRODUCTION

Food is primarily referred to as the substance required for a number of life-sustaining processes, including the creation of energy, provision of nutrients, support of numerous metabolic processes, as well as the development and maintenance of the body. Nutrition science's focus at the turn of the 20th century was on body development and avoiding deficits (Derenski et al., 2016). Since the previous two decades, there has been a significant growth in our understanding of how nutrition affects our health and well-being, which has prompted the development of new, healthier meals that lower the chance of developing a number of chronic illnesses (Welch & Graham, 1999). Functional foods are traditional foods that have been changed to provide health advantages over unmodified counterparts. These foods are created in this fashion and are known as functional foods (Enkhmaa et al., 2018). The phrase "functional food," which describes processed meals that include components that support certain bodily processes in addition to being nutrient-dense, was originally used in Japan in the 1980s (Tank et al., 2010). As of this writing, Japan is the only country that has developed a unique regulatory clearance process for functional foods. FOSHU, which stands for "Food for Specified Health Effect," was initially used by the Japanese. According to Weststrate et al., functional meals should primarily be intended for function enhancement or (longer-term) illness risk reduction for "healthy" individuals rather than for the scientifically appropriate disease treatment of "sick" individuals (Booth et al., 2012). Growth, development, and differentiation; substrate metabolism; protection against reactive oxidant species; the cardiovascular system; gastrointestinal physiology and function; and behavior and psychological functions may all be affected by functional augmentation (Koletzko et al., 1998). Researchers have found a link between upper body obesity, diabetes, and hyperlipidemia and a higher risk of cardiovascular disease (CVD) since the early 1920s, and the term "metabolic syndrome" (MetS) was first used to characterize the collection of abnormalities in 1977 (Alkhatib et al., 2021; Despres et al., 1990). Heller et al. highlighted the relationship between type-2 diabetes, obesity, hyperlipoproteinemia, hyperuricemia, and hepatic steatosis as accumulative risk factors for atherosclerosis (Alkhatib et al., 2021). The association between obesity, gout, type 2 diabetes, and hypertension with hyperlipoproteinemia was also discussed in the same year. The idea was expanded upon a year later by Phillips et al., who proposed a link between heart disease, aging, and obesity and risk factors for myocardial infarction, such as glucose intolerance, hypertriglyceridemia, hypercholesterolemia, hyperinsulinemia, and high blood pressure (Gulliford et al., 2005; Wang et al., 2020). As a collection of connected abnormalities, including hyperglycemia, dyslipidemia, and high blood pressure that may result in CVD, MetS, also known as "syndrome X," was originally described in 1988 (Prasad, 2014). It was suggested that the root cause of the aforementioned issues may be underlying insulin resistance. The collection of anomalies that often result in CVD and type-2 diabetes has been referred to by a variety of names, including MetS, American syndrome, syndrome X, and insulin resistance syndrome. MetS in children has recently been redefined by Flemming et al. using methods of metabolic syndrome early diagnosis (Alkhatib et al., 2021). The term "metabolic syndrome" refers to a grouping of at least three of the following five medical conditions: abdominal obesity, hypertension, increased fasting plasma glucose, elevated serum triglyceride levels, and low levels of high-density lipoprotein (Amihaesei & Chelaru, 2014).

9.2 PROBLEMS ASSOCIATED WITH METABOLIC SYNDROME

9.2.1 *INSULIN RESISTANCE*

A number of diseases can result in diabetes, heart disease, and stroke. High blood pressure, high blood sugar, extra body fat around the waist, and abnormal cholesterol levels are the hallmarks of metabolic syndrome (Bray & Bellanger, 2006). A heart attack or stroke is more likely to occur as a result of the disorder. Apart from a large waist circumference, the majority of diseases linked to metabolic syndrome do not exhibit any symptoms (Johnson et al., 2009). Exercise, a healthy diet, losing weight, and quitting smoking may all be beneficial. Additionally, medication may be recommended. Insulin resistance is related to diabetes, glucose intolerance, dyslipidemia, hyperuricemia, and hypertension (Kendall & Harmel, 2002). In actuality, the limited epidemiological studies that have been carried out have only examined NIDDM or impaired glucose tolerance (IGT) (Feskens et al., 1995). As a consequence, we still don't fully grasp how widespread insulin resistance is in the most common metabolic diseases.

Type 2 diabetes and prediabetes are linked to insulin resistance. When the body is unable to react against the quantity of insulin generated, it may result in insulin resistance (Arnold et al., 2018). One of the organs in the body, the pancreas, produces insulin. It prevents your body from absorbing excessive amounts of sugar (glucose). You may get energy from the carbohydrate glucose (Röder et al., 2016). On the other hand, if you eat too much sugar, it might be harmful to your health. Unless a blood test is done, the majority of individuals are unaware that they have insulin resistance (Tobey et al., 1981). The main causes of insulin resistance are obesity (especially belly fat), a sedentary lifestyle, and a high-carbohydrate diet. During pregnancy, some women experience insulin resistance. Gestational diabetes is the name for this condition (Ten & Maclaren, 2004). Many illnesses, including polycystic ovarian syndrome, heart disease, and non-alcoholic fatty liver disease, are linked to insulin resistance (Baranova et al., 2011).

9.2.2 *ABDOMINAL OBESITY*

Blood lipid problems, inflammation, insulin resistance, full-blown diabetes, and an elevated risk of cardiovascular disease are all characteristics of the metabolic syndrome (Haffner, 2006). Although the scientific importance of metabolic syndrome is still up for debate, the recommended criteria for identifying those with the condition have significantly advanced preventive medicine (Després & Lemieux, 2006). The risk of cardiovascular disease globally cannot be predicted just by metabolic syndrome. However, the clinical diagnosis of metabolic syndrome must consider abdominal obesity, the most prevalent symptom, which is a marker of "dysfunctional adipose tissue" (Després & Lemieux, 2006).

9.2.2.1 ASIDE FROM BEING OVERWEIGHT

Despite the fact that obesity is a risk factor for both type 2 diabetes and insulin resistance, as well as a significant risk factor for both illnesses, not all obese patients are insulin resistant or at high risk for diabetes and cardiovascular disease (Abbasi et al., 2002). This explains why, compared to other modifiable risk factors for CVD including hypertension, smoking, and cholesterol (high low-density lipoprotein (LDL)/low HDL), obesity has been a poorly identified modifiable CVD risk factor (Ren et al., 2010). For any given level of total body fat, however, the subset of patients with a selective excess of intra-abdominal, or visceral, adipose tissue is at a noticeably elevated risk of insulin resistance and symptoms of the metabolic syndrome (Hamdy et al., 2006). Although elevated visceral fat has been linked to a number of atherogenic and diabetogenic abnormalities, it is unclear whether elevated visceral fat is a cause or merely a marker of a dysmetabolic profile (Després & Lemieux, 2006).

9.2.2.2 PATHOPHYSIOLOGY OF VISCERAL OBESITY

Excessive visceral fat development, which may be linked to the symptoms of insulin resistance, may also be caused by unhealthy adipose tissue that is unable to retain the extra energy (Paniagua, 2016). According to this view, a person's ability to handle an excess of calories—whether from a high-calorie diet, a sedentary lifestyle or—as is frequently the case—a combination of the two factors—may determine their susceptibility to metabolic syndrome (Després & Lemieux, 2006). Evidence indicates that even if a person has a positive energy balance, they will still be protected from developing metabolic syndrome if the extra energy is focused toward insulin-sensitive subcutaneous adipose tissue (Elks & Francis, 2010). When adipose tissue is absent, inadequate, or insulin resistant, extra triacylglycerol can collect in unfavorable regions such as the liver, heart, skeletal muscle, and visceral adipose tissue (Heilbronn et al., 2004). This condition is known as ectopic fat deposition. Smoking, the well-established hereditary propensity to visceral obesity, and a neuroendocrine profile linked to an adverse response to stress are among the factors linked to a preferred deposition of visceral fat and indications of insulin resistance (Després & Lemieux, 2006; Scott et al., 2012). Visceral obesity, insulin resistance, atherogenic dyslipidemia, and an inflammatory, pro-thrombotic profile are among the metabolic repercussions of this "defect" in energy partitioning (Pershadsingh, 2006). These traits describe the metabolic syndrome. Clinical criteria for metabolic syndrome, with the two most important ones being the presence of hypertriglyceridemia in the waist and high fasting triacylglycerol levels (Després & Lemieux, 2006).

9.2.3 DYSLIPIDEMIA

The metabolic syndrome is a group of illnesses that significantly increases the chance of developing type 2 diabetes and cardiovascular disease (CVD). Many, if not all, of the abnormalities associated with insulin-mediated glucose disposal resistance and compensatory hyperinsulinemia are shared by metabolic syndrome and diabetes. Atherogenic dyslipidemia is one of the diseases associated with metabolic syndrome, which also includes abdominal obesity, insulin resistance (with or without glucose tolerance), high blood pressure, and prothrombotic and proinflammatory variables (Table 9.1).

TABLE 9.1 The Metabolic Syndrome According to Adult Treatment Panel III

Sl. No.	Risk Factor	Defining Level
1.	Abdominal obesity (waist circumference):	
	Men	>102 cm
	Women	>88 cm
	Triglycerides	≥150 cm
2.	HDL cholesterol:	
	Men	<40 mg/dl
	Women	<50 mg/dl
3.	Blood pressure	≥130/>85 mmHg
4.	Fasting glucose	≥100 mg/dl

Increased fasting and postprandial triglyceride-rich lipoproteins (TRLs), decreased HDL, and increased small, LDL particles are the three components of dyslipidemia that result from insulin resistance (Ruotolo & Howard, 2002). It is probable that a single underlying metabolic defect is to blame for all of the lipoprotein changes identified in insulin resistance dyslipidemia since the metabolism of all lipoproteins is so linked (DeFronzo & Ferrannini, 1991; Figure 9.1). In individuals with insulin resistance, their independent occurrence is quite rare.

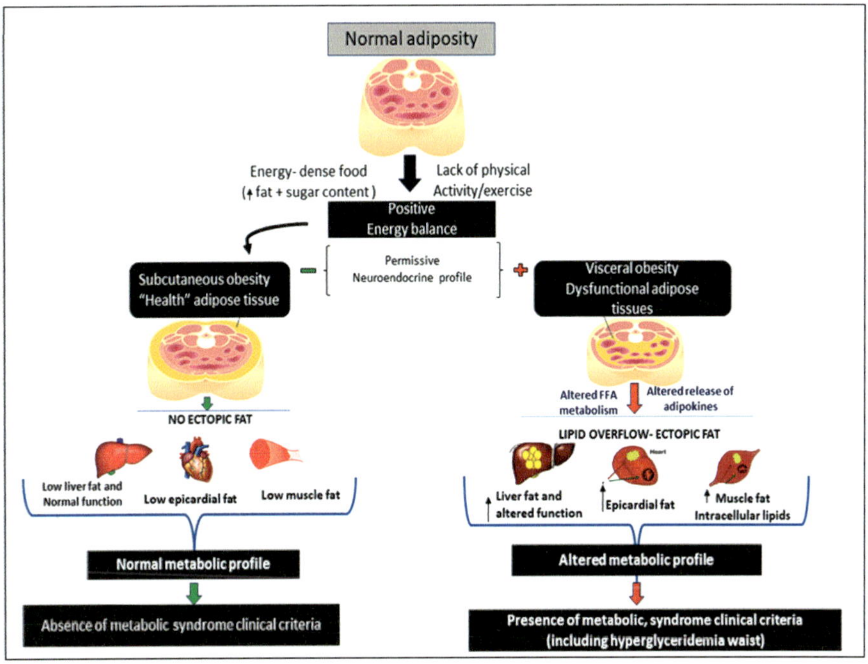

FIGURE 9.1 Schematic representation of visceral obesity.

9.2.4 *CARDIOVASCULAR DISEASE AND HYPERTENSION*

High blood pressure is more common in obese individuals than in lean individuals. Additionally, high blood pressure is a significant risk factor for CVD (Torrance et al., 2007). However, compared to lean people, obese people with high blood pressure have a lower risk of developing CVD. It seems that the cardiovascular system is not substantially affected by obesity-induced hypertension (Kotsis et al., 2018). This strategy is not generally accepted by the hypertension community, and the Framingham Heart Study did not support it (Mahmood et al., 2014).

The largest global cause of sickness and death is cardiovascular disease. According to epidemiological studies, the aging population will cause 23.3 million people to die from cardiovascular illnesses by the year 2030 (Mathers & Loncar, 2006). Many patients do not get positive clinical results from management and treatments, despite intensive therapy for cardiovascular disorders (Baddour et al., 2005). The increasing prevalence of obesity and type 2 diabetes may make it more difficult to provide proper treatment for cardiovascular disease. Obesity, diabetes mellitus, dyslipidemia, and hypertension are frequently identified as the main factors of cardiovascular disease incidence: The risk of cardiovascular mortality as a whole may rise noticeably with even a minor rise in body weight (DeFronzo & Ferrannini, 1991). A collection of risk factors all connected to metabolism is consulted as the metabolic syndrome. Since metabolic syndrome was first mentioned in medical terminology a few decades ago, the incidence of its cardiovascular effects has been quickly increasing around the globe (Saklayen, 2018). The current definition of metabolic syndrome includes a range of clinical signs, such as a large waist circumference, dyslipidemia, hypertension, hyperglycemia, and insulin resistance (Kilpatrick et al., 2007). These symptoms are all connected to an increased incidence of type 2 diabetes and obesity. Patients who have one or more metabolic syndrome signs, such as obesity and sedentary behavior, may also have generalized clinical symptoms (Stone & Saxon, 2005).

9.3 DIFFERENT TYPES OF NUTRACEUTICALS AND THEIR MARKETED PRODUCTS

Nutraceuticals are foods or dietary supplements that have beneficial medical or health effects, such as the treatment or prevention of disease (Prabu et al., 2012). Since they are natural dietary supplements, non-toxic, and have fewer side effects than medications, nutraceuticals have an edge over such products. Nutraceuticals are divided into three primary categories depending on their chemical composition, classifications, and natural sources of nutrition such as herbs, dietary supplements, dietary fiber, and so on (Das et al., 2012). The industry's fastest-growing segment was dietary supplements, products that are natural or herbal (at a rate of 19.5% annually) (11.6% per year). A projected USD 117 billion would be spent on the worldwide nutraceutical sector (Kumar et al., 2018). The FDA regulates dietary supplements to ensure their safety, using supplements like meals. According to the

Indian government, the Food Safety and Standard Act was established in 2006 to oversee the nutraceutical sector (Santini et al., 2018). Herbal use of nutraceuticals (Keservani et al., 2010a, b) is a potent method for preserving health and avoiding disease, ensuring the best possible health by preventing and treating acute and long-term ailments brought on by a bad diet (Sen & Chakraborty, 2011). Stephen Derelict, MD, who founded and served as chairman of the Foundation for Innovation in Medicine (FIM) in Cranford, New Jersey, combined the terms "nutrition" and "pharmaceutical" to create the term "nutraceuticals" in 1989 (Singh, 2020). Let food be your medicine, Hippocrates, the Greek physician who is sometimes referred to as the "father of medicine," told his patients. Its guiding idea is "Focus on Prevention" (Majeed et al., 2011). In this context, terminology like dietary supplements, multifunctional foods, and functional foods are frequently utilized. Functional foods are traditional foods that also have nutritional benefits and include elements or chemicals that have therapeutic or health benefits (Bordbar et al., 2011).

Nutritional supplements are commodities designed to complement the diet that carry or include one or more of the following dietary components, according to the Dietary Supplement Health and Education Act (DSHEA) (Jiang, 2009). A concentration, metabolite, component, extract, or combination of any one of the following: an amino acid, a vitamin, a mineral, an herb or other botanical, a supplement used by people to increase daily consumption of certain nutrients, or a vitamin, mineral, herb, or botanical (Fitzpatrick, 2003). It comes in liquid, tablet, and capsule form for pills. It is not meant to be consumed as traditional cuisine or as the only food group during meals or as part of a diet. The label describes it as a "dietary supplement" (Stipanuk & Caudill, 2018).

Foods that are intended to be consumed as a regular component of a diet but also provide health advantages above and beyond just providing basic nourishment are referred to as "functional foods" (Tables 9.2–9.5; Hasler, 2000).

In nutritional therapy, a complementary medical strategy, foods, or nutraceuticals are used. This kind of treatment is founded on the idea that food, in addition to giving us nourishment and energy, may also be medicinal (Brown et al., 2003). The use of such nutraceuticals to assist in the body's detoxification, prevent vitamin and mineral shortages, and restore normal digestion and eating practices (Martins et al., 2014) according to the theory underlying nutraceuticals and nutritional therapy, helps to achieve this goal. Plant compounds known as phytonutrients have unique biological effects

TABLE 9.2 Classification of Nutraceuticals

Sl. No.	Class	Examples
1.	Inorganic mineral supplements	Minerals
2.	Vitamin supplements	Vitamins
3.	Digestive enzymes	Enzymes
4.	Probiotics	Lactobacillus acidophilus
5.	Prebiotics	Digestive enzymes
6.	Herbs as a functional food	Soya proteins
7.	Cereals and grains	Fibers
8.	Dietary fibers	Fibers
9.	Antioxidants	Vitamin C
10.	Phytochemicals	Carotenoids
11.	Health drinks	Fruits juice

TABLE 9.3 Various Types of Vitamins and Their Health Benefits

Sl. No.	Name of Vitamin	Sources	Health Benefits
1.	Vitamin A1	Fish liver oil, liver.	Antioxidants maintenance of healthy skin, and vision
2.	Vitamin A2	Cheese, butter carrots, spinach, pumpkins, papaya.	Mucous membrane.
3.	Vitamin D	Fish liver oil, wheat germ oil, egg yolk, milk, butter.	Essential for the formation of bones and teeth, helps the body absorb and use calcium.
4.	Vitamin E	Wheat germ oil, cotton seed oil, peanut oil.	Antioxidant helps blood cells, muscles, lungs, and nerve tissue, boost the immune system.
5.	Vitamin K	Cabbage, cauliflower, tomatoes.	Essential for blood clotting.
6.	Vitamin B1	Cereals, pulses	Essential in neurologic.
7.	Vitamin B2	Nuts, yeast	Helps in energy production.
8.	Vitamin B3 (pantothenic)	Liver, meat, yeast	Helps to convert food into energy and maintain proper brain function.
9.	Folic acid	Green vegetables	Essential in pregnancy, helps in RBC formation.
10.	Nicotinic acid (B5)	Yeast, egg, milk	Required for various nervous system functions.

TABLE 9.4 Represents the Common Herbals and Nutraceuticals and Their Health Benefits

Sl. No.	Common Name	Biological Name	Constituents	Health Benefits
1.	Garlic	Dried bulbs of Allium sativum (Liliaceae).	Allin and allicin	Anti-inflammatory, antibacterial, antigout, nerine tonic.
2.	Maidenhair tree	Leaves of Ginkgo biloba (Ginkgoaceae).	Ginkgolide and bilobalide	PAF antagonist, memory enhancer, antioxidant.
3.	Ginger	Rhizomes of Zingiber officinale (Zingiberaceae).	Zingiberene and gingerols	Stimulant, chronic bronchitis, hyperglycemia, and throat ache.
4.	Echinacea	Dried herb of Echinacea purpurea (Asteraceae).	Alkylamide and echinacoside	Anti-inflammatory, immunomodulator, antiviral.
5.	Ginseng	The dried root of Panax ginseng (Araliaceae).	Ginsenosides and panaxosides.	Stimulating immune and nervous system and adaptogenic properties.
6.	Liquorice	Dried root of Glycyrrhiza glabra (Leguminosae)	Glycyrrhizin and liquirtin	Anti-inflammatory and anti-allergic, expectorant.
7.	St. John's wort	The dried aerial part of Hypericum perforatum (Hypericaceae).	Hypericin and hyperforin	Antidepressant, against HIV and hepatitis C virus.
8.	Turmeric	Rhizome of Curcuma longa (Zingiberaceae).	Curcumin	Anti-inflammatory, antiarthritic, anticancer, and antiseptic.
9.	Onion	Dried bulb of Allum cepa Linn. (Liliaceae)	Allicin and Allin	Hypoglycemic activity, antibiotics, and anti-atherosclerosis.
10.	Valeriana	Dried root Valeriana officinals linn. (Valerianaceae).	Valerenic acid and valerate	Tranquilizer, migraine, menstrual pain, intestinal cramps, bronchial spasms.
11.	Aloes	Dried juice of leaves Aloes barbadensis mill. (Liliaceae).	Aloins and aloesin	Dilates capillaries, anti-inflammatory, emollient, and wound healing properties.
12.	Goldenseal	Dried root of Hydrastis Canadensis. (Ranunculaceae).	Hydrastine and berberine	Antimicrobial, astringent, antihemorrhagic, treatment of mucosal inflammation.
13.	Senna	Dried leaves of Cassia angustifolia (Leguminosae).	Sennosides	Purgative
14.	Asafetida	Oleo gum resin of Ferula assafetida L. (umbelliferae)	Ferulic acid and umbellic acid.	Stimulant, carminative, expectorant.
15.	Bael	Unripe fruits of Aegle marmelos corr. (Rutaceae)	Marmelosin	Digestive appetizer, treatment of diarrhea and dysentery.
16.	Brahmi	Herbs of Centella asiatica (umbelliferae)	Asiaticoside and madecassoside.	Nervine tonic, spasmolytic, anti-anxiety.

TABLE 9.5 List of Marketed Nutraceutical Products

Sl. No.	Products	Category	Contents	Manufacturer
1.	Calcirol D-3	Calcium supplement	Calcium and vitamins	Cedilla Healthcare Limited, Ahmedabad, India
2.	GRD (23–25)	Nutritional supplement	Proteins, vitamins, minerals, and carbohydrates.	Zydus Cadila Ltd. Ahmedabad, India
3.	Proteinex®	Protein supplement	Predigested protein, vitamins, minerals, and carbohydrates.	Pfizer Ltd., Mumbai, India
4.	Coral calcium	Calcium supplement	Calcium and trace minerals.	Nature's Answer, Hauppauge, NY, USA.
5.	Chyawanprash	Immune booster	Amla, ashwagandha, pippali	Dabur India Ltd.
6.	Omega woman	Immune supplement	Antioxidants, vitamins, and phytochemicals (e.g., lycopene and resveratrol).	Wassen, Surrey, U.K.
7.	Celestial health tone	Immune booster	Dry fruit extract	Celestial Biolabs Limited
8.	Amiriprash (Gold)	Good immunomodulator	Chyawanprash avalena, swarnabhasma, and RasSindur	UapPharma Pvt. Ltd.

that improve human health (Zhao, 2007). The phytochemicals function in the following manner:

- Biochemical reaction substrate.
- Enzymatic reaction cofactors.
- Enzyme reaction inhibitors.
- Absorbents that bind to and remove harmful substances from the intestine.
- Enhance vital nutrient absorption and/or stability.
- Beneficial bacteria-specific growth factor.
- Beneficial bacteria ferment on this substrate.
- Selective inhibitors of pathogenic bacteria in the intestine.
- Selective inhibitors of harmful bacteria in the intestine.
- Ligands that activate or inhibit intracellular or cell surface receptors.
- The category of nutraceuticals.
- Vitamins, fatty acids, amino acids, and minerals are a few examples of the compounds known as nutrients.

- Herbals are concentrated forms of plants or their extracts (Dillard & German, 2000).
- Other-source reagents (such as pyruvate, chondroitin sulfate, and steroid hormone precursors) that are used for specific purposes include meal replacements, weight-loss supplements, fortified traditional meals, and sports nutrition (Manikandaselvi & Nithya, 2011). Numerous categories exist for dividing up nutraceuticals, such as food sources, modes of action, chemical makeup, and so forth.

9.4 THE CONTRIBUTION OF DIETARY SUPPLEMENTS TO THE PREVENTION AND TREATMENT OF METABOLIC SYNDROME AND ASSOCIATED DISEASES

Due to poor dietary practices that favor meals high in fat and sugar, lack of physical exercise, or a sedentary lifestyle, metabolic disorders including diabetes mellitus and obesity are fast rising in the Westernized world (Mitra et al., 2020). Conversely, due to its limited long-term effectiveness and safety concerns, pharmaceutical intervention for obesity is still a contentious topic. The primary underlying cause of metabolic syndrome is obesity (Smyth & Heron, 2006). Over the last 20 years, obesity has been spreading rapidly worldwide. According to a WHO assessment classifying obesity as a growing pandemic (Gilman, 2008), millions of people may face catastrophic weight-related problems if prompt action is not taken. Obesity is one of the biggest health issues and most prevalent chronic diseases. In 2005, 24.2% of men and 23.5% of women who participated in health surveys in the United States were classified as obese (Jackson et al., 2005). An imbalance between energy intake (food consumption), which is primarily stored as triglycerides, and energy expenditure is the main factor contributing to obesity (basal metabolic rate and biochemical processes) (Hassan & El-Gharib, 2015).

A type of excess energy known as triglycerides is often retained in adipose tissue. When adipose tissue function is compromised due to obesity, there is an excessive deposit of fat in the liver, other organs, and adipose tissue, which increases the risk of metabolic changes that increase overall morbidity (Abranches et al., 2015). Given that nutritional therapy and pharmaceutical intervention are the mainstays in treating metabolic syndrome and its effects on health, researchers have been compelled to investigate any potential drug-nutrient or drug-food interactions in this area (McCabe et al., 2003). When another food, drug, or beverage is present or when certain chemical substances in the environment are present, the effects of one drug are said to interact

(Koziolek et al., 2019). Inadvertent interactions between food and drugs may result in therapeutic failure (such as hyperglycemia in the case of diabetes mellitus) or an increase in undesirable effects (i.e., hypoglycemia in the case of diabetes mellitus) (Harrigan et al., 2001). The traditional alterations in medication bioavailability brought on by food are what lead to clinically significant food-drug interactions (Schmidt & Dalhoff, 2002). Thus, in the context of metabolic disorders where nutrition plays a substantial role in overall therapy, the potential impact of food and nutrient consumption on pharmaceutical therapeutic efficacy may be crucial (Sokoła-Wysoczańska et al., 2018).

A nutraceutical is a food (or part of a meal) with medicinal or health benefits, such as the prevention or treatment of illness (Dudeja & Gupta, 2017). Nutraceuticals are a wide range of products that are produced by the food industry, the herbal and dietary supplement industry, and the pharmaceutical industry (Pandey et al., 2010). Nutritional supplements cover the majority of therapeutic areas, including those relating to sleep, digestion, cold and cough, cancer prevention, blood pressure, analgesics, depression, hyperglycemia, and hypoglycemia (Singh & Sinha, 2012). Depending on the ease of understanding and uses, such as for clinical trial design, academic education, and functional foods, nutraceuticals may be arranged in a variety of ways (Bröring et al., 2006).

9.4.1 ANTIOXIDANT NUTRACEUTICALS AND VITAMIN C

Antioxidant vitamins. According to animal studies, eating enough dietary antioxidants may prevent or delay diabetic complications like renal and neurological dysfunction by preventing oxidative stress (Sharifi-Rad et al., 2020). However, there is a dearth of conclusive human evidence. Vitamin C in the form of ascorbic acid is a chain-breaking antioxidant that directly neutralizes Reactive Oxygen Species (ROS) and prevents the progression of chain reactions that would otherwise lower protein glycation (Hamid et al., 2010). In mice with diabetes, vitamin C also reduces sorbitol accumulation and lipid peroxides in erythrocytes. Patients with type 2 diabetes and low vitamin C levels get 800 mg of vitamin C daily; however, neither endothelial dysfunction nor insulin resistance are improved (Matough et al., 2012).

9.4.2 VITAMIN E (α-TOCOPHEROL)

Protects membranes from lipid peroxidation by directly reacting with singlet oxygen, peroxyl, and superoxide radicals as a part of the overall peroxyl radical-trapping antioxidant system (Bendich et al., 1986). As a component of the overall peroxyl radical-trapping antioxidant system, protects membranes from lipid peroxidation by directly interacting with singlet oxygen, peroxyl, and superoxide radicals (Sies et al., 1992). When vitamin E levels are low, more peroxides and aldehydes are present in many tissues. There have been conflicting findings about the amounts of vitamin E in diabetics (Seven et al., 2004). In order to ascertain if lipid peroxidation and platelet activation in type 2 diabetes are reversible, we looked at the effects of short-term vitamin E supplementation (600 mg per day for 2 weeks) on the excretion of 8-iso-PGF2 and 11-dehydro-TXB2 in the urine (Holt, 2000). With vitamin E supplementation, 8-iso-PGF2 excretion nearly returned to baseline while plasma vitamin E levels underwent discernible alterations (Samoylenko et al., 2013). The increases in F2-isoprostane generation, which were followed by equivalent decreases in thromboxane metabolite excretion, also suggest a cause-and-effect relationship between elevated lipid peroxidation and persistent platelet activation in this circumstance (Ferroni et al., 2012). Observational, prospective cohort studies suggest that higher dietary antioxidant intake or supplementation (including vitamins A, C, E, folic acid, niacin, alpha-carotene, selenium, and zinc) may lower the risk of cardiovascular disease and death (Berkowitz, 2003). In light of these findings, the American Heart Association suggested consuming a balanced diet with an emphasis on fruits, vegetables, and whole grains that are strong in antioxidants (Tribble, 1999). However, the results of controlled clinical trials that used randomization have not been able to demonstrate a consistent protective effect of any one antioxidant or antioxidant combination (vitamins C, E, and beta-carotene) in the primary or secondary prevention of cardiovascular events (Jensen et al., 2008). Additionally, taking supplements of the vitamins C, E, and/or beta-carotene was connected to an increased risk of dying from any cause in multiple research studies (Enstrom et al., 1992). Further, vitamin B supplementation was connected to a quicker drop-in glomerular filtration rate and an increase in vascular events in people with diabetic nephropathy when compared to placebo (Thornalley & Rabbani, 2010).

Recently, vitamin E was administered instead of a placebo to non-diabetic patients with non-alcoholic steatohepatitis, a disorder closely related to insulin resistance (Caldwell, 2017). Through research in healthy volunteers, the baseline rate of lipid peroxidation has been established as a critical factor influencing the response to vitamin E delivery (Chiarelli et al., 2002). This theory is confirmed by research showing that patients with different rates of lipid peroxidation may respond differently to the same dose of vitamin E's antioxidant effects (Roob et al., 2000). We found a linear relationship between the baseline rate of 8-iso-PGF2 excretion and the slope of changes in this indication of lipid peroxidation following short-term 600 mg/day therapy in a variety of clinical settings (Pallantza et al., 2010). Difficulties with dosage and treatment duration may also affect how well vitamin E supplements work. A strong linear trend between vitamin E dosage and % change in plasma concentrations of F2-isoprostanes has been seen in dose-ranging research; however, the magnitude was only significant at doses of 1,600 and 3,200 I.U./day (Roberts II et al., 2007). Furthermore, time-course research showed that after 16 weeks of supplementation, the plasma F2-isoprostane concentrations were at their highest level of suppression (Davì et al., 2010). Together, these elements may have effects on how vitamin E is studied in diabetic people as well as how clinical trials of antioxidant intervention are planned and conducted (Steinberg & Witztum, 2002).

9.4.3 α-LIPOIC ACID

A powerful ROS scavenger, α-Lipoic acid is a naturally occurring antioxidant. In its oxidized state, it has the peculiar virtue of being a ROS scavenger, quenching multiple radicals (Nimesh & Ashwlayan, 2018). In addition to their ability to chelate transition metals and regenerate other antioxidants like glutathione, vitamin C, and vitamin E, α-Lipoic Acid and Dihydrolipoic Acid function as a redox pair (an electron-donating molecule and its oxidized version) (Flora, 2009). In those with type 2 diabetes, α-lipoic acid raises insulin sensitivity by about 18–20%. A review of clinical trials using α-lipoic acid to treat diabetic neuropathy found positive effects on both acute symptoms and the course of the disease (Jacob et al., 1999).

A powerful ROS scavenger, α-Lipoic acid is a naturally occurring antioxidant. In its oxidized state, it has the peculiar virtue of being a ROS scavenger, quenching multiple radicals (Zorov et al., 2014). In addition to their ability to chelate transition metals and regenerate other antioxidants like glutathione, vitamin C, and vitamin E, α-Lipoic Acid and Dihydrolipoic Acid function as a redox pair (an electron-donating molecule and its oxidized version) (Parfenov & Zaikov, 2018). *In vivo* and *in vitro* studies have demonstrated that α-Lipoic Acid shields the retina from ischemia-reperfusion damage. Ischemic damage to the retina, which develops in diabetic retinopathy, is thought to be one of the main causes of vision loss. In those with type 2 diabetes, lipoic acid raises insulin sensitivity by about 18–20% (Khalilpour et al., 2017).

9.5 PLANT EXTRACTS USED IN THE MANAGEMENT OF METABOLIC SYNDROME AND RELATED DISORDERS

9.5.1 *TRIGONELLA FOENUM-GRACEUM*

Fenugreek is a leguminous plant that is often grown in Northern Africa and India, and its seeds are used as a spice and culinary component all over the globe (Acharya et al., 2008). Fenugreek seeds are rich in protein and fiber and have been shown to lower blood sugar and cholesterol levels in mice, rats, dogs, and people (Madar & Stark, 2002). Fenugreek seeds have hypoglycemic properties because of their high neutral and soluble fiber content, which delays stomach emptying and lowers post-meal blood glucose levels (Cassidy et al., 2018). Other gastrointestinally active substances found in the seeds include steroidal saponins, which may prolong stomach emptying, and the alkaloid trigonelline, which may lessen glycosuria (Srinivasan, 2006).

9.5.1.1 *ANTIDIABETIC EFFECT OF TRIGONELLA*

Diabetes mellitus (DM) is characterized by elevated glucose levels and abnormal glucose metabolism. Elevated blood glucose is ascribed to insulin insufficiency or resistance, which leads to decreased glucose absorption by insulin-dependent organs such as the liver and muscle cells (Olokoba et al., 2012). On the other hand, insulin-dependent tissues such as heart tissue, blood vessels, peripheral nerves, renal medulla, and lens experience persistent hyperglycemia-induced glucose overutilization (CHAUHAN). Blood glucose control is widely acknowledged as the most effective way to prevent diabetes-related tissue damage and consequent issues such as cardiovascular ailments including micro- and macro-angiopathy, nephropathy, neuropathy, and retinopathy (Adeghate & Singh, 2014). However, managing blood glucose levels is challenging and there is no medication available to help. Numerous investigations have demonstrated that various Trigonella extractions, both crude and refined, dramatically reduced blood glucose levels in both diabetic individuals and laboratory animals (Nagulapalli et al., 2017). Trigonella has a number of known therapeutic properties, but its hypoglycemic or antihyperglycemic impact has drawn the most attention, and diabetes patients also utilize it for this reason (Zia et al., 2001).

Different Trigonella extract types have been employed by many researchers in experimental models to show that they have hypoglycemic effects. The most current references have been handled here (Baquer et al.,

2011). Soluble Dietary Fiber (SDF) from Trigonella seeds was administered orally to type-2 diabetic rats daily for 28 days. This treatment increased liver glycogen stores and enhanced overall antioxidant status without changing blood insulin levels or insulin production (Hannan et al., 2007). In cultured 3T3-L1 adipocytes, Trigonella improved glucose transport and insulin action. According to these findings, the antidiabetic effects of *T. foenum*-graecum seed-derived SDF are mediated by inhibiting the digestion and absorption of carbohydrates and by increasing peripheral insulin activity (Yadav & Baquer, 2014). It is hypothesized that SDF fraction prevented mice with type 2 diabetes and non-diabetic diabetes from experiencing an increase in blood sugar after consuming oral sucrose (Yadav & Baquer, 2014).

Kannappan and Anuradha found that the insulin-sensitizing properties of polyphenols produced from fenugreek seeds were comparable to those of the well-known diabetic drug metformin in a rat model (Yadav & Baquer, 2014). Experimental rats fed fructose experienced increased levels of glucose, insulin, triglycerides, and free fatty acids, as well as changes in the insulin sensitivity indices, enzyme activity, and glycogen content (Rector et al., 2008). Further evidence that the tyrosine phosphorylation status of these rats has declined comes from the fact that a diet high in fructose causes an increase in Protein Tyrosine Phosphatase (PTP) and a decrease in Protein Tyrosine Kinase (PTK) activities (Jung et al., 2013). The injection of Fenugreek Seed Polyphenolic Extract (FPEt) improved insulin sensitivity and tyrosine phosphorylation status in fructose-fed animals compared to metformin-treated rats. This implies that FPEt improved insulin signaling and sensitivity and supported the cellular functions of insulin (Kilambi & Shah, 2021).

An elevated glucose level has a direct causal link to atherosclerotic changes in diabetics. In a previous investigation (Haffner, 1998), Trigonella leaf extract was found to have a beneficial vascular effect. This investigation looked at how Trigonella leaf extract may change the vascular pathophysiology in diabetic rats. In diabetic rats given Trigonella extract (200 mg/kg; i.p.) every other day for a month, the thoracic aorta's contractile response to KCl and noradrenaline as well as the relaxation response to acetylcholine (ACh) were evaluated (Vaez Mahdavi et al., 2008). When compared to control rats, diabetic rats showed a noticeably higher maximum contractile response to KCl and Na and a significantly lower maximum relaxation response to ACh (Shi et al., 2007). These alterations were dramatically reversed after treatment with Trigonella extract, indicating that it has beneficial effects on the vascular system in diabetic rats (Kumar et al., 2012). The information presented above suggests that Trigonella not only controls glucose levels but also prevents the emergence of further diabetes problems (Yadav & Baquer, 2014). However, these outcomes could be related to improved blood glucose management, which stops the emergence of supplementary problems. Therefore, it would seem that Trigonella's hypoglycemic qualities might be the source of its anti-diabetic benefits (Yadav & Baquer, 2014).

A significant worldwide health problem is the rising prevalence of obesity and the accompanying emergence of several lifestyle diseases that make up metabolic syndrome (Ginsberg & MacCallum, 2009). Obesity is linked to the contemporary urban lifestyle, which includes a calorie-rich diet, a sedentary lifestyle, and a lack of physical exercise. These factors contribute to the build-up of extra fat and abnormal fat metabolism (Willett & Skerrett, 2017). The risk of many chronic inflammatory illnesses, which are brought on by low-grade inflammation linked to obesity, is thought to be considerably reduced by controlling lipid levels, especially those of LDL cholesterol and triglycerides (Friedewald et al., 2009). Trigonella has been shown to modulate lipid levels in experimental models. Fenugreek showed lower blood triglyceride (TG), total cholesterol, and liver lipid contents (Friedewald et al., 2009). Three months of 2.5 g twice daily fenugreek administration to healthy subjects had no impact on blood lipid levels, fasting blood sugar, or postprandial blood sugar (Bordia et al., 1997). However, fenugreek significantly lowered blood lipids, including total cholesterol and triglycerides, when administered in a comparable manner to CVD patients with or without type-2 diabetes, with no impact on HDL cholesterol (Fedacko et al., 2016). In a different experiment, Trigonella-derived SDF improved dyslipidemia and had a propensity to reduce platelet aggregation in type-2 diabetic rats (Yadav & Baquer, 2014). In SDF-fed rats, atherogenic lipids—triglycerides, cholesterol, and LDL cholesterol—significantly decreased while HDL cholesterol rose. Fenugreek seeds' capacity to modulate the activity of many glucose and lipid metabolism enzymes or to increase biliary cholesterol excretion may be responsible for the fenugreek seeds' ability to reduce hepatic lipids (Yadav & Baquer, 2014).

Lipid peroxides (LPO), which are produced during the metabolism of cholesterol and lipid membranes, are involved in the pathogenesis of many illnesses of the aging brain (Vani & Devi, 2005). The concurrent administration of fenugreek seeds powder or extract for five months increased levels of lactate dehydrogenase (LDH) activities and LPO in the posterior brain, liver, and plasma, while reversing total cholesterol, TG, and LDL-cholesterol levels (Yadav & Baquer, 2014). This suggests an antioxidative role in the brain that may be attributed to its modulatory effect on plasma lipid metabolism (Yadav & Baquer, 2014).

Additionally, ethanol extract of Trigonella seed fed to hypercholesterolemic rats caused plasma cholesterol levels to drop by 18 to 26% and liver cholesterol concentrations to drop, indicating a hypocholesterolemia effect (Stark & Madar, 1993). The researchers hypothesized that bile salts in the gastrointestinal tract may have interacted with saponin-like active ingredients in the ethanol extract of fenugreek seeds to change lipid metabolism (Beier & Nigg, 2019). Steroid saponins from fenugreek seeds also altered eating behavior by increasing food intake and incentive to eat as well as lowering plasma cholesterol levels (Petit et al., 1995). Fenugreek has also been shown in recent research to enhance the excretion of total bile acids and cholesterol into the stool while decreasing the levels of hepatic TG and total cholesterol in a dose-dependent manner (Muraki et al., 2011). The liver, plasma TG, and plasma cholesterol concentrations are all known to be impacted by saponins' effects on lipid metabolism. Along with numerous alkaloids, flavonoids (Keservani & Sharma, 2014), and polyphenols, fenugreek seeds also contain saponins (Nagulapalli Venkata et al., 2017). Although the precise chemical mechanism through which fenugreek impacts lipid metabolism is still not understood, it was hypothesized that fenugreek could treat dyslipidemia by lowering the hepatic lipid content in diabetic mice through diosgenin, a saponin derived from Trigonella seeds. This compound prevented TG accumulation and the expression of lipogenic genes in a hepatic cell line (HepG2 cells) by inhibiting the transactivation of the liver X receptor (Naicker, 2017). Further discussion focused on the effects of fenugreek on glycemia and lipidemia, as well as its potential as a functional food and nutraceutical. Researchers claimed that the gum found in fenugreek seeds was associated with hypocholesterolemia (Khorshidian et al., 2016).

Fenugreek or methi, also known as *Trigonella foenum-graecum* L. (family: Fabaceae), is a legume that is frequently used as a condiment to improve the flavor and taste of food (Yadav et al., 2019). Its water-soluble compound GII extract from the seeds increased the amount of glycogen in the liver and muscles and stimulated the activity of several enzymes, including hexokinase, glucokinase, pyruvate kinase, malic enzyme, glucose-6-phosphate dehydrogenase, and superoxide dismutase, in sub-diabetic and moderately diabetic rabbits for 15 days and in severely diabetic rabbit. Pancreatic cells that had been partially damaged were also repaired after treatment with GII (Pomeranz & Meloan, 1994). Trigonelline, nicotinic acid, and coumarin are anti-diabetic phytochemicals that were extracted from fenugreek seeds.

These three antidiabetic substances from fenugreek showed excellent results in rabbit models of severe and mild diabetes that were induced by alloxan (Khan et al., 2018). According to a meta-analysis of 10 clinical studies on type 2 diabetes patients, fenugreek may significantly improve glycemic management by modifying indicators, such as fasting blood glucose level by–0.96 mmol/l, HbA1c value by–0.85%, and 2-hour postprandial glucose level by –2.19 mmol/l (DeFronzo, 1999). In a 2-month double-blind placebo-controlled trial on 25 subjects with type 2 diabetes mellitus, hydroalcoholic extract of fenugreek seed decreased insulin resistance compared to the control, as shown by an increase in insulin sensitivity percentage (112.9% vs 92.2%, respectively) and beta-cell secretion percentage (86.3% vs 70.1%, respectively) through the HOMA-IR test (Bashtian et al., 2013).

9.5.2 *CAMELLIA SINENSIS* (WHITE TEA)

White tea and other forms of tea are produced by the *Camellia sinensis* tea plant (green, oolong, and black). White tea is made only once a year, in the spring, from freshly harvested tea leaves (Ahmed & Stepp, 2013). When growing, immature tea leaves may be protected from the sun to produce less chlorophyll and produce white tea (Ahmed & Stepp, 2013). White tea has a broad variety of physiological and pharmacological effects, including antioxidant, anti-inflammatory, and anticancer capabilities (Hinojosa-Nogueria, 2021). There were reports of anti-atherogenic, anti-hypertensive, hypolipidemic, and hypocholesterolemic effects (Velayutham et al., 2008). According to some research, oolong tea and black tea may help mice with alcoholic fatty liver disease by controlling their gut flora. Proteins, minerals, and amino acids are all present in white tea. The primary ingredients in white tea are gallic acid, caffeine, and catechins (Jiang et al., 2019).

9.5.2.1 EFFECT OF WHITE TEA AND ITS CONSTITUENTS ON OBESITY

White, green, and black tea have reportedly been shown to suppress pancreatic lipase activity. Compared to the other varieties, white tea was more efficient. Flavan-3-ol content in white and green teas is about equal. Flavanols are abundant in green tea. Additionally, white tea contains considerable amounts of strictinin, trigalloyl glucose, and digalloyl glucose (Sajilata et al., 2008).

Preadipocytes were incubated with 0.1%, 0.25%, 0.5%, and 0.75% white tea extract, which significantly decreased TG throughout adipogenesis without affecting cell viability. Tea extract also showed lipolytic activity by increasing the amount of free glycerol (32 g/ml) in treated cells in comparison to control cells (Lahrita, 2018). Tea extract decreased the expression of SIRT1 mRNA and ADD1/SREBP-1c protein during adipogenesis when compared to control cells (Söhle et al., 2009). These results show that white tea greatly inhibits adipogenesis and boosts lipolysis activity. White tea extract (2%) with a high catechin content reduced glucose and cholesterol absorption while increasing HDL levels and LDL receptor binding activity (Nishiumi et al., 2010). It has also been demonstrated that tea extract can successfully lower TG levels and lipase activity in HepG2 cell lines (Marrelli et al., 2016). Aqueous white tea extract (1.5%) for 30 days drastically decreased blood levels of glucose, LDL, cholesterol, and TG while raising levels of HDL when compared to control diabetic rats (Juárez-Rojop et al., 2012).

We investigated the impact of teas on the plasma bile acid profile (BAs). White, green, and oolong tea consumption increased plasma levels of muri-cholic acid, glycocholic acid, taurochenodeoxycholic acid, glycodeoxycholic acid, tauromuricholic acid, tauroursodeoxycholic acid, and taurocholic acid in comparison to controls while lowering levels of isolithocholic acid and taurolithocholic acid (Anaeigoudari et al., 2021). The bile acid metabolism was changed by teas, and this modification may have contributed to the health benefits of teas (Mai et al., 2004). White tea extract (0.5%) was administered to male mice that were fed a high-fat diet and saw a reduction in blood TG. White tea extract reduces oxidative stress in the liver and adipose tissue. Additionally, tea extract did not aid animals in consuming less food or losing weight (Bae et al., 2018).

The effects of white tea polysaccharide and polyphenol (400 or 800 mg/kg) were studied on rats fed a high-fat diet for six weeks. These components slowed the accumulation of body fat and weight gain (Wu et al., 2018). In addition, polyphenols and polysaccharides raised blood lipid and antioxidant index levels, lowered serum leptin levels, and enhanced the expression of the IL-6 and TNF-α genes (Xu et al., 2015).

In lowering blood leptin levels, polysaccharides and polyphenols also show synergistic benefits. These findings suggest that a possible treatment for obesity would include combining polysaccharides and polyphenols (Chen et al., 2016).

After receiving either low- or high-fat supplemented meals (5% and 30% triglyceride, respectively) for a month, mice's body weight, visceral fat, and hepatic fat accumulation, as well as the onset of hyperinsulinemia and hyperleptinemia, all significantly decreased (Rahman et al., 2017). Additionally, catechin treatment significantly increased the mRNA expression and oxidation activity of the liver's acyl-CoA oxidase and medium-chain acyl-CoA dehydrogenases (Hiršová, 2013). When compared to the starting point, the 12-week administration of catechins (118.5 and 483.0 mg/day) to healthy male subjects aged 27 to 47 resulted in significant decreases in BMI, waist circumference, body fat ratio, abdominal fat, total cholesterol, glucose, and plasminogen activator inhibitor-1 (PAI-1) in the serum (Hase et al., 2001).

Treatment of an overweight participant (n = 107) with a beverage containing 625 mg of catechins and 39 mg of caffeine resulted in a bodyweight decrease over the course of 12 weeks compared to the control group (39 mg of caffeine). The catechin group experienced greater percentage changes in fasting serum TG, total abdominal fat, and subcutaneous abdominal fat compared to the control group (Maki et al., 2009).

9.5.2.2 EFFECT OF WHITE TEA AND ITS CONSTITUENT ON DIABETES

Aqueous white tea extracts (0.5%) administered to normal control or diabetic control rats dramatically enhanced drink consumption (Al-Shiekh et al., 2014). Tea extracts significantly lowered blood glucose levels and improved glucose tolerance when compared to the diabetic group (Aybar et al., 2001). The white tea group had much lower total and LDL cholesterol compared to the diabetic rats, but liver weight and glycogen were considerably increased (Islam, 2011). The mRNA and protein expression levels of the glucose transporters GLUT1 and GLUT3 in the cardiac tissue of prediabetic rats were markedly increased by consuming white tea (1%). Additionally, administration of white tea raised cardiac acetate and alanine levels, ferric's antioxidant power, lactate dehydrogenase (LDH) expression and activity, and ferric's antioxidant capacity (Dias, 2019). The regular intake of white tea (1%) increased glucose tolerance and insulin sensitivity. Additionally, tea extract decreased the expression levels of the proteins GLUT1 and GLUT3 in the brains of prediabetic rats (Nunes et al., 2015). Additionally, tea extract increased antioxidant activity and lowered lipid peroxidation and protein oxidation in the cortex of prediabetic rats.

Diabetic rats fed with white tea extract (2%) exhibited significantly greater blood and liver levels of glutathione peroxidase (GSH-px), superoxide dismutase (SOD), and catalase (CAT) compared to the diabetic control group (Zidan et al., 2019). The effect of white tea ethanolic extract (WTE) on this decrease was investigated in diabetic rats by intravenous administration of WTE (100 mg/kg, BW) for 14 days (Prabhu et al., 2009). These advantages are brought about by catechins, a flavonoid molecule found in tea extract. When rats with diabetes were given catechins (25 and 50 mg/kg), the rodents' body weight changed. Catechins significantly reduced heart hypertrophy, matrix metallopeptidase 9 (MMP-9) levels, and plasma glucose levels (Velayutham et al., 2008). Additionally, catechin decreased the indicators of neuronal oxidative stress. (+)-catechin (0.2, 1.0, and 5.0 mmol/L) significantly reduced renal dysfunction and exhibited protective effects against structural nephropathies when administered to type 2 diabetic mice for 16 weeks (Vatharajan, 2016). Additionally, in diabetic mice, catechin decreased NF-B p65 phosphorylation and pro-inflammatory mediators including TNF-α and IL-1β.

Giving type 2 diabetes patients 96.3 mg of beverages high in catechins daily for 12 weeks was found to significantly reduce waist circumference when compared to the control group in a double-blind controlled study (Suzuki et al., 2016). Additionally, catechin markedly increased adiponectin and insulin levels in comparison to the control group. Drinking beverages containing catechin (540–588 mg) for 12 weeks significantly reduced body weight, waist circumference, visceral fat, and visceral fat area in six human investigations (n = 921, 505 men) (Wolfram, 2007). These results suggested that white tea and catechin may reduce the risk of metabolic syndrome by reducing abdominal fat (MetS) (Yang et al., 2016). Healthy postmenopausal women who drank catechin-rich beverages (615 mg/350 ml) daily for four weeks had postprandial glucose levels and serum postprandial thioredoxin drop by 3% and 5%, respectively, in comparison to the placebo group (Di Lorenzo et al., 2017). Furthermore, catechins increased antioxidant activity and reduced protein oxidation.

9.5.3 *CINNAMOMUM CASSIA*

In addition to blood glucose, cinnamon has also been shown to have favorable effects on other indicators of metabolic syndrome. Both spontaneously hypertensive rats and individuals with metabolic syndrome (22 men and women given a 500 mg extract daily for 12 weeks) effectively used cinnamon extract to reduce their blood pressure (Roussel et al., 2009). Additionally,

Wistar rats on a high-fructose diet and some clinical studies revealed that cinnamon has triglyceride-lowering benefits (Aguiar et al., 2019). For instance, serum triglycerides, LDL-cholesterol, and total cholesterol were all significantly reduced in the trial in Pakistani patients with type 2 diabetes described in the preceding paragraph (Graf et al., 2010), despite the fact that these effects were not supported by findings from a trial in a less severely diabetic European population that received a similar dose of cinnamon.

In their experiments, Cao et al. looked into the impact of *C. burmannii* extract and cinnamon polyphenols (CP) on the expression of the insulin receptor, glucose transporter 4 (GLUT4), and tristetraprolin (TTP/ZFP36) in adipocytes. Aqueous extract and CP both increased the expression of GLUT4 and TTP in the lipid tissues, according to Western blotting, which also showed that CP increased IR levels (Al-Dhubiab, 2012). Real-time PCR analysis demonstrates that aqueous extracts (100 g/mL) rapidly increase adipocyte TTP mRNA by a factor of about 6. At higher *C. burmannii* concentrations, IR protein and mRNA levels were actually decreased. The study concluded that the plant may be able to enhance various metabolic processes, including insulin response, glucose transmembrane transport, and anti-inflammatory properties. According to Sheng et al.'s research, cinnamon temporarily and competitively inhibits the alpha-glucosidase enzyme, which helps to lessen the signs and symptoms of streptozotocin-induced diabetes in rats. The anti-diabetic activities of cinnamon are thought to be a result of the B and A type procyanidins oligomers that are prevalent in the extracts of *C. cassia* and *C. tammala* (Udrea et al., 2021), according to studies by Chen et al. They discovered that the two cinnamon extracts had anti-diabetic properties in this investigation utilizing the diabetic (db/db) mouse model, which is a typical animal model for type 2 diabetes. Studies on the histopathology of the pancreas, liver, and adipose tissue revealed that *C. cassia* encouraged lipid build-up in the liver and adipose tissue whereas *C. tammala* increased the blood's concentration of insulin and the pancreas' ability to produce it (Aggarwal & Heber, 2014).

While conflicting results were still being observed regarding evidence from only a few clinical trials, Ranasinghe et al. and Bandara et al. conducted a systematic review on the effects of *Cinnamon zeylanicum* and *Cinnamon aromaticum* on diabetes mellitus and found a number of beneficial effects both *in vitro* and *in vivo* (Medagama, 2015). *C. zeylanicum* reduced intestinal glucose absorption by inhibiting the actions of α-glucosidase and β-amylase *in vitro*. By directly expressing the glucose transporter-4, it also encourages insulin release, prevents gluconeogenesis, and improves cellular glucose absorption

(Rivera-Yañez et al., 2020). The body benefits from *C. zeylanicum*, which also raises insulin levels, raises HDL cholesterol, lowers fasting blood sugar, and prevents diabetes-related weight loss (Governa et al., 2018). *C. zeylanicum* also effectively reduced metabolic issues connected to insulin resistance and the consequences of diabetic neuropathy and nephropathy without the adverse effects of drug-induced liver destruction (Arozal et al., 2020).

Additionally, 58 people with type 2 diabetes who had HbA1c levels higher than 7% took part in a placebo-controlled, double-blind clinical study during which they received a placebo, hypoglycemic drugs, and 2 g of cinnamon every day for 12 weeks. At the end of the trial, HbA1c was significantly lower in the cinnamon group (8.22–7.86%) than in the placebo group (8.55–8.68%). Systolic and diastolic blood pressure in the cinnamon-treated group were lower on average than in the placebo group (SBP = 132.6–129.2 mmHg; DBP = 85.2–80.2 mmHg).

Waist circumference, fasting plasma glucose, and body mass index all decreased statistically significantly in the cinnamon group at month three compared to baseline; however, the changes were similar to those observed in the placebo group, and there were no discernible differences in the total lipid profiles (Borzoei et al., 2018). A distinct clinical experiment revealed the efficiency and safety of a novel bioactive chemical (DLBS3233) produced from *Lagerstroemia speciosa* and *Cinnamomum burmannii* in enhancing insulin sensitivity and cell physiological function in people with impaired glucose tolerance (Arozal et al., 2020). The HOMA-IR index's lower value signifies that DLBS3233 treated insulin resistance more well than the placebo did. Restoration of the two-phase insulin secretion was consistently better in the DLBS3233 group (Arozal et al., 2020). Additionally, DLBS3233 has no known adverse side effects and produces a significantly higher oral disposition index than the placebo. The opposite result was found in a second double-blind, randomized, and placebo-controlled clinical experiment with patients with type 2 diabetes who either took a 3 g/day cinnamon supplement or a control group. At the end of the intervention, neither group's insulin, HbA1c, carboxymethyl lysine, total antioxidant capacity, nor group differences in malondialdehyde levels were significantly different from one another (Candidate et al., 2018).

9.5.4 *MURRAYA KOENIGII*

Curry leaves are the common name for Murraya koenigii (M. koenigii; L. spreng; Family: Rutaceae). M. koenigii is widely distributed across the world's tropical and subtropical climates. Only two of the 14 Murraya species found worldwide, M. koenigii and M. paniculata, may be found in India (Ibrahim et al., 2022). Due to its broad range of traditional medicinal characteristics, M. koenigii is highly significant. This plant, also known as "krishnanimba," has been utilized for ages in a variety of ways and occupies a special position in Indian Ayurvedic treatment (Suthar et al., 2021). Among its various parts, M. koenigii's leaves, roots, bark, and fruit are known to support a number of biological functions. The flavor and other qualities of the aromatic bioactive components in M. koenigii leaves are maintained even after drying. The leaves of M. koenigii have a somewhat acidic flavor and aroma and a little bitter taste. In Indian cuisine, they are employed as anthelmintics, analgesics, digestives, and appetizers. The green leaves of M. koenigii are used to treat edema, bruising, piles, diarrhea, inflammation, itching, and new wounds. Somewhat purgative are the roots. They are energizing and used to treat typical bodily ailments. Snake bites may be treated using the bark (Vidhya et al., 2021). The essential oil extracted from M. koenigii leaves has been shown in experiments on animal models to have antioxidative, hepatoprotective, antibacterial, antifungal, anti-inflammatory, and nephroprotective activities. The therapeutic qualities of M. koenigii have been attributed to the chemical makeup of several carbazole alkaloids and other important metabolites, such as terpenoids, flavonoids, phenolics, carbohydrates, carotenoids, vitamins, and nicotinic acid from various portions of the M. koenigii plant (Khan, 2017).

The use of M. koenigii in conventional medications and DIY treatments has received more attention in recent years. However, little investigation has been done to determine the medicinal and pharmacological effectiveness of M. koenigii in promoting health benefits and treating illness (Abeysinghe et al., 2021). This review will go over the pharmacological effects of M. koenigii's bioactive components and traditional medicinal usage. In order to provide information on the most recent findings that might guide future research, this review seeks to provide a well-managed synthesis of the available studies together with potential recommendations. Therefore, the present review will describe and cover prior and current key works on M. koenigii linked to the themes chosen rather than covering a small number of carefully chosen studies over a short period of time. The information will be methodically sorted, contrasted, and summarized, including phytochemical screening, identification, and pharmacological actions. We predict that all of these efforts will result in a useful synthesis of pharmacological activity that will start off future views in the clearest possible way (Sen & Samanta, 2014).

Due to their affordability, medicinal herbs are most often used in underdeveloped nations to manage diabetes mellitus. Diabetes mellitus is a metabolic disorder that poses a serious risk to human health. In recent years, a variety of plant phytochemicals with anti-diabetic effects have been discovered (Patel et al., 2012). Alkaloids from M. koenigii leaves have been studied for their potential to extend anti-diabetic effects and have been found to inhibit the aldose reductase enzyme, glucose utilization, and other enzyme systems (Malode et al., 2021). M. koenigii was examined for its ability to block α-glucosidase, and this ability was discovered. Patients with type 2 diabetes often get therapy with alpha-glucosidase inhibitors. According to research, M. koenigii's ethanolic extract significantly lowered blood sugar levels. M. koenigii's ability to reduce blood sugar levels is mediated by its antioxidant properties and insulin-like actions. Additionally, M. koenigii showed a potent antioxidant effect by reducing malondialdehyde (MDA), increasing glutathione (GSH), and significantly reducing the homeostatic model assessment (HOMA)-insulin resistance index. Overall, it is evident that M. koenigii has antidiabetic and antioxidant benefits in rats.

9.5.5 *PUNICA GRANATUM (POMEGRANATE)*

9.5.5.1 *EFFECTS OF POMEGRANATE ON T2DM DYSLIPIDEMIA IS TYPICAL FEATURE OF TYPE 2 DIABETES*

Increased ectopic triglyceride accumulation in peripheral tissues as a result of increased FFA, which mostly comes from lipolytic adipose tissue or high-calorie intake, furthered the development of insulin resistance (Fabbrini et al., 2010). Pomegranate extracts showed the largest effect on these levels among a variety of fruit extracts, including apple, strawberry, guava, papaya, and orange. Pomegranate ellagic acid was shown to lower plasma total cholesterol and triglyceride levels in rats given the HFD in a dose-dependent manner (Hou et al., 2019a). Additionally, it was demonstrated that pomegranate flower extracts reduced blood total cholesterol, triglycerides, LDL-C, and VLDL-C while increasing HDL-C in diabetic rats receiving the medication streptozotocin (STZ). Despite the fact that pomegranate seed extract did not appear to improve dyslipidemia in T2DM, the administration of pomegranate seed oil, which contains 9-cis, 11-trans, and 13-cis conjugated linolenic acid, reduced the accumulated hepatic triacylglycerol in Otsuka Long-Evans Tokushima Fatty (OLETF) rats and significantly increased insulin sensitivity (Hou et al., 2019a). This effect may be a result of the considerable distinctions between humans and other animals, especially those in physiology and metabolism, but it also paves the way for future therapeutic research on pomegranates (Turrini et al., 2015).

In type 2 diabetic rats, only pomegranate seed oil significantly reduced insulin resistance, and the advantages were on par with those of the medicine serving as the positive control, rosiglitazone. This is held for pomegranate bloom, peel, and seed extracts (Duke, 2009). Since adipose tissue is an important site for energy storage and a significant source of plasma FFA, it plays a significant role in determining total insulin sensitivity (Ruan & Lodish, 2003). The processes of lipogenesis and lipolysis in adipocytes influence triacylglycerol synthesis and breakdown in addition to serving as two regulatory targets for a number of pharmaceuticals or herbal remedies used to treat type 2 diabetes. Some T2DM treatments prevent excessive lipid accumulation by blocking adipocyte lipolysis, which also prevents ectopic lipid storage and insulin resistance (Boren et al., 2013). In the adipose tissue of obese rats given an HFD, ingestion of pomegranate vinegar decreased the levels of mRNA expression for the protein's sterol regulatory element binding protein-1c (SREBP-1c) and peroxisome proliferator-activated receptor (PPAR) (Choi et al., 2020). Pomegranate juice suppressed both lipogenesis and lipolysis in human adipose tissue and adipocytes from mice and people, according to Les and colleagues.

Furthermore, it was found in the same study that punicalagin and ellagic acid only suppressed lipolysis in a dose-dependent manner. According to these findings, pomegranate extracts control the lipid metabolism in adipose tissue, and the variations in outcomes show that different pomegranate active ingredients serve a variety of purposes. The same researchers then found that decreasing triglyceride levels and the expression of genes essential for adipocyte formation in 3T3-L1 mouse pre-adipocytes led to the discovery that urolithin A, an ellagic acid metabolite produced by colon microflora, had anti-adipogenic properties (Johanningsmeier & Harris, 2011). Urolithin A, a chemical that affects the gut flora physiologically, is likely to be produced by an active component in pomegranate extracts. Diabetes causes an increase in fatty acid intake and oxidation in the heart, which causes cardiac fat to accumulate and eventually cause cardiac dysfunction. In Zucker diabetic rats, oral administration of pomegranate flower extracts decreased cardiac mRNA expression levels of the enzyme's carnitine palmitoyl transferase 1 and PPAR, as well as heart triglyceride content, plasma triglyceride, and total cholesterol (CPT-1) (Xu et al., 2009). The results also showed that, in contrast to gallic and ursolic acids, only oleanolic acid, one of the primary components of pomegranate flower extracts, had PPAR activator capabilities. This study implies that PPAR activation and the reduction of myocardial lipid uptake in diabetes are related to the beneficial effects of pomegranate flower extracts (Katz et al., 2007). Additionally, it has been demonstrated that pomegranate extracts containing 40% punicalagin enhance mitochondrial function and activate cardiac AMPK signaling in rats receiving the HFD, which lowers cardiac triglyceride, total cholesterol, and myocardial damage (AlMatar et al., 2018).

9.5.6 *LAGENARIA SICERARIA*

In India and other tropical and subtropical areas of the globe, *Lagenaria siceraria*, often known as bottle gourd and a member of the Cucurbitaceae family, is widely cultivated. The bottle gourd contains phytoconstituents, minerals, vitamins, fiber, and other nutrients that have powerful nutraceutical and therapeutic effects (Mustafa, 2020). The plant's specific portions are used to cure conditions including headaches and baldness, among others. According to reports, *L. siceraria* has hepatoprotective, immunomodulatory, analgesic, anti-inflammatory, anti-hyperlipidemic, antioxidant, and anti-hyperglycemic effects on people. There are many recognized varieties of *L. siceraria*; the sweet version is often used as a vegetable and to make sweets and pickles, while the wild species is favored for medicinal purposes. One method used in India to treat issues linked to obesity is to consume one or two glasses of raw bottled gourd juice in the morning on an empty stomach (Saeed et al., 2022).

The effectiveness of vacuum-dried fruit juice extract and methanol extract as diuretics was studied in albino rats. Evaluation of a variety of factors, including total urine volume and electrolyte concentrations in urine such as sodium, potassium, and chloride. Rats treated with vacuum-dried juice extract and methanol extract (100–200 mg/kg; p.o.) showed larger urine contents when compared to the comparable controls. Electrolyte excretion increased dose-dependently in both juice and methanol extract when compared to controls. It was statistically significant that juice and methanol extract both exhibited more diuretic potential than the regularly used diuretic medicine furosemide (20 mg/kg; i.p.).

9.5.7 *EMBLICA OFFICINALIS*

Protein, fat, and minerals like iron, calcium, and phosphorus are all present in amla fruits in varying amounts (2.0–4.5, 2.1–3.1, and 0.2–0.6 g/100 g DW, respectively). More than 70 g/100 g of the dry weight (DW) of amla fruits include carbohydrates. Another crucial element is fiber (7.2–16.5 g/100 g DW). Numerous studies have linked the cultivar to variations in the amla fruit's chemical makeup. Ascorbic acid is a further crucial element present in amla fruit (vitamin C). Various studies evaluating various amla varieties have found values ranging from 193 to 720 mg/100 g (Carr et al., 2021; Hussain et al., 2021; Jain et al., 2004; Saeed et al., 2022; Tarwadi et al., 2007). Despite the fact that the ideal recommended daily intake has not yet been established due to the urgency of new factors from modern society, many governmental health authorities around the world established Recommended Dietary Allowance (minimum level to meet the needs of a healthy person for a day), which ranges between 40 and 110 mg vitamin C/day (Nampoothiri et al., 2011). Furthermore, the health authorities in China and Australia have recommended a daily intake of 190–220 mg. This means that consuming a serving size of at least 100 g of fresh amla fruits (2–3 pieces) from any of the varieties listed in Table 9.1 will provide the daily requirement for vitamin C. *P. emblica* L. juice may have more vitamin C than other fruits like apple, lime, pomegranate, and some varieties of grapes (188,189). Other nutrients in amla fruits include calcium, iron, and vitamins A, B1, and E (290 IU, 30 mg/100 g, and 0.17 mg/100 g, respectively) (Ansari et al., 2014).

Diabetes Prevention Diabetes protection has been linked to the naturally occurring chemicals in *P. Emblica* L. According to *in vitro* research, major enzymes involved in the digestion of glucose, namely amylase and glucosidase, were less active when the principal phytochemicals contained in amlas, such as ellagic acid and ascorbic acid, were present. The benefits of diabetes prevention have also been demonstrated in animals. When fed 1.25 g/kg of a freeze-dried *P. emblica* L. aqueous extract, diabetic long Evan male mice (induced by streptozotocin) exhibited decreased levels of blood glucose and triglycerides (Ansari et al., 2014). Similar to this, Patel & Goyal (2011) pointed out the antidiabetic potential of *P. emblica* L. juice (1 mL/kg/day) due to the fact that the animals with induced diabetes experienced a more gradual rise in blood glucose levels. In a second experiment, dosages of 250 and 500 mg/kg of ellagic acid-rich *P. emblica* L. extract dramatically reduced blood glucose levels and increased serum insulin levels in diabetic mice (Fatima et al., 2017). In the experiment run by Nain et al., the phytochemical extracted from *P. emblica* L. leaves produced similar findings (Nain et al., 2012). According to these scientists, diabetic mice received daily doses of between 100 and 400 mg/kg, which caused an increase in serum insulin and a commensurate drop in blood glucose. Clinical studies also indicate the benefits of amla phytochemicals for diabetes patients' health.

For instance, diabetic individuals receiving daily doses of up to 3 g of *P. emblica* L. powder extract after 21 days of the study exhibited decreased blood glucose levels (Akhtar et al., 2011). After discovering that daily administration of 10 g of amla powder for 90 days dramatically reduced blood glucose levels in diabetic individuals, Walia et al. (2015) found a similar outcome. Additionally, a flavonoid-rich extract from *P. emblica* L. reduced the prevalence of neuropathy in diabetics (Kumar et al., 2015). The bioactive ingredients in amla seem to be essential for treating diabetes, especially for assisting in restoring insulin and glucose levels.

9.5.8 *VIGNA MUNGO*

The mung bean (*Vigna radiata* L.) is a significant pulse that is consumed all over the world but is most popular in Asian countries. It has a long history of use in traditional medicine. It is a well-liked functional food for promoting excellent health because it is a well-known wonderful source of protein, dietary fiber, minerals, vitamins, and significant amounts of bioactive components, such as polyphenols, polysaccharides, and peptides (Zaidel et al., 2021). According to research, the mung bean possesses hepatoprotective and immunomodulatory qualities, the capacity to lower hyperglycemia, hyperlipemia, and hypertension, as well as the ability to prevent cancer and melanogenesis. These health benefits are primarily brought about by the quantity and kind of active compounds present in mung beans (Zhang et al., 2022). Vitexin and isovitexin are the two primary polyphenols contained in mung beans, and peptides with hydrophobic amino acid residues and low molecular weight have higher bioactivity. Considering the surge in interest in using grain legumes currently (Hou et al., 2019b).

Hyperlipidemia and atherosclerosis are currently the two main causes of heart disease and mortality. A key risk factor for the emergence of hyperlipidemia and coronary heart disease is a high plasma cholesterol level. Maintaining the body's regular functions requires lowering the elevated serum cholesterol to an appropriate level. Mung bean consumption has been connected in studies to altered lipid metabolism (Connor & Connor, 1972). In hamsters fed a high-cholesterol diet, mung bean protein was found to dose-dependently lower plasma lipid levels, including total cholesterol (TC), triglycerides (TG), and non-high-density lipoprotein cholesterol (non-HDL-C) (Hou et al., 2019b). This effect was partially mediated by the up-regulation of 3-hydroxy-3-methyl glutaryl coenzyme A reductase and cholesterol-7-hydroxylase (CYP7A1). According to one theory, mung bean protein lowers cholesterol by reducing cholesterol synthesis and absorption while increasing bile acid and sterol excretion in feces (Macarulla et al., 2001). In a different study, it was discovered that the mung bean's vitexin, isovitexin, and ethanolic extracts significantly decreased fat accumulation in both *in vitro* and animal studies by lowering the expression of genes linked to fat storage, such as acetyl-CoA carboxylase, a rate-limiting enzyme of fatty acid synthesis, peroxisome proliferator-activated receptor, and CCAAT/ enhancer binding protein alpha, a liver-enriched (Mehta et al., 2021). It was hypothesized that the activation of the MEK/ERK signaling pathway served as a mediator for the suppression of adipogenic gene expression.

9.5.9 *MOMORDICA CHARANTIA*

M. charantia, a flowering vine in the Cucurbitaceae family, is also referred to as bitter melon or bitter gourd. Because of its extremely bitter fruits, which are frequently used in cooking and as a natural remedy for diabetes, this tropical plant is widely grown throughout Asia, India, East Africa, and South America (Abasca et al., 2005). It is a perennial climbing plant with elongated fruits that have a knobby surface and an average height of 5 meters. It is one of the best plants for treating diabetes and a beneficial dietary and medicinal plant for human health (Kinara et al., 2016).

Diabetes has been successfully treated throughout the globe using plant-based medication. In fact, this may be the only kind of treatment accessible to diabetes patients in many regions of the globe, particularly in developing nations (Smokovski et al., 2015). There are several evaluations of herbal remedies for diabetes written by various writers. Numerous plants that are utilized as herbal medicines are described in Ayurveda and other traditional medical systems for the treatment of diabetes. Due to their cheap cost and lack of adverse effects, they thus play a significant part in alternative medicine. According to reports, the active ingredients found in medicinal plants have the ability to regenerate pancreas cells, release insulin, and combat the issue of insulin resistance. The etiology of the emergence of diabetic complications includes hyperglycemia (Tiwari & Rao, 2002). Herbs that lower blood sugar levels promote insulin secretion, improve adipose or muscle tissue's ability to absorb glucose and reduce the liver's ability to produce glucose. The main treatment tools continue to be insulin and oral hypoglycemic medications such as sulfonylureas and biguanides, although efforts are being made to create more potent anti-diabetic drugs. Numerous conventional herbal therapies have been used to treat diabetes in Asia and other developing countries. *M. charantia* is one of the plants that has been thoroughly investigated for the treatment of diabetes. *M. charantia*, one of the most promising plants for diabetes currently, has a long history of use that is supported by the latest scientific studies on its beneficial effects. According to studies on the traditional use of *M. charantia* in India, it is one of the most important plants for lowering blood glucose levels in diabetic patients (Zhang et al., 2016).

9.5.10 LAGERSTROEMIA SPECIOSE

A shrub to a big tree belonging to the Lythraceae family, *Lagerstroemia speciosa* has several stems or trunks that branch out slightly above the ground. Carlos Linnaeus provided the first description of the genus *Lagerstroemia.* The term Lagerstroemia honors Swedish scientist Magnus von Lagerstroem, who sent Linnaeus samples from the East (Harrison, 2009). The popular names for *Lagerstroemia speciosa* in the Philippines are Banaba plant, huge crape myrtle, and queen's crape myrtle. It also goes by the name "pride of India." In the Philippines, India, and Malaysia, Banaba is readily available (Mathias, 1985). The fruits are subglobose capsule-shaped and range in length from 2.2 to 3.0 cm. Ellagitannins and similar substances found in the leaves and fruits of *Lagerstroemia speciosa* are among its chemical components. Methionine, isoleucine, alpha-amino butyric acid, and alanine are all present in leaf extracts, but no alkaloids, glucosides, sterols, or flavonoids are (Bijauliya et al., 2017). Additionally, 3-O-methylellagic acid, new tannin-lager tannin, ellagic acid, 3,3,4-tri-O-methylellagic acid, beta-sitosterol, and amyl alcohol are present in the leaves. A person with diabetes has high blood sugar levels as a result of either insufficient pancreatic insulin synthesis or inefficient cell responses to insulin. The leaves of the *Lagerstroemia speciosa* plant have a great deal of therapeutic promise, especially for the treatment of diabetes. The leaves are 10–20 cm long, acuminate, and elliptic or oblong-lanceolate. Extracts from the leaves of *Lagerstroemia speciosa* have been used in traditional medicine to treat diabetes since they were first made public in a study published in 1940. According to authorities, obesity is one of the most serious public health problems of the 21st century because it is a leading preventable cause of death worldwide and is becoming more common in both adults and children (Çakmur, 2017). Banaba extracts have no negative side effects and are a potent anti-obesity action. As a result of the search for a treatment for various ailments, including diabetes and obesity, among others, several therapeutic agents have been created. Ironically, though, their usage was restricted due to their many negative side effects and ineffectiveness. The hunt for more powerful agents is still ongoing, and the Lagerstroemia species is one among them (Tundis et al., 2010).

Hypoglycemic and anti-diabetic effects. Murakami et al. examined *Lagerstroemia speciosa* in the Ehrlich ascites of the tumor cells in 1993. They found that corosolic acid reduced blood sugar levels generally by activating glucose transport. The potential for treating type 2 diabetes was investigated by Judy et al. in 2003 using a standardized extract (glucosol) from the leaves of Lagerstroemia speciosa. Models that have a dose-response structure (Oboh et al., 2021). They discovered that two weeks of daily glucosol doses of 32 mg and 48 mg resulted in a considerable drop in blood glucose levels. Tanquilut et al. (2009) investigated the hypoglycemic effects of *Lagerstroemia speciosa* pers on alloxan-induced diabetic mice. Studies indicate that *Lagerstroemia speciosa* has a favorable antihyperglycemic effect that aids in controlling the high glucose levels in mice with alloxan-induced diabetes (Tanquilut et al., 2009). Saha et al. in 2009 looked into the mechanism of action of the hypoglycemic effect of *Lagerstroemia speciosa* leaf extract on streptozotocin-induced diabetic rats. They concluded that the strong hypoglycemic action of the hot water extract of *Lagerstroemia speciosa* leaves on experimental diabetic rats was caused by the inhibition of gluconeogenesis and the activation of glucose oxidation through the pentose phosphate pathway (Stohs et al., 2012). In a study by Amornnat et al. in 2009, diabetic rats underwent an experiment, and the researchers discovered that water extract from *Lagerstroemia speciosa* leaves may lower the rats' fasting blood glucose levels. An investigation on the increase of glucose absorption in L8 myotubes by the extract from *Lagerstroemia speciosa* was conducted by Niwat & Juntipa in 2009. The findings imply that the activity of *Lagerstroemia speciosa* leaves may be predominantly mediated by the production of novel transporters and may include both insulin-dependent and independent pathways. *Lagerstroemia speciosa* (Banaba), according to Cheolin Park & Jae-Sik Lee in 2011, is a natural treatment for diabetic patients because it is crucial in controlling the blood levels of insulin and sugar. The antidiabetic action was thus established (Kotnala et al., 2013). Banaba (Lagerstroemia speciosa) and its active ingredient, corosolic acid, were used in Miura et al. (2012) research on managing diabetes and its complications. They discovered that corosolic acid had antioxidant and antihyperlipidemic properties in addition to lowering blood sugar levels in humans within 60 minutes (Stohs et al., 2012).

9.6 DIFFERENT TYPES OF PHYTOCHEMICAL COMPOUNDS USED IN THE MANAGEMENT OF METABOLIC SYNDROME AND RELATED DISORDERS

9.6.1 *BETANIN*

The water-soluble red pigment betanin, also known as phytolaccamin ($C_{24}H_{27}N_2O_{13}$), is found in the roots of beetroot, Beta vulgaris L. It is identified as a food additive by its E number. When exposed to light, heat, and oxygen, betanin degrades; hence it is used in frozen items, perishable goods, and products that are sold in dry form. The hue of betanin is determined between a pH of 4 and 5. At first bright bluish-red, it gradually turns blue-violet as the pH increases. As the pH increases to alkaline values, betanin is hydrolyzed. Beetroot, an annual or biennial cultivar of *Beta vulgaris* subsp. *Vulgaris conditiva* which has spread over the world from the Americas to Europe and Asia, includes a variety of delectable taproots produced in the Middle East. It is considered to be a rich and nutritious source with health-promoting properties, including antioxidant and anti-inflammatory effects, anticarcinogenic and antidiabetic activities, hepatoprotective, hypotensive, and wound healing capacities. Beetroot is being employed as a useful ingredient in the production of numerous dishes as a result (Şanlier et al., 2019). Notably, the bulk of current studies on beetroot supplementation, particularly those concentrating on its hypotensive and ergogenic properties, underlined the critical role of inorganic NO_3 in the therapeutic influence of this crop and its byproducts (Lim, 2016). Numerous interventional studies from a small body of literature have examined the effects of beetroot and its byproducts on systolic and diastolic blood pressure, vascular and endothelial function, insulin, and glucose responses in the context of glycemic homeostasis, and the abundance of microbiota (dos Santos Baião et al., 2017). In the end, it was found that the results were generally unpredictable. The hypotensive and hypoglycemic effects of beet juice consumption have also not been conclusively connected to a single, fundamental causal mechanism; a similar analytical perspective was also evident in the microbiological and renal investigation. Several physiologically active phytochemicals, including betalains, flavonoids, polyphenols, saponins, and inorganic nitrate, are present in beetroot (NO_3) (Haley, 1979). A variety of minerals, including potassium, sodium, phosphorus, calcium, magnesium, copper, iron, zinc, and manganese, are also abundant in it. It is frequently consumed in the form of added juice, powder, bread, gel, boiled, oven-dried, pickled, pureed, or jam-processed items across a variety of culinary traditions. Effects of beetroot on insulin and glucose regulation. The potential hypoglycemic effects of beet juice have been studied in the past in both healthy individuals and patients with a variety of diseases. Five human studies and two animal studies were looked at in this study (Mirmiran et al., 2020). P value equals 0.004. The considerable reduction in blood glucose levels and the positive impact on the glycemic and insulin responses were both largely attributed to many routes and the major participation of bioactive components (such as polyphenols, flavonoids, nitrate, etc.).

Since it plays a complementary function in the occurrence of diabetic problems, the lipid profile was also briefly addressed in connection with this issue. An observational study on the phytochemical composition of 225 mL of beetroot juice and the related postprandial period involved 16 healthy participants. Three samples of 50 g of readily accessible carbs were given; the first sample included lemon; the second sample was a matched control drink and contained sucrose, fructose, and glucose; and the third sample had glucose. The glycemic and insulin responses to the two drinks in the first sample were positively correlated, according to this research (Anderson & Woodend, 2003). The post-beetroot juice glycemic responses of the first and second drinks were found to be significantly lower than those of the third. Between beetroot juice and the control beverage, a much-reduced insulin response was evoked although it was not statistically significant. In this regard, it is proposed that the late increase in the early postprandial glucose or insulin responses may be attributed to the polyphenol-rich beetroot juice. According to the findings of a recent study on 30 healthy participants, longer-term consumption of a 10% beet juice solution within 4 weeks caused a further trend downward shift in blood glucose levels of 34.5% when compared to the baseline and washout period (Castellani). However, this difference was not visible within 2 weeks of the interventional phase.

Due to the significant absorption from the hypotensive action, it might be argued that regular consumption of beetroot juice is necessary to sustain long-lasting effects on blood glucose and insulin responses. The delivery of 270 mL of beetroot juice to healthy participants in a randomized cross-over study was shown to be advantageous since it decreased the sustainability and peak of blood glucose levels in comparison to a sugar-matched control drink and stalled the post-glycemic response. Among obese and non-obese people with glucose tolerance, Beals et al. have examined the escalating interference of concurrent consumption of dietary fiber-rich beetroot juice and 25 g of glucose (75 g total carbohydrate load). At baseline, participants received 500 mL of beetroot solution (17 mmol nitrate and 25 g glucose), followed by doses of glucose at intervals of 5, 45, 60, and 90 minutes, and a combination of glucose solution and insulin at 10, 20, 30, and 120 minutes (Murray, 2007). It was shown that inhibiting nitrate reductase activity increased insulin resistance (= 0.009) and masked insulin sensitivity in obese people, in addition to reducing the demand for metabolic reactions to beetroot juice mixed with glucose (Tweedie, 2015).

Unlikely, co-ingesting glucose and beet juice increased blood glucose levels at 60 and 90 minutes in obese people more than nonobese adults ($p = 0.004$). Thus, it was shown that nitrate-rich diets may be advantageous for obese adults who have a greater chance of developing insulin resistance. Multiple pathways were proposed among studies in this review that were consistent with the blood-glucose-lowering action of Beta vulgaris. Some studies highlighted the significance of bioactive substances, such as ethanol's function in the activity of beet juice after an ethanolic extraction (EEBT). Additionally, the role of commensal bacteria in the nitrite-nitrate pathway was discussed. Inhibiting α-amylase and α-glucosidase, increasing paraoxonase 1, and altering intracellular signal transduction are additional processes that help meals and hormones lower blood sugar levels (PON1). Blood cortisol levels increase after eating beetroot since it is a stress hormone and an important factor in enhancing gluconeogenesis (Mirmiran et al., 2020). There is a drop in glucose levels that goes along with this. This occurrence could be caused by the adrenal cortex's ability to produce Adrenocorticotropic Hormone (ACTH) or by the way that it works there. The consumption of beetroot juice decreased blood sugar levels in comparison to the control and placebo beverages. It is believed that the causes of this are the polyphenols, betanins, and neobetanin, a consequence of betanin breakdown, as well as the ethanol concentration, nitrite-nitrate route, and the suppression of hormone reductase activity. In addition to the beverage's capacity to lower blood sugar levels, certain research highlighted the beneficial effects of beetroot juice on lipid profile and its indices (TC, TG, HDL, and LDL), which are directly related to the incidence of T2DM (Mirmiran et al., 2020).

In this regard, one randomized, double-blind trial investigated the effects of beet juice 2 hours after consumption on plasma glucose and lipid status. The only parameter related to it that was shown to be significantly greater in the intervention group was TG at pre-treatment levels (Mirmiran et al., 2020).

In any event, it was found that the preadministration of beet juice reduced the 2HPP when compared to the control. When the lipid profile measures were evaluated after therapy, all but HDL showed significantly lower values than those in the control group. However, it was still unclear if these implications were related to the antioxidant content of Beta vulgaris and lipoic acid, or if there were additional factors at work (Sahebkar et al., 2016).

9.6.2 CURCUMIN

Turmeric rhizomes contain a polyphenol called curcumin, which has a number of biological properties (*Curcuma longa* L.). Desmethoxycurcumin and bisdemethoxycurcumin are two other analogs of curcumin, often known as curcuminoids, that are present in turmeric (Jyotirmayee & Mahalik, 2022). Due to poor intestinal absorption and quick metabolism, curcumin and curcuminoids have low oral bioavailability. Clinical research has shown that curcumin has the potential to treat a variety of human ailments by exerting anti-inflammatory, anticancer, hypoglycemic, antioxidant, antiviral, and antibacterial effects (Epstein et al., 2010). Various cell signaling molecules connected to cancer, inflammation, and other disorders have been demonstrated to directly interact with curcumin. Various transcription factors, growth factors, inflammatory cytokines, protein kinases, and other enzymes are also affected by curcumin (Kunnumakkara et al., 2008). Numerous clinical studies have examined the use of curcumin in the MetS components. Yang et al. studied the effects of 1,950 mg per day of curcumin extract (95% curcuminoids) on the weight, glucose, and lipid profiles of people with MetS in a randomized double-blind controlled experiment. After a 12-week course of therapy, HDL-C levels sharply increased and LDL-C levels sharply decreased (Shivappa, 2014). In a previous randomized double-blind controlled study, supplementing with curcumin did not significantly improve total cholesterol, LDL-C, HDL-C, or TGs in patients with acute coronary syndrome. Melo et al. demonstrated in a comprehensive review and meta-analysis that supplementing with curcuminoids and/or curcumin lowered HbA1c concentrations without changing the homeostatic model evaluation of insulin resistance (HOMA-IR) (Hankinson et al., 2021). Individuals with dysglycemia (pre-diabetes, diabetes, or metabolic syndrome) may drop their fasting blood glucose levels by taking a single curcumin or a combination of curcuminoids; however, non-diabetic or euglycemic people cannot.

The usage of turmeric extracts failed to produce any positive results in this meta-analysis, unlike curcumin and curcuminoids (Binns, 2015). Curcumin was given in conjunction with piperine or as phytosomes to increase its absorption. Piperine may enhance curcumin bioavailability by decreasing liver conjugation and, as a result, its urine excretion. Phytosomes are phospholipid and bioactive natural chemical complexes. Phospholipids' amphipathic properties increase their bioavailability and shield the bioactive compounds from being broken down in the gastrointestinal system (Siviero et al., 2015). Around 50 diabetic patients were given curcumin (1,000 mg/day) and piperine (10 mg/day) for 3 months. According to this study by Panahi et al., when compared to the placebo group, blood levels of glucose, HbA1c, C-peptide, and transaminases significantly decreased (Francini-Pesenti et al., 2019). Cicero et al. recently administered daily treatments of 200 mg of phytosomal curcumin and 8 mg of piperine to 80 overweight participants. The blood pressure, TG, HDL-C, waist circumference, aspartate aminotransferase (AST), HOMA-IR, alanine aminotransferase (ALT), gamma-glutamyl transferase, and serum cortisol were significantly improved from the baseline.

9.6.3 CAPSAICIN

First isolated in 1876, capsaicin's structure was determined in 1919, and it was chemically synthesized in 1930. Capsaicin, dihydrocapsaicin, nordihydrocapsaicin, homocapsaicin, and homodihydrocapsaicin are some of the capsaicinoids. Capsaicin and dihydrocapsaicin make up over 90% of the capsaicinoids in any fruit from the Capsicum genus, with capsaicin making up about 70% to 80% (Krajewska, 1984). Capsaicin is a hot chemical that is highly absorbed, influences thermoregulation, and triggers autonomic responses. Capsaicin is marketed as creams and patches for the treatment of pain in neuralgias and neuropathies. As a potential treatment for rheumatoid arthritis, surgical discomfort, persistent neuropathic pain, and musculoskeletal pain, phase III clinical investigations are now being developed. We will discuss capsaicin's pharmacological capacity to reduce metabolic syndrome in this section. Capsaicin acts through the transmembrane cation channel TRPV1, which has six putative transmembrane domains and a calcium-permeable pore region. TRPV1 prefers Ca^{2+} to Na^{+}.

The channel may open as a result of a variety of stimuli, including temperature, stretch, osmotic sensing, taste, low pH, pressure, vibration, and endogenous and exogenous substances. In 3T3-L1 adipocytes, capsaicin's effects on calcium influx and the inhibition of adipogenesis were lessened when TRPV1 was precisely silenced by targeted RNA interference. The receptor for capsaicin is TRPV1. TRPV1 has been discovered in a number of tissues since it was first detected on sensory nerve fibers. The tissues having the largest concentrations include the trigeminal ganglia, dorsal root ganglia, neurons, urine bladder, and testis. Adipocytes, smooth muscle cells, endothelial cells, pancreatic beta-cells, liver, heart, skeletal muscle, and kidney all express it. Nutrients 2018, 10, x for peer review 2 of 21 discusses calcium influx and adipogenesis inhibition in 3T3-L1 adipocytes. The trigeminal ganglia, dorsal root ganglia, neurons, urine bladder, and testis express TRPV1 at the highest levels, despite the fact that it was initially detected on sensory nerve fibers. Adipocytes, smooth muscle cells, endothelial cells, pancreatic beta-cells, liver, heart, skeletal muscle, and kidney are additional tissues that express TRPV1 (Nilius et al., 2008).

9.6.4 CONJUGATED LINOLEIC ACID (CLAS)

Conjugated linoleic acids (CLAs), a type of polyunsaturated fatty acid, are present in foods derived from ruminant animals by nature. To create at least 28 known isomers of CLA, the two conjugated double bonds are positioned in different geometric (i.e., cis or trans) and positional locations. 18:2cis-9, trans-11 (9,11 CLA, or rumenic acid) and 18:2trans-10, cis-12 (10,12 CLA) (Murrieta, 2007), which make up around 85% and 10% of all naturally occurring CLA isomers, respectively, are the most common of them. By producing linoleic acid isomerase, which contains a sizable portion of ruminant microorganisms, bacteria that create linoleic acid (18:2cis-9, cis-12) biohydrogenate linoleic acid into CLAs (more details are provided in the section on the biohydrogenation of CLA) (Harfoot, 1997). Foods produced from ruminants, such as beef, lamb, butter, and dairy products, are therefore inherently abundant in CLA. CLA can also be manufactured synthetically from linoleic acid-rich oils, such as safflower, sunflower, maize, and soybean oils, using the same alkaline-catalyzed process that converts linoleic acid into CLA. This synthetic preparation results in a variable ratio of the most common CLA isomers, with 40%–45% of 9,11 CLA and 40%–45% of 10,12 CLA, and the remaining proportion is made up of trace amounts of other CLA isomers (Bauman et al., 2020).

9.6.4.1 CLA EFFECTS ON OBESITY IN ANIMAL MODELS

Researchers have studied the significant effect CLA has on adiposity for the past 20 years. According to preliminary research, male and female ICR mice fed a chow diet supplemented with mixed CLA (0.5% w/w) experienced a 60% increase in fat loss over the course of 30 days. Increased fat oxidation and lipolysis were blamed for this outcome. A prior study in Sprague-Dawley rats demonstrated a dose-dependent reduction in the levels of triglycerides and non-esterified fatty acids in white adipose tissue after three weeks of mixed CLA diet (Evans et al., 2002). Importantly, none of these first observations was made prior to a change in body weight that could be seen. Later research revealed that 10,12 CLA was the CLA isomer that was active in lowering adiposity. In several mouse models as well as those using rats, hamsters, and pigs, mixed CLA has been shown to initially reduce obesity. However, it's possible that various species, like mice and rats, respond differently to CLA treatment. In contrast to obese Zucker rats, lean Zucker rats had decreased adiposity when given a 0.5% mixed CLA-containing diet for five weeks. Although the cause of this species difference is unclear, it may be related to variations in research designs (DeLany et al., 1999). There has been a lot of interest in figuring out the mechanism(s) through which 10,12 CLA promotes fat loss in mice models. Early studies demonstrated that 10,12 CLA promotes the oxidation of fat stores by assessing the gene expression of peroxisome proliferation-activated receptor alpha (Ppara) and its downstream targets acyl-coenzyme A oxidase (Acox1) and carnitine palmitoyl transferase-1 (Cpt1). Studies reported that 10,12 CLA greatly increases the conversion of radiolabeled fatty acids like palmitate and oleate into carbon dioxide in cultured adipocytes, a marker of accelerated fatty acid oxidation. Furthermore, we demonstrated *in vivo* that mice supplemented with 10,12 CLA had considerably greater levels of acylcarnitine, which are crucial fatty acid byproducts. According to recent studies, browning of white adipose tissue is a method for fat mobilization that could aid in weight loss and fat reduction (Flux, 2004).

In the first study, Wendel et al. demonstrated that CLA (1.5% mixed isomer) increased UCP1 expression in white adipose tissue using ob/ob mice, a mouse model of spontaneous obesity induced by the absence of the leptin gene. It is interesting that only the epididymal (visceral) portion of white adipose tissue showed browning in this study, and that the effects of CLA were only discernible during the obesogenic stage (Li et al., 2008). The next group used Sv129 mice and administered low doses of CLA isomers to thoroughly examine the effects of CLA on browning. Under the guidance of Michael McIntosh, this team showed that multiple low doses of 10,12 CLA (0.03%, 0.13%, and 0.33%) promoted the enhanced synthesis of uncoupling protein 1 (UCP1) from both inguinal (subcutaneous) and epididymal (visceral) white adipose tissue in lean mice. This group went on to show that eating a low-fat diet and taking 10,12 CLA at a dosage of 0.1% may similarly stimulate the browning of white adipose tissue (Shen et al., 2013).

Although Shen et al.'s study employed a dosage of 10,12 CLA that was almost six times lower than the amount used in Wendel et al.'s trial, it nonetheless improved the browning of both epididymal (visceral) and inguinal (subcutaneous) white adipose tissue with only very little adverse effects on liver weight. More recently, our team has shown that 10,12 CLA (1%), in a mouse model with phenotypes resembling the human metabolic syndrome (Ldlr/mice fed a diet high in sucrose and saturated fat), promotes the significant browning of white adipose tissue in obese mice, with concomitantly increased energy expenditure. Additionally, the mice were better able to maintain their core body temperatures when exposed to cold, suggesting that the browning of white adipose tissue may aid in thermogenesis. Therefore, further research is required to ascertain if the weight reduction benefits of 10,12 CLA are caused by its browning effects. Adiponectin is a hormone released by adipocytes that possess anti-inflammatory, anti-atherogenic, and anti-diabetic characteristics (McNeill et al., 2021).

Several studies have shown that CLA supplementation lowers the levels of adiponectin in the bloodstream. It has recently been shown that although CLA supplementation decreases fat storage, it also significantly lowers the levels of circulating adiponectin in mice. This discovery may contribute to the understanding of how altered glucose metabolism is related to weight loss caused by CLA (Gray et al., 2013). It is unknown what causes this adiponectin loss, but a recent study by our team suggests that co-treatment with the thiazolidinedione rosiglitazone, a PPAR gamma (PPAR) agonist that directly upregulates adiponectin, can improve glucose metabolism while still enabling CLA-mediated weight loss by at least partially restoring the adiponectin levels. The majority of the research to date indicates that CLA reduces PPAR mRNA expression, activation, and downstream targets, despite some studies suggesting that it is a PPAR agonist. Because of this, the lower PPAR activity and adiponectin levels imply that CLA promotes a particular type of weight loss that is not especially advantageous for metabolism. Co-treatments that minimize the negative impact on glucose metabolism help to ameliorate this mechanism-based way.

9.6.5 POLYUNSATURATED FATTY ACIDS

Plant-derived omega-3 polyunsaturated fatty acids: numerous clinical research and meta-analyses have demonstrated the lipid-lowering effects of omega-3 polyunsaturated fatty acids (PUFAs), although the vast majority of these investigations used marine omega-3 PUFAs (De Lorgeril & Salen, 2012). The primary omega-3 fatty acid in plants, alpha-linolenic acid (ALA), is abundant in almonds, green leafy vegetables, linseed, flaxseed, walnuts, and vegetable oils like canola, soybean, and hemp oil. Additionally, the diatom *Odontella aurita* is very high in docosahexaenoic acid (DHA), as are other microalgae. Prostaglandins are produced more readily, ACE activity is suppressed, angiotensin II production is reduced, nitric oxide (NO) is produced more readily, and TGF-beta expression is suppressed by omega-3 PUFAs (Cicero & Colletti, 2016).

ALA has a hypotensive effect since it is a precursor to eicosanoids, which may create prostaglandins and leukotrienes and reduce vascular tone. Alpha-linolenic acid appears to have favorable effects on MetS and type 2 diabetes due to its effects on dyslipidemia, inflammation, hypertension, platelet aggregation, and prothrombotic effects, as well as its capacity to reduce the risk factors for cardiovascular disease. The cardioprotective effects of ALA have been associated with its role as a precursor in the body's conversion to EPA (Cicero & Colletti, 2016). Systolic blood pressure, insulin levels, total and LDL cholesterol, as well as body weight, decreased in both groups ($P < 0.05$) in a clinical trial evaluating the effectiveness of a 6-month hypoenergetic diet enriched with a high MUFA content and an ALA intake of 3.5 g/diet in patients with metabolic syndrome. Diastolic blood pressure and serum TAG, however, were significantly decreased after the high ALA intake, but not in the control group (Only by supplementation can one regularly acquire the 2 to 4 g/diet amounts of omega-3 PUFAs needed to decrease cholesterol).

The triglyceride-lowering effects of eicosapentaenoic acid (EPA) and docosahexaenoic acid (DHA) seem to be comparable at the moment; however, in comparison trials, DHA induced more TG reduction and a rise in LDLC and HDL-C than EPA (Assad et al., 2021). In addition, ALA decreases LDL-C levels slightly but momentarily and enhances insulin sensitivity in hyperlipidemic people. Comparatively speaking, EPA and DHA have more noticeable short-term impacts than ALA, notwithstanding the possibility that ALA serves a longer-term dietary purpose. The biological effects of 0.3 g/day of long-chain-3 PUFA appear to be equal to those of 4 g/day of ALA consumption. Omega-3 PUFAs may also have a moderate, dose-dependent hypotensive effect, the strength of which may depend on the severity of hypertension, according to certain animal and human studies (Colussi et al., 2007).

9.6.6 BERBERINE

Berberine is an alkaloid with strong pharmacological effects that is currently the subject of a lot of attention. Berberine is a plant extract that has historically been used in traditional medicine; however, modern research methods have revealed that berberine may be a possible treatment for modern diseases. A recent study has established the significance of its anticancer action and its value in treating neurological, metabolic, and cardiovascular issues. The medication has been tested in numerous clinical studies on individuals with metabolic syndrome (Nautiyal, 2007).

9.6.6.1 ANTIDIABETIC ACTION OF BERBERINE

Among other things, metabolic syndrome is characterized as the etiology of central obesity, glucose intolerance, and insulin resistance. A rising number of younger patients are now affected by the battle against insulin resistance and obesity. It has also emerged as a crucial issue in the struggle against infertility. The antidiabetic effect of berberine has been shown *in vivo*, and it has been known to have antidiabetic qualities in T2DM since 1986. The most well-researched possible medicinal use of berberine is its anti-diabetic action (Gurib-Fakim, 2006). Unfortunately, although having positive benefits and a strong safety profile, its low bioavailability continues to restrict its use in clinical settings. According to earlier studies, berberine helps individuals with type 2 diabetes reduce their levels of alanine and aspartate transaminase and reduce insulin resistance. Additionally, it was demonstrated that berberine improved levels of fasting and postprandial blood glucose as well as glycosylated hemoglobin while reducing insulin resistance (Zhang et al., 2008).

Berberine stimulates glycolysis by enhancing insulin synthesis, raising glucokinase activity, and suppressing gluconeogenesis and adipogenesis in the liver. Turning on 5-adenosine monophosphate kinase encourages the translocation of the glucose-4 transporter into the plasma and increases insulin sensitivity in individuals with insulin resistance (AMPK). It has also been observed that in individuals with insulin resistance, where the protein kinase B (Akt) signaling pathway is weakened, berberine increases Akt phosphorylation and, therefore, activates Akt, specifically via the activation of AMPK. The most likely mechanism by which berberine controls glucose absorption is the activation of the AMPK pathway, according to research publications (Huang et al., 2021). The AMPK-dependent adipose tissue triglyceride lipase is one of the mechanisms of action in the prevention of obesity and is positively associated with long-term weight loss, and berberine promotes its expression. It has also been demonstrated that berberine boosts the amount of insulin produced in response to glucose. The chemical increases the level of glucagon-like peptide-1 in islet cells, which enhances the release of insulin, as demonstrated both *in vitro* and *in vivo* (GLP-1) (Feng et al., 2012). Because it inhibits glycosidase, berberine may reduce the amount of glucose that is transported through the intestinal epithelium. As a result, it could have antihyperglycemic effects. Following oral therapy, only plasma concentrations that are barely nanomolar in value can be found in both people and animals.

It is comparable to metformin because of its great therapeutic potential. Berberine has various benefits in its usage, including in individuals who cannot take metformin treatment, due to its excellent effectiveness and safety profile (An et al., 2014). Berberine not only seems to regulate blood glucose much better than metformin, but it also outperforms the advantages of rosiglitazone by enhancing fasting blood glucose levels. The mechanism of berberine's effectiveness in cases of obesity, particularly those with T2DM, is currently the subject of in-depth research. Clinical evaluation of berberine's impact on insulin resistance in obese women with polycystic ovarian syndrome revealed improved insulin resistance. Improvements in lipid markers (total cholesterol, LDL, TG, the cholesterol/HDL ratio, and the TG/HDL ratio), weight reduction, and fat mass decrease were seen in obese individuals with cardiometabolic syndrome risk factors. The development of insulin resistance in ischemic situations in obese people is regulated by c-Jun N-terminal kinases (JNK) and excitotoxic neurotransmitters (Di Daniele et al., 2013). In addition to acting as a neuroprotectant, berberine affects the lipid metabolic pathways that these kinases are in charge of. This activity also has the anticancer consequences that are described below. A number of human-confirmed routes have also demonstrated an impact on body mass, which is partially connected to its anti-diabetic benefits. *In vitro* tests revealed that berberine markedly decreased the number and size of lipid droplets present in the 3T3-L1 adipocyte cell lines. According to clinical research, berberine inhibits α-glycosidase. By lowering the expression of liver X receptor alpha, peroxisome proliferator-activated receptor (PPAR), and sterol element-binding protein 1 receptor, there was also a clinically shown inhibitory impact on adipocyte development (SREBP). Through the PPAR and CCAAT/enhancer-binding protein pathways, berberine also promotes basal triglyceride lipolysis in adipocytes and prevents the separation and augmentation of preadipocytes and adipocytes (Davidson, 2006).

These mechanisms serve as the foundation for comprehending berberine's effects on the treatment and prevention of obesity. Research on berberine's efficacy in treating polycystic ovarian syndrome is now underway, and the findings will be important for treating those who suffer from this condition. Research shows the tremendous potential of berberine supplementation in people with polycystic ovarian syndrome due to its capacity to reduce insulin resistance and improve ovulation. Three months of treatment with 500 mg of berberine in 26 patients with polycystic ovary syndrome resulted in a significant improvement in the lipid profile, an increase in pregnancy rates, and a decrease in the signs and symptoms of severe ovarian hyperstimulation syndrome (Calcaterra et al., 2021). When berberine was used instead of metformin, these people's side effects, lipid metrics, and body mass index (BMI) all dropped. Further research showed that berberine and Yasmin significantly increased sex hormones and carbohydrate metabolism.

Additionally, in women with polycystic ovarian syndrome and insulin resistance, berberine, and letrozole work together synergistically to stimulate ovulation. The results are better than when metformin and letrozole are combined. Berberine has the potential to significantly raise ovulation rates. The combination of letrozole and berberine did not, however, significantly improve fertility in patients with polycystic ovarian syndrome, according to a different study (Xie et al., 2019). Researchers are currently paying close attention to the role that nutraceuticals play in T2DM, and several of them are being carefully explored. There is evidence that certain dietary supplements reduce the plasma levels of postprandial and fasting glucose, glycated hemoglobin, and fasting plasma insulin. Nutraceutical berberine, in combination with chromium picolinate, inositol, curcumin, and Banaba, has been positively associated with a reduction in inflammation in patients with dysglycemia, as well as an improvement in glycometabolic compensation, triglycerides, and cholesterol levels, according to a number of clinical studies and additional research (Adapa et al., 2018). Studies have shown that individuals with fasting dysglycemia had lower levels of high-sensitivity C-reactive protein (CRP) after three months of combination nutraceutical therapy. When given jointly, berberine and Bifidobacteria further established their supportive roles in the treatment of diabetes in patients with pre-diabetes and diabetes mellitus.

9.6.7 PSYLLIUM FIBERS

The botanical name for the native tropical plant known as Psyllium is Plantago (family Plantaginaceae). The Plantago genus contains more than 200 species, and psyllium is a common name for them. It is also known as isabgol and ispaghula in the local Indian tongue. Isabgol, which refers to the shape of the Psyllium seed, is derived from the Persian word "band ghoul," which means "horse flower" (Noutchang, 2018). Persia was home to the psyllium plant. This perennial herb, which normally has short stems between 10 and 18 inches long, is also known as isabgol, aspaghol, ashwagolam, bazarqutuna, aspagol, and blond psyllium depending on the region. This plant is commonly cultivated throughout several continents. The majority of the time, psyllium is grown for its mucilage, a white fibrous material with hydrophilic properties. *Plantago ovata* and *Plantago psyllium* species are frequently cultivated for commercial purposes to make mucilage. The psyllium husk (seed coat) is also employed professionally in the food industry, including bakeries, ice cream shops, and confectioneries (Kumar et al., 2017).

A useful food is psyllium. Psyllium is employed in a number of commercial sectors, including the food and pharmaceutical industries. Due to its many physicochemical qualities, psyllium is often added to functional food items such as meal replacements, morning cereals, biscuits, bread, and bakery goods. To increase the fiber content of the diet, it is frequently added to shakes, juices, yogurt, syrups, soups, and even ice creams. Additionally, it thickens beverages and frozen desserts (Gelroth & Ranhotra, 2001). The additional minerals and phytochemicals in psyllium dietary fiber allow it to be consumed as a complete meal and fill the fiber gap. To increase psyllium's use in food and safety, numerous initiatives are being made to improve its physicochemical, biological, sensory, and functional qualities. Psyllium cannot be disseminated in water or aqueous solutions due to its strong water absorption capability. Many studies have worked on psyllium, offering many methods to enhance its functioning. In 1998, the Food and Drug Administration (FDA) suggested that by consuming more fiber each day (Tosif et al., 2021), cholesterol might be reduced or maintained at a sufficient level. The mucilage found in seed husks has valuable qualities as a thickening agent that may be used in the food industry. It is a culinary additive that may be used in chocolate and other dishes. In ice cream, it may serve as the primary stabilizer. By making liquids or flavored drinks richer and more consistent, it enhances their flavor and mouthfeel. Due to its tasty flavor and exceptional storage durability, fiber supplements are in high demand. It may be used for sizing purposes and as a foundation for cosmetics. The psyllium husk may be utilized as an excellent binder and can be broken down into compressed tablets since it has a strong binding ability (Chawla & Patil, 2010). When psyllium is treated with hot caustic soda, it forms a jelly-like structure that might be used in place of agar-agar gel. Germicidal lubricating gel and dry dentifrice powder have both been made using psyllium seed gum. Additionally, it may be a component of petroleum. When a cow is breastfeeding, it may be utilized as cattle feed or combined with jaggery. About 69% of the weight of the whole seed harvest is a de-husked seed that may be utilized as bird food.

Psyllium may be administered in varied doses for hypercholesterolemia while considering males's and women's hormonal conditions, including pre- and postmenopausal women. While no substantial reduction in total cholesterol was shown in premenopausal women (Pei, 2008), postmenopausal women may dramatically lower their total cholesterol levels and lower their risk of coronary heart disease by taking roughly 15 gm of psyllium daily. The amount of psyllium taken by pre- and postmenopausal women had no effect on their triglyceride, apolipoprotein A1, or apolipoprotein B concentrations. Due to the higher glucose levels in diabetic patients and the increased polysaccharide content in hyperlipidemia, psyllium is added to processed foods to help people manage their weight (Salem et al., 2020). The bioactive component arabinoxylan found in fiber increases the medicinal potential and quality of bakery goods. Psyllium is added to bread dough with a 93% acceptance rate in celiac disease patients, compared to a 97% acceptance rate in non-celiac disease patients. Psyllium may substitute for gluten when creating bread dough items with a chemical makeup that is less than 42.3% fat and fewer than 32% calories. In this manner, psyllium fiber-based goods have fewer calories and less fat.

Additionally, while making milk solid dessert from low-fat cow milk, this mucilage powder is used. The created herbal dessert product may include nutrients that are low in carbohydrates, rich in protein and dietary fiber, devoid of trans fats, and high in saturated fats. Additionally, it has the ability to relieve acidity and constipation. Mucilage and psyllium gum are examples of naturally occurring biopolymers. Their uses in the biotechnological, pharmacological, and nutraceutical (Keservani et al., 2017, 2020) areas are expanding daily. Psyllium has been successfully used for many years in the food and pharmaceutical industries as a thickening agent, colloidal stabilizer, and gelling agent (Verma & Mogra, 2013).

Psyllium mucilage has characteristics that make it unique for usage as a matrix for the delivery and/or trapping of different drug types, proteins, and cells. Given that it is a natural polysaccharide, it is essential for industrial uses. As a prebiotic, psyllium provides the nutrients required for the probiotics to flourish as healthy microbial colonies in the gut. The basis of the crucial microbiome of the colon is provided by these intestinal bacteria. A healthy gut bacterial colony is also essential for a robust immune system and aids in the body's ability to effectively fight off illness, maintain healthy cells and tissues, and minimize inflammation (Douglas, 2018). Additionally, prebiotics promote softer bowel motions in people who are constipated. Psyllium husk promotes the health of gut flora and the microbiota, especially in people who have constipation. Psyllium increases the production of short-chain fatty acids like propionate and butyrate, which are crucial for microbial health. The capacity of psyllium to retain water in the small intestine increases the amount of water that enters the ascending colon (Havenaar, 2011).

9.7 DIFFERENT TYPES OF NUTRACEUTICALS OF ANIMAL ORIGIN USED FOR THE MANAGEMENT OF METABOLIC SYNDROME AND RELATED DISORDERS

9.7.1 L. CARNITINE

The creation of energy and the metabolism of fatty acids both depend heavily on the vitamin carnitine, which is only conditionally required. Compared to meat eaters, vegetarians have a higher bioavailability (Newson). Distinct shortages result from either genetic mutation in the carnitine transporters or co-occurring conditions such as liver or renal illness. In diseases including cardiomyopathy, malnutrition, sepsis, cirrhosis, diabetes, endocrine disorders, and aging, aberrations of carnitine regulation lead to carnitine shortage. L-carnitine is the physiologically active form of carnitine, and nutritional supplementation with it is advantageous for those who are uremic. It may also improve nerve conduction, neuropathic pain, and immunological function in diabetics while being lifesaving for those who have primary carnitine deficiency (Andrea Moura et al., 2015). Alzheimer's disease, hepatic encephalopathy, and other excruciating neuropathies are just a few of the neurological conditions that carnitine has shown to have great promise in treating in clinical settings. Topical therapy for dry eye provides osmoprotection and control mechanisms for inflammatory and immunological responses. There is increasing evidence that carnitine supplementation may help treat obesity, improve glucose intolerance, and raise total energy expenditure in addition to being recognized as a dietary supplement in the treatment of cardiovascular disease (Flanagan et al., 2010).

9.7.1.1 HEART DISORDERS AND SUPPLEMENTATION IN CARDIOVASCULAR DISEASE

Since human skeletal and cardiac muscles are unable to produce carnitine, they have comparatively high plasma quantities of the substance. One of the most vulnerable organs to a carnitine-acylcarnitine carrier (CAC) deficit is the heart. CAC enables the import of fatty acyl moieties into the mitochondria where they are oxidized via the β-oxidation pathway by facilitating the carnitine/acylcarnitine exchange. The majority of the heart's energy comes from this route. The effects of CAC deficiency include cardiomyopathy, cardiac arrhythmia (perhaps brought on by the buildup of long-chain fatty acids and acylcarnitine that cannot be oxidized), cardiac insufficiency, and respiratory distress. Heart failure has been linked to a carnitine deficit. The mechanism(s) behind L-(LC) carnitine's effects on cardiovascular disorders remain unclear. In a rat model, Miguel-Carrasco et al. showed that prolonged administration of LC lowers blood pressure and lessens the inflammatory response connected to arterial hypertension (Guzmán-Guillén et al., 2017). Carnitine was shown to impede the recovery of contractile function after transient ischemia, contradicting the known positive benefits of carnitine excess.

Additionally, immediately after reperfusion, supplementing with carnitine enhanced the heart's contractility. Carnitine supplementation affects both damage and recovery of contractile function following brief ischemia in perfused rat hearts, according to Diaz and colleagues, under circumstances where it does not promote glucose oxidation. Patients with severe cardiovascular conditions such as coronary heart disease, chronic heart failure, and peripheral vascular disease have been proven to benefit from the use of L-carnitine (Furnary et al., 2003). L-carnitine supplementation for a period of 12 months reduced the incidence of chronic heart failure and mortality in individuals with chronic heart disease by lowering left ventricular dilatation and preventing ventricular remodeling. L-carnitine helps prevent cardiac damage in ischemia mostly by enhancing glucose metabolism and lowering the toxicity of elevated free fatty acid levels. L-carnitine has been shown to be protective against ST-elevation myocardial infarction (Xue et al., 2007). Prompt L-carnitine treatment and ongoing maintenance therapy reduce progressive left ventricular dilatation after an acute myocardial infarction. Despite not lowering the overall risk of death or heart failure at six months, L-carnitine lowers early mortality. Additional benefits of L-carnitine supplementation include the prevention of ventricular hypertrophy and dysfunction, a decrease in the size of the infarct and cardiac biomarkers, and a reduction in the overall frequency of cardiac events, such as fatal and nonfatal infarction. According to Xue and colleagues, the restoration of myocardial energy stores and the resumed normal oxidative metabolism are what cause L-positive carnitine's benefits in cardiovascular disease. As a supplement for cardiovascular illness, carnitine has received a lot of endorsements. Carnitine supplementation, however, should be highlighted as it was previously reported since it affects both damage and recovery of contractile function following temporary ischemia in the perfused rat heart under circumstances when it does not promote glucose oxidation (Di Lisa et al., 1998).

9.7.2 BOVINE COLOSTRUM

All mammals give their babies colostrum, also known as beestings, bisnings, or first milk, within the first 24 to 48 hours after delivery. The majority of animals produce colostrum immediately before giving birth. Only the first few hours after birth can human neonates get colostrum from their mothers, and this lays the groundwork for lifelong immunity. Bovine and human colostrum (BC) is a viscous, yellowish liquid that is thick, and sticky and contains more antibodies than regular milk. Colostrum delivers naturally generated nutrients in a highly concentrated low-volume form since newborns have relatively tiny and undeveloped GI systems. It acts as a laxative in neonates and aids in the passage of the infant's first feces, known as meconium. It also aids in the removal of excess bilirubin from the infant's body to avoid jaundice (Bagwe-Parab et al., 2020). Neonates are protected from infectious infections by the antibodies found in colostrum, which also provides passive immunity and growth factors for GI development. Colostrum's health advantages have been well-known for decades. Additionally, studies have revealed that the active ingredients in bovine (cow and buffalo) colostrum are 100–1,000 times more effective than those in human colostrum.

9.7.2.1 ROLE OF BOVINE COLOSTRUM IN THE MANAGEMENT OF DIABETES

Diabetes (type-1 or insulin-dependent diabetes), which is assumed to be brought on by an autoimmune disease, is thought to be primarily caused by a strong allergic reaction to the protein Glutamic Acid Decarboxylase (GAD), which is present in cow's milk (Harrison & Honeyman, 1999). This autoimmune condition and other comparable allergies may be controlled and inhibited thanks to the many bioactive substances included in colostrum. Colostrum contains immunoglobulin IGF-1, which can bind to insulin and IGF-1 receptors located in target cells of the human body (Bagwe et al., 2015). Additionally, BC was shown to lower glucose and malondialdehyde levels in rats with diabetes induced by alloxan. Similar research using mice revealed that both BC and HBC were capable of significantly lowering cholesterol and glucose levels, with HBC coming out on top.

9.8 CONCLUSION

A healthy lifestyle based on proper nutrition, adequate sleep, and exercise is the best method to prevent metabolic diseases. Several factors including food quality, timing of food consumption, food quantity, medication intake, and light exposure may play a key role in human health. This study highlighted the problems associated with metabolic diseases and the importance of different nutraceuticals in human health. Additionally, the study highlighted the role of several plant extracts in the management of metabolic syndrome.

ACKNOWLEDGMENT

The authors thank Dr. Alka Lohani, IFTM University Moradabad, India for providing the opportunity to contribute to her research. Also, thanks to ISF College of Pharmacy, Moga India for providing an excellent platform to complete this work.

KEYWORDS

- **cardiovascular diseases**
- **functional foods**
- **herbal remedies**
- **metabolic diseases**
- **metabolic syndrome**
- **plant extracts**
- **polyunsaturated fatty acids**
- **spices**

REFERENCES

Abbasi, F., Brown, B. W., Lamendola, C., McLaughlin, T., & Reaven, G. M. (2002). Relationship between obesity, insulin resistance, and coronary heart disease risk. *Journal of the American College of Cardiology, 40*(5), 937–943. https://doi.org/10.1016/S0735-1097(02)02051-X.

Abeysinghe, D., Alwis, D., Kumara, K., & Chandrika, U. (2021). Nutritive importance and therapeutics uses of three different varieties (*Murraya koenigii*, *Micromelum minutum*, and *Clausena indica*) of curry leaves: An updated review. *Evidence-Based Complementary and Alternative Medicine, 2021*, Article ID 9980934. https://doi.org/10.1155/2021/9980934.

Abranches, M. V., de Oliveira, F. C. E., da Conceição, L. L., & Peluzio, M. d. C. G. (2015). Obesity and diabetes: The link between adipose tissue dysfunction and glucose homeostasis. *Nutrition Research Reviews, 28*(2), 121–132. https://doi.org/10.1017/S0954422415000060.

Acharya, S., Thomas, J., & Basu, S. (2008). Fenugreek, an alternative crop for semiarid regions of North America. *Crop Science, 48*(3), 841–853. https://doi.org/10.2135/cropsci2007.07.0401.

Adeghate, E., & Singh, J. (2014). Structural changes in the myocardium during diabetes-induced cardiomyopathy. *Heart Failure Reviews, 19*(1), 15–23. https://doi.org/10.1007/s10741-013-9388-7.

Aggarwal, B. B., & Heber, D. (2014). Spices and dietary supplements with anti-inflammatory activity. In N. S. Bidlack, J. F. Rodriguez-Proteau, & M. C. Omaye (Eds.), *Immunonutrition: Interactions of Diet, Genetics, and Inflammation* (pp. 317–333). CRC Press.

Aguiar, L. M., Geraldi, M. V., Cazarin, C. B. B., & Junior, M. R. M. (2019). Functional food consumption and its physiological effects. In V. R. Preedy (Ed.), *Bioactive Compounds* (pp. 205–225). Elsevier.

Ahmed, S., & Stepp, J. R. (2013). Green tea: The plants, processing, manufacturing and production. In V. R. Preedy & R. R. Watson (Eds.), *Tea in Health and Disease Prevention* (pp. 19–31). Academic Press.

Al-Dhubiab, B. E. (2012). Pharmaceutical applications and phytochemical profile of *Cinnamomum burmannii*. *Pharmacognosy Reviews, 6*(12), 125–131. https://doi.org/10.4103/0973-7847.96533.

Al-Shiekh, A. A., Al-Shati, A. A., & Sarhan, M. A. (2014). Effect of white tea extract on antioxidant enzyme activities of streptozotocin-induced diabetic rats. *Egyptian Academic Journal of Biological Sciences. C, Physiology and Molecular Biology, 6*(2), 17–30.

Alkhatib, D. H., Jaleel, A., Tariq, M. N. M., Feehan, J., Apostolopoulos, V., Cheikh Ismail, L., & Dhaheri, A. S. A. (2021). The role of bioactive compounds from dietary spices in the management of metabolic syndrome: An overview. *Nutrients, 14*(1), Article 175. https://doi.org/10.3390/nu14010175.

AlMatar, M., Islam, M. R., Albarri, O., Var, I., & Koksal, F. (2018). Pomegranate as a possible treatment in reducing risk of developing wound healing, obesity, neurodegenerative disorders, and diabetes mellitus. *Mini Reviews in Medicinal Chemistry, 18*(6), 507–526. https://doi.org/10.2174/1389557518666180305122058.

AMIHAESEI, I. C., & Chelaru, L. (2014). Metabolic syndrome: A widespread threatening condition; risk factors, diagnostic criteria, therapeutic options, prevention and controversies: An overview. *The Medical-Surgical Journal, 118*(4), 896–900.

An, Y., Sun, Z., Zhang, Y., Liu, B., Guan, Y., & Lu, M. (2014). The use of berberine for women with polycystic ovary syndrome undergoing IVF treatment. *Clinical Endocrinology, 80*(3), 425–431. https://doi.org/10.1111/cen.12301.

Anaeigoudari, A., Safari, H., & Khazdair, M. R. (2021). Effects of *Nigella sativa*, *Camellia sinensis*, and *Allium sativum* as food additive on metabolic disorders, a literature review. *Frontiers in Pharmacology, 12*, Article 3155. https://doi.org/10.3389/fphar.2021.63155.

Anderson, G. H., & Woodend, D. (2003). Consumption of sugars and the regulation of short-term satiety and food intake. *The American Journal of Clinical Nutrition, 78*(4), 843S–849S. https://doi.org/10.1093/ajcn/78.4.843S.

Andrea Moura, F., Queiroz de Andrade, K., Celia Farias dos Santos, J., & Oliveira Fonseca Goulart, M. (2015). Lipoic acid: Its antioxidant and anti-inflammatory role and clinical applications. *Current Topics in Medicinal Chemistry, 15*(5), 458–483. https://doi.org/10.2174/1568026615666150202150235.

Arnold, S. E., Arvanitakis, Z., Macauley-Rambach, S. L., Koenig, A. M., Wang, H. Y., Ahima, R. S., & Stoeckel, L. E. (2018). Brain insulin resistance in type 2 diabetes and Alzheimer disease: Concepts and conundrums. *Nature Reviews Neurology, 14*(3), 168–181. https://doi.org/10.1038/nrneurol.2017.185.

Arozal, W., Louisa, M., & Soetikno, V. (2020). Selected Indonesian medicinal plants for the management of metabolic syndrome: Molecular basis and recent studies. *Frontiers in Cardiovascular Medicine, 7*, Article 82. https://doi.org/10.3389/fcvm.2020.00082.

Assad, V., Saraiva, J. F. K., Faludi, A. A., Moreira, A. S. B., Geloneze, B., Magnoni, C. D., & Cintra, D. E. C. (2021). Position statement on fat consumption and cardiovascular health–2021. *Arquivos Brasileiros de Cardiologia, 116*(1), 160–212. https://doi.org/10.36660/abc.20210125.

Aybar, M. J., Riera, A. N. S., Grau, A., & Sánchez, S. S. (2001). Hypoglycemic effect of the water extract of *Smallanthus sonchifolius* (yacon) leaves in normal and diabetic rats. *Journal of Ethnopharmacology, 74*(2), 125–132. https://doi.org/10.1016/S0378-8741(00)00361-1.

Baddour, L. M., Wilson, W. R., Bayer, A. S., Fowler Jr, V. G., Bolger, A. F., Levison, M. E., & Gewitz, M. H. (2005). Infective endocarditis: Diagnosis, antimicrobial therapy, and management of complications: A statement for healthcare professionals from the Committee on Rheumatic Fever, Endocarditis, and Kawasaki Disease, Council on Cardiovascular Disease in the Young, and the Councils on Clinical Cardiology, Stroke, and Cardiovascular Surgery and Anesthesia, American Heart Association: Endorsed by the Infectious Diseases Society of America. *Circulation, 111*(23), e394–e434. https://doi.org/10.1161/CIRCULATIONAHA.105.165564.

Bae, U. J., Park, J., Park, I. W., Chae, B. M., Oh, M. R., Jung, S. J., Ryu, G. S., Chae, S. W., & Park, B. H. (2018). Epigallocatechin-3-gallate-rich green tea extract ameliorates fatty liver and weight gain in mice fed a high fat diet by activating the sirtuin 1 and AMP activating protein kinase pathway. The American Journal of Chinese Medicine, 46(03), 617–632. https://doi.org/10.1142/S0192415X18500393.

Bagwe-Parab, S., Yadav, P., Kaur, G., Tuli, H. S., & Buttar, H. S. (2020). Therapeutic applications of human and bovine colostrum in the treatment of gastrointestinal diseases and distinctive cancer types: The current evidence. Frontiers in Pharmacology, 11, Article 1100. https://doi.org/10.3389/fphar.2020.01100.

Bagwe, S., Tharappel, L. J., Kaur, G., & Buttar, H. S. (2015). Bovine colostrum: An emerging nutraceutical. Journal of Complementary and Integrative Medicine, 12(3), 175–185. https://doi.org/10.1515/jcim-2014-0062.

Baquer, N. Z., Kumar, P., Taha, A., Kale, R., Cowsik, S., & McLean, P. (2011). Metabolic and molecular action of Trigonella foenum-graecum (fenugreek) and trace metals in experimental diabetic tissues. Journal of Biosciences, 36(2), 383–396. https://doi.org/10.1007/s12038-011-9038-0.

Baranova, A., Tran, T., Birerdinc, A., & Younossi, Z. (2011). Systematic review: Association of polycystic ovary syndrome with metabolic syndrome and non-alcoholic fatty liver disease. Alimentary Pharmacology & Therapeutics, 33(7), 801–814. https://doi.org/10.1111/j.1365-2036.2011.04607.x.

Bashtian, M. H., Emami, S. A., Mousavifar, N., Esmaily, H. A., Mahmoudi, M., & Poor, A. H. M. (2013). Evaluation of fenugreek (Trigonella foenum-graceum L.) seeds extract on insulin resistance in women with polycystic ovarian syndrome. Iranian Journal of Pharmaceutical Research: IJPR, 12(2), 475–481.

Basu, B., Bagadiya, A., Makwana, S., Vipul, V., Batt, D., & Dharamsi, A., (2011). Formulation and evaluation of fast dissolving tablets of cinnarizine using superdisintegrant blends and subliming material. Journal of Advanced Pharmaceutical Technology & Research, 2(4), 266–273.

Bauman, D. E., Corl, B. A., & Peterson, D. G. (2020). The biology of conjugated linoleic acids in ruminants. In L. J. Beaulieu & K. J. S. Krishnan (Eds.), Advances in Conjugated Linoleic Acid Research (pp. 146–173). CRC Press.

Beier, R. C., & Nigg, H. N. (2019). Toxicology of naturally occurring chemicals in food. In H. A. Pakade & C. V. O. Omonhinmin (Eds.), Foodborne Disease Handbook (pp. 37–186). CRC Press.

Bendich, A., Machlin, L., Scandurra, O., Burton, G., & Wayner, D. (1986). The antioxidant role of vitamin C. Advances in Free Radical Biology & Medicine, 2(2), 419–444. https://doi.org/10.1016/8755-9668(86)90019-7.

Berkowitz, J. M., 2003. User's Guide Natural Allergy Relief. Basic Health Publications, Inc.

Bijauliya, R. K., Alok, S., Kumar, M., Chanchal, D. K., & Yadav, S. (2017). A comprehensive review on herbal cosmetics. International Journal of Pharmaceutical Sciences and Research, 8(12), 4930–4949.

Binns, S. E. (2015). Combining curcumin and alpha lipoic acid to treat cardiometabolic syndrome. Colorado State University.

Booth, F. W., Roberts, C. K., & Laye, M. J. (2012). Lack of exercise is a major cause of chronic diseases. Comprehensive Physiology, 2(2), 1143–1211. https://doi.org/10.1002/cphy.c110025.

Bordbar, S., Anwar, F., & Saari, N. (2011). High-value components and bioactives from sea cucumbers for functional foods—A review. Marine Drugs, 9(10), 1761–1805. https://doi.org/10.3390/md9101761.

Bordia, A., Verma, S., & Srivastava, K. (1997). Effect of ginger (Zingiber officinale Rosc.) and fenugreek (Trigonella foenum-graecum L.) on blood lipids, blood sugar and platelet aggregation in patients with coronary artery disease. Prostaglandins, Leukotrienes and Essential Fatty Acids, 56(5), 379–384. https://doi.org/10.1016/S0952-3278(97)90511-5.

Boren, J., Taskinen, M. R., Olofsson, S. O., & Levin, M. (2013). Ectopic lipid storage and insulin resistance: A harmful relationship. Journal of Internal Medicine, 274(1), 25–40. https://doi.org/10.1111/joim.12075.

Borzoei, A., Rafraf, M., & Asghari-Jafarabadi, M. (2018). Cinnamon improves metabolic factors without detectable effects on adiponectin in women with polycystic ovary syndrome.

Asia Pacific Journal of Clinical Nutrition, 27(3), 556–563. https://doi.org/10.6133/apjcn.032017.04.
Bray, G. A., & Bellanger, T. (2006). Epidemiology, trends, and morbidities of obesity and the metabolic syndrome. Endocrine, 29(1), 109–117. https://doi.org/10.1385/ENDO:29:1:109.
Bröring, S., Martin Cloutier, L., & Leker, J. (2006). The front end of innovation in an era of industry convergence: Evidence from nutraceuticals and functional foods. R&D Management, 36(5), 487–498. https://doi.org/10.1111/j.1467-9310.2006.00450.x.
Brown, J. K., Byers, T., Doyle, C., Courneya, K. S., Demark-Wahnefried, W., Kushi, L. H., & Aziz, N. (2003). Nutrition and physical activity during and after cancer treatment: An American Cancer Society guide for informed choices. CA: A Cancer Journal for Clinicians, 53(5), 268–291. https://doi.org/10.3322/canjclin.53.5.268.
Caballero-García, A., Noriega-González, D. C., Roche, E., Drobnic, F. & Córdova, A., (2023). Effects of L-Carnitine Intake on Exercise-Induced Muscle Damage and Oxidative Stress: A Narrative Scoping Review. Nutrients, 15(11), p.2587.
Çakmur, H. (2017). Obesity as a growing public health problem. In P. R. Preedy (Ed.), Adiposity-Epidemiology and Treatment Modalities. Springer.
Calcaterra, V., Verduci, E., Cena, H., Magenes, V. C., Todisco, C. F., Tenuta, E., & Di Profio, E. (2021). Polycystic ovary syndrome in insulin-resistant adolescents with obesity: The role of nutrition therapy and food supplements as a strategy to protect fertility. Nutrients, 13(6), Article 1848.
Caldwell, S. (2017). NASH therapy: Omega 3 supplementation, vitamin E, insulin sensitizers and statin drugs. Clinical and Molecular Hepatology, 23(2), 103–108.
Candidate, S. Y. P., Candidate, J. S. P., Nissa Mazzola PharmD, C. (2018). Nutritional supplements for the prevention of diabetes mellitus and its complications. *Journal of Nutrition & Intermediary Metabolism, 14*, 16–21.
Cassidy, Y. M., McSorley, E. M., Allsopp, P. J. (2018). Effect of soluble dietary fiber on postprandial blood glucose response and its potential as a functional food ingredient. *Journal of Functional Foods, 46*, 423–439.
Castellani, J. W., & Tipton, M. J., (2015). Cold stress effects on exposure tolerance and exercise performance. Compr Physiol, 6(1), 443–469.
Chauhan, A. Proteins. *International Journal of Inventions in Pharmaceutical Sciences, 4*(6).
Chawla, R., Patil, G. (2010). Soluble dietary fiber. *Comprehensive Reviews in Food Science and Food Safety, 9*(2), 178–196.
Chen, G., Yuan, Q., Saeeduddin, M., Ou, S., Zeng, X., Ye, H. (2016). Recent advances in tea polysaccharides: Extraction, purification, physicochemical characterization and bioactivities. *Carbohydrate Polymers, 153*, 663–678.
Cheng, Z., Blackford, J., Wang, Q., & Yu, L. L., (2009). Acid treatment to improve psyllium functionality. Journal of Functional Foods, 1(1), 44–49.
Chiarelli, F., Cipollone, F., Mohn, A., Marini, M., Iezzi, A., Fazia, M., Tumini, S., De Cesare, D., Pomilio, M., Pierdomenico, S. D. (2002). Circulating monocyte chemoattractant protein-1 and early development of nephropathy in type 1 diabetes. *Diabetes Care, 25*(10), 1829–1834.
Choi, J.-H., Kim, M.-K., Yeo, S.-H., Kim, S. (2020). Short-term Cudrania tricuspidata fruit vinegar administration attenuates obesity in high-fat diet-fed mice by improving fat accumulation and metabolic parameters. *Scientific Reports, 10*(1), 1–19.
Cicero, A. F., Colletti, A. (2016). Role of phytochemicals in the management of metabolic syndrome. *Phytomedicine, 23*(11), 1134–1144.

Colussi, G., Catena, C., Baroselli, S., Nadalini, E., Lapenna, R., Chiuch, A., Sechi, L. A. (2007). Omega-3 fatty acids: From biochemistry to their clinical use in the prevention of cardiovascular disease. *Recent Patents on Cardiovascular Drug Discovery (Discontinued), 2*(1), 13–21.

Connor, W. E., Connor, S. L. (1972). The key role of nutritional factors in the prevention of coronary heart disease. *Preventive Medicine, 1*(1–2), 49–83.

Das, L., Bhaumik, E., Raychaudhuri, U., Chakraborty, R. (2012). Role of nutraceuticals in human health. *Journal of Food Science and Technology, 49*(2), 173–183.

Davì, G., Santilli, F., Patrono, C. (2010). Nutraceuticals in diabetes and metabolic syndrome. *Cardiovascular Therapeutics, 28*(4), 216–226.

Davidson, M. H. (2006). Mechanisms for the hypotriglyceridemic effect of marine omega-3 fatty acids. *The American Journal of Cardiology, 98*(4), 27–33.

De Lorgeril, M., Salen, P. (2012). New insights into the health effects of dietary saturated and omega-6 and omega-3 polyunsaturated fatty acids. *BMC Medicine, 10*(1), 1–5.

DeFronzo, R. A. (1999). Pharmacologic therapy for type 2 diabetes mellitus. *Annals of Internal Medicine, 131*(4), 281–303.

DeFronzo, R. A., Ferrannini, E. (1991). Insulin resistance: A multifaceted syndrome responsible for NIDDM, obesity, hypertension, dyslipidemia, and atherosclerotic cardiovascular disease. *Diabetes Care, 14*(3), 173–194.

DeLany, J. P., Blohm, F., Truett, A. A., Scimeca, J. A., West, D. B. (1999). Conjugated linoleic acid rapidly reduces body fat content in mice without affecting energy intake. *American Journal of Physiology-Regulatory, Integrative and Comparative Physiology, 276*(4), R1172–R1179.

Derenski, K., Catlin, J., Allen, L. (2016). Parenteral nutrition basics for the clinician caring for the adult patient. *Nutrition in Clinical Practice, 31*(5), 578–595.

Després, J. P., Lemieux, I. (2006). Abdominal obesity and metabolic syndrome. *Nature, 444*(7121), 881–887.

Despres, J.-P., Moorjani, S., Lupien, P. J., Tremblay, A., Nadeau, A., Bouchard, C. (1990). Regional distribution of body fat, plasma lipoproteins, and cardiovascular disease. *Arteriosclerosis: An Official Journal of the American Heart Association, Inc., 10*(4), 497–511.

Di Daniele, N., Petramala, L., Di Renzo, L., Sarlo, F., Della Rocca, D. G., Rizzo, M., Fondacaro, V., Iacopino, L., Pepine, C. J., De Lorenzo, A. (2013). Body composition changes and cardiometabolic benefits of a balanced Italian Mediterranean Diet in obese patients with metabolic syndrome. *Acta Diabetologica, 50*(3), 409–416.

Di Lisa, F., Menabo, R., Canton, M., Petronilli, V. (1998). The role of mitochondria in the salvage and the injury of the ischemic myocardium. *Biochimica et Biophysica Acta (BBA)-Bioenergetics, 1366*(1–2), 69–78.

Di Lorenzo, A., Curti, V., C Tenore, G., M Nabavi, S., Daglia, M. (2017). Effects of tea and coffee consumption on cardiovascular diseases and relative risk factors: An update. *Current Pharmaceutical Design, 23*(17), 2474–2487.

Dias, T. I. R. A., (2019). Effect of White Tea on the Reproductive Function of Diabetic or Prediabetic Individuals (Doctoral dissertation, Universidade da Beira Interior (Portugal).

Dillard, C. J., & German, J. B. (2000). Phytochemicals: Nutraceuticals and human health. Journal of the Science of Food and Agriculture, 80(12), 1744–1756.

dos Santos Baião, D., Silva de Freitas, C., Paes Gomes, L., Da Silva, D., Carolina NTF Correa, A., Ribeiro Pereira, P., Mere Del Aguila, E., Margaret Flosi Paschoalin, V. (2017).

Polyphenols from root, tubercles and grains cropped in Brazil: Chemical and nutritional characterization and their effects on human health and diseases. Nutrients, 9(9), 1044.

Douglas, A. E. (2018). Fundamentals of Microbiome Science: How Microbes Shape Animal Biology. Princeton University Press.

Dudeja, P., & Gupta, R. (2017). Nutraceuticals. In Food Safety in the 21st Century (pp. 491–496). Elsevier.

Duke, J. A. (2009). The Green Pharmacy Guide to Healing Foods: Proven Natural Remedies to Treat and Prevent More Than 80 Common Health Concerns. Rodale Books.

Elks, C. M., & Francis, J. (2010). Central adiposity, systemic inflammation, and the metabolic syndrome. Current Hypertension Reports, 12(2), 99–104.

Enkhmaa, B., Surampudi, P., Anuurad, E., & Berglund, L. (2018). Lifestyle changes: effect of diet, exercise, functional food, and obesity treatment on lipids and lipoproteins. Endotext [Internet].

Enstrom, J. E., Kanim, L. E., & Klein, M. A. (1992). Vitamin C intake and mortality among a sample of the United States population. Epidemiology, 103(11), 194–202.

Epstein, J., Sanderson, I. R., & MacDonald, T. T. (2010). Curcumin as a therapeutic agent: The evidence from in vitro, animal and human studies. British Journal of Nutrition, 103(11), 1545–1557.

Evans, M. E., Brown, J. M., & McIntosh, M. K. (2002). Isomer-specific effects of conjugated linoleic acid (CLA) on adiposity and lipid metabolism. The Journal of Nutritional Biochemistry, 13(9), 508–516.

Fabbrini, E., Sullivan, S., & Klein, S. (2010). Obesity and nonalcoholic fatty liver disease: Biochemical, metabolic, and clinical implications. Hepatology, 51(2), 679–689.

Fedacko, J., Singh, R., Niaz, M., Ghosh, S., Fedackova, P., Tripathi, A., Etharat, A., Onsaard, E., Singh, V., & Shastun, S. (2016). Fenugreek seeds decrease blood cholesterol and blood glucose as adjunct to diet therapy in patients with hypercholesterolemia. *World Heart Journal, 8*(3), 239.

Feng, X.-T., Leng, J., Xie, Z., Li, S.-L., Zhao, W., Tang, Q.-L. (2012). GPR40: A therapeutic target for mediating insulin secretion. International Journal of Molecular Medicine, 30(6), 1261–1266.

Ferroni, P., Vazzana, N., Riondino, S., Cuccurullo, C., Guadagni, F., Davi, G. (2012). Platelet function in health and disease: From molecular mechanisms, redox considerations to novel therapeutic opportunities. Antioxidants & Redox Signaling, 17(10), 1447–1485.

Feskens, E. J., Virtanen, S. M., Räsänen, L., Tuomilehto, J., Stengård, J., Pekkanen, J., Nissinen, A., Kromhout, D. (1995). Dietary factors determining diabetes and impaired glucose tolerance: A 20-year follow-up of the Finnish and Dutch cohorts of the Seven Countries Study. Diabetes Care, 18(8), 1104–1112.

Fitzpatrick, L. A. (2003). Phytoestrogens—Mechanism of action and effect on bone markers and bone mineral density. Endocrinology and Metabolism Clinics, 32(1), 233–252.

Flanagan, J. L., Simmons, P. A., Vehige, J., Willcox, M. D., Garrett, Q. (2010). Role of carnitine in disease. Nutrition & Metabolism, 7(1), 1–14.

Flora, S. J. (2009). Structural, chemical and biological aspects of antioxidants for strategies against metal and metalloid exposure. Oxidative Medicine and Cellular Longevity, 2(4), 191–206.

Flux, C. L. (2004). The effect of conjugated linoleic acid on lipid metabolism in the hamster and the sheep. University of Nottingham.

Francini-Pesenti, F., Spinella, P., Calò, L. A. (2019). Potential role of phytochemicals in metabolic syndrome prevention and therapy. Diabetes, Metabolic Syndrome and Obesity: Targets and Therapy, 12(1987), 1987–2002.

Friedewald, V. E., Kornman, K. S., Beck, J. D., Genco, R., Goldfine, A., Libby, P., Offenbacher, S., Ridker, P. M., Van Dyke, T. E., Roberts, W. C. (2009). The American Journal of Cardiology and Journal of Periodontology editors' consensus: Periodontitis and atherosclerotic cardiovascular disease. Journal of Periodontology, 80(7), 1021–1032.

Furnary, A. P., Gao, G., Grunkemeier, G. L., Wu, Y., Zerr, K. J., Bookin, S. O., Floten, H. S., Starr, A. (2003). Continuous insulin infusion reduces mortality in patients with diabetes undergoing coronary artery bypass grafting. The Journal of Thoracic and Cardiovascular Surgery, 125(5), 1007–1021.

Gelroth, J., Ranhotra, G. S. (2001). Food uses of fiber. In G. A. Spiller (Ed.), Handbook of Dietary Fiber (pp. 435–451). CRC Press.

Gilman, S. L. (2008). Fat: A Cultural History of Obesity. Polity.

Ginsberg, H. N., MacCallum, P. R. (2009). The obesity, metabolic syndrome, and type 2 diabetes mellitus pandemic: Part I. Increased cardiovascular disease risk and the importance of atherogenic dyslipidemia in persons with the metabolic syndrome and type 2 diabetes mellitus. Journal of the Cardiometabolic Syndrome, 4(2), 113–119.

Governa, P., Baini, G., Borgonetti, V., Cettolin, G., Giachetti, D., Magnano, A. R., Miraldi, E., & Biagi, M. (2018). Phytotherapy in the management of diabetes: A review. *Molecules, 23*(1), 105. https://doi.org/10.3390/molecules23010105.

Graf, B. L., Raskin, I., Cefalu, W. T., & Ribnicky, D. M. (2010). Plant-derived therapeutics for the treatment of metabolic syndrome. *Current Opinion in Investigational Drugs, 11*(10), 1107.

Gray, B., Steyn, F., Davies, P., & Vitetta, L. (2013). Omega-3 fatty acids: A review of the effects on adiponectin and leptin and potential implications for obesity management. *European Journal of Clinical Nutrition, 67*(12), 1234–1242. https://doi.org/10.1038/ejcn.2013.197.

Gulliford, M. C., Charlton, J., & Latinovic, R. (2005). Increased utilization of primary care 5 years before diagnosis of type 2 diabetes: A matched cohort study. *Diabetes Care, 28*(1), 47–52. https://doi.org/10.2337/diacare.28.1.47.

Gurib-Fakim, A. (2006). Medicinal plants: Traditions of yesterday and drugs of tomorrow. *Molecular Aspects of Medicine, 27*(1), 1–93. https://doi.org/10.1016/j.mam.2005.07.008.

Guzmán-Guillén, R., Puerto, M., Gutiérrez-Praena, D., Prieto, A. I., Pichardo, S., Jos, Á., Campos, A., Vasconcelos, V., & Cameán, A. M. (2017). Potential use of chemoprotectants against the toxic effects of cyanotoxins: A review. *Toxins, 9*(6), 175. https://doi.org/10.3390/toxins9060175.

Haffner, S. M. (1998). The importance of hyperglycemia in the nonfasting state to the development of cardiovascular disease. *Endocrine Reviews, 19*(5), 583–592. https://doi.org/10.1210/edrv.19.5.0344.

Haffner, S. M. (2006). Relationship of metabolic risk factors and development of cardiovascular disease and diabetes. *Obesity, 14*(S6), 121S–127S. https://doi.org/10.1038/oby.2006.282.

Haley, T. J. (1979). Review of the toxicology of paraquat (1, 1′-dimethyl-4, 4′-bipyridinium chloride). *Clinical Toxicology, 14*(1), 1–46. https://doi.org/10.3109/15563657908987984.

Hamdy, O., Porramatikul, S., & Al-Ozairi, E. (2006). Metabolic obesity: The paradox between visceral and subcutaneous fat. *Current Diabetes Reviews, 2*(4), 367–373. https://doi.org/10.2174/1573399810602040367.

Hamid, A., Aiyelaagbe, O., Usman, L., Ameen, O., & Lawal, A. (2010). Antioxidants: Its medicinal and pharmacological applications. *African Journal of Pure and Applied Chemistry, 4*(8), 142–151.
Hankinson, S. J., Miller, M., & Freeman, A. M. (2021). Lifestyle approaches to lowering triglycerides. In M. Harrison (Ed.), *Prevention and Treatment of Cardiovascular Disease* (pp. 211–223). Springer.
Hannan, J., Ali, L., Rokeya, B., Khaleque, J., Akhter, M., Flatt, P., & Abdel-Wahab, Y. (2007). Soluble dietary fibre fraction of Trigonella foenum-graecum (fenugreek) seed improves glucose homeostasis in animal models of type 1 and type 2 diabetes by delaying carbohydrate digestion and absorption, and enhancing insulin action. *British Journal of Nutrition, 97*(3), 514–521. https://doi.org/10.1017/S0007114507312319.
Harfoot, C., & Hazlewood, G. P. (1997). The rumen microbial ecosystem. *382*.
Harrigan, R. A., Nathan, M. S., & Beattie, P. (2001). Oral agents for the treatment of type 2 diabetes mellitus: Pharmacology, toxicity, and treatment. *Annals of Emergency Medicine, 38*(1), 68–78. https://doi.org/10.1067/mem.2001.115128.
Harrison, L. C., & Honeyman, M. C. (1999). Cow's milk and type 1 diabetes: The real debate is about mucosal immune function. *Diabetes, 48*(8), 1501–1507. https://doi.org/10.2337/diabetes.48.8.1501.
Harrison, M. (2009). *Flowering Shrubs and Small Trees for the South*. Pineapple Press Inc.
Hase, T., Komine, Y., Meguro, S., Takeda, Y., Takahashi, H., Matsui, Y., Inaoka, S., Katsuragi, Y., Tokimitsu, I., & Shimasaki, H. (2001). Anti-obesity effects of tea catechins in humans. *Journal of Oleo Science, 50*(7), 599–605. https://doi.org/10.5650/jos.50.599.
Hasler, C. M. (2000). The changing face of functional foods. *Journal of the American College of Nutrition, 19*(sup5), 499S–506S. https://doi.org/10.1080/07315724.2000.10718968.
Hassan, H. A., & El-Gharib, N. E. (2015). Obesity and clinical riskiness relationship: Therapeutic management by dietary antioxidant supplementation—A review. *Applied Biochemistry and Biotechnology, 176*(3), 647–669. https://doi.org/10.1007/s12010-015-1660-2.
Havenaar, R. (2011). Intestinal health functions of colonic microbial metabolites: A review. *Beneficial Microbes, 2*(2), 103–114. https://doi.org/10.3920/BM2010.0042.
Heilbronn, L., Smith, S., & Ravussin, E. (2004). Failure of fat cell proliferation, mitochondrial function and fat oxidation results in ectopic fat storage, insulin resistance and type II diabetes mellitus. *International Journal of Obesity, 28*(4), S12–S21. https://doi.org/10.1038/sj.ijo.0802850.
Holt, S. G. (2000). Oxidant stress as a regulator of renal function in disease. University of London, Royal Free Hospital School of Medicine (United Kingdom).
Hou, C., Zhang, W., Li, J., Du, L., Lv, O., Zhao, S., & Li, J. (2019a). Beneficial effects of pomegranate on lipid metabolism in metabolic disorders. *Molecular Nutrition & Food Research, 63*(16), 1800773. https://doi.org/10.1002/mnfr.201800773.
Hou, D., Yousaf, L., Xue, Y., Hu, J., Wu, J., Hu, X., Feng, N., & Shen, Q. (2019b). Mung bean (Vigna radiata L.): Bioactive polyphenols, polysaccharides, peptides, and health benefits. *Nutrients, 11*(6), 1238. https://doi.org/10.3390/nu11061238.
Huang, J., Feng, W., Li, S., Tang, H., Qin, S., Li, W., Gong, Y., Fang, Y., Liu, Y., & Wang, S. (2021). Berberine exerts anti-cancer activity by modulating adenosine monophosphate-activated protein kinase (AMPK) and the phosphatidylinositol 3-kinase/protein kinase B (PI3K/AKT) signaling pathways. *Current Pharmaceutical Design, 27*(4), 565–574. https://doi.org/10.2174/1381612827666201217143538.

Ibrahim, N. D., Seow, L. J., Sekar, M., Rani, N. N. I. M., & Lum, P. T. (2022). Ten commonly available medicinal plants in Malaysia with potential sun protection factor and antioxidant properties–A review. *Pharmacognosy Journal, 14*(2), 444–455.

Islam, M. S. (2011). Effects of the aqueous extract of white tea (Camellia sinensis) in a streptozotocin-induced diabetes model of rats. *Phytomedicine, 19*(1), 25–31. https://doi.org/10.1016/j.phymed.2011.07.013.

Jackson, J. E., Doescher, M. P., Jerant, A. F., & Hart, L. G. (2005). A national study of obesity prevalence and trends by type of rural county. *The Journal of Rural Health, 21*(2), 140–148. https://doi.org/10.1111/j.1748-0361.2005.tb00078.x.

Jacob, S., Ruus, P., Hermann, R., Tritschler, H., Maerker, E., Renn, W., Augustin, H., Dietze, G., & Rett, K. (1999). Oral administration of RAC-α-lipoic acid modulates insulin sensitivity in patients with type-2 diabetes mellitus: A placebo-controlled pilot trial. *Free Radical Biology and Medicine, 27*(3–4), 309–314. https://doi.org/10.1016/S0891-5849(99)00090-6.

Jensen, G. S., Wu, X., Patterson, K. M., Barnes, J., Carter, S. G., Scherwitz, L., Beaman, R., Endres, J. R., & Schauss, A. G. (2008). In vitro and in vivo antioxidant and anti-inflammatory capacities of an antioxidant-rich fruit and berry juice blend. Results of a pilot and randomized, double-blinded, placebo-controlled, crossover study. *Journal of Agricultural and Food Chemistry, 56*(18), 8326–8333. https://doi.org/10.1021/jf800738j.

Jiang, H., Yu, F., Qin, L., Zhang, N., Cao, Q., Schwab, W., Li, D., & Song, C. (2019). Dynamic change in amino acids, catechins, alkaloids, and gallic acid in six types of tea processed from the same batch of fresh tea (Camellia sinensis L.) leaves. *Journal of Food Composition and Analysis, 77*, 28–38. https://doi.org/10.1016/j.jfca.2019.01.010.

Jiang, T. (2009). Re-thinking the dietary supplement laws and regulations 14 years after the Dietary Supplement Health and Education Act implementation. *International Journal of Food Sciences and Nutrition, 60*(4), 293–301. https://doi.org/10.1080/09637480801991124.

Johanningsmeier, S. D., & Harris, G. K. (2011). Pomegranate as a functional food and nutraceutical source. *Annual Review of Food Science and Technology, 2*, 181–201. https://doi.org/10.1146/annurev-food-030810-153709.

Johnson, W. D., Kroon, J. J., Greenway, F. L., Bouchard, C., Ryan, D., & Katzmarzyk, P. T. (2009). Prevalence of risk factors for metabolic syndrome in adolescents: National Health and Nutrition Examination Survey (NHANES), 2001–2006. *Archives of Pediatrics & Adolescent Medicine, 163*(4), 371–377. https://doi.org/10.1001/archpediatrics.2009.3.

Juárez-Rojop, I. E., Díaz-Zagoya, J. C., Ble-Castillo, J. L., Miranda-Osorio, P. H., Castell-Rodríguez, A. E., Tovilla-Zárate, C. A., Rodríguez-Hernández, A., Aguilar-Mariscal, H., Ramón-Frías, T., & Bermúdez-Ocaña, D. Y. (2012). Hypoglycemic effect of Carica papaya leaves in streptozotocin-induced diabetic rats. *BMC Complementary and Alternative Medicine, 12*(1), 1–11. https://doi.org/10.1186/1472-6882-12-236.

Jung, K. J., Kim, D. H., Lee, E. K., Song, C. W., Yu, B. P., & Chung, H. Y. (2013). Oxidative stress induces inactivation of protein phosphatase 2A, promoting proinflammatory NF-κB in aged rat kidney. *Free Radical Biology and Medicine, 61*, 206–217. https://doi.org/10.1016/j.freeradbiomed.2013.04.021.

Jyotirmayee, B., & Mahalik, G. (2022). A review on selected pharmacological activities of Curcuma longa L. *International Journal of Food Properties, 25*(1), 1377–1398. https://doi.org/10.1080/10942912.2022.2112746.

Katz, S. R., Newman, R. A., & Lansky, E. P. (2007). Punica granatum: Heuristic treatment for diabetes mellitus. *Journal of Medicinal Food, 10*(2), 213–217. https://doi.org/10.1089/jmf.2006.234.

Kendall, D. M., & Harmel, A. P. (2002). The metabolic syndrome, type 2 diabetes, and cardiovascular disease: Understanding the role of insulin resistance. *American Journal of Managed Care, 8*(20 Suppl), S635–S653.

Keservani, R. K., & Sharma, A. K. (2014). Flavonoids: Emerging trends and potential health benefits. *Journal of Chinese Pharmaceutical Sciences, 23*(12), 815.

Keservani, R. K., Kesharwani, R. K., Sharma, A. K., Vyas, N., & Chadoker, A. (2010b). Nutritional supplements: An overview. *International Journal of Current Pharmaceutical Review and Research, 1*(1), 59–75.

Keservani, R. K., Kesharwani, R. K., Vyas, N., Jain, S., Raghuvanshi, R., & Sharma, A. K. (2010a). Nutraceutical and functional food as future food: A review. *Der Pharmacia Lettre, 2*(1), 106–116.

Keservani, R. K., Sharma, A. K., & Kesharwani, R. K. (2017). An overview and therapeutic applications of nutraceutical and functional foods. In *Recent Advances in Drug Delivery Technology* (pp. 160–201). ISBN: 9781522507543.

Keservani, R. K., Sharma, A. K., & Kesharwani, R. K. (Eds.). (2020). *Nutraceuticals and Dietary Supplements: Applications in Health Improvement and Disease Management*, 35–56. CRC Press. ISBN: 9781771888738.

Khalilpour, S., Latifi, S., Behnammanesh, G., Majid, A. M. S. A., Majid, A. S. A., & Tamayol, A. (2017). Ischemic optic neuropathy as a model of neurodegenerative disorder: A review of pathogenic mechanism of axonal degeneration and the role of neuroprotection. *Journal of the Neurological Sciences, 375*, 430–441. https://doi.org/10.1016/j.jns.2017.02.046.

Khan, A. S. (2017). *Medicinally Important Trees*. Springer.

Khan, F., Negi, K., & Kumar, T. (2018). Effect of sprouted fenugreek seeds on various diseases: A review. *Journal of Diabetes & Metabolic Disorders Control, 5*, 119–125. https://doi.org/10.15406/jdmdc.2018.05.00154.

Khorshidian, N., Yousefi Asli, M., Arab, M., Adeli Mirzaie, A., & Mortazavian, A. M. (2016). Fenugreek: Potential applications as a functional food and nutraceutical. Nutrition and Food Sciences Research, 3(1), 5–16.

Kilambi, P., & Shah, P. A. (2021). Fenugreek: A wonder spice with versatile pharmacological activities and clinical applications. In Fenugreek (pp. 395–445). Springer. https://doi.org/10.1007/978-3-030-59369-6_18.

Kilpatrick, E. S., Rigby, A. S., & Atkin, S. L. (2007). Insulin resistance, the metabolic syndrome, and complication risk in type 1 diabetes: "Double diabetes" in the Diabetes Control and Complications Trial. Diabetes Care, 30(3), 707–712. https://doi.org/10.2337/dc06-1982.

Kinara, M., Hazarika, I., John, M., Methew, A., Chandy, V., & Das, A. (2016). Phytochemical screening and antidiabetic activity of Momordica charantia fruit extract. European Journal of Pharmaceutical and Medical Research, 3(10), 297–303.

Koletzko, B., Aggett, P. J., Bindels, J., Bung, P., Ferre, P., Gil, A., Lentze, M. J., Roberfroid, M., & Strobel, S. (1998). Growth, development and differentiation: A functional food science approach. British Journal of Nutrition, 80(S1), S5–S45. https://doi.org/10.1079/BJN19980101.

Kotnala, M., Chakraborthy, G., & Mazumder, A. (2013). Lagerstroemia species: A current review. International Journal of PharmTech Research, 5(2), 906–909.

Kotsis, V., Tsioufis, K., Antza, C., Seravalle, G., Coca, A., Sierra, C., Lurbe, E., Stabouli, S., Jelakovic, B., & Redon, J. (2018). Obesity and cardiovascular risk: A call for action from the European Society of Hypertension Working Group of Obesity, Diabetes and the High-risk

Patient and European Association for the Study of Obesity: Part B: Obesity-induced cardiovascular disease, early prevention strategies and future research directions. Journal of Hypertension, 36(7), 1441–1455. https://doi.org/10.1097/HJH.0000000000001731.

Koziolek, M., Alcaro, S., Augustijns, P., Basit, A. W., Grimm, M., Hens, B., Hoad, C. L., Jedamzik, P., Madla, C. M., & Maliepaard, M. (2019). The mechanisms of pharmacokinetic food-drug interactions–A perspective from the UNGAP group. European Journal of Pharmaceutical Sciences, 134, 31–59. https://doi.org/10.1016/j.ejps.2019.04.003.

Krajewska, A. M. (1984). Isolation, identification and sensory evaluation of capsaicinoids. University of Georgia.

Kumar, C. G., Sripada, S., & Poornachandra, Y. (2018). Status and future prospects of fructooligosaccharides as nutraceuticals. In Role of Materials Science in Food Bioengineering (pp. 451–503). https://doi.org/10.1016/B978-0-12-811448-3.00014-6.

Kumar, D., Pandey, J., Kumar, P., & Raj, V. (2017). Psyllium mucilage and its use in pharmaceutical field: An overview. Current Synthetic and Systems Biology, 5(134), 2332–0737.

Kumar, P., Taha, A., Kale, R., McLean, P., & Baquer, N. Z. (2012). Beneficial effects of Trigonella foenum-graecum and sodium orthovanadate on metabolic parameters in experimental diabetes. Cell Biochemistry and Function, 30(6), 464–473. https://doi.org/10.1002/cbf.2833.

Kunnumakkara, A. B., Anand, P., & Aggarwal, B. B. (2008). Curcumin inhibits proliferation, invasion, angiogenesis and metastasis of different cancers through interaction with multiple cells signaling proteins. Cancer Letters, 269(2), 199–225. https://doi.org/10.1016/j.canlet.2008.03.009.

Lahrita, L. (2018). Anti-Obesity Study of Indonesian Medicinal Plants: An In Vitro Study in Adipocytes. Hokkaido University.

Li, J. J., Huang, C. J., & Xie, D. (2008). Anti-obesity effects of conjugated linoleic acid, docosahexaenoic acid, and eicosatetraenoic acid. Molecular Nutrition & Food Research, 52(6), 631–645. https://doi.org/10.1002/mnfr.200700205.

Lim, T. (2016). Beta vulgaris. In Edible Medicinal and Non-Medicinal Plants (pp. 26–68). Springer. https://doi.org/10.1007/978-94-017-7191-7_3.

Macarulla, M. T., Medina, C., De Diego, M. A., Chavarri, M., Zulet, M. Á., Martínez, J. A., Noèel-Suberville, C., Higueret, P., & Portillo, M. P. (2001). Effects of the whole seed and a protein isolate of faba bean (Vicia faba) on the cholesterol metabolism of hypercholesterolaemic rats. British Journal of Nutrition, 85(5), 607–614. https://doi.org/10.1079/BJN2001327.

Madar, Z., & Stark, A. H. (2002). New legume sources as therapeutic agents. British Journal of Nutrition, 88(S3), 287–292. https://doi.org/10.1079/BJN2002684.

Mahmood, S. S., Levy, D., Vasan, R. S., & Wang, T. J. (2014). The Framingham Heart Study and the epidemiology of cardiovascular disease: A historical perspective. The Lancet, 383(9921), 999–1008. https://doi.org/10.1016/S0140-6736(13)61752-3.

Mai, V., Katki, H. A., Harmsen, H., Gallaher, D., Schatzkin, A., Baer, D. J., & Clevidence, B. (2004). Effects of a controlled diet and black tea drinking on the fecal microflora composition and the fecal bile acid profile of human volunteers in a double-blinded randomized feeding study. The Journal of Nutrition, 134(2), 473–478. https://doi.org/10.1093/jn/134.2.473.

Maki, K. C., Reeves, M. S., Farmer, M., Yasunaga, K., Matsuo, N., Katsuragi, Y., Komikado, M., Tokimitsu, I., Wilder, D., & Jones, F. (2009). Green tea catechin consumption enhances

exercise-induced abdominal fat loss in overweight and obese adults. The Journal of Nutrition, 139(2), 264–270. https://doi.org/10.3945/jn.108.098293.
Malode, G. P., Parbat, A. Y., Shaikh, A. R., Panchale, W. A., Manwar, J. V., & Bakal, R. L. (2021). Phytochemistry, pharmacology and botanical aspects of Murraya koenigii in the search for molecules with bioactive potential: A review. GSC Advanced Research and Reviews, 6(3), 143–155. https://doi.org/10.30574/gscarr.2021.6.3.0096.
Malve, H. & Bhalerao, P., (2023). Past, present, and likely future of Nutraceuticals in India: Evolving role of pharmaceutical physicians. Journal of Pharmacy and Bioallied Sciences, 15(2), 68–74.
Manikandaselvi, S., & Nithya, V. (2011). Development and biochemical analysis of iron supplementary nutraceuticals from Moringa oleifera and Amaranthus polygonoides. Advances in Pharmacology and Toxicology, 12(3), 47.
Marrelli, M., Conforti, F., Araniti, F., & Statti, G. A. (2016). Effects of saponins on lipid metabolism: A review of potential health benefits in the treatment of obesity. Molecules, 21(10), 1404. https://doi.org/10.3390/molecules21101404.
Martins, N., Ferreira, I. C., Barros, L., & Silva, S., Henriques, M. (2014). Candidiasis: Predisposing factors, prevention, diagnosis, and alternative treatment. Mycopathologia, 177(5), 223–240. https://doi.org/10.1007/s11046-014-9749-1.
Mathers, C. D., & Loncar, D. (2006). Projections of global mortality and burden of disease from 2002 to 2030. PLoS Medicine, 3(11), e442. https://doi.org/10.1371/journal.pmed.0030442.
Mathias, M. E. (1985). Flowering Plants in the Landscape. University of California Press.
Matough, F. A., Budin, S. B., Hamid, Z. A., Alwahaibi, N., & Mohamed, J. (2012). The role of oxidative stress and antioxidants in diabetic complications. Sultan Qaboos University Medical Journal, 12(1), 5.
McCabe, B. J., Frankel, E. H., & Wolfe, J. J. (2003). Monitoring nutritional status in drug regimens. In McCabe, B. J., Frankel, E. H., & Wolfe, J. J. (Eds.), Handbook of Food-Drug Interactions (pp. 73–108). CRC Press.
McNeill, B. T., Suchacki, K. J., & Stimson, R. H. (2021). Mechanisms in endocrinology: Human brown adipose tissue as a therapeutic target: Warming up or cooling down? European Journal of Endocrinology, 184(6), R243–R259. https://doi.org/10.1530/EJE-20-1288.
Medagama, A. B. (2015). The glycaemic outcomes of cinnamon: A review of the experimental evidence and clinical trials. Nutrition Journal, 14(1), 1–12. https://doi.org/10.1186/s12937-015-0038-2.
Mehta, N., Rao, P., & Saini, R. (2021). A review on metabolites and pharmaceutical potential of food legume crop mung bean (Vigna radiata L. Wilczek). BioTechnologia: Journal of Biotechnology, Computational Biology and Bionanotechnology, 102(4), 425–435.
Mirmiran, P., Houshialsadat, Z., Gaeini, Z., Bahadoran, Z., & Azizi, F. (2020). Functional properties of beetroot (Beta vulgaris) in management of cardio-metabolic diseases. Nutrition & Metabolism, 17(1), 1–15. https://doi.org/10.1186/s12986-020-00480-3.
Mitra, S., De, A., & Chowdhury, A. (2020). Epidemiology of non-alcoholic and alcoholic fatty liver diseases. Translational Gastroenterology and Hepatology, 5, 16. https://doi.org/10.21037/tgh.2019.09.08.
Muraki, E., Hayashi, Y., Chiba, H., Tsunoda, N., & Kasono, K. (2011). Dose-dependent effects, safety, and tolerability of fenugreek in diet-induced metabolic disorders in rats. Lipids in Health and Disease, 10(1), 1–6. https://doi.org/10.1186/1476-511X-10-240.
Murray, F. (2007). Natural Supplements for Diabetes: Practical and Proven Health Suggestions for Types 1 and 2 Diabetes. Basic Health Publications, Inc.

Murrieta, C. M. (2007). Lipogenic enzyme mRNA of milk and adipose tissue of lactating beef cows and their calves: Influence of day of lactation, maternal dietary fat supplementation, and body condition score. University of Wyoming.

Mustafa, N. M. A. (2020). Physicochemical properties and fatty acids composition of oil extracted from bottle gourd (Lagenaria siceraria) seeds. University of Gezira.

Nagulapalli Venkata, K. C., Swaroop, A., Bagchi, D., & Bishayee, A. (2017). A small plant with big benefits: Fenugreek (Trigonella foenum-graecum Linn.) for disease prevention and health promotion. Molecular Nutrition & Food Research, 61(6), 1600950. https://doi.org/10.1002/mnfr.201600950.

Naicker, N., (2017). An Investigation of the Anti-Hyperglycaemic, Biochemical and Molecular Effects of 4-Hydroxyisoleucine and Fenugreek Seed Extract in Comparison to Metformin in vitro and in vivo (Doctoral dissertation).

Nilius, B., Vennekens, R., & Owsianik, G. (2008). Vanilloid transient receptor potential cation channels: An overview. Current Pharmaceutical Design, 14(1), 18–31. https://doi.org/10.2174/138161208783330850.

Nimesh, S., & Ashwlayan, V. (2018). Nutraceuticals in the management of diabetes mellitus. Pharm Pharmacol Int J, 6(2), 114–120. https://doi.org/10.15406/ppij.2018.06.00160.

Nishiumi, S., Bessyo, H., Kubo, M., Aoki, Y., Tanaka, A., Yoshida, K.-I., & Ashida, H. (2010). Green and black tea suppress hyperglycemia and insulin resistance by retaining the expression of glucose transporter 4 in muscle of high-fat diet-fed C57BL/6J mice. Journal of Agricultural and Food Chemistry, 58(24), 12916–12923. https://doi.org/10.1021/jf103103f.

Nunes, A. R., Alves, M. G., Tomás, G. D., Conde, V. R., Cristóvao, A. C., Moreira, P. I., Oliveira, P. F., & Silva, B. M. (2015). Daily consumption of white tea (Camellia sinensis (L.)) improves the cerebral cortex metabolic and oxidative profile in prediabetic Wistar rats. British Journal of Nutrition, 113(5), 832–842. https://doi.org/10.1017/S0007114514004251.

Oboh, M., Govender, L., Siwela, M., & Mkhwanazi, B. N. (2021). Anti-diabetic potential of plant-based pentacyclic triterpene derivatives: Progress made to improve efficacy and bioavailability. *Molecules, 26*(23), 7243. https://doi.org/10.3390/molecules26237243.

Olokoba, A. B., Obateru, O. A., & Olokoba, L. B. (2012). Type 2 diabetes mellitus: a review of current trends. *Oman Medical Journal, 27*(4), 269. https://doi.org/10.5001/omj.2012.68.

Pallantza, Z., Kozanitou, M., Papageorgiou, N., Vlachopoulou, A., Tsekoura, M., Kontou, H., Karaferi, A., Tousoulis, D., & Bossinakou, E. (2010). The impact of the G58A polymorphism on fibrinogen a-chain gene on factors V, X and thrombin in patients with advanced atherosclerosis. *Haematologica-The Hematology Journal*. Ferrata Storti Foundation via Giuseppe Belli 4, 27100 Pavia, Italy, pp. 758–758.

Pandey, M., Verma, R. K., & Saraf, S. A. (2010). Nutraceuticals: New era of medicine and health. *Asian Journal of Pharmaceutical and Clinical Research, 3*(1), 11–15.

Paniagua, J. A. (2016). Nutrition, insulin resistance and dysfunctional adipose tissue determine the different components of metabolic syndrome. *World Journal of Diabetes, 7*(19), 483. https://doi.org/10.4239/wjd.v7.i19.483.

Parfenov, E. A., (2018). Biotic Type Antioxidants: The Prospective Search Area For Novel Chemical Drugs. Routledge.

Patel, D., Kumar, R., Laloo, D., & Hemalatha, S. (2012). Natural medicines from plant source used for therapy of diabetes mellitus: An overview of its pharmacological aspects. *Asian Pacific Journal of Tropical Disease, 2*(3), 239–250. https://doi.org/10.1016/S2222-1808(12)60055-6.

Patel, S., (2015). Functional food relevance of whey protein: A review of recent findings and scopes ahead. Journal of Functional Foods, 19, 308–319.

Pershadsingh, H. A. (2006). Treating the metabolic syndrome using angiotensin receptor antagonists that selectively modulate peroxisome proliferator-activated receptor-γ. *The International Journal of Biochemistry & Cell Biology, 38*(5–6), 766–781. https://doi.org/10.1016/j.biocel.2005.12.005.

Petit, P. R., Sauvaire, Y. D., Hillaire-Buys, D. M., Leconte, O. M., Baissac, Y. G., Ponsin, G. R., & Ribes, G. R. (1995). Steroid saponins from fenugreek seeds: Extraction, purification, and pharmacological investigation on feeding behavior and plasma cholesterol. *Steroids, 60*(10), 674–680. https://doi.org/10.1016/0039-128X(95)00094-V.

Pomeranz, Y., & Meloan, C. E. (1994). Enzymatic methods. In *Food Analysis* (pp. 506–531). Springer.

Prabhu, K., Lobo, R., Shirwaikar, A., & Shirwaikar, A. (2009). Ocimum gratissimum: A review of its chemical, pharmacological and ethnomedicinal properties. *The Open Complementary Medicine Journal, 1*(1), 1–15.

Prabu, S. L., SuriyaPrakash, T., Kumar, C. D., SureshKumar, S., & Ragavendran, T. (2012). Nutraceuticals: A review. *Elixir Pharmacy, 46*, 8372–8377.

Prasad, G. R. (2014). Metabolic syndrome and chronic kidney disease: Current status and future directions. *World Journal of Nephrology, 3*(4), 210. https://doi.org/10.5527/wjn.v3.i4.210.

Rahimi-Madiseh, M., Lorigoini, Z., Zamani-Gharaghoshi, H. & Rafieian-Kopaei, M., (2017). Berberis vulgaris: specifications and traditional uses. Iranian Journal of Basic Medical Sciences, 20(5), 569.

Rahman, H. A., Sahib, N. G., Saari, N., Abas, F., Ismail, A., Mumtaz, M. W., & Hamid, A. A. (2017). Anti-obesity effect of ethanolic extract from Cosmos caudatus Kunth leaf in lean rats fed a high fat diet. *BMC Complementary and Alternative Medicine, 17*(1), 1–17. https://doi.org/10.1186/s12906-017-1570-y.

Rector, R. S., Thyfault, J. P., Morris, R. T., Laye, M. J., Borengasser, S. J., Booth, F. W., & Ibdah, J. A. (2008). Daily exercise increases hepatic fatty acid oxidation and prevents steatosis in Otsuka Long-Evans Tokushima Fatty rats. *American Journal of Physiology-Gastrointestinal and Liver Physiology, 294*(3), G619–G626. https://doi.org/10.1152/ajpgi.00045.2007.

Rekha, U. V., Bhuminathan, S., & Shankar, P. R., (2021). Anti–Diabetic Activity of Murraya koenigii–A Comprehensive Review. Journal of Pharmaceutical Research International, 33(58B), 462–470.

Ren, J., Grundy, S. M., Liu, J., Wang, W., Wang, M., Sun, J., Liu, J., Li, Y., Wu, Z., & Zhao, D. (2010). Long-term coronary heart disease risk associated with very-low-density lipoprotein cholesterol in Chinese: The results of a 15-Year Chinese Multi-Provincial Cohort Study (CMCS). *Atherosclerosis, 211*(1), 327–332. https://doi.org/10.1016/j.atherosclerosis.2010.01.037.

Rivera-Yañez, N., Rivera-Yañez, C. R., Pozo-Molina, G., Méndez-Catalá, C. F., Méndez-Cruz, A. R., & Nieto-Yañez, O. (2020). Biomedical properties of propolis on diverse chronic diseases and its potential applications and health benefits. *Nutrients, 13*(1), 78. https://doi.org/10.3390/nu13010078.

Roberts II, L. J., Oates, J. A., Linton, M. F., Fazio, S., Meador, B. P., Gross, M. D., Shyr, Y., & Morrow, J. D. (2007). The relationship between dose of vitamin E and suppression of oxidative stress in humans. *Free Radical Biology and Medicine, 43*(10), 1388–1393. https://doi.org/10.1016/j.freeradbiomed.2007.07.010.

Röder, P. V., Wu, B., Liu, Y., & Han, W. (2016). Pancreatic regulation of glucose homeostasis. *Experimental & Molecular Medicine, 48*(3), e219–e219. https://doi.org/10.1038/emm.2016.6.

Roob, J. M., Khoschsorur, G., Tiran, A., Horina, J. H., Holzer, H., & Winklhofer-Roob, B. M. (2000). Vitamin E attenuates oxidative stress induced by intravenous iron in patients on hemodialysis. *Journal of the American Society of Nephrology, 11*(3), 539–549.

Roussel, A.-M., Hininger, I., Benaraba, R., Ziegenfuss, T. N., & Anderson, R. A. (2009). Antioxidant effects of a cinnamon extract in people with impaired fasting glucose that are overweight or obese. *Journal of the American College of Nutrition, 28*(1), 16–21. https://doi.org/10.1080/07315724.2009.10719761.

Ruan, H., & Lodish, H. F. (2003). Insulin resistance in adipose tissue: Direct and indirect effects of tumor necrosis factor-α. *Cytokine & Growth Factor Reviews, 14*(5), 447–455. https://doi.org/10.1016/S1359-6101(03)00052-2.

Ruotolo, G., & Howard, B. V. (2002). Dyslipidemia of the metabolic syndrome. *Current Cardiology Reports, 4*(6), 494–500. https://doi.org/10.1007/s11886-002-0090-7.

Sahebkar, A., Serban, M.-C., Gluba-Brzózka, A., Mikhailidis, D. P., Cicero, A. F., Rysz, J., & Banach, M. (2016). Lipid-modifying effects of nutraceuticals: An evidence-based approach. *Nutrition, 32*(11–12), 1179–1192. https://doi.org/10.1016/j.nut.2016.03.008.

Sajilata, M., Bajaj, P. R., & Singhal, R. (2008). Tea polyphenols as nutraceuticals. *Comprehensive Reviews in Food Science and Food Safety, 7*(3), 229–254. https://doi.org/10.1111/j.1541-4337.2008.00042.x.

Saklayen, M. G. (2018). The global epidemic of the metabolic syndrome. *Current Hypertension Reports, 20*(2), 1–8. https://doi.org/10.1007/s11906-018-0812-z.

Salem, M. A., Hamdan, D. I., Mostafa, I., Adel, R., Elissawy, A., & El-Shazly, A. (2020). Natural products, the new intervention regime of metabolic disorders. In *Natural Products in Clinical Trials* (pp. 32–122). Atta-ur-Rahman, Shazia Anjum, & Hesham R. El-Seedi (Eds.).

Samoylenko, A., Hossain, J. A., Mennerich, D., Kellokumpu, S., Hiltunen, J. K., & Kietzmann, T. (2013). Nutritional countermeasures targeting reactive oxygen species in cancer: From mechanisms to biomarkers and clinical evidence. *Antioxidants & Redox Signaling, 19*(17), 2157–2196. https://doi.org/10.1089/ars.2013.5370.

Şanlier, N., Gökcen, B. B., & Sezgin, A. C. (2019). Health benefits of fermented foods. *Critical Reviews in Food Science and Nutrition, 59*(3), 506–527. https://doi.org/10.1080/10408398.2017.1383355.

Santini, A., Cammarata, S. M., Capone, G., Ianaro, A., Tenore, G. C., Pani, L., & Novellino, E. (2018). Nutraceuticals: Opening the debate for a regulatory framework. *British Journal of Clinical Pharmacology, 84*(4), 659–672. https://doi.org/10.1111/bcp.13496.

Schmidt, L. E., & Dalhoff, K. (2002). Food-drug interactions. *Drugs, 62*(10), 1481–1502. https://doi.org/10.2165/00003495-200262100-00004.

Scott, K. A., Melhorn, S. J., & Sakai, R. R. (2012). Effects of chronic social stress on obesity. *Current Obesity Reports, 1*(1), 16–25. https://doi.org/10.1007/s13679-011-0003-5.

Sen, S., & Chakraborty, R. (2011). The role of antioxidants in human health. In *Oxidative Stress: Diagnostics, Prevention, and Therapy* (pp. 1–37). ACS Publications. https://doi.org/10.1021/bk-2011-1083.ch001.

Sen, T., & Samanta, S. K. (2014). Medicinal plants, human health and biodiversity: A broad review. In *Biotechnological Applications of Biodiversity* (pp. 59–110). Springer. https://doi.org/10.1007/978-81-322-1683-4_4.

Seven, A., Güzel, S., Seymen, O., Civelek, S., Bolayırlı, M., Uncu, M., & Burçak, G. (2004). Effects of vitamin E supplementation on oxidative stress in streptozotocin induced diabetic rats: Investigation of liver and plasma. *Yonsei Medical Journal, 45*(4), 703–710. https://doi.org/10.3349/ymj.2004.45.4.703.

Sharifi-Rad, M., Anil Kumar, N. V., Zucca, P., Varoni, E. M., Dini, L., Panzarini, E., Rajkovic, J., Tsouh Fokou, P. V., Azzini, E., & Peluso, I. (2020). Lifestyle, oxidative stress, and antioxidants: Back and forth in the pathophysiology of chronic diseases. *Frontiers in Physiology, 11*, 694. https://doi.org/10.3389/fphys.2020.00694.

Shen, W., Chuang, C.-C., Martinez, K., Reid, T., Brown, J. M., Xi, L., Hixson, L., Hopkins, R., Starnes, J., & McIntosh, M. (2013). Conjugated linoleic acid reduces adiposity and increases markers of browning and inflammation in white adipose tissue of mice. *Journal of Lipid Research, 54*(4), 909–922. https://doi.org/10.1194/jlr.M034520.

Shi, Y., Feletou, M., Ku, D., Man, R., & Vanhoutte, P. (2007). The calcium ionophore A23187 induces endothelium-dependent contractions in femoral arteries from rats with streptozotocin-induced diabetes. *British Journal of Pharmacology, 150*(5), 624–632. https://doi.org/10.1038/sj.bjp.0707132.

Shi, Z., Zhu, J. X., Guo, Y. M., Niu, M., Zhang, L., Tu, C., Huang, Y., Li, P. Y., Zhao, X., Zhang, Z. T. and Bai, Z. F., 2021. Epigallocatechin gallate during dietary restriction—potential mechanisms of enhanced liver injury. Frontiers in Pharmacology, 11, p.609378.

Shivappa, N. (2014). Dietary inflammatory index and its relationship with inflammation, metabolic biomarkers and mortality. University of South Carolina.

Sies, H., Stahl, W., & Sundquist, A. R. (1992). Antioxidant functions of vitamins: Vitamins E and C, beta-carotene, and other carotenoids. *Annals of the New York Academy of Sciences, 669*(1), 7–20. https://doi.org/10.1111/j.1749-6632.1992.tb17086.x.

Singh, J., & Sinha, S. (2012). Classification, regulatory acts and applications of nutraceuticals for health. *International Journal of Pharma and Bio Sciences, 2*(1), 177–187.

Singh, M. (2020). Emerging trends in food preservation. In *Emerging Approaches in Food, Biotechnology & Pharmaceutical Technology Development* (p. 44). https://doi.org/10.1016/b978-0-12-819329-6.00004-6.

Siviero, A., Gallo, E., Maggini, V., Gori, L., Mugelli, A., Firenzuoli, F., & Vannacci, A. (2015). Curcumin, a golden spice with a low bioavailability. *Journal of Herbal Medicine, 5*(2), 57–70. https://doi.org/10.1016/j.hermed.2015.03.001.

Smokovski, I., Milenkovic, T., Trapp, C., & Mitov, A. (2015). Diabetes care in Republic of Macedonia: Challenges and opportunities. *Annals of Global Health, 81*(6), 792–802. https://doi.org/10.1016/j.aogh.2015.12.013.

Smyth, S., & Heron, A. (2006). Diabetes and obesity: The twin epidemics. *Nature Medicine, 12*(1), 75–80. https://doi.org/10.1038/nm0106-75.

Söhle, J., Knott, A., Holtzmann, U., Siegner, R., Grönniger, E., Schepky, A., Gallinat, S., Wenck, H., Stäb, F., & Winnefeld, M. (2009). White tea extract induces lipolytic activity and inhibits adipogenesis in human subcutaneous (pre)-adipocytes. *Nutrition & Metabolism, 6*(1), 1–10. https://doi.org/10.1186/1743-7075-6-20.

Sokoła-Wysoczańska, E., Wysoczański, T., Wagner, J., Czyż, K., Bodkowski, R., Lochyński, S., & Patkowska-Sokoła, B. (2018). Polyunsaturated fatty acids and their potential therapeutic role in cardiovascular system disorders—A review. *Nutrients, 10*(10), 1561. https://doi.org/10.3390/nu10101561.

Srinivasan, K. (2006). Fenugreek (Trigonella foenum-graecum): A review of health beneficial physiological effects. *Food Reviews International, 22*(2), 203–224. https://doi.org/10.1080/87559120600586315.

Stark, A., & Madar, Z. (1993). The effect of an ethanol extract derived from fenugreek (Trigonella foenum-graecum) on bile acid absorption and cholesterol levels in rats. *British Journal of Nutrition, 69*(1), 277–287. https://doi.org/10.1079/BJN19930031.

Steinberg, D., & Witztum, J. L. (2002). Is the oxidative modification hypothesis relevant to human atherosclerosis? Do the antioxidant trials conducted to date refute the hypothesis? *Circulation, 105*(17), 2107–2111. https://doi.org/10.1161/01.CIR.0000015464.47778.22.

Stipanuk, M. H., & Caudill, M. A. (2018). *Biochemical, Physiological, and Molecular Aspects of Human Nutrition-E-Book*. Elsevier Health Sciences. https://doi.org/10.1016/C2015-0-01159-1.

Stohs, S. J., Miller, H., & Kaats, G. R. (2012). A review of the efficacy and safety of banaba (Lagerstroemia speciosa L.) and coprozoic acid. *Phytotherapy Research, 26*(3), 317–324. https://doi.org/10.1002/ptr.3597.

Stone, N. J., & Saxon, D. (2005). Approach to treatment of the patient with metabolic syndrome: Lifestyle therapy. *The American Journal of Cardiology, 96*(4), 15–21. https://doi.org/10.1016/j.amjcard.2005.03.010.

Suthar, P., Kumar, S., Kumar, V., Vaidya, D., Sharma, A., & Sharma, A. (2021). Murraya koenigii (L.) Spreng: Speculative ethnobotanical perspectives of ubiquitous herb with versatile nutra/functional properties. *South African Journal of Botany*, 145, 111–134. https://doi.org/10.1016/j.sajb.2021.03.009.

Suzuki, T., Pervin, M., Goto, S., Isemura, M., & Nakamura, Y. (2016). Beneficial effects of tea and the green tea catechin epigallocatechin-3-gallate on obesity. *Molecules, 21*(10), 1305. https://doi.org/10.3390/molecules21101305.

Tank Dharti, S., Gandhi, S., & Shah, M. (2010). Nutraceuticals-portmanteau of science and nature. *International Journal of Pharmaceutical Sciences Review and Research, 5*(3), 33–38. https://doi.org/10.26452/ijpsrr.v5i3.2370.

Tanquilut, N., Tanquilut, M., Estacio, M., Torres, E., Rosario, J., & Reyes, B. (2009). Hypoglycemic effect of Lagerstroemia speciosa (L.) Pers. on alloxan-induced diabetic mice. *Journal of Medicinal Plants Research, 3*(12), 1066–1071.

Ten, S., & Maclaren, N. (2004). Insulin resistance syndrome in children. *The Journal of Clinical Endocrinology & Metabolism, 89*(6), 2526–2539. https://doi.org/10.1210/jc.2004-0315.

Thornalley, P. J., & Rabbani, N. (2010). Vitamin B6, B9 and B12 in diabetic nephropathy—beware. *Nature Reviews Endocrinology, 6*(9), 477–478. https://doi.org/10.1038/nrendo.2010.117.

Tiwari, A. K., & Rao, J. M. (2002). Diabetes mellitus and multiple therapeutic approaches of phytochemicals: Present status and future prospects. *Current Science, 83*(1), 30–38.

Tobey, T. A., Greenfield, M., Kraemer, F., & Reaven, G. M. (1981). Relationship between insulin resistance, insulin secretion, very low-density lipoprotein kinetics, and plasma triglyceride levels in norm triglyceridemic man. *Metabolism, 30*(2), 165–171. https://doi.org/10.1016/0026-0495(81)90130-3.

Torrance, B., McGuire, K. A., Lewanczuk, R., & McGavock, J. (2007). Overweight, physical activity and high blood pressure in children: A review of the literature. *Vascular Health and Risk Management, 3*(1), 139–149. https://doi.org/10.2147/vhrm.2007.3.1.139.

Tosif, M. M., Najda, A., Bains, A., Kaushik, R., Dhull, S. B., Chawla, P., & Walasek-Janusz, M. (2021). A comprehensive review on plant-derived mucilage: Characterization, functional properties, applications, and its utilization for nanocarrier fabrication. *Polymers, 13*(7), 1066. https://doi.org/10.3390/polym13071066.

Tribble, D. L. (1999). Antioxidant consumption and risk of coronary heart disease: Emphasis on vitamin C, vitamin E, and β-carotene: A statement for healthcare professionals from the American Heart Association. *Circulation, 99*(4), 591–595. https://doi.org/10.1161/01.CIR.99.4.591.

Tundis, R., Loizzo, M., & Menichini, F. (2010). Natural products as α-amylase and α-glucosidase inhibitors and their hypoglycaemic potential in the treatment of diabetes: An update. *Mini Reviews in Medicinal Chemistry, 10*(4), 315–331. https://doi.org/10.2174/138955710791331028.

Turrini, E., Ferruzzi, L., & Fimognari, C. (2015). Potential effects of pomegranate polyphenols in cancer prevention and therapy. *Oxidative Medicine and Cellular Longevity, 2015*, 938475. https://doi.org/10.1155/2015/938475.

Tweedie, S. J. (2015). Effects of beetroot juice, protein supplementation, and resistance training on strength in older adults (Doctoral dissertation, Wake Forest University).

Udrea, A. M., Gradisteanu Pircalabioru, G., Boboc, A. A., Mares, C., Dinache, A., Mernea, M., & Avram, S. (2021). Advanced bioinformatics tools in the pharmacokinetic profiles of natural and synthetic compounds with anti-diabetic activity. *Biomolecules, 11*(11), 1692. https://doi.org/10.3390/biom11111692.

Vaez Mahdavi, M., Roghani, M., & Baluchnejadmojarad, T. (2008). The role of nitric oxide and prostaglandins in the effects of alcoholic Trigonella foenum-graecum seed extract on aortic reactivity in streptozotocin-diabetic rats. *Daru, 16*(1), 29–34.

Vani, G., & Devi, C. S. S. (2005). Protective effect of bacoside A on cigarette smoking-induced brain mitochondrial dysfunction in rats. *Journal of Environmental Pathology, Toxicology and Oncology, 24*(3), 225–234. https://doi.org/10.1615/JEnvPathToxOncol.v24.i3.40.

Varatharajan, R. (2016). Dose-and time dependent effects of oil-palm (Elaeis guineensis) leaf extract in streptozocin-induced oxidative stress and renal damage in diabetic rats (Doctoral dissertation, University of Malaya).

Velayutham, P., Babu, A., & Liu, D. (2008). Green tea catechins and cardiovascular health: An update. *Current Medicinal Chemistry, 15*(18), 1840–1850. https://doi.org/10.2174/092986708785132979.

Verma, A., & Mogra, R. (2013). Psyllium (Plantago ovata) husk: A wonder food for good health. *International Journal of Science and Research, 4*(9), 1581–1585. https://doi.org/10.26452/ijrps.v9i1.1230.

VSS, P., Adapa, D., Vana, D. R., Choudhury, A., Jahangir, M. A., & Chatterjee, A. (2018). Nutritional components relevant to type-2-diabetes: Dietary sources, metabolic functions and glycaemic effects. Journal of Research in Medical and Dental Science, 6(5), 52–75.

Wang, H. H., Lee, D. K., Liu, M., Portincasa, P., & Wang, D. Q.-H. (2020). Novel insights into the pathogenesis and management of the metabolic syndrome. Pediatric Gastroenterology, Hepatology & Nutrition, 23(3), 189.

Welch, R. M., & Graham, R. D. (1999). A new paradigm for world agriculture: Meeting human needs: Productive, sustainable, nutritious. Field Crops Research, 60(1–2), 1–10.

Willett, W., & Skerrett, P. J. (2017). Eat, Drink, and Be Healthy: The Harvard Medical School Guide to Healthy Eating. Simon and Schuster.

Wolfram, S. (2007). Effects of green tea and EGCG on cardiovascular and metabolic health. Journal of the American College of Nutrition, 26(4), 373S–388S.

Wu, T., Xu, J., Chen, Y., Liu, R., & Zhang, M. (2018). Oolong tea polysaccharide and polyphenols prevent obesity development in Sprague–Dawley rats. Food & Nutrition Research, 62 (pp. 12–19).

Xie, L., Zhang, D., Ma, H., He, H., Xia, Q., Shen, W., & Cong, J. (2019). The effect of berberine on reproduction and metabolism in women with polycystic ovary syndrome: A systematic review and meta-analysis of randomized control trials. Evidence-Based Complementary and Alternative Medicine, 2019 (p. 7918631).

Xu, K. Z.-Y., Zhu, C., Kim, M. S., Yamahara, J., & Li, Y. (2009). Pomegranate flower ameliorates fatty liver in an animal model of type 2 diabetes and obesity. Journal of Ethnopharmacology, 123(2), 280–287.

Xu, Y., Zhang, M., Wu, T., Dai, S., Xu, J., & Zhou, Z. (2015). The anti-obesity effect of green tea polysaccharides, polyphenols and caffeine in rats fed with a high-fat diet. Food & Function, 6(1), 296–303.

Xue, Y. Z., Wang, L. X., Liu, H. Z., Qi, X. W., Wang, X. H., & Ren, H. Z. (2007). L-carnitine as an adjunct therapy to percutaneous coronary intervention for non-ST elevation myocardial infarction. Cardiovascular Drugs and Therapy, 21(6), 445–448.

Yadav, S. R., Biyani, D. M., & Umekar, M. J. (2019). Trigonella foenum-graecum: An herbal plant review. World Journal of Pharmaceutical Research, 8(12), 402–419.

Yadav, U. C., & Baquer, N. Z. (2014). Pharmacological effects of Trigonella foenum-graecum L. in health and disease. Pharmaceutical Biology, 52(2), 243–254.

Yang, C. S., Zhang, J., Zhang, L., Huang, J., & Wang, Y. (2016). Mechanisms of body weight reduction and metabolic syndrome alleviation by tea. Molecular Nutrition & Food Research, 60(1), 160–174.

Zaidel, D. N. A., Muhamad, I. I., Hashim, Z., Jusoh, Y. M. M., & Salleh, E. (2021). Innovation and challenges in the development of functional and medicinal beverages. In D. N. A. Zaidel, S. N. Hasnain, & S. Hasan (Eds.), Functional Foods and Nutraceuticals for Human Health (pp. 137–198). Apple Academic Press.

Zhang, A., Fu, L., Zuo, F., & Qian, L. (2022). HPLC analysis of vitexin and isovitexin content changes during mung bean germination. Journal of Food Measurement and Characterization, 1–8, 3302–3309.

Zhang, F., Lin, L., & Xie, J. (2016). A mini-review of chemical and biological properties of polysaccharides from Momordica charantia. International Journal of Biological Macromolecules, 92(246–253).

Zhang, Y., Li, X., Zou, D., Liu, W., Yang, J., Zhu, N., & Wu, P. (2008). Treatment of type 2 diabetes and dyslipidemia with the natural plant alkaloid berberine. The Journal of Clinical Endocrinology & Metabolism, 93(7), 2559–2565.

Zhao, J. (2007). Nutraceuticals, nutritional therapy, phytonutrients, and phytotherapy for improvement of human health: A perspective on plant biotechnology application. Recent Patents on Biotechnology, 1(1), 75–97.

Zia, T., Hasnain, S. N., & Hasan, S. (2001). Evaluation of the oral hypoglycaemic effect of Trigonella foenum-graecum L. (methi) in normal mice. Journal of Ethnopharmacology, 75(2–3), 191–195.

Zidan, Y., Bouderbala, S., Hayet, C., & Malika, B., (2020). The protective effect of olive cake treatment on oxidant/antioxidant biomarkers, on serum, red blood cells and liver, in streptozotocin-induced diabetic rats fed cholesterol-enriched diet. Nutrition & Food Science, 50(4), 785–798.

Zorov, D. B., Juhaszova, M., & Sollott, S. J. (2014). Mitochondrial reactive oxygen species (ROS) and ROS-induced ROS release. Physiological Reviews, 94(3), 909–950.

PART IV

MICRONUTRIENTS, POLYPHENOLS, AND OTHERS IN OBESITY

CHAPTER 10

ROLE OF MICRONUTRIENTS IN OBESITY AND WEIGHT MANAGEMENT

RASHMI SAXENA PAL,[1] SARANYA PUNNIYAKOTTI,[1] MANINDERJIT KAUR,[1] and YOGENDRA PAL[2]

[1]*School of Pharmaceutical Sciences, Lovely Professional University, Phagwara, Punjab, India*

[2]*Bharat College of Pharmacy, Nakodar, Jalandhar, Punjab, India*

ABSTRACT

Public health is concerned about the prevalence of obesity and weight control because it mirrors the general inability to achieve and maintain a healthy body weight worldwide. The main problem is that obesity and overweight are associated with a wide range of comorbidities, which are risk factors for many fatal conditions like diabetes, cancer, and other heart-rclated illnesses. In monitoring obesity and managing weight, diet, exercise, and behavioral changes all matter a lot. Obese people are known to improperly consume vitamins and minerals. No single diet that focuses on managing weight loss has been completely effective in addressing obesity and optimizing metabolic parameters. The maintenance of a healthy body weight is a challenging endeavor because there are many controlling criteria, mostly varying from person to person's body type. Across all age groups, micronutrient deficiencies have been discovered in obese people, and the impacts on human functioning have been extensively researched in many populations. The hypothesis of micronutrient deficits impacting obese populations has little supporting facts and data. An analysis of the literature that has been

Nutraceuticals in Obesity Management and Control. Raj K. Keservani & Alka Lohani (Eds.)

assembled from diverse sources indicates links between vitamin deficits and obesity in various populations. Concerning correlations and possible contrivances of deficiencies' metabolic effects include their stimulation of leptin and insulin metabolism. It would be helpful to conduct more research to clarify how certain micronutrient deficits relate to obesity. Obesity is influenced by a variety of internal and external factors, all of which are complicated, dynamic, and constant. This chapter will go over the importance of micronutrients and how they relate to managing weight and preventing obesity.

10.1 INTRODUCTION

The body requires vitamins and minerals in extremely small amounts, which are known as micronutrients. The creation of energy, improvement of immunity, blood coagulation, and other biological processes all depend on vitamins. Minerals are important for various physiological functions, including development, bone health overall, bodily fluid balance, and others (Morris et al., 2022). However, their influence on the body's general health is fragile, and a lack of any one of them can result in serious—even life-threatening—circumstances. Deficits in obese persons have been noticed in various regions of the world, and it is obvious that these may affect several metabolic processes, harm the immune system, and increase the risk of comorbidities (Garcia et al., 2009). Micronutrient deficiencies have been associated in many populations with obesity, and it has been discovered that these deficiencies might influence leptin and insulin metabolism. A lack of micronutrients can affect how your body regulates your appetite and how you utilize energy. This is demonstrated by numerous metabolic pathways (Plows et al., 2009). Obesity-related micronutrient insufficiency may result from altered metabolic and excretory characteristics in addition to insufficient dietary intake. This means that the optimal status of vitamins, minerals, and trace elements in overweight individuals needs to be addressed. Many obese individuals do not consume enough vitamins and minerals, leading to deficiencies in iron, calcium, magnesium, zinc, copper, folate, vitamins A, B12, C, D, and E. Inadequate intake of fruits, vegetables, legumes, and whole grains, coupled with excessive consumption of high-calorie foods and processed sugars, are other challenges they face. Micronutrient deficiencies and poor diet quality increase the risk of developing various chronic diseases, such as cancer, cardiovascular disease, diabetes, and osteoporosis, while also compromising immunity and cognitive function. It has been found that strategies like food supplementation and the use of multivitamins and mineral supplements can help address insufficient micronutrient intake. Some studies have shown that weight loss efforts emphasizing a healthy, balanced diet can improve micronutrient levels. Research published in the International Journal of Obesity compared a 29-component multivitamin and mineral supplement with a low-calcium dietary supplement and a placebo over 26 weeks, yielding positive results. The study revealed that supplementing with micronutrients significantly reduced body weight and fat mass, lowered blood pressure, and improved lipid profiles. However, supplementing with calcium alone only positively affected blood lipids. According to Li et al.'s study, low vitamin D levels may encourage weight gain, obesity, and metabolic syndrome (Li et al., 2010). Therefore, it is well known that excess body fat in the form of dominant adiposity is associated with insulin resistance and an increase in mixed lipid absorption, both of which play a substantial role in type 2 diabetes and hyperlipidemia. When compared to non-obese people, it has been found that overweight people have lower blood levels of vitamins and minerals. Food enrichment projects are being supported in an effort to promote nutrient intake among the population worldwide and to raise awareness of the negative effects of a lack of various micronutrients. For instance, adding iodine to salt eliminated goiter (The National Academies Press, 2003). By examining the physiological mechanisms that can cause these correlations, awareness of the related connection may be sustained. For instance, it has been discovered that various antioxidant, vitamin, and mineral applications are related to serum leptin levels. By controlling energy expenditure and food intake, leptin maintains the consistency of adipose tissue. It also regulates components of the inflammatory response, which are risk factors for obesity (Obradovic et al., 2021). It notifies the hypothalamus that it is full, which lowers calorie intake and fat storage while increasing energy use and glucose metabolism and halting further weight gain. The effects of micronutrient deficiencies and their connection to obesity are examined in this chapter, along with any potential links between vitamin and mineral deficiency and the prevalence of obesity and associated body fat deposition.

10.2 PRESENT SCENARIO

Lack of nutrients such as antioxidants, vitamin A, vitamin D, B-complex, calcium, iron, and zinc are linked to obesity. The emergence of diabetes and other illnesses in obese people is attributed to high rates of nutritional deficiencies. Diabetes may develop in the obese population if certain vitamins and minerals, which are crucial for insulin signaling and glucose metabolism, are deficient. Obesity is also influenced by behavioral, environmental, and genetic factors. The availability of low-cost, high-calorie, nutrient-poor foods has expanded over the past 40 years, which is one of the main causes of the global rise in obesity. The micronutrient content of typical foods has decreased somewhat as a result of contemporary farming and food processing techniques, including frozen and preserved foods. It has been discovered that different uses of serum leptin are associated with concentrations of certain antioxidants, vitamins, and minerals. Since the altered expression of this hormone is a key factor in the difficulties associated with obesity, it suppresses appetite and its relationship to obesity. Increased dietary fiber has been shown in studies using fiber supplements to offer a wide range of health advantages. Obesity and diabetes are related to one another in a complex way. There is growing clinical evidence that supports this theory on the metabolic effects of particular deficiencies, such as those in vitamin D, chromium, biotin, thiamine, and vitamin C.

10.3 MICRONUTRIENTS AND THEIR ROLE

Obesity is the result of a number of causes, including fewer opportunities for exercise, a rise in the amount of high-calorie meals, and the occurrence of genes that raise the likelihood of obesity. But ultimately, ingesting more calories leads to obesity. Diabetes may occur in the obese population as a result of deficiencies in certain minerals and vitamins that are crucial for insulin signaling pathways and glucose metabolism. Micronutrients are essential for metabolism and the protection of tissue function, but increasing consumption will not have any effect on diseases that may not be caused by a lack of these nutrients. There is a universal deficiency in the percentage of certain micronutrients in obese people as mentioned in Table 10.1.

TABLE 10.1 Individual Micronutrient Deficiencies in Obese Individuals

Micronutrient	Percentage Deficiency
Vitamin C	35–45%
Vitamin A	17%
Thiamine	3–8%
Copper	68%
Zinc	14–30%
Folate	3–4%
Vitamin D	80–90%
Vitamin B12	9.5%

10.3.1 VITAMIN

10.3.1.1 VITAMIN D

Obesity and other elements of the dysmetabolic state associated with adiposity are closely related to vitamin D insufficiency. Given the volumetric diffusion of vitamin D into the greater capabilities of fat, serum, liver, and muscle, the extraordinary prevalence of vitamin D shortfall in obese issues is a well-expected conclusion. Numerous investigations have confirmed the link between its insufficiency and obesity. Regarding the inverse correlation between elevated adiposity, specifically abdominal obesity, as well as its decreased plasma concentrations, there are numerous feasible causes (Vranić et al., 2019). On the other hand, leptin, which is produced mostly by vitamin D, is a crucial component in the development and spread of obesity. Therefore, a vitamin D deficiency can cause obesity by causing an increase in appetite. Numerous studies have demonstrated that insufficient vitamin D levels increase the probability of obesity in women, are common in youngsters, and are connected with aging, obesity, and increasing age (Yao et al., 2015). The majority of nations diagnose vitamin D deficiency in children and adolescents, alongside the increased proportion of metabolic disease and obesity in pediatric patients. The hormonal monitoring of glucose metabolism, the synthesis of adipokines by fat tissue, and the necessary vitamin D intake across ages are some of the non-calcemic effects of vitamin D that are significant as mentioned in Table 10.2. The regulation of insulin secretion mechanisms and glucose homeostasis depends heavily on vitamin D. The accumulation of inactive forms and lower bioavailability of vitamin D is caused by excessive metabolic processes, enzymatic abnormalities, or decreased activity of alpha-hydroxylase, the crucial enzyme in the biotransformation of calciferol in a liver packed with fat. Vitamin D has an impact on systemic inflammation, insulin secretion, and tissue sensitivity to insulin in obese people. The direct and indirect effects of vitamin D cause local 1,25(OH)2D production, CYP27B1 expression, and VDR activation in pancreatic β cells (Maestro et al., 2013). The daily requirement for vitamin D intake is recommended by the Institute of Medicine of the National Academy of Sciences as shown in Table 10.2.

10.3.1.2 VITAMIN A

Studies on people have demonstrated a link between vitamin A consumption and obesity. Utilizing its metabolites, vitamin A may be crucial in

TABLE 10.2 Recommended Amount of Vitamin D Across Age

Sl. No.	Age (Years)	Vit D Requirement (mcg)
1.	Up to 6 months	10
2.	7–12 months	10
3.	1–3	15
4.	4–8	15
5.	9–70	15
6.	>70	20
	Special Population	
7.	Pregnant and breastfeeding women	15

controlling obesity. In healthy people 18 to 22 years old, there is an inverse connection between vitamin A intake and obesity. Every age group of people needs optimal quantities of vitamin A as mentioned in Table 10.3. People who were overweight or obese had lower serum levels of retinol. Weight and serum retinol concentration are adversely correlated (Jeyakumar & Vajreswari, 2015). According to case-control studies conducted in Brazil, vitamin A insufficiency, as indicated by low blood levels of retinol, is common in overweight children and is strongly linked to insulin resistance in adults with extreme obesity. In another study, it was discovered that other populations had higher rates of obesity when their dietary consumption of vitamin A was low. When their food level of vitamin A is not considerably different, obese people have lower amounts of this vitamin than eutrophic people. A "silent" vitamin A deficit brought on by obesity is characterized by decreased liver levels and signaling in several organs. For the first time, it was shown that obesity results in a sharp decline in vitamin concentration, even when the diet contains an acceptable amount of vitamin A. Additionally, vitamin A has been linked to a number of other physiological functions (Frey & Vogel, 2011). Excess energy accumulates as fat in adipose tissue as a result of a variety of hereditary and lifestyle factors, which leads to obesity and accompanying comorbidities like diabetes, hypertension, and cardiovascular disease. Retinaldehyde and retinoic acid, two vitamin A metabolites, and their role in controlling the metabolism of adipose tissue have been clarified by recent research (Zile, 2001). Vitamin A is a significant fat-soluble micronutrient essential for neuronal cells, reproduction, the immune system, eyesight, and other processes, etc. Vitamin A performs a variety of physiological roles, but during the last two decades, intensive research has identified it as a crucial controller of adipocyte biology. Recent research (ALDH, CRBP, LRAT,

RBP4, RDH, BCMO, STRA6, and RetSat) addressing the involvement of the vitamin A metabolic route to many physiological processes through gene knockout models highlights the wide range of events that vitamin A regulates (Yasmeen et al., 2012). The Institute of Medicine, National Academy of Sciences, suggested the daily need for vitamin A consumption as shown in Table 10.3.

TABLE 10.3 Recommended Amount of Vitamin A Across Age

SL. No.	Age (Years)	Vit A Requirement (IU)
1.	1–3	600 IU
2.	4–8	600 IU
3.	9–18	600 IU
4.	19–49	600 IU
	Special Population	
5.	Pregnant and breastfeeding women	800 IU

10.3.1.3 VITAMIN C

Practices that focus on antioxidants may be a worthwhile endeavor to address the problems associated with obesity and fat storage. It has been shown that consuming vitamin C negatively affects the development of obesity in both people and animals, as well as hypertension, gallbladder disease, stroke, cancer, and atherosclerosis. It has been proposed that ascorbic acid may have the following positive impacts on systems connected to obesity:

- Regulate lipolysis of adipose cells;
- Modulate secretion of glucocorticoids from adrenal glands;
- Stop the metabolism of glucose and secretion of leptin in isolated adipose cells (Garcia-Diaz et al., 2014).

Citrus fruits, tomatoes, and tomato juice, and potatoes are the main sources of vitamin C. Other sources include red and green peppers, kiwifruit, broccoli, strawberries, Brussels sprouts, and cantaloupe. Even though vitamin C is not generally present in grains, which is why it is added to some fortified breakfast cereals. The Institute of Medicine, National Academy of Sciences, suggested the daily requirement consumption of vitamin C as mentioned in Table 10.4.

TABLE 10.4 Recommended Amount of Vitamin C Across Age

Sl. No.	Age (Years)	Vit C Requirement (mg)
1.	1–3	15 mg
2.	4–8	25 mg
3.	9–13	45 mg
4.	14–18	70 mg
5.	19 and above	85 mg
	Special Population	
6.	Pregnant and breastfeeding women	80 mg

10.3.1.4 VITAMIN E

In the 1920s, three study groups one after the other reported that rats fed an almost refined diet became infertile, but quickly regained fertility after adding green leaves or whole grains to their diet. These early studies allowed researchers to describe and refine an important nutritional element for the breeding of experimental animals, later called vitamin E. Vitamin E is a combination of eight different lipophilic molecular forms namely alpha, beta, gamma, and delta (α, β, γ, and δ) tocopherol and tocotrienol. Among these α-tocopherol and γ-tocopherol are more commonly available in the food we eat. Some of the foods fortified with vitamin E include vegetable oils (sunflower oil, safflower oil, also corn and soybean oil), nuts (almonds, groundnuts, hazelnuts), seeds (sunflower seeds), whole grains, and green leafy vegetables (broccoli, spinach).

Studies that showed inhibition of hydrogen peroxide-induced erythrocyte hemolysis in men were reviewed, and the Institute of Medicine of the United States (US) has estimated the average requirement of vitamin E at 12 mg/day. The daily requirement of vitamin E across different ages is shown in Table 10.5. Busso et al. (2021) mentioned that the consumption of alpha-tocopherol by women in the US (98%) and Spain (82%) is below the estimated average requirement level. Clinical signs and symptoms of vitamin E deficiency are not common. Neurological symptoms were reported in patients with genetic mutations in alpha-tocopherol transfer protein, mutations of the genes involved in the metabolism of lipoproteins, malabsorption of fats, or hematologic disorders. Although there are rare clinical manifestations of vitamin E deficiency, the beneficial effects of vitamin E supplements in patients with chronic diseases like obesity, fatty liver disease, and metabolic syndrome demonstrate that subclinical deficiency of vitamin E also requires attention. The Institute of Medicine, National Academy of Sciences, recommends the daily intake requirement of vitamin E as shown in Table 10.5.

TABLE 10.5 Recommended Amount of Vitamin E Across Age

Sl. No.	Age (Years)	Vit E Requirement (mg)
1.	Up to 6 months	4
2.	7–12 months	5
3.	1–3	6
4.	4–8	7
5.	9–13	11
6.	14–18	15
7.	>18	15
	Special Population	
8.	Pregnant women	15
9.	Breastfeeding women	19

Vitamin E is a fat-soluble vitamin with antioxidant activity that plays a significant role in energy metabolism based on the expression of a number of genes. In addition to its antioxidant activity, the anti-inflammatory activities of vitamin E are also reported. Inflammatory mediators like tumor necrosis factor and interleukins can reduce insulin sensitivity and pave the way to obesity. The antioxidant activity of vitamin E could play a major role here by decreasing pro-inflammatory cytokines and scavenging free radicals. Garcia et al. (2009) mentioned that blood concentrations of vitamin E were low in obese individuals compared to non-obese individuals. Similar results have been reported by many researchers (Figure 10.1).

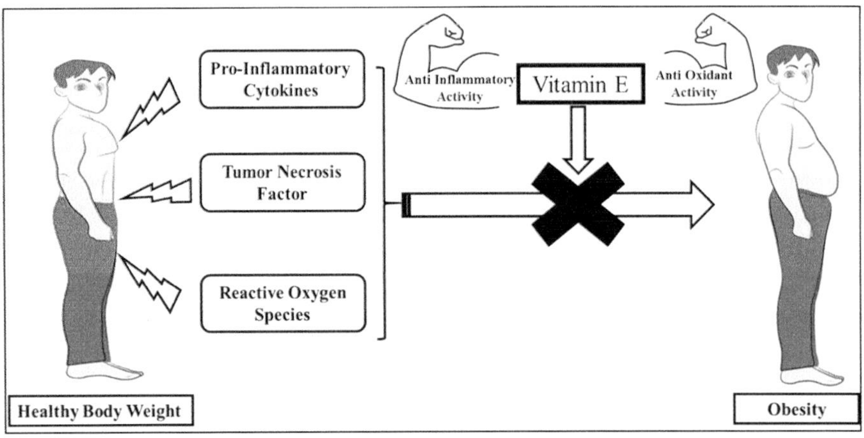

FIGURE 10.1 Role of vitamin E in reduction of obesity.

During the oxidation of fats, vitamin E inhibits the creation of reactive oxygen species molecules. The role of vitamin E in preventing or reducing insulin resistance has been studied extensively, and the reports are controversial and not consistent. Manning et al. in 2004 studied the impact of high-dose vitamin E in an overweight population and reported that it is associated with reduced insulin resistance and other inflammatory mediators, including free fatty acids. In a study of the effects of vitamin E on body weight and fat metabolism conducted in rats (Azman et al., 2001), the authors concluded that vitamin E plays a vital role in weight gain and that higher doses of vitamin E can lead to obesity in female rats. In contrast to this study, another report stated that there was neither significant weight gain nor weight loss among male rats that were supplemented with two different doses of vitamin E (Yee et al., 1998).

Balbi et al. in 2018 conducted a meta-analysis to study the association between vitamin E supplementation and blood sugar levels in patients with diabetes. Their findings report that vitamin E, when supplemented in addition to the antidiabetic treatment the diabetic patients receive, has a tendency to reduce the complications of diabetes and also shows improved antioxidant activity. Wong et al. (2017) recommend vitamin E supplementation for potential reduction in metabolic syndrome and weight gain. The results of Marfianti et al. (2020) were in line with Wong et al. (2017); in their report, they stated that vitamin E is a promising method to enhance improvement in metabolism and increase insulin sensitivity, reducing insulin resistance in obese subjects. A positive correlation between central adiposity and vitamin E concentrations was reported by Wallstrom et al. (2001) in a cross-sectional study conducted among 253 men and 276 women.

10.3.1.5 VITAMIN K

Vitamin K is the common name of a group of compounds that are similar in structure to 2-methyl-1,4-naphthoquinone, which is the common form of this fat-soluble vitamin in natural sources of food and food supplements. The Vitamin K group of compounds includes phylloquinone (vitamin K1) and the menaquinone (MK) series (MK4-MK13). Depending on the size of the unsaturated isoprenyl side chains, the MK series is designated. The primary form of vitamin K in green leafy vegetables and the significant dietary form is phylloquinone. Dietary sources of phylloquinone include green leafy vegetables, vegetable oils, and some fruits. Menaquinones are produced by the intestinal flora within the human body. However, a small amount is present in many animal-based fermented foods. Eggs, dairy products, and meats contain a small amount of menaquinone and traces of phylloquinone. All menaquinone series are primarily of bacterial origin, except MK4. MK4 is synthesized within the body by converting phylloquinone through a process that does not involve bacteria.

The enzyme, vitamin K-dependent carboxylase, is involved in the protein synthesis of those proteins that are essential in the process of blood clotting, bone metabolism, and various other physiological functions. Vitamin K acts as a coenzyme to Vitamin K-dependent carboxylase and is involved in blood clotting and bone mineralization. Vitamin K is also a fat-soluble vitamin. Unlike other fat-soluble vitamins, it is present in low levels in the circulating blood. Vitamin K is present in the liver, heart, brain, pancreas, and bone. The evidence to determine the estimated average requirement of vitamin K is inadequate, and hence the Food and Nutrition Board (FNB) at the Institute of Medicine of the National Academies established the adequate intake (AI) of vitamin K. Table 10.6 shows the AI of vitamin K across age and gender.

TABLE 10.6 Recommended Adequate Intake of Vitamin K

Sl. No.	Age (Years)	Vitamin K Requirement (mcg)	
		Male	Female
1.	Up to 6 months	2	2
2.	7–12 months	2.5	2.5
3.	1–3	30	30
4.	4–8	55	55
5.	9–13	60	60
6.	14–18	75	75
7.	>18	120	90
		Special Population	
8.	Pregnancy		75
9.	Lactation		90

We can understand that vitamin K plays a major role in blood clotting and bone mineralization. Deficiency of vitamin K is rare and is clinically significant only when prothrombin time is increased, where it could result in internal bleeding due to interrupted blood clotting mechanisms. However, internal bleeding and hemorrhage are the classical signs of vitamin K deficiency that could be observed in people with malabsorption and those taking drugs that interact with vitamin K metabolism. Vitamin K deficiency can also lead to osteoporosis due to decreased bone mineralization. However, these clinical presentations are rare in adults unless they have disrupted food absorption mechanisms or are consuming drugs that interfere with the metabolism of vitamin K. The transport of vitamin K through the placenta is less, increasing the risk of its deficiency among neonates. A condition called vitamin K deficiency bleeding (VKDB) can occur in neonates during their first few days of life after birth due to the deficiency of vitamin K. As a prophylaxis to VKDB, 0.5–1 mg of vitamin K1 is administered intramuscularly at birth as per the recommendations of the American Academy of Pediatrics.

Vitamin K is reported to be associated with body fat and its metabolic implications. Research states that vitamin K improves the lipid profile and helps prevent cardiovascular diseases. Additionally, it plays a significant role in glucose metabolism, improves insulin sensitivity, and decreases the risk of developing diabetes mellitus. Santos et al. (2019) mentioned in their research that a relationship exists between vitamin K intake, body fat, lipid profile, and blood sugar markers' homeostasis in adults and the elderly. They added that the probable mechanism for the effect of vitamin K on body weight could be because it directly acts on cellular functions. Shea et al. (2010) stated that there is not much evidence supporting the association between vitamin K and adiposity. They found high concentrations of vitamin K1 in the adipose tissues of mice. The authors report that high adiposity may be associated with vitamin K deficiency and further studies are required to provide more insights about the role of vitamin K in obesity-related health outcomes.

10.3.1.6 VITAMIN B1

Thiamine is one of the water-soluble vitamins, also called vitamin B1. It is found naturally in whole grains, meat, and fish, and is also fortified in breads, cereals, and infant formula foods. Heating foods can lead to a partial loss of thiamine. This vitamin plays an important role in cellular functions, and energy metabolism, and is vital for the growth and development of cells. Thiamine has a short half-life and therefore requires a continuous supply through food. Vitamin B1 is stored in small amounts in the liver of the human body. The majority (80%) of vitamin B1 in the human body exists as thiamine diphosphate (TDP), a metabolically active form of vitamin B1, also known as thiamine pyrophosphate. The Institute of Medicine, National Academy of Sciences, recommends the daily intake requirement of vitamin B1 as shown in Table 10.7.

TABLE 10.7 Recommended Adequate Intake of Vitamin B1

SL. No.	Age (Years)	Vit B1 Requirement (mg)	
		Male	Female
1.	Up to 6 months	0.2	0.2
2.	7–12 months	0.3	0.3
3.	1–3	0.5	0.5
4.	4–8	0.6	0.6
5.	9–13	0.9	0.9
6.	14–18	1.2	1.0
7.	19–50	1.2	1.1
8.	51+	1.2	1.1
	Special Population		
9.	Pregnancy		1.4
10.	Lactation		1.4

Deficiency of thiamine occurs due to decreased absorption and enhanced excretion rates in a few conditions like AIDS, alcohol dependence, the elderly, diabetes, etc. Weight loss and anorexia, confusion, short-term memory loss, other neurological signs and symptoms, muscle weakness, and cardiovascular signs like cardiomegaly are the early manifestations of thiamine deficiency. The popular effect of thiamine deficiency is beriberi. Patients with beriberi present with sensory, motor, and reflex function impairment, peripheral neuropathy, and wasting.

Vitamin B1 deficiencies in obese patients were reported by researchers who studied their associations. Taleban et al. (2019) mentioned that there is a positive association between the increased prevalence of obesity and long-term consumption of obesity among US citizens. Zhou et al. reported that when vitamin B-fortified foods were introduced in China, the prevalence of obesity increased drastically. The possible causes of vitamin B1 deficiency in obese patients are shown in Figure 10.2.

Densupsoontorn et al. observed that centrally and morbidly obese groups of patients studied had thiamine deficiency when compared to individuals with normal body weight, but they did not find any statistical significance between these groups. The authors recommend individuals to maintain healthy body weight, reduce body weight to appropriate scale if overweight, reduce high intake of carbohydrates or foods highly dense in energy, cook fish and shellfish thoroughly before consuming, avoid consuming the same or similar food repeatedly or try a variety of foods, and avoid overcooked foods in order to prevent thiamine deficiency.

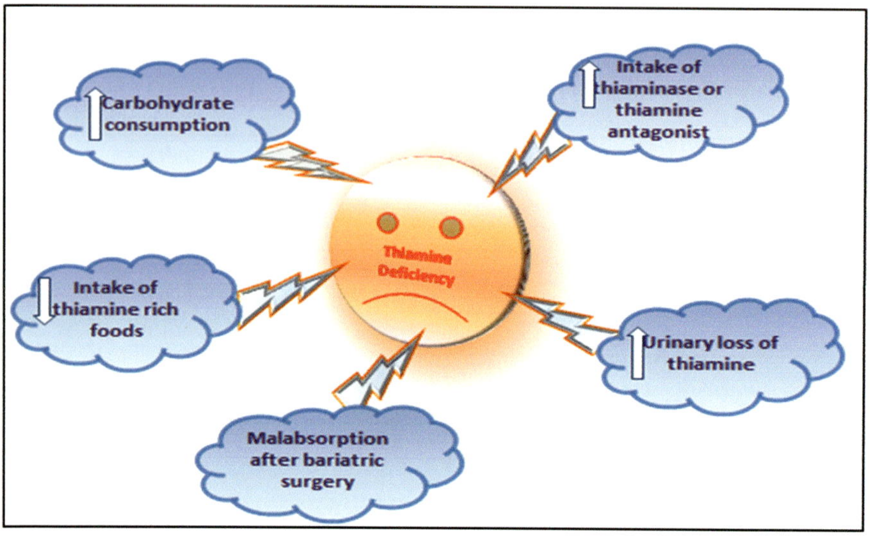

FIGURE 10.2 Possible causes of vitamin B1 deficiency in obese patients.

10.3.1.7 VITAMIN B12

Vitamin B12 is a water-soluble vitamin, also called cobalamin because of the presence of cobalt in it. The metabolically active forms of vitamin B12 are methylcobalamin and 5-deoxyadenosylcobalamin. Cyanocobalamin and hydroxocobalamin are the other two forms of vitamin B12 that are activated biologically into methylcobalamin and 5-adenosylcobalamin. Cobalamin is naturally present in some foods, especially of animal origin including fish, meat, eggs, and dairy products, and also fortified in nutritional yeasts, available as dietary supplements and also on prescription for chronic disease patients.

Vitamin B12 plays an active role in the function of the central nervous system, the production of red blood cells, and the synthesis of DNA. It also plays a significant role in the synthesis of S-adenosylmethionine by acting as a cofactor for the enzymes, L-methylmalonyl-CoA mutase, and methionine synthase. The recommended dietary allowances of cobalamin are shown in Table 10.8.

Deficiency of cobalamin is caused by impaired absorption of vitamin B12 from food, surgery in the gastrointestinal tract, long-term use of some medicines like metformin, inadequate supplementation from food, and lack of intrinsic factors in the case of pernicious anemia. The signs and symptoms

TABLE 10.8 Recommended Dietary Intake of Vitamin B12

Sl. No.	Age (Years)	Vit B12 Requirement (mcg)	
		Male	Female
1.	Up to 6 months	0.4	0.4
2.	7–12 months	0.5	0.5
3.	1–3	0.9	0.9
4.	4–8	1.2	1.2
5.	9–13	1.8	1.8
6.	14–18	2.4	2.4
7.	19+	2.4	2.4
		Special Population	
8.	Pregnancy		2.6
9.	Lactation		2.8

of cobalamin deficiency include megaloblastic anemia, leukopenia, thrombocytopenia, pancytopenia, glossitis, pallor, weight loss, dementia, and infertility. Neurological manifestations of vitamin B12 deficiency are numbness and paresthesia in the hands and feet. Baltaci et al. (2012) stated that there are controversial statements published by researchers regarding the dual association of cobalamin deficiency and obesity. The authors reported that overweight and obesity contribute to cobalamin deficiency and individuals should be monitored for vitamin B12 levels even when they are not symptomatic. Dursun et al. (2018) mentioned that vitamin B12 levels are low in obese children. The authors also reported a strong negative correlation between obesity and low levels of cobalamin among the children studied in their research. In a study published in 2020, the authors observed a strong negative correlation between low levels of cobalamin and increased body mass index. They also studied the association between cobalamin levels and gender, and across age, but did not observe any significant differences (Salameh et al., 2020).

10.3.1.8 FOLIC ACID

Folic acid is also called Vitamin B9, a water-soluble vitamin found in natural food sources and also available as dietary supplements and prescription medicine. Folic acid is naturally available as folate and plays many important roles in the human body. It helps in protein metabolism, formation of DNA and RNA, producing healthy red blood cells, growth and development, fetal development and pregnancy, immune function, and breakdown of homocysteine. Tetrahydrofolate (THF) is a biologically active form of folic acid. Folate deficiency is commonly seen compared to other vitamins, which could be due to its increased requirement/demand, insufficient intake, and impaired absorption. Vitamin B9 is abundantly found in green leafy vegetables, beans, wheat germ, fresh fruits, sunflower seeds, and yeast. Animal sources of folic acid include eggs, milk, and dairy products. The natural sources of folic acid are shown in Figure 10.3.

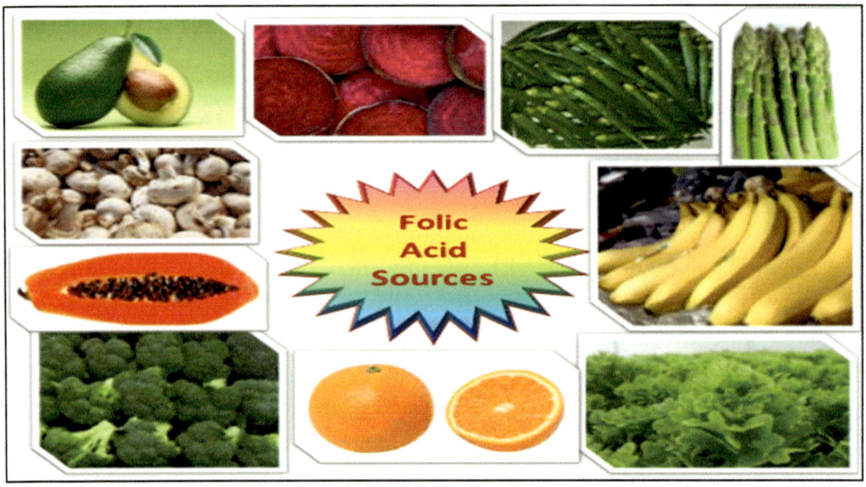

FIGURE 10.3 Sources of folic acid.

Folate absorption is impaired in patients with disorders of the gastrointestinal system including celiac disease, short bowel syndrome, or gastric bypass. Drugs that antagonize the effect of folate include methotrexate, sulfasalazine, phenytoin, and trimethoprim. A deficiency of folic acid can lead to neural tube defects, megaloblastic anemia, pancytopenia, oral ulcers, glossitis, and neurological impairment like irritability, depression, declined cognition, psychosis, and insomnia. The normal serum levels of folic acid should be >4 ng/ml. Concentrations <2 ng/ml are considered a deficiency in folic acid. Other investigations to confirm the diagnosis of folic acid deficiency (based on its serum level) include elevated levels of methylmalonic acid and homocysteine levels.

In a study (van der et al., 2021) conducted among obese and non-obese women receiving folate through diet and supplements in a controlled manner, the blood levels of folic acid were observed to be low in obese women when compared to non-obese women. The author mentions that the low levels of folate in obese women could be because of altered processes of metabolism and chronic low-grade inflammation in obese women. The author also stated that an adequate intake of folic acid of around 0.4 mg/day by women of higher weight categories did not reduce the risk of neural tube defects. Parker et al. reported that the risk of neural tube defects was higher in obese women irrespective of their adequate intake of folic acid. The National Health and Nutrition Examination Survey in 2004 observed that there was an association between low folic acid levels and increased body mass index in women.

Folate deficiency can affect the metabolism of lipids and energy. Insulin resistance, metabolic syndrome, fatty liver disease, and an imbalanced lipoprotein profile are all linked to altered metabolism and dysregulation of folate metabolism. Mlodzik-Czyzewska et al. (2020) mentioned that though many studies have reported an association between obesity and folate deficiency, the role of folate in obesity is still unexplained. Bird et al. in their study observed that obesity was positively associated with red blood cell folate. The authors also add that further research is required to find how obesity alters the status of folate in serum levels and red blood cells. The recommended dietary intake of folic acid is mentioned in Table 10.9.

TABLE 10.9 Recommended Dietary Intake of Folic Acid

SL. No.	Age (Years)	Folic Acid Requirement (mcg)	
		Male	Female
1.	Up to 6 months	65	65
2.	7–12 months	80	80
3.	1–3	150	150
4.	4–8	200	200
5.	9–13	300	300
6.	14–18	400	400
7.	19+	400	400
	Special Population		
8.	Pregnancy		600
9.	Lactation		500

10.3.2 ZINC

Zinc is an essential micronutrient that plays a significant role in cellular functions, immunity, growth and development in childhood and pregnancy, protein synthesis, as a catalyst for around 100 enzymes, DNA synthesis, and wound healing. It is an important micronutrient that is not stored by the body and necessitates regular intake of adequate amounts in our diet. Zinc is available in many natural food sources and is also available in fortified foods, as dietary supplements, and as prescription medicines. The daily requirements of zinc vary across age and gender. The recommended average level of zinc required to meet the nutrient requirement is shown in Table 10.10.

TABLE 10.10 Recommended Dietary Intake of Zinc

Sl. No.	Age (Years)	Zinc Requirement (mg)	
		Male	Female
1.	Up to 6 months	2	2
2.	7–12 months	3	3
3.	1–3	3	3
4.	4–8	5	5
5.	9–13	8	8
6.	14–18	11	9
7.	19+	11	8
Special Population			
8.	Pregnancy		11
9.	Lactation		12

Beans, whole grains, nuts, seafood like lobster and crabs, oysters, red meat, and poultry are the natural sources of zinc. The main source of zinc with maximum absorption is oysters and animal-source foods when compared to natural plant sources. The compound phytates present in whole grains, and other foods like legumes and cereals, bind zinc and prevent it from being absorbed. Hence, the bioavailability of zinc is lower in foods from plant sources and higher in animal sources. Deficiency of zinc as a micronutrient can cause growth retardation, loss of appetite, taste impairment, lower immunity, delayed wound healing, hair loss, diarrhea, eye and skin lesions, weight loss, lethargy, and impotence. Obesity and its related inflammations are observed in individuals with micronutrient deficiencies. Zinc is also studied extensively in this aspect to explore the association between zinc and obesity. Many researchers have reported that the plasma levels of zinc and its absorption from food are lower in obese individuals. In a study, the researchers observed that a daily intake of 30 mg of zinc gluconate for a period of one month resulted in a significant loss in body weight and body mass index (Payoo et al.). Zinc has multiple roles in cellular functions. It possesses anti-inflammatory activity, regulates appetite, improves insulin sensitivity, and reduces insulin resistance. Khorsandi et al. (2019) mentioned that supplementing zinc with a diet restricted in calories regulates appetite, reduces anthropometric measurements, and inflammatory markers in patients with obesity, and also added that Zinc may play an important role in the management of obesity. Although many studies report a positive association between zinc supplementation and insulin sensitivity, controversial results are also reported by a few researchers (between non-diabetic obese and non-obese individuals) (Marreiro et al., 2004; Obeid et al., 2008). Zaky et al. (2013) observed that there was an inverse association between plasma zinc levels and BMI, LDL cholesterol; and a positive association with HDL cholesterol. Another researcher, in line with the previous study, concludes that diabetic obese individuals had lower serum zinc concentrations when compared with non-obese patients (Ramya et al., 2020).

10.3.3 IRON

Iron is a basic element in human history, from the commencement of civilization to modern days. It is an important micronutrient present in many foods, particularly red meats, and is essential for the human body's healthy physical and mental development (Al-Fartusie & Mohssan, 2017). Young people's bodies contain 3–4 grams of iron, of which about 2/3 are typically stored as hemoglobin, and the remaining 30%–40% are found as iron-binding proteins like ferritin and transferrin (Anderson & Frazer, 2017). It has also played a crucial role in a variety of significant macromolecules, including those involved in metabolism, respiration, DNA synthesis, and energy production. Nearly all living things require it as a cofactor. Due to iron's role in processes involving free radicals, iron levels must be tightly managed (Cappellini et al., 2020). Global health issues including obesity and iron insufficiency affect billions of people (Chooi et al., 2019; Cappellini et al., 2020). Early in the 1960s, studies on adolescents found a link between decreasing serum iron levels and obesity (Seltzer & Mayer, 1963; Wenzel et al., 1962). Obesity and being overweight are major risk factors for many chronic illnesses, including diabetes, heart disease, and some types of cancer (Gregg & Shaw, 2017; Camaschella, 2017). Iron deficiency, also known as hypoferremia, is the most common single micronutrient deficiency on a global scale (Camaschella, 2017).

One of the risk factors for iron homeostasis disruption, which causes iron deficiency anemia or hypoferremia, is obesity. In the entire world, it is the most pervasive single micronutrient deficit. A shortage of iron or the appearance of obesity in conjunction with iron deficiency, which is frequently seen in people of different ages and sexes, suggests a strong connection between obesity and the body's iron levels. The association could be explained by elevated hepcidin levels induced by persistent inflammation. A little peptide hormone called hepcidin controls the intestinal absorption of iron in a negative manner. Significant body weight loss improves iron status by increasing iron absorption in overweight and obese people by reducing chronic inflammation and serum hepcidin levels. To confirm this impact, additional randomized controlled trials are necessary (Naseem et al., 2021). During pregnancy, obesity, and hyperglycemia have become major problems. Although obesity prevalence varies by age and is reported to be between 40 and 60% in some communities. Insulin resistance is associated with obesity and metabolic syndrome (MS). As is known, a BMI greater than 25 is defined as overweight, and greater than 30 is defined as obesity (Chambers et al., 2006). The recommended dietary intake of iron is mentioned in Table 10.11.

TABLE 10.11 Recommended Dietary Intake of Iron

Sl. No.	Age (Years)	Iron Requirement (mg)	
		Male	Female
1.	Up to 6 months	0.27	0.27
2.	7–12 months	11	11
3.	1–3	7	7
4.	4–8	10	10
5.	9–13	8	8
6.	14–18	11	15
7.	19+	8	18
		Special Population	
8.	Pregnancy		27
9.	Lactation		10

Iron-rich food includes spinach, liver and other organ meats, legumes, red meat, pumpkin seeds, quinoa, and turkey.

10.3.4 CALCIUM

Calcium is a crucial mineral that has recently garnered recognition for its ability to control body weight and the distribution of body fat. While it is not a silver bullet in the struggle against obesity, even being a small nutrient, it plays a large role (Çayan & Jale, 2020). Numerous biological processes, including skeletal mineralization, muscular contraction, cell division, and glycogen metabolism, depend on calcium (Pravina et al., 2013). Negative feedback systems such as intestine absorption, renal reabsorption, and bone storage can regulate calcium metabolism in the human body (Peacock, 2010). Following a low calcium intake, the adipocyte cell experiences an increase in intracellular calcium. This model predicts a rise in serum vitamin D due to the activation of calcium-sensitive receptors in fatty tissue. This may be described by the combined effect of enhanced lipogenic marker activity and decreased lipolytic enzyme activation (Villarroel et al., 2014). The link between calcium consumption and obesity may be explained by calcium's impact on thermogenesis and adipocyte calcium metabolism. Low intracellular [Ca^{2+}] concentrations in response to low plasma calcium concentrations associated with low calcium intake can be mediated by calcitriol (1,25-dihydroxy vitamin D) (Gruff & Gropper, 2000).

The anti-obesity mechanism of calcium as a micronutrient is related to the amount of intracellular Ca^{2+} in fat cells, which is controlled by 1,25-dihydroxyvitamin D (1,25-(OH)2-D), which plays a role in promoting lipogenesis and stimulating intracellular Ca^{2+} in the fat cells, resulting in lipolysis (Cifuentes et al., 2005; Zemel, 2002). When 1,25-dihydroxyvitamin D (1,25-(OH)2-D) is suppressed, intracellular Ca^{2+} concentration in adipose tissue lowers, which results in increased lipolytic property and decreased lipogenesis, the anti-obesity effect is explained in high calcium diets (Yaldız, 2015). The recommended dietary intake of Calcium is mentioned in Table 10.12.

TABLE 10.12 Recommended Dietary Intake of Calcium

Sl. No.	Age (Years)	Calcium Requirement (mg)
1.	0–1 Year	525 mg
2.	1–3	350 mg
3.	4–6	450 mg
4.	7–10	550 mg
5.	11–18	900 mg
6.	19–50	700 mg
7.	50+	700 mg
	Special Population	
8.	Pregnancy	1,000 mg
9.	Lactation	1,250 mg

Calcium-rich foods are Dairy products like milk, yogurt, and cheese, Soybeans, dark green vegetables, canned salmon, figs, flour tortillas, and canned baked beans.

10.3.5 MAGNESIUM

Beans, nuts, green leafy vegetables, and whole grains are the rich source of magnesium. It is one of the four major macroelements as cations, along with sodium, potassium, calcium, and magnesium, and the second most important intracellular element after potassium. The magnesium content of an adult human body is approximately 24–30 g (1,000 mmol/L), of which roughly 60% is found in bones, 25%–30% in muscles, 6%–8% in soft tissues (brain, heart, liver, kidneys), and just 1% is present in intracellular fluids, including plasma (Geiger & Wanner, 2012; Belin & He, 2007; Naithani et al., 2014; De Baaij, 2015). Magnesium (Mg^{2+}) is the second most prevalent intracellular cation and the fourth most prevalent cation in the human body. Bones contain about 60%, soft tissues about 40% of the body's magnesium and the remaining 1% is found in body fluids like blood. It acts as a cofactor in numerous enzymatic reactions, affecting the substrates and the enzymes as a structural or catalytic component. Mg^{2+} is important for the formation of macromolecules in the intermediate catabolism and essential Mg^{2+}-dependent processes are muscle movements, regular neuropsychiatric function, and the release of chemical messengers (Jahnen-Dechent & Ketteler, 2012). The daily requirement of magnesium is 420 and 320 mg per day for adult males and females, respectively (Volpe, 2013). The normal quantity of magnesium in serum is 1.5–2.3 mg/dL or 0.62–0.95 mmol/L (Kratz et al., 2015). There are three states of the existence of magnesium in the serum. The essential protein is approximately one-third bound to serum magnesium, 25% to albumin, 8% to globulin, and two-thirds to serum magnesium 92% free, and 8% complexed with phosphates, citrates, and other molecules (Insel et al., 2009). In obese persons, low magnesium level occurs commonly and leads to the stimulation of inflaming pathways (Liana, 2010).

- Calcium entry into cells and preparation of Phagocytic cells to respond;
- Stimulation of defined receptors by the opening of calcium channels;
- Liberation of neurochemicals: substance P;
- Stimulation of nuclear factor kappa B (NFkB) by oxidation of cell membrane.

The degree of obesity is inversely correlated with serum magnesium levels and is directly proportional to adverse values of serum lipid parameters in obese children and adults, indicating higher systemic blood pressure (Zaakouk et al., 2016). Obesity and chronic magnesium deficiency are interrelated. Two conditions, metabolic syndrome and type 2 diabetes, commonly associated with obesity, specifically abdominal obesity, have been linked to decreased concentrations of magnesium in the blood. Even in individuals with normal magnesium concentrations, appropriate magnesium supplementation increases insulin sensitivity in obese, nondiabetic subjects, emphasizing the importance of optimizing magnesium levels early to prevent insulin resistance and type 2 diabetes later (Takaya et al., 2003; Mooren, 2011; Hadjistavri et al., 2010; Watson et al., 2013). The recommended intake of magnesium in the diet is mentioned in Table 10.13.

TABLE 10.13 Recommended Dietary Intake of Magnesium

Sl. No.	Age (Years)	Magnesium Requirement (mg)	
		Male	Female
1.	Up to 6 months	30	30
2.	7–12 months	75	75
3.	1–3	80	80
4.	4–8	130	130
5.	9–13	240	240
6.	14–18	410	360
7.	19+	420	320
	Special Population		
8.	Pregnancy		350
9.	Lactation		320

The richest dietary magnesium sources include pumpkin seeds, almonds, dry spinach, cashews, pumpkin seeds, and peanuts.

10.3.6 CHROMIUM

An essential micronutrient found in a typical diet is chromium (Cefalu & Hu, 2004). Numerous foods naturally contain trivalent chromium, such as eggs, cereals, nuts, and vegetables (Anderson & Kozlovsky, 1985). It is required for the metabolism of lipids and carbohydrates in human tissues (Albarracin et al., 2008). To create stable complexes with glutathione, picolinic acid, dinicotinic acid, chlorine, niacin, yeast, and amino acids like glycine, trivalent chromium is used in the food business (Sahin et al., 2011).

Numerous mechanisms have been proposed for how chromium may help people lose weight. It is said to improve insulin sensitivity (Anderson, 1998), and chromium, when attached to a low-molecular-weight oligopeptide, can improve how insulin interacts with its receptor (Vincent, 1998). Additionally, chromium has been linked to both a decrease in food cravings (Attenburrow et al., 2002) and an increase in metabolic rate (Onakpoya et al., 2011).

An important nutrient called chromium (Cr) is involved in the control of lipid and carbohydrate metabolism (Anderson, 1998). Humans typically consume less chromium than is ideal through diet (Anderson, 1998; Diez et al., 2007). Additionally, it has been noted that chromium influences glucose, insulin, and lipid metabolism to enhance lean body mass (LBM) and decrease the percentage of body fat, which may result in weight loss in people. Animal studies back the chromium's effects on body composition, which are contentious (Page et al., 1993; Lindermann et al., 1995; Kornegay et al., 1997; Min et al., 1997; Mooney et al., 1997; Ward et al., 1997; Fekete et al., 2001). The recommended dietary intake of chromium is mentioned in Table 10.14.

TABLE 10.14 Recommended Dietary Intake of Chromium

SL. No.	Age (Years)	Chromium Requirement (mcg)	
		Male	Female
1.	Up to 6 months	0.2	0.2
2.	7–12 months	5.5	5.5
3.	1–3	11	11
4.	4–8	15	15
5.	9–13	25	21
6.	14–18	35	24
7.	19+	35	25
	Special Population		
8.	Pregnancy		30
9.	Lactation		45

Vegetables like broccoli, potatoes, and green beans, whole-grain foods, beef, and chicken, fruits like apples and bananas, grape juice, milk, and dairy products are some of the best sources of dietary chromium.

10.3.7 COPPER

A microelement called copper is crucial for maintaining human health. Cu levels in cells and tissues must be tightly controlled for optimal physiological functions. It is a co-factor of enzymes involved in a variety of processes, including antioxidative, inflammatory, and mitochondrial. Cu is said to have a significant part in the metabolism of fat. Rats develop non-alcoholic fatty liver disease (NAFLD) when their diets are low in copper (Song et al., 2013). According to the third National Health and Nutrition Survey, an adult's daily dietary consumption of copper ranges between 1.0 and 1.6 mg (Trumbo et al., 2001). Numerous pathologic diseases, including inflammation, obesity, hypercholesterolemia, and fatty liver with Cu imbalance, have been identified (Aigner et al., 2010; Lefevre et al., 1986). When a sizable amount of the stomach and proximal small bowel is skipped, copper, which is absorbed in the stomach, duodenum, and possibly the proximal jejunum, may not be sufficiently absorbed from the food. As with most minerals, copper's absolute absorption rises straight with dose, but copper's relative bioavailability falls with dose. The amount of copper absorbed varies depending on the diet's composition and copper concentration, with fractional copper absorption reflecting dietary consumption and body reserves. At a dietary dose of 2 mg per day, the absorption is anticipated to be around 35%, whereas serum biomarkers are impressively consistent across dietary intakes of 0.8 and 7.5 mg per day (Turnlund et al., 1990, 1998). Cu levels are higher in the blood, as well as locally in the liver and adipose tissue of obese people. Body mass index (BMI) and SSAO activity in adipose tissue both positively correlate with copper levels in serum and fat tissue. Obese patients had higher levels of serum SSAO and Cp. It is also observed that Cu levels have a positive link with insulin, leptin, and leptin/BMI, recommending a safe role in obesity. The suggested intake of copper in a day is mentioned in Table 10.15.

TABLE 10.15 Recommended Dietary Intake of Copper

Sl. No.	Age (Years)	Copper Requirement (mcg)	
		Male	Female
1.	Up to 6 months	200	200
2.	7–12 months	200	200
3.	1–3	340	340
4.	4–8	440	440
5.	9–13	700	700
6.	14–18	890	890
7.	19+	900	900
	Special Population		
8.	Pregnancy		1,000
9.	Lactation		1,300

Some of the richest dietary sources of copper are shellfish, seeds and nuts, organ meats, wheat-bran cereals, whole-grain products, and chocolate.

10.3.8 *BIOTIN*

A water-soluble vitamin called biotin functions as a cofactor for a set of carboxylases. Biotin modulates gene expression and has a diverse range of effects on systemic processes including development and immunology, independent of its function as a carboxylase prosthetic group (Watanabe & Endo, 1990; Watanabe, 1996). While vitamin B7/biotin has not been well studied in severe obesity (Hill, 1997), impaired bacterial synthesis of B vitamins can alter human metabolism and inflammation (Yoshii et al., 2019; Hayashi et al., 2017). It is unclear whether a dysbiotic gut microbiota profile can affect the host's biotin status and whether severe obesity alters the metabolism of biotin-producing bacteria. Despite being underutilized, biotin is essential for host physiological processes like lipid and glucose metabolism (Fernandez-Mejia, 2005). Biotin plays a crucial role in fatty acid production and mitochondrial oxidation in human fat tissue (Tong, 2013). The recommended dietary intake of biotin is mentioned in Table 10.16.

TABLE 10.16 Recommended Dietary Intake of Biotin

Sl. No.	Age (Years)	Biotin Requirement (mcg)	
		Male	Female
1.	Up to 6 months	5	5
2.	7–12 months	6	6
3.	1–3	8	8
4.	4–8	12	12
5.	9–13	20	20
6.	14–18	25	25
7.	19+	30	30
	Special Population		
8.	Pregnancy		30
9.	Lactation		35

Foods rich in biotin include dark green leafy vegetables such as turnip greens, spinach, romaine lettuce, asparagus, Brussels sprouts, broccoli, beans, peanuts, sunflower seeds, fresh fruit, fruit juices, whole grains, liver, seafood, and eggs.

10.4 CONCLUSION

We should look forward to properly planned and designed randomized studies that consider the effect of micronutrient supplementation on various groups, taking into account factors such as age, gender, and the degree of obesity. The strategic change for obesity should include lifestyle changes, healthy food choices, and nutritive food choices as part of a comprehensive method to anticipate the progression of type 2 diabetes. The incorporation of various vitamins can be considered. In a scenario where few weight loss chemicals are readily available, the timely possibility that micronutrient supplementation may be essential for body weight control is important. It is also necessary to address the dietary gaps in our diet. We should anticipate well-planned, randomized studies that consider the impact of micronutrient supplementation on different groups, taking into account various aspects such as age, gender, and the degree of obesity. As part of a planned strategy to anticipate the progression of type 2 diabetes, the strategic change for obesity should involve lifestyle modifications, healthy food choices, and nutritious food choices. The inclusion of different vitamins can be considered. Any of these micronutrient deficiencies have the potential to affect glucose metabolism and obesity.

KEYWORDS

- **diet**
- **micronutrients**
- **minerals**
- **nutrition**
- **obesity**
- **vitamins**
- **weight**

REFERENCES

Aasheim, E. T., Hofso, D., Hjelmesaeth, J., Birkeland, K. I., & Bohmer, T. (2008). Vitamin status in morbidly obese patients: A cross-sectional study. *American Journal of Clinical Nutrition, 87*, 362–369.

Aigner, E., et al. (2010). A role for low hepatic copper concentrations in nonalcoholic fatty liver disease. *American Journal of Gastroenterology, 105*(9), 1978–1985.

Al Fartusie, F. S., & Mohssan, S. N. (2017). Essential trace elements and their vital roles in human body. *Indian Journal of Advanced Chemical Science, 5*(3), 127–136.

Albarracin, C. A., Fuqua, B. C., Evans, J. L., & Goldfine, I. D. (2008). Chromium picolinate and biotin combination improves glucose metabolism in treated, uncontrolled overweight to obese patients with type 2 diabetes. *Diabetes/Metabolism Research and Reviews, 24*(1), 41–51.

Alcala, M., Calderon-Dominguez, M., Serra, D., Herrero, L., Ramos, M. P., & Viana, M. (2017). Short-term vitamin E treatment impairs reactive oxygen species signaling required for adipose tissue expansion, resulting in fatty liver and insulin resistance in obese mice. *PLoS One, 12*(10), e0186579.

Alshwaiyat, N. M., Ahmad, A., Wan Hassan, W. M. R., & Al-Jamal, H. A. N. (2021). Association between obesity and iron deficiency (Review). *Experimental and Therapeutic Medicine, 22*(5), 1268.

Anderson, G. J., & Frazer, D. M. (2017). Current understanding of iron homeostasis. *American Journal of Clinical Nutrition, 106*(6), 1559S–1566S.

Anderson, R. A. (1998). Chromium, glucose intolerance and diabetes. *Journal of the American College of Nutrition, 17*, 548–555.

Anderson, R. A. (1998). Effects of chromium on body composition and weight loss. *Nutrition Reviews, 56*, 266–270.

Anderson, R. A., & Kozlovsky, A. S. (1985). Chromium intake, absorption and excretion of subjects consuming self-selected diets. *American Journal of Clinical Nutrition, 41*(6), 1177–1183.

Astrup, A., & Bügel, S. (2010). Micronutrient deficiency in the aetiology of obesity. *International Journal of Obesity, 34*, 947–948.

Attenburrow, M. J., Odontiadis, J., Murray, B. J., Cowen, P. J., & Franklin, M. (2002). Chromium treatment decreases the sensitivity of 5-HT2A receptors. *Psychopharmacology (Berl), 159*, 432–436.

Azman, A., Khalid, B. A. K., & Ima-Nirwana, S. (2001). The effects of vitamin E on bodyweight and fat mass in intact and ovariectomized female rats. *Medical Journal of Islamic Academy of Sciences, 14*(4), 125–138.

Báez-Saldaña, A., & Ortega, E. (2004). Biotin deficiency accelerates thymus involution, blocks thymocyte maturation and decreases nose-rump length in mice. *Journal of Nutrition, 134*, 1979–1987.

Báez-Saldaña, A., Díaz, G., Espinoza, B., & Ortega, E. (1998). Biotin deficiency induces changes in subpopulations of spleen lymphocytes in mice. *American Journal of Nutrition, 64*, 431–437.

Balbi, M. E., Tonin, F. S., Mendes, A. M., Borba, H. H., Wiens, A., Fernandez-Llimos, F., & Pontarolo, R. (2018). Antioxidant effects of vitamins in type 2 diabetes: A meta-analysis of randomized controlled trials. *Diabetology and Metabolic Syndrome, 10*, 18.

Baltaci, D., Kutlucan, A., Turker, Y., Yilmaz, A., Karacam, S., Deler, H., Ucgun, T., & Kara, I. H. (2013). Association of vitamin B12 with obesity, overweight, insulin resistance and metabolic syndrome, and body fat composition; primary care-based study. *Medicinski Glasnik (Zenica), 10*(2), 203–210.

Belin, R. J., & He, K. (2007). Magnesium physiology and pathogenic mechanisms that contribute to the development of the metabolic syndrome. *Magnesium Research, 20*(2), 107–129.

Bird, J. K., Ronnenberg, A. G., Choi, S. W., Du, F., Mason, J. B., & Liu, Z. (2015). Obesity is associated with increased red blood cell folate despite lower dietary intakes and serum concentrations. *Journal of Nutrition, 145*(1), 79–86.

Booth, S. L. (2012). Vitamin K: Food composition and dietary intakes. *Food & Nutrition Research, 56*, 1–5. https://doi.org/10.3402/fnr.v56i0.5505.

Busso, D., David, A., Penailillo, R., Echeverría, G., Rigotti, A., Kovalskys, I., Gómez, G., Cortés Sanabria, L. Y., Yépez García, M. C., Pareja, R. G., Herrera-Cuenca, M., Fisberg, M., & On Behalf of The Elans Study Group. (2021). Intake of vitamin E and C in women of reproductive age: Results from the Latin American Study of Nutrition and Health (ELANS). *Nutrients, 13*(6), 1954.

Camaschella, C. (2017). New insights into iron deficiency and iron deficiency anemia. *Blood Reviews, 31*(4), 225–233.

Cappellini, M. D., Musallam, K. M., & Taher, A. T. (2020). Iron deficiency anaemia revisited. *Journal of Internal Medicine, 287*(2), 153–170.

Çayan Kuytak, J., & Çatak, J. (2020). The relationship between calcium and obesity. *Dicle Medical Journal, 6*(1), 41–45.

Cefalu, W. T., & Hu, F. B. (2004). Role of chromium in human health and in diabetes. *Diabetes Care, 27*(11), 2741–2751.

Chambers, E. C., Heshka, S., Gallagher, D., Wang, J., Pi-Sunyer, F. X., & Pierson, R. N. Jr. (2006). Serum iron and body fat distribution in a multiethnic cohort of adults living in New York City. *Journal of the American Dietetic Association, 106*, 680–684.

Chooi, Y. C., Ding, C., & Magkos, F. (2019). The epidemiology of obesity. *Metabolism, 92*, 6–10.

Cifuentes, M., Albala, C., & Rojas, C. (2005). Calcium-sensing receptor expression in human adipocytes. *Endocrinology, 146*, 2176–2179.

Dakshinamurti, K., & Chauhan, J. (1994). Biotin-binding proteins. In K. Dakshinamurti (Ed.), *Vitamin Receptors: Vitamins as Ligands in Cell Communication* (Vol. 1, pp. 200–249). Cambridge University Press.

Damms-Machado, A., Weser, G., & Bischoff, S. C. (2012). Micronutrient deficiency in obese subjects undergoing low calorie diet. *Nutrition Journal, 11*, 34.

Datta, M., & Vitolins, M. Z. (2016). Food fortification and supplement use: Are there health implications? *Critical Reviews in Food Science and Nutrition, 56*(13), 2149–2159.

de Baaij, J. H. F., Hoenderop, J. G. J., & Bindels, R. J. M. (2015). Magnesium in man: implications for health and disease. *Physiological Reviews, 95*, 1–46.

Densupsoontorn, N., Srisawat, C., Chotipanang, K., Junnu, S., Kunnangja, S., Wongarn, R., et al. (2019). Prevalence of and factors associated with thiamin deficiency in obese Thai children. *Asia Pacific Journal of Clinical Nutrition, 28*(1), 116–121.

Diaz, M. L., Watkins, B. A., Li, Y., Anderson, R. A., & Campbell, W. W. (2008). Chromium picolinate and conjugated linoleic acid do not synergistically influence diet- and exercise-induced changes in body composition and health indexes in overweight women. *Journal of Nutrition and Biochemistry, 19*(1), 61–68.

Dursun, F., & Gerenli, N. (2019). Relationship between insulin resistance and vitamin B12 deficiency in obese children. *Haydarpasa Numune Medical Journal, 59*(1), 84–87.

EFSA Panel on Dietetic Products, Nutrition and Allergies (NDA). (2015). Scientific Opinion on Dietary Reference Values for magnesium. *EFSA Journal, 13*(7), 4186.

Fekete, S., Szakall, I., Kosa, E., Andrasofszky, E., Fodor, K., Hidas, A., & Tozser, J. (2001). Alteration of body composition in rats: effect of organic chromium and L-carnitine. *Acta Veterinaria Hungarica, 49*, 385–398.

Fernández-Mejía, C (2005). Pharmacological effects of biotin. *Journal of Nutritional Biochemistry, 16*(7), 424–427.

Frey, S. K., & Vogel, S. (2011). Vitamin A metabolism and adipose tissue biology. *Nutrients, 3*, 27–39.
García, O. P., Long, K. Z., & Rosado, J. L. (2009). Impact of micronutrient deficiencies on obesity. *Nutrition Reviews, 67*, 559–572.
Garcia-Diaz, D. F., Lopez-Legarrea, P., Quintero, P., & Martinez, J. A. (2014). Vitamin C in the treatment and/or prevention of obesity. *Journal of Nutritional Science and Vitaminology, 60*(6), 367–379.
Geiger, H., & Wanner, C. (2012). Magnesium in disease. *Clinical Kidney Journal, 5*(Suppl 1), 25–38.
Gregg, E. W., & Shaw, J. E. (2017). Global health effects of overweight and obesity. *New England Journal of Medicine, 377*(1), 80–81.
Gropper, S. S., & Smith, J. L. (2020). Advanced Nutrition and Human Metabolism. Belmont, CA: Wadsworth Publishing.
Hadjistavri, L. S., Sarafidis, P. A., Georgianos, P. I., et al. (2010). Beneficial effects of oral magnesium supplementation on insulin sensitivity and serum lipid profile. *Medical Science Monitor, 16*(6), 307–312.
Hayashi, A., Mikami, Y., Miyamoto, K., et al. (2017). Intestinal dysbiosis and biotin deprivation induce alopecia through overgrowth of Lactobacillus murinus in mice. *Cell Reports, 20*, 1513–1524.
Hill, M. J. (1997). Intestinal flora and endogenous vitamin synthesis. *European Journal of Cancer Prevention, 6*(Suppl 1), S43–S45.
Insel, P., Turner, R. E., & Ross, D. (2009). Water and minerals: The ocean within. In P Insel, RE Turner, D Ross (Eds.), *Discovering Nutrition* (3rd ed., pp. 420–421). Jones & Bartlett Learning.
Jahnen-Dechent, W., & Ketteler, M. (2012). Magnesium basics. *Clinical Kidney Journal, 5*(Suppl 1), 3–14.
Jeyakumar, S. M., & Vajreswari, A. (2015). Vitamin A as a key regulator of obesity & its associated disorders: Evidences from an obese rat model. *Indian Journal of Medical Research, 141*(3), 275–284.
Jeyakumar, S. M., & Vajreswari, A. (2015). Vitamin A as a key regulator of obesity & its associated disorders: Evidences from an obese rat model. *Indian Journal of Medical Research, 141*(3), 275–284.
Kerns, J. C., Arundel, C., & Chawla, L. S. (2015). Thiamin deficiency in people with obesity. *Advances in Nutrition, 6*, 147–153.
Khan, K. M., & Jialal, I. (2022). Folic Acid Deficiency. In: StatPearls [Internet]. Treasure Island (FL): StatPearls Publishing. Available from: https://www.ncbi.nlm.nih.gov/books/NBK535377/ (accessed on 15 June 2024).
Khorsandi, H., Nikpayam, O., Yousefi, R., Parandoosh, M., Hosseinzadeh, N., Saidpour, A., & Ghorbani, A. (2019). Zinc supplementation improves body weight management, inflammatory biomarkers and insulin resistance in individuals with obesity: A randomized, placebo-controlled, double-blind trial. *Diabetology & Metabolic Syndrome, 11*, 101.
Kimmons, J. E., Blanck, H. M., Tohill, B. C., Zhang, J., & Khan, L. K. (2006). Associations between body mass index and the prevalence of low micronutrient levels among US adults. *MedGenMed, 8*(4), 59.
Kornegay, E. T., Wang, Z., Wood, C. M., & Lindemann, M. D. (1997). Supplemental chromium picolinate influences nitrogen balance, dry matter digestibility, and carcass traits in growing-finishing pigs. *Journal of Animal Science, 75*, 1319–1323.

Kratz, A., Pesce, M. A., Basner, R. C., & Einstein, A. J. (2015). Laboratory values of clinical importance. In AS Fauci, DL Kasper, SL Hauser, DL Longo, JL Jameson, J Loscalzo (Eds.), *Harrison's Principles of Internal Medicine* (19th ed., pp. 2761). McGraw-Hill Education.

Lefevre, M., Keen, C. L., Lonnerdal, B., Hurley, L. S., & Schneeman, B. O. (1986). Copper deficiency-induced hypercholesterolemia: effects on HDL subfractions and hepatic lipoprotein receptor activity in the rat. *Journal of Nutrition, 116*(9), 1735–1746.

Li, Y., Wang, C., Zhu, K., Feng, R. N., & Sun, C. H. (2010). Effects of multivitamin and mineral supplementation on adiposity, energy expenditure and lipid profiles in obese Chinese women. *International Journal of Obesity, 34*(6), 1070–1077.

Liana, A., Miu, R. M., & Andreica, M. (2010). Obesity and magnesium deficiency: is oxidative stress involved? *Clujul Medical, 83*(4), 581–583.

Lindermann, M. D., Wood, C. M., & Harper, A. F. (1995). Dietary chromium picolinate additions improve gain: feed and carcass characteristics in growing-finishing pigs and increase litter size in reproducing sows. *Journal of Animal Science, 73*, 457–465.

Lo Menzo, E., Cappellani, A., Zanghì, A., Di Vita, M., Berretta, M., & Szomstein, S. (2014). Nutritional implications of obesity: Before and after bariatric surgery. *Bariatric Surgery Practice and Patient Care, 9*(1), 9–17.

Maestro, B., Davila, N., Carranza, M. C., & Calle, C. (2003). Identification of a vitamin D response element in the human insulin receptor gene promoter. *Journal of Steroid Biochemistry and Molecular Biology, 84*, 223–230.

Magnúsdóttir, S., Ravcheev, D., de Crécy-Lagard, V., et al. (2015). Systematic genome assessment of B-vitamin biosynthesis suggests cooperation among gut microbes. *Frontiers in Genetics, 6*, 148.

Manning, P. J., Sutherland, W. H. F., Walker, R. J., Williams, S. M., De Jong, S. A., Ryalls, A. R., & Berry EA. (2004). Effect of high-dose vitamin E on insulin resistance and associated parameters in overweight subjects. *Diabetes Care, 27*(9), 2166–2171.

Marreiro, D. N., Fisberg, M., & Cozzolino, S. M. (2004). Zinc nutritional status and its relationships with hyperinsulinemia in obese children and adolescents. *Biological Trace Element Research, 100*, 137–149.

Min, J. K., Kim, W. Y., & Chae, B. J. (1997). Effects of chromium picolinate (CrPic) on growth performance, carcass characteristics, and serum traits in growing-finishing pigs. *Asian-Australasian Journal of Animal Sciences, 10*, 81–111.

Mlodzik-Czyzewska, M. A., Malinowska, A. M., & Chmurzynska, A. (2020). Low folate intake and serum levels are associated with higher body mass index and abdominal fat accumulation: A case control study. *Nutrition Journal, 19*, 53.

Mooney, K. W., & Cromwell, G. L. (1997). Effects of Cr chloride as potential carcass modifiers in swine. *Journal of Animal Science, 75*, 2661–2671.

Mooren, F. C., Krüger, K., Völker, K., Golf, S. W., Wadepuhl, M., & Kraus, A. (2011). Oral magnesium supplementation reduces insulin resistance in non-diabetic subjects – A double-blind, placebo-controlled, randomized trial. *Diabetes, Obesity & Metabolism, 13*(3), 281–284.

Morris, A. L., & Mohiuddin, S. S. Biochemistry, Nutrients. [Updated 2022 May 8]. In: StatPearls [Internet]. Treasure Island (FL): StatPearls Publishing; 2022.

Naithani, M., Bharadwaj, J., & Singh, V. S. (2014). Magnesium: The fifth electrolyte. *Journal of Medical Nutrition and Nutraceuticals, 3*, 66–72.

National Institutes of Health. (n.d.). *Thiamin – Health Professional Fact Sheet*. Retrieved from: https://ods.od.nih.gov/factsheets/Thiamin-HealthProfessional/ (accessed on 15 June 2024).

National Institutes of Health. (n.d.). *Vitamin B12 – Health Professional Fact Sheet*. Retrieved from: https://ods.od.nih.gov/factsheets/Vitaminb12-HealthProfessional/ (accessed on 15 June 2024).

National Institutes of Health. (n.d.). *Vitamin K – Health Professional Fact Sheet*. Retrieved from: https://ods.od.nih.gov/factsheets/VitaminK-HealthProfessional/ (accessed on 15 June 2024).

National Institutes of Health. (n.d.). *Zinc – Health Professional Fact Sheet*. Retrieved from: https://ods.od.nih.gov/factsheets/Zinc-HealthProfessional/ (accessed on 15 June 2024).

Obeid, O., Elfakhani, M., Hlais, S., Iskandar, M., Batal, M., Mouneimne, Y., Adra, N., & Hwalla, N. (2008). Plasma copper, zinc, and selenium levels and correlates with metabolic syndrome components of Lebanese adults. *Biological Trace Element Research, 123*, 58–65.

Onakpoya, I. J., Wider, B., Pittler, M. H., & Ernst, E. (2011). Food supplements for body weight reduction: a systematic review of systematic reviews. *Obesity Reviews, 19*, 239–244.

Page, T. G., Southern, L. L., Ward, T. L., & Thompson, D. L. Jr. (1993). Effects of chromium picolinate on growth and serum and carcass traits of growing-finishing pigs. *Journal of Animal Science, 71*, 656–662.

Pascual, R. W., Phelan, S., La Frano, M. R., Pilolla, K. D., Griffiths, Z., & Foster, G. D. (2019). Diet quality and micronutrient intake among long-term weight loss maintainers. *Nutrients, 11*(12), 3046.

Payahoo, L., Ostadrahimi, A., Mobasseri, M., Khaje Bishak, Y., Farrin, N., Asghari Jafarabadi, M., & Mahluji, S. (2013). Effects of zinc supplementation on the anthropometric measurements, lipid profiles and fasting blood glucose in healthy obese adults. *Advanced Pharmaceutical Bulletin, 3*(1), 161–165.

Peacock, M. (2010). Calcium metabolism in health and disease. *Clinical Journal of the American Society of Nephrology, 5*, 23–30.

Plows, J. F., Stanley, J. L., Baker, P. N., Reynolds, C. M., & Vickers, M. H. (2018). The pathophysiology of gestational diabetes mellitus. *International Journal of Molecular Sciences, 19*(11), 3342.

Pravina, P., Sayaji, D., & Avinash, M. (2013). Calcium and its role in human body. *International Journal of Research in Pharmacy and Biomedical Sciences, 4*, 659–668.

Ramya, S., & Ponsuganthi, K. (2020). A study of serum zinc and copper in obese and non-obese type 2 diabetic patients. *MedPulse International Journal of Biochemistry, 16*(1), 01–05.

Rodriguez-Melendez, R., & Zempleni, J. (2003). Regulation of gene expression by biotin. *Journal of Nutritional Biochemistry, 14*(12), 680–690.

Sahin, K., Tuzcu, M., Orhan, C., et al. (2011). The effects of chromium complex and level on glucose metabolism and memory acquisition in rats fed high-fat diet. *Biological Trace Element Research, 143*(2), 1018–1030.

Salameh, A. A. B., Dalala'h, K. M. A. L., Bdour, K. M., Hamad, Y. S. B., Alzu'bi, A. B., & Al-Najdawi, M. S. (2020). The relationship between serum vitamin B12 level, obesity, and age: A cross-sectional study. *Journal of the Royal Medical Services, 27*(2), 10.

Seltzer, C. C., & Mayer, J. (1963). Serum iron and iron-binding capacity in adolescents. II. Comparison of obese and nonobese subjects. *American Journal of Clinical Nutrition, 13*, 354–361.

Shea, M. K., Booth, S. L., Gundberg, C. M., Peterson, J. W., Waddell, C., Dawson-Hughes, B., & Saltzman, E. (2010). Adulthood obesity is positively associated with adipose tissue concentrations of vitamin K and inversely associated with circulating indicators of vitamin K status in men and women. *The Journal of Nutrition, 140*(5), 1029–1034.

Song, M., Schuschke, D. A., Zhou, Z., et al. (2013). Modest fructose beverage intake causes liver injury and fat accumulation in marginal copper deficient rats. *Obesity, 21*, 1669–1675.

Takaya, J., Higashino, H., Kotera, F., & Kobayashi, Y. (2003). Intracellular magnesium of platelets in children with diabetes and obesity. *Metabolism, 52*(4), 468–471.

Taleban, R., Heidari-Beni, M., Qorbani, M., Motlagh, M. E., Fazel-Tabar Malekshah, A., Moafi, M., et al. (2019). Is dietary vitamin B intake associated with weight disorders in children and adolescents? The weight disorders survey of the CASPIAN-IV Study. *Health Promotion Perspectives, 9*(4), 290–306.

The National Academies Press. (2003). *Dietary Reference Intakes: Guiding Principles for Nutrition Labeling and Fortification*. Washington, DC.

Tong, L. (2013). Structure and function of biotin-dependent carboxylases. *Cellular and Molecular Life Sciences, 70*(5), 863–891.

Trumbo, P., Yates, A. A., Schlicker, S., & Poos, M. (2001). Dietary reference intakes: vitamin A, vitamin K, arsenic, boron, chromium, copper, iodine, iron, manganese, molybdenum nickel, silicon, vanadium, and zinc. *Journal of the American Dietetic Association, 101*(3), 294–301.

Turnlund, J. R., Keen, C. L., & Smith, R. G. (1990). Copper status and urinary and salivary copper in young men at three levels of dietary copper. *American Journal of Clinical Nutrition, 51*, 658–664.

Turnlund, J. R., Keyes, W. R., Peiffer, G. L., & Scott, K. C. (1998). Copper absorption, excretion, and retention by young men consuming low dietary copper determined by using the stable isotope 65Cu. *American Journal of Clinical Nutrition, 67*, 1219–1225.

van der Windt, M., Schoenmakers, S., van Rijn, B., Galjaard, S., Steegers-Theunissen, R., & van Rossem, L. (2021). Epidemiology and (Patho)Physiology of Folic Acid Supplement Use in Obese Women before and during Pregnancy. *Nutrients, 13*(2), 331.

Via, M. (2012). The malnutrition of obesity: Micronutrient deficiencies that promote diabetes. *ISRN Endocrinology, 2012*, 103472.

Villarroel, P., Villalobos, E., Reyes, M., & Cifuentes, M. (2014). Calcium, obesity, and the role of the calcium-sensing receptor. *Nutrition Reviews, 72*, 627–637.

Vincent, J. B. (1999). Mechanisms of chromium action: low-molecular weight chromium-binding substance. *Journal of the American College of Nutrition, 18*, 6–12.

Volpe, S. L. (2013). Magnesium in disease prevention and overall health. *Advances in Nutrition, 4*, 378–383.

Vranić, L., Mikolašević, I., & Milić, S. (2019). Vitamin D deficiency: Consequence or cause of obesity? *Medicina (Kaunas), 55*(9), 541.

Wallstrom, P., Wirfalt, E., Lahmann, P. H., Gullberg, B., Janzon, L., & Berglund, G. (2001). Serum concentrations of beta-carotene and alpha-tocopherol are associated with diet, smoking, and general and central adiposity. *American Journal of Clinical Nutrition, 73*, 777–785.

Ward, T. L., Southern, L. L., & Bidner, T. D. (1997). Interactive effects of dietary chromium tripicolinate and crude protein level in growing-finishing pigs provided inadequate and adequate floor space. *Journal of Animal Science, 75*, 1001–1005.

Watanabe, T. (1996). Morphological and biochemical effects of excessive amounts of biotin on embryonic development in mice. *Experientia, 52*, 149–154.

Watanabe, T., & Endo, A. (1990). Teratogenic effects of maternal biotin deficiency on mouse embryos examined at midgestation. *Teratology, 42*, 295–300.

Watson, R. R., Preedy, V. R., & Zibadi, S. (Eds.). (2013). *Magnesium in Human Health and Disease*. New York: Humana Press.

Wenzel, B. J., Stults, H. B., & Mayer, J. (1962). Hypoferraemia in obese adolescents. *Lancet, 2*(7251), 327–328.

Wong, S. K., Chin, K. Y., Suhaimi, F. H., Ahmad, F., & Ima-Nirwana, S. (2017). Vitamin E as a potential interventional treatment for metabolic syndrome: Evidence from animal and human studies. *Frontiers in Pharmacology, 8*, 444.

Yao, Y., Zhu, L., He, L., Duan, Y., Liang, W., Nie, Z., Jin, Y., Wu, X., & Fang, Y. (2015). A meta-analysis of the relationship between vitamin D deficiency and obesity. *International Journal of Clinical and Experimental Medicine, 8*(9), 14977–14984.

Yasmeen, R., Jeyakumar, S. M., Reichert, B., Yang, F., & Ziouzenkova, O. (2012). The contribution of vitamin A to autocrine regulation of fat depots. *Biochimica et Biophysica Acta (BBA) – Molecular and Cell Biology of Lipids, 1821*, 190–197.

Yee, J. K., & Ima-Nirwana, S. (1998). Palm vitamin E protects against ferric nitriloacetate-induced impairment of bone calcification. *Asia Pacific Journal of Pharmacology, 13*, 1–7.

Yoshii, K., Hosomi, K., Sawane, K., et al. (2019). Metabolism of dietary and microbial vitamin B family in the regulation of host immunity. *Frontiers in Nutrition, 6*, 48.

Zaakouk, A. M., Hassan, M. A., & Tolba, O. A. (2016). Serum magnesium status among obese children and adolescents. *Egyptian Pediatric Association Gazette, 64*, 32–37.

Zaky, D. S. E., Sultan, E. A., Salim, M. F., & Dawod, R. S. (2013). Zinc level and obesity. *Egyptian Journal of Internal Medicine, 25*, 209–212.

Zeitz, U., Weber, K., Soegiarto, D. W., Wolf, E., Balling, R., & Erben, R. G. (2003). Impaired insulin secretory capacity in mice lacking a functional vitamin D receptor. *The FASEB Journal, 17*, 509–511.

Zemel, M. B. (2002). Regulation of adiposity and obesity risk by dietary calcium: mechanisms and implications. *Journal of the American College of Nutrition, 21*, 146–151.

Zhou, S. S., & Zhou, Y. (2014). Excess vitamin intake: An unrecognized risk factor for obesity. *World Journal of Diabetes, 5*(1), 1.

Zhou, S. S., Li, D., Zhou, Y. M., Sun, W. P., & Liu, Q. G. (2010). B-vitamin consumption and the prevalence of diabetes and obesity among the US adults: Population based ecological study. *BMC Public Health, 10*, 746.

Zile, M. H. (2001). Function of vitamin A in vertebrate embryonic development. *Journal of Nutrition, 131*, 705–708.

Ziouzenkova, O., Orasanu, G., Sharlach, M., Akiyama, T. E., Berger, J. P., Viereck, J., & Plutzky, J. (2007). Retinaldehyde represses adipogenesis and diet-induced obesity. *Nature Medicine, 13*, 695–702.

CHAPTER 11

POLYPHENOL DERIVATIVES IN OBESITY MANAGEMENT

PRAGYA,[1] VAIBHAV RASTOGI,[2] RITIKA SAXENA,[3] AFREEN HASHMI,[4] and ANURAG VERMA[2]

[1]*Department of Pharmaceutics, Amity Institute of Pharmacy, Amity University Uttar Pradesh, Lucknow Campus, Uttar Pradesh, India*

[2]*Teerthanker Mahaveer College of Pharmacy, Teerthanker Mahaveer University, Moradabad, Uttar Pradesh, India*

[3]*School of Biotechnology, IFTM University, Moradabad, Uttar Pradesh, India*

[4]*Faculty of Pharmacy, Babu Banarasi Das Northern India Institute of Technology, Lucknow, Uttar Pradesh, India*

ABSTRACT

A severe issue impacting millions of individuals is excessive weight gain (obesity). The past few decades have witnessed a consecutive rise in the count of overweight/obese people all across the world. Traditional methods of treating obesity and the accompanying complications include consuming a nutritious and well-balanced diet, engaging in physical activity, modifying lifestyle, the use of synthetic anti-obesity medicines, and surgical treatments (bariatric surgery). However, these methods have a number of drawbacks, such as the patient's non-compliance, inability to adhere to a balanced diet, harmful adverse effects of synthetic drugs, and the possibility of relapse with a serious outcome. So there is a rising worldwide trend toward employing natural substances for obesity therapy. It has been found that secondary

Nutraceuticals in Obesity Management and Control. Raj K. Keservani & Alka Lohani (Eds.)

plant metabolites such as phenolics, flavonoids (flavones, anthocyanins, flavonols, etc.), lignans, stilbenes, and terpenoids, as well as others, have potent anti-obesity effects. Specifically, this chapter focuses on the effects of polyphenols on preventing obesity, including their classifications, sources, and anti-obesity mechanisms. The findings of current studies on polyphenols, their usage as an anti-obesity drug, and the mechanisms by which they reduce obesity are also discussed in this chapter. The underlying mechanisms of polyphenols in the management of obesity need to be confirmed in future research, which can then potentially contribute to the evidence-based use of these compounds in the field of human health.

11.1 INTRODUCTION

Obesity is a chronic, multifaceted medical disorder that has a significant detrimental impact on human health (Hu, 2007). The definition of overweight and obesity is "abnormal or excessive fat buildup that poses a risk to health." Overweight is defined as having a body mass index (BMI) over 25, and obesity as having a BMI over 30. According to the global burden of disease, the problem has reached epidemic proportions, with over 4 million people per year dying as a result of being overweight or obese in 2017 (Obesity [Online]).

In both adults and children, the incidences of overweight and/or obesity are exponentially rising. Globally, the percentage of overweight or obesity among children and adolescents aged 5 to 19 more than quadrupled from 4% to 18% between 1975 and 2016. Over 1 billion people are obese worldwide, including 650 million adults, 340 million teenagers, and 39 million children, according to a recent study (Obesity [Online]). This number is still increasing. At 36.2%, the obesity rate in the United States is the 12th highest in the world (Obesity rates by country 2022 [Online]).

With its detrimental effects on mortality, morbidity, and healthcare expenses, obesity is growing in importance as a public health issue. Obesity is commonly stigmatized and connected to the false idea that it is primarily attributed to a lack of will resulting in poor eating choices and inactivity. However, a large body of research-based literature depicts obesity as a complicated, chronic illness caused by the interaction of various genetic, environmental, metabolic, and behavioral variables. The prevalence of other diseases known as comorbidities, such as cardiovascular disease, diabetes, hyperlipidemia, stroke, non-alcoholic fatty liver disease, malignancies, osteoarthritis, pulmonary disease, and polycystic ovarian syndrome (PCOS), has increased in tandem with the prevalence of obesity (Upadhyay et al., 2018; Cawley & Meyerhoefer, 2012).

The globe faces a serious public health concern in the 21st century: the management and prevention of overweight and obesity. The loss of body weight is always inextricably linked to the treatment of obesity.

Recent literature has evidenced a number of approaches to address this challenge, such as healthy lifestyle choices (diet and exercise), restoring a healthy lipid metabolism, using medications, or having bariatric surgery (Torres-Fuentes et al., 2015). Recent research has demonstrated that several dietary elements that are naturally occurring can affect body weight and are a reliable method for preventing obesity. Particularly, consuming foods high in polyphenols can aid in lowering the physiological excess weight that gradually happens in the general population (Boccellino & D'Angelo, 2020).

A suppression in food intake, declined lipogenesis, elevated lipolysis, depressed fatty acid oxidation, and suppressed adipogenesis and apoptosis have all been associated with dietary polyphenols (Keservani & Sharma, 2014; Keservani et al., 2016a, b). The most significant factors in the treatment of obesity are these pharmacological effects, particularly lipid metabolism and adipogenesis (Wang et al., 2014). It is thought that polyphenols have subtle effects through a variety of processes and biochemical targets, which together have significant health advantages (Li et al., 2018). This suggests that polyphenols may be effective in treating obesity and that they can be added to certain foods to potentially have this effect. Finding polyphenolic substances for the treatment of obesity that have high efficacy and few adverse effects is a research area that is receiving more attention (Singh et al., 2020).

In this perspective, this chapter discusses how polyphenolic derivatives might assist in preventing obesity. It outlines various ways in which polyphenols exert their anti-obesity potential and aid in the prevention of both disease and its associated complications. Additionally, it includes summaries of recent studies on polyphenols that demonstrate their significance in weight loss prevention.

11.2 OBESITY

According to The Centers for Disease Control and Prevention, obesity is defined as a body mass index (BMI) over the 95th percentile (Flegal et al.,

2009). Obesity is a long-term condition with a complicated pathophysiology that is defined by adipose tissue hypertrophy and hyperplasia, which leads to an unbalanced energy situation. On the other hand, it is a condition that will enhance the probability of developing non-communicable diseases and mental health illnesses in a wide range (Banerjee et al., 2020). This is most clearly visible during the COVID-19 pandemic (COVID-19 and obesity: The 2021 atlas [Online]). Additionally, there is evidence linking obesity to influenza and other respiratory viral infections (Moser et al., 2019). Obesity did not receive much prioritization of its prevalence and effects, which are growing gradually in emerging economies (COVID-19 and obesity: The 2021 atlas [Online]).

Combinations of many factors are responsible for the childhood obesity epidemic. Although several factors, namely socioeconomic status, emotional and mental stress, anxiety, and social ignorance, accumulate results in childhood obesity, the main culprit is the intake of high-calorie food accompanied by little or no physical activity. Additionally, some people are obese due to their genetic makeup, but most of them become obese only because of the imbalance between calorie consumption and expenditure. Some studies reported that with advancements in economic conditions, there is an increased demand for fat-rich food, resulting in more energy intake that ultimately causes children to become more obese. In fact, obese children are at greater risk of acquiring diseases such as cardiovascular diseases, diabetes, and types of cancer including endometrial, colon, and breast cancer (Buoncristiano et al., 2021).

The frequency of obesity is more reported among females when compared with males worldwide, equally in developed and developing nations. This is evident from the global data that on the scale of obesity, 15% of women are more obese as compared to 11% of men. Women are more vulnerable than men to becoming obese due to the fact that women physiologically store a higher amount of fat and hold relatively bigger adipose stores and a higher total percentage of body fat. During the reproductive age, women are more susceptible to becoming obese, which is attributed to weight gain during gestational years, post-pregnancy weight gain and retention, as well as unfavorable and stressful lifestyle risk aspects during pregnancy in the postpartum period. This obesity causes women to develop gynecological cancers which include breast, cervical, and ovarian cancer (Flegal et al., 2009).

Strategies that can be undertaken to prevent obesity among children include primary prevention of obesity itself and secondly, following the avoidance of weight regain after weight loss (Dehghan et al., 2005). Looking at women, their problems need to be addressed quickly, and multi-faceted obesity prevention and mitigation must be considered (Flegal et al., 2009).

11.3 POLYPHENOLS

A large class of bioactive substances known as polyphenols are found in plants as secondary metabolites. Natural sources of polyphenols include plants, vegetables, and their derivative products (Table 11.1), and they are of great importance because they affect the flavor, appearance, and nutritional qualities of these foods. They naturally occur in human diets, and research indicates that consuming them may have positive effects on a variety of health-related factors. It is widely acknowledged that dietary polyphenols from fruits, vegetables, and other plant-based foods may offer a variety of health advantages (Boccellino et al., 2019; Giudice et al., 2017; Saberi-Karimian et al., 2019; Motti et al., 2018; D'Angelo et al., 2019). Products including wine, onions, tea, grapes, chocolates, and coffee are demonstrated to be rich in polyphenols, although it is challenging to quantify the total polyphenol content in foods due to the variety of chemical structures (Boccellino & D'Angelo, 2020).

Chemically speaking, polyphenols are phenolic compounds having additional functional groups such as glycosides, methyl ethers, and esters attached to their chemical structure as well as at least one or more aromatic rings containing a hydroxyl group (Bhuyan & Basu, 2017). Polyphenols are typically divided into flavonoids (flavanols, flavonols, flavones, isoflavones, anthocyanins) and non-flavonoids depending on the chemical structure (phenolic acids, stilbenes, lignans, others) and complexity (i.e., the number of phenolic rings and substitution groups) (Naczk & Shahidi, 2006; Pandey & Rizvi, 2009; Bhardwaj et al., 2021).

11.3.1 FLAVONOIDS

Nearly 9,000 structurally distinct flavonoids have been recognized in nature. Furthermore, a heterogeneous subgroup consists of a variety of phenolic molecules with a common 15-carbon flavan structure (diphenyl-propane skeleton (C6–C3–C6)) in their skeleton containing two aromatic and one heterocyclic ring (Tsao, 2010). There are several classes of flavonoids, classified according to their carbon structure and level of oxidation. The

TABLE 11.1 Main Classes of Polyphenols, Their Food Sources, and General Chemical Structure

Polyphenol	Subgroup	Food Source	General Structure
Flavonoids	Flavonols	Red onion, Mexican oregano, spinach, saffron.	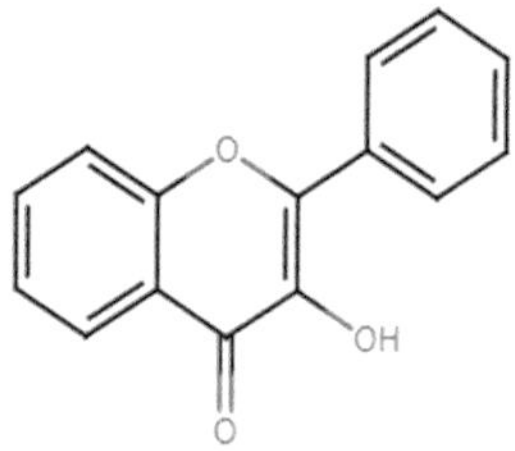
	Flavones	Peppermint, celery leaves and seeds, common verbena	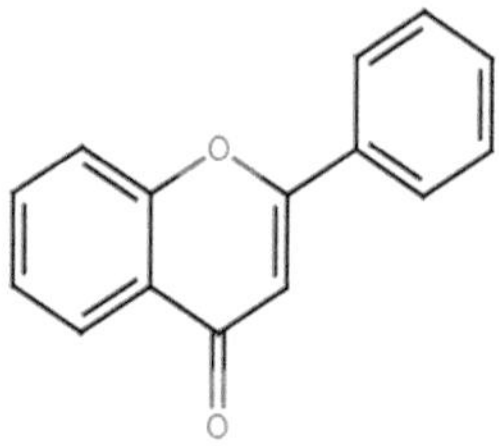
	Isoflavones	Soy flour, paste, soybean	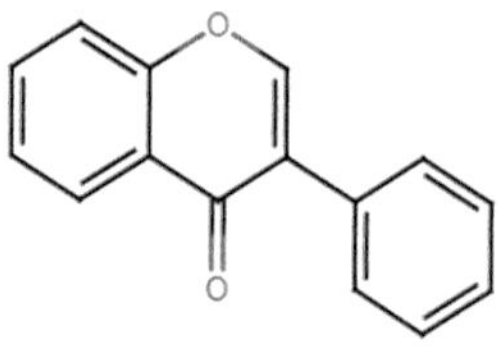
	Flavanones	Grapefruit, orange, rosemary	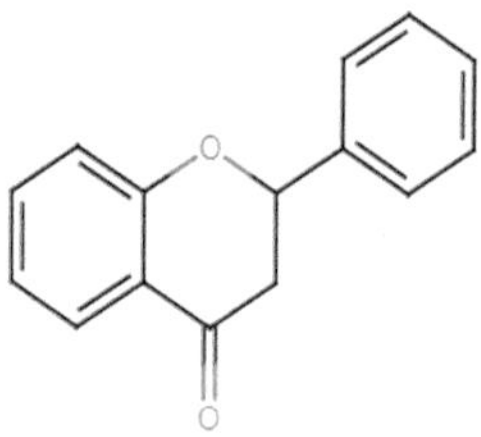
	Anthocyanidins	Black elderberry, blackberry, black currant	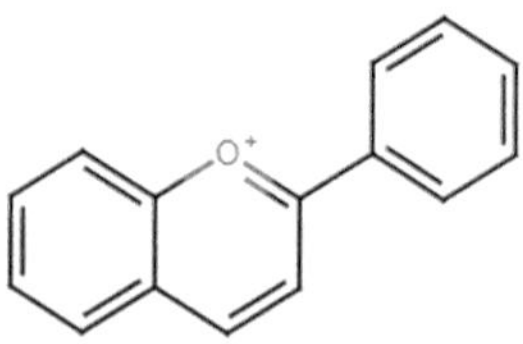
	Flavanols	Black tea, green tea, chocolate, cocoa	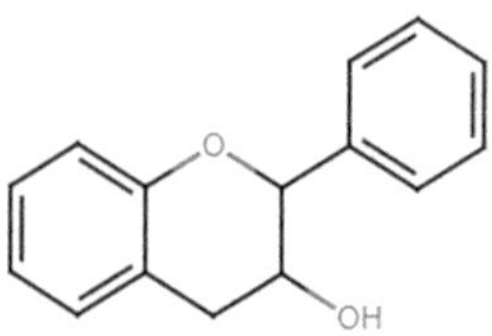

TABLE 11.1 *(Continued)*

Polyphenol	Subgroup	Food Source	General Structure
Lignans	–	Flaxseeds, black sesame oil, virgin olive oil, whole grain rye-flour	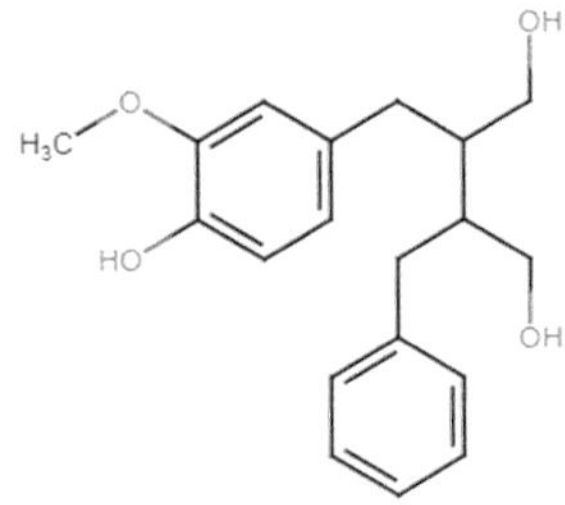
Phenolic acids	Benzoic acid	Raspberries, pomegranates, cranberries, chestnuts, cloves, star anise	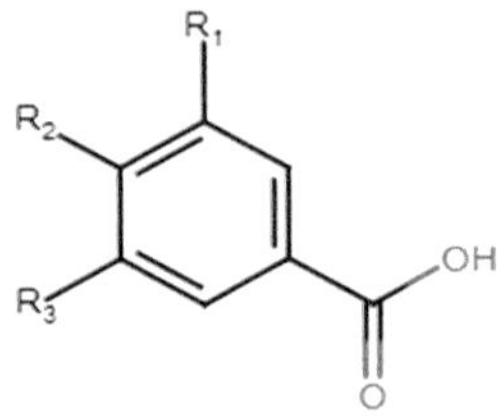
	Cinnamic acid	Coffee, maize oil, potato, dried rosemary	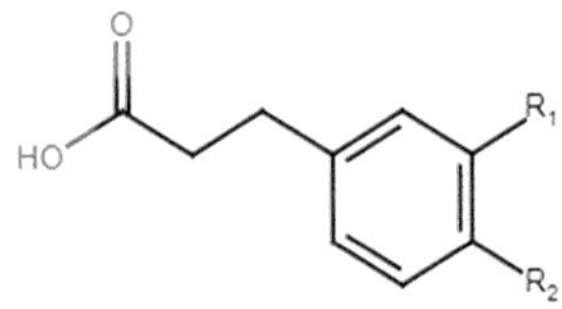
Stilbenes	Resveratrol	Red wine, grapes, nuts	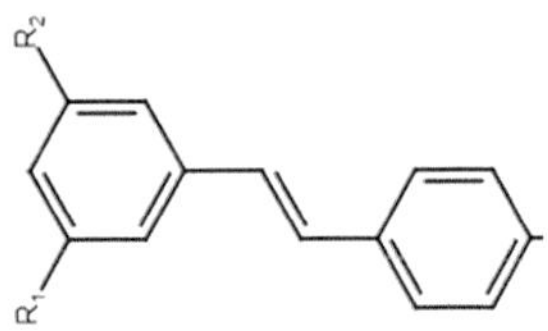

Source: Mrduljaš et al. (2017); Flavonoids: Chemical Structure, Classification, and Examples [Online].

flavonoids are classified into 13 classes viz. flavonols, flavanols, flavones, isoflavones, anthocyanidins or anthocyanins, and flavanones (Scalbert & Williamson, 2000), as shown in Table 11.1. It's interesting to note that the antioxidant and radical scavenger effect is caused by the aromatic rings' substitution sequence (Kumar & Pandey, 2013). Additionally, the quantity and availability of free hydroxyl groups in their skeleton affect the antioxidant capacity (Bravo, 1998; Manach et al., 2004).

Through the control of food intake/absorption, boosting energy expenditure, inhibiting energy storage, or influencing lipid oxidation through thermogenesis, flavonoids may contribute to obesity (Schwartz et al., 2000).

The most prevalent subclass of flavonoids in the typical human diet is called a flavonol, which is a 3-hydroxy derivative of a flavanone. The most popular flavonols include myricetin, kaempferol, and quercetin. The number of distinct glycosidic pairings for quercetin and kaempferol is at least 279 and 347, respectively (Tsao, 2010).

Flavones are distinguished by the presence of a double bond between C2 and C3 in the flavonoid skeleton, with no substitution at the C3 position and oxidation at the C4 position (Hostetler et al., 2017). Acacetin, apigenin, diosmetin, luteolin, and chrysoeriol, as well as their derivatives, are the most prevalent flavone aglycones. In numerous *in vivo* and *in vitro* investigations, flavones demonstrated antioxidant, antiproliferative, anticancer, antibacterial, estrogenic, and anti-inflammatory properties (Singh et al., 2014).

The lack of a double bond between carbons 2 and 3 and the presence of a chiral center at carbon 2 are characteristics of flavanones. Due to their high reactivity, these compounds are vulnerable to several O- and/or C-substitutions at the A- or B-ring (Khan et al., 2014). Hesperetin and (4′-methoxy-5,7,3′-trihydroxyflavanone) (5,7,4′-trihydroxy flavanone) are the two main flavanone aglycones; among others, its glycosides, hesperidin (hesperetin 7-rutinoside) and naringin (naringenin-7-neohesperidoside) have also been found to be effective. Intestinal microbiotas hydrolyze or deglycosylate flavanone glycosides in the small intestine and colon to produce the corresponding active aglycones. The released aglycones of flavanones are changed into their corresponding glucuronides, sulfates, and sulfoglucuronides when they pass through the small intestine and liver during the absorption process. The produced substances are released into plasma, dispersed to various tissues, and eliminated in urine (Matsumoto et al., 2004).

Water-soluble polyphenols known as anthocyanins (ACNs) have a strong antioxidant capacity and can block or reduce free radicals by giving or transferring electrons from hydrogen atoms. Aglycone-anthocyanidins and their glycosides are ACNs. The positions and numbers of hydroxyl groups, level of methylation, quantity of monoglycosides, diglycosides, and triglycosides, type of sugars (the most prevalent sugars are glucose, galactose, and arabinose), and number and type of aliphatic or aromatic acids (i.e., p-coumaric, caffeic, and ferulic acids) are all parameters on the basis of which they are differentiated (Pastor-Villaescusa et al., 2018; Mrduljaš et al., 2017). Depending on the pH and the structural composition of the tissues, this subclass of flavonoids gives plant tissues (flowers, leaves, fruits, and roots) colors ranging from blue, purple, and red. With more than 600 different chemicals discovered in nature, anthocyanidins are regarded as the most significant category of flavonoids in plants (Riaz et al., 2016). Depending on their chemical structure, ACNs have been demonstrated to have gut microbiota-modulating properties and also function as antioxidants, prebiotics, and anti-inflammatory agents (Vendrame et al., 2016).

The subclass of flavonoids known as flavanols is the most complicated, ranging from basic monomers (such as catechin and its isomer epicatechin) to oligomers and polymers (such as proanthocyanidins) and other derived chemicals (such as theaflavins and thearubigins) (Mena et al., 2014). Catechins, also known as flavanols or flavan-3-ols, are widely used. The key structural distinction between flavanols and other flavonoids is the lack of a double bond connecting C2 and C3 and the absence of a C4 carbonyl in the ring C. Additionally, flavanols can have two chiral centers on their molecules (placed on C2 and C3) thanks to the hydroxylation at C3, leading to four potential diastereoisomers.

Condensed tannins, or proanthocyanidins (PAs), are a class of flavonoids generated from flavan-3-ols, which are prevalent in the human diet. They are regarded as the second most common class of natural phenolics, behind lignins. Although higher-molecular-weight polymers are frequently encountered, PAs can also form as monomers, dimers, trimers, and oligomers of 20 or more units (Wang et al., 2011).

11.3.2 NONFLAVONOIDS

The non-flavonoids consist of phenolic acids, such as benzoic and hydroxycinnamic acids, as well as stilbenes. Gallotannins, ellagitannins, stilbene oligomers, and lignans are other non-flavonoids that may be discovered in nature (Manach et al., 2004, 2005). With a wide range of chemical structures that are accountable for their various qualities, non-flavonoids make up a significant category of polyphenols. These include phenolic acids, stilbenes, lignans, and curcuminoids. Compounds of phenolic acid are distinguished by the presence of a benzenic ring, a carboxyl moiety, and a variable number of hydroxyl and/or methoxyl groups in their basic structure (Yang et al., 2001).

The two primary categories of phenolic acids are benzoic and cinnamic acids, as well as their derivatives. The simplest phenolic acids in nature are the benzoic acids, which contain seven carbon atoms. Cinnamic acids, on the other hand, have nine carbon atoms and are seldom seen in plants in their natural form. Gallic acid and ellagic acid are two of the most significant benzoic acid derivatives. Another component of intricate structures, such as hydrolyzable tannins, is hydroxybenzoic acid (gallotannins and ellagitannins (Manach et al., 2004).

A significant antioxidant activity that is dependent on the quantity of hydroxyl groups present in the molecule is a characteristic of phenolic acids, according to Yang et al. (2001), which make up around 1/3rd of the phenolic portion in the individual's diet (Yang et al., 2001; Piazzon et al., 2012). Usually, hydroxylated cinnamic acids are superior to benzoic acids in terms of efficacy.

Plants respond to stress, infection, and other adversities by producing phytoalexins called stilbenes. The estrogenic activity and the potential to alter the estrogen receptor signaling pathway are distinctive features of this class of polyphenols. Only resveratrol is thought to be significant for human health despite its modest levels in the human diet. The most important stilbene is resveratrol (3,5,4′-trihydroxystilbene), which gets its name from the plant source utilized for separation (a resinous polyphenol derived from resorcinol that is found in Veratrum species and includes hydroxyl (eOH) groups (-ol)) (Park & Pezzuto, 2015).

Resveratrol has demonstrated anti-inflammatory, antioxidant, and cardio-protective properties as well as anti-diabetic and anti-obesity properties (Nohr et al., 2016). Although it is present in both cis and transforms, the trans isomer functions as an antioxidant more effectively (Mikulski et al., 2010). The uneven effects of resveratrol on obesity-related morbidities may be caused by variations in experimental design and settings (patient type, dosage, timing of intervention, and resveratrol molecular structure) (Kjaer et al., 2017). One study suggests that specific metabolic pathways, particularly those involved in steroid metabolism and the gut microbiome, crucially perform a substantial role in the mechanism by which resveratrol reduces obesity and that these metabolic pathways may be the subject of resveratrol's effects in future clinical trials (Korsholm et al., 2017).

Lignans are formed of two phenylpropane units found in numerous plants and are structurally parallel to 17-estradiol belonging to the phytoestrogens group (Terens et al., 2013). Their estrogenic activity is credited to the presence of two cinnamic acid residues. Lignans act as a feast for colonic bacteria resulting in healthy proliferations ascribing to metabolized into enterolignans, enterodiol, and enterolactone subsequent to ingestion (Borriello et al., 1985).

Lignans have been reported to have a wide spectrum of health-promoting properties, comprising protective assets against oncogenesis, osteoporosis, and coronary heart disease (Adlercreutz, 2007) and antidiabetic and antiobesity effects (Bhathena & Velasquez, 2002).

11.4 MECHANISM OF ACTION OF POLYPHENOLS AS ANTI-OBESITY AGENT

The impact of polyphenols on obesity has been studied in several cellular and animal research, as well as certain human studies. According to the findings of these studies, polyphenols provide anti-obesity functions via a number of different mechanisms. Polyphenols exhibit their anti-obesity potential either alone or in a particular combination of mechanisms (Singh et al., 2020). The different mechanisms by which polyphenols impart their anti-obesity action are mentioned in subsections (Figure 11.1).

11.4.1 INCREASED ENERGY CONSUMPTION

Increased adiposity is caused by an energy imbalance, in which the negative effects of excessive food intake are not counterbalanced by increased energy expenditure. Weight loss is only possible when energy consumption surpasses its expenditure, leading to a negative energy balance. The daily energy consumption can be accounted for and regulated in terms of Basal metabolic rate, physical activity, and thermic effect of food (Balaji et al., 2016). Thermogenic regulation and energy expenditure can be improved by polyphenolic substances. Through non-shivering thermogenesis, brown adipose tissue significantly contributes to the regulation of obesity. Uncoupling protein 1 (UCP1) controls thermogenesis by reducing the proton gradient and separating oxidation from ATP production (Cannon & Nedergaard, 2004). In response to nutrition and other stimuli, sympathetic pathways via β-adrenoreceptors activate BAT (Wood Dos Santos et al., 2018). Through the control of leptin, thyroid hormones, and β-adrenergic agonists, UCP3, which is related to UCP1, also promotes thermogenesis and may have anti-obesity effects (Gong et al., 1997). As a result, controlling energy expenditure by activating BAT and modulating UCP is a biologically sound method of reducing obesity (Lowell & Spiegelman, 2000).

By interfering with AMPK, SIRT1, PGC1, catechol-O-methyltransferase (COMT), and sympathetic nervous system (SNS), which are key players in the transcriptional regulation and physiology of adipose tissue, phenolic compounds such as curcumin, quercetin, resveratrol, isoflavones, gallic acid, and flavonol stimulate thermogenesis (Mele et al., 2017).

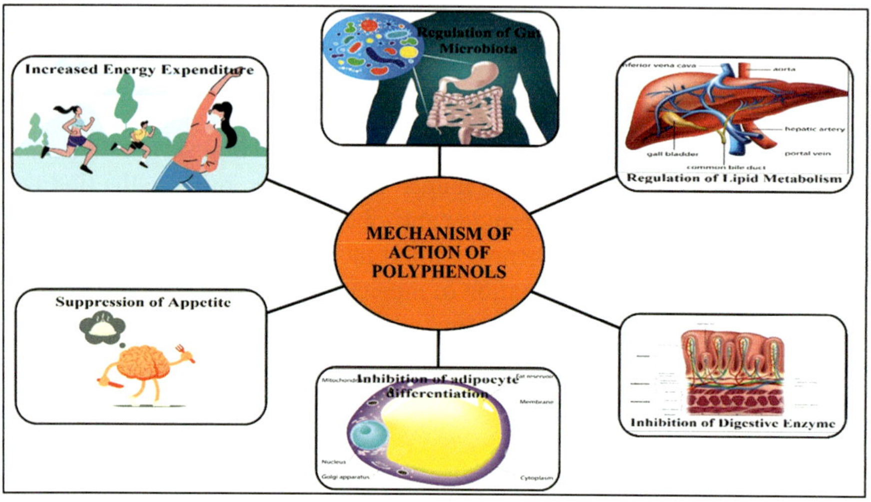

FIGURE 11.1 Mechanism of action of polyphenols.

Source: Adapted from Singh et al., 2020

11.4.2 SUPPRESSED APPETITE

Appetite regulation comprises neurological and hormonal systems that facilitate obesity prevention. Dopamine, serotonin, and histamine are hormones associated with appetite management (Chantre & Lairon, 2002). By interacting with the brainstem and other brain reward systems, the hypothalamus is crucial in controlling appetite (Roh et al., 2016). Adiponectin, leptin, and apelin are all bioactive adipokines produced by adipose tissue that control energy balance and glucose homeostasis (Kalupahana et al., 2012). Additionally, a variety of neuropeptides and neurotransmitters in the hypothalamus assist in regulating the homeostatic management of energy balance by regulating energy intake (Ashrafi, 2007). Melanin-concentrating hormone (MCH) receptor antagonists may serve as a substitute strategy for suppressing appetite (Bays, 2004). MCH, an endogenous hormone that stimulates appetite, and its receptors have been related to a decline in body weight in mice (Yu & Kim, 2012).

Plant-derived phenolic compounds reduce appetite either by suppressing the release of hormones that cause hunger, by altering MCH receptors, or by deactivating appetite sensors (Geoffroy et al., 2011). Therefore, the aptitude of natural polyphenols as an effective anti-obesity agent for the control of obesity can be explored. Apart from the above mechanism, polyphenols also exert their appetite suppression effect by regulating various gut hormones such as GLP-1 (glucagon-like peptide 1), pancreatic polypeptide, cholecystokinin, peptide tyrosine-tyrosine, and oxyntomodulin which are involved in transmitting the satiety signals to the brain.

11.4.3 INHIBITION OF ADIPOCYTE DIFFERENTIATION

The primary biological component of adipose tissue, the adipocyte, is crucial for maintaining homeostasis in terms of lipids and energy balance. While extra energy from food is stored in the white adipose tissue (WAT) as triglyceride droplets, the brown adipose tissue (BAT) makes use of stored energy when thermogenesis calls for it (Tong & Hotamisligil, 2001). Increased adipogenesis and adipocyte differentiation result in an accumulation of a large number of adipocytes, which leads to obesity (Ali et al., 2013). There are multiple phases to adipocyte differentiation, and any of these stages can be effectively interfered with by a variety of transcriptional factors to treat obesity (Lefterova & Lazar, 2009). Members of the proliferator-activated receptor (PPAR), CCAAT/enhancer binding protein (C/EBP), and sterol regulatory element binding proteins (SREBP) classes are among some of the crucial transcription factors involved in adipocyte development (Brey et al., 2009).

Resveratrol, curcumin, and other polyphenols disrupt or inhibit one or more steps of adipogenesis (Mohamed et al., 2014). These phytochemicals can change the adipocyte life cycle by inhibiting adipocyte differentiation and adipogenesis, suppressing preadipocyte growth and mitogenesis, and inducing mature adipocyte apoptosis. Such physiological processes can be modified to create effective methods for managing and controlling obesity (Wang et al., 2014).

11.4.4 INHIBITION OF DIGESTIVE ENZYMES

Amylase, glucosidase, and lipase, three important digestive enzymes, are known to be inhibited by polyphenols. This results in less efficient digestion of carbohydrates and lipids, which lowers calorie intake. The primary enzymes for the breakdown of starch are amylase and glucosidase. Carbohydrate breakdown produces glucose, which, when in excess, leads to elevated glucose levels in the blood. This stimulates the pancreas to release insulin in order to maintain the glucose amount in the blood. Glycolysis, which breaks down glucose, glycogenesis in the liver and muscles, which turns glucose into glycogen, and de novo lipogenesis in the liver and adipose tissue are the three glucose-utilizing mechanisms that are started at this point (Wong et al., 2016). De novo lipogenesis refers to the production of fatty acids from carbohydrates that are later esterified to form triglycerides for adipose tissue storage. The digestive enzyme lipase breaks down phospholipids, triglycerides, and fats. Humans have two different forms of lipases: extra-duodenal, which is made up of pancreatic, hepatic, lipoprotein, and endothelial lipase, and pre-duodenal, which comprises lingual and gastric. Dietary fats are hydrolyzed by lipase and transformed into monoglycerides and fatty acids. These simpler fatty compounds enter the enterocytes as mixed micelles. Triglycerides are produced in enterocytes and build up in adipose tissue for energy production. Thus, extra carbohydrates and fats that the body cannot use for energy are converted to triglycerides and fatty acids and accumulate in adipose tissue, which causes obesity (Birari & Bhutani, 2007). Hence, one of the most efficient ways to treat obesity is by suppressing these digestive enzymes. Various flavonoids (proanthocyanidins) and non-flavonoids (gallic acid, ellagitannins, epigallocatechin, epigallocatechin gallate, quercetin) have been reported to exhibit an inhibitory effect on digestive enzymes (Liu et al., 2018; McDougall et al., 2009; Ganjayi et al., 2017; Liu et al., 2013).

11.4.5 REGULATION OF LIPID METABOLISM

A plethora of enzymes and hormones are engaged in the multi-step process of lipid metabolism, which produces, stores, and degrades fatty acids, triglycerides, and cholesterol. Lipid metabolism is divided into two categories: cholesterol metabolism and fatty acid and triglyceride metabolism. As the primary modulator of lipid synthesis pathways, Adenosine Monophosphate-Activated Protein Kinase (AMPK) has the power to suppress the production of fatty acids by interfering with sterol-regulatory-element-binding-protein-1c (SREBP-1c) and fatty acid synthase. Inhibiting the production of cholesterol, AMPK activation promotes fatty acid oxidation in the liver (Srivastava et al., 2012). Similarly, carnitine palmitoyl transferase 1A (CPT1A) can expedite fatty acid oxidation and lower liver triglyceride levels. The breakdown of cholesterol and the oxidation of fatty acids are two processes that can be controlled by the peroxisome proliferator-activated receptor (PPAR) (Takei et al., 2017). In order to prevent obesity, these parameters can be modulated in a way that affects lipid metabolism.

Activating AMPK and PPAR, which might result in the inhibition of acetyl-CoA carboxylase (ACC) and fatty acid synthase, are two mechanisms by which polyphenols have been claimed to prevent obesity. By reducing fatty acid synthesis and increasing fatty acid oxidation, these activities collectively reduce lipid build-up and oxidative stress. Researchers have reported that the polyphenols in hibiscus, blueberries, quercetin, epigallocatechin-3-gallate, resveratrol, curcumin, green tea, and other plants have the aforementioned mechanism (Jiao et al., 2018; Wang et al., 2018; Peng et al., 2020; Herranz-Lopez et al., 2019).

11.4.6 REGULATION OF GUT MICROBIOTA

The trillions of microorganisms that live in the gut together form a sophisticated microbial ecosystem. According to a study, bacteria from three major divisions Firmicutes (Gram-positive), Bacteroidetes (Gram-negative), and Actinobacteria (Gram-positive) combine to make up more than 90% of the total bacteria present in the gut of an adult person. When Bäckhed et al. (2004) transplanted the microbiota from normally growing mice to germ-free (GF) mice, they discovered the first evidence connecting gut microbiota to the onset of obesity. They discovered that GF mice were shielded from the onset of obesity when kept on a high-fat diet (HFD). The host's physiological functioning, metabolic rate, and energy depot are all influenced by the gut microorganisms in different ways, which makes the host more prone to obesity. Energy harvesting from indigestible food, influence on fatty acid oxidation, influence on the fasting-induced adipose factor (FIAF), bile acids, satiety, lipogenesis, metabolic endotoxinemia, and the endocannabinoid system are all part of the mechanism. However, it is still unclear how these processes interact with one another and how this affects a person's overall metabolic condition (Kumar Singh et al., 2019; Dahiya et al., 2017).

11.5 ANTI-OBESITY ACTION OF SOME POLYPHENOLIC PLANT SOURCES

Azlan et al. (2020) investigated the impact of crocin, the main constituent of saffron extract (*Crocus sativus* L.), on a model of induced obesity in rats. Their research aims to better understand the therapeutic effects of saffron extract and crocin by examining and comparing the metabolite alterations in obese individuals and obese individuals administered with saffron extract and crocin. The obese rats were fed a high-fat diet (HFD) for eight weeks at two different dosages (40 and 80 mg/kg) of crocin and saffron extracts. Proton nuclear magnetic resonance was used to examine how the serum's metabolite profiles had changed (1H-NMR). Multivariate data analysis (MVDA) pattern recognition revealed that saffron extract plus crocin at 80 mg/kg was the most effective dose when compared to 40 mg/kg. Additionally, it demonstrated that both therapies operate along separate routes, particularly when it comes to the metabolism of glucose, lipids, and creatinine. They concluded that saffron extract was found to be superior to crocin in treating obesity; this data indicated that saffron extract can be taken into consideration as an alternative to crocin (Ramli et al., 2020).

Numerous investigations revealed that an onion peel water extract is a high source of flavonoids such as cyanidin, caffeic, sinapinic, ferulic, sinapinic, and tannic acids (Chia et al., 2019; Kumar et al., 2022). Onion peels have a greater concentration of flavonoids than the edible portions of the onion (Sagar et al., 2020). Therefore, since onion peels contain a high concentration of flavonoids, they may be effective in improving obesity. The anti-obesity properties of onion peel extract (OPE) were examined *in vitro* and *in vivo* by Yu et al. (2021) using 3T3-L1 pre-adipocytes and C57BL/6J mice on a high-fat diet (HFD). By lowering the expression of lipogenesis-related genes such as peroxisome proliferator-activated receptor-, CCAAT/enhancer binding protein, fatty acid synthase, and acetyl CoA carboxylase, OPE drastically lowered the lipids of 3T3-L1 cells and blocked lipid formation. OPE-treated animals weighed much less than mice on the HFD. In comparison to mice on the HFD, animals treated with OPE exhibited reduced levels of triglycerides, total cholesterol, and low-density lipoprotein cholesterol in their blood. After OPE therapy, the expression levels of the genes involved in adipogenesis dramatically reduced. The findings demonstrated that OPE suppressed lipid accumulation by reducing the expression of the adipogenesis gene and decreased adipose tissue hypertrophy. These findings showed that OPE could have anti-obesity benefits and may offer a source of OPE for the creation of naturally anti-obesity foods and dietary supplements (Yu et al., 2021).

In another study, Song & Seo (2022) utilized red onion extract treatment to validate the alterations in the genes linked to pancreatic lipase activity and pre-adipocyte cell development their research. 3T3-L1 adipocytes were used to assess the impact of red onion extract therapy on pre-adipocyte differentiation, and Real-Time PCR was used to validate the gene activity. The experiment's findings show that pancreatic lipase activity is inhibited by red onion extract in a concentration-dependent way. The activity of the genes C/EBPα, C/EBPβ, and PPARγ, which are linked to adipocyte growth, was also demonstrated to be inhibited, along with adipocyte differentiation. According to the findings of this study, it is possible to create red onion extract as a high-potential substance with anti-obesity effectiveness by reducing adipocyte development by manipulating genes involved in adipocyte differentiation (Song & Seo, 2022).

Spinacia oleracea, also known as spinach, is a leafy green vegetable high in flavonoids, polyphenols, carotenoids, and vitamins, all of which have antioxidant properties. Flavonoid-rich fruits and vegetables are believed to inhibit weight gain by promoting satiety. Panda & Shinde (2017) investigated the potential of a spinach leaf extract (SOE) which is high in flavonoids to reduce appetite in rats. The SOE was subjected to HPTLC in order to identify flavonoids. For a period of 14 days, rats were given SOE through p.o. the route in a dose of 200 mg/kg and 400 mg/kg, respectively, and fluoxetine in a dose of 6 mg/kg through the i.p. route as a pre-meal. Daily weight gain and food consumption were tracked throughout the course of the treatment. In order to examine the satiety-inducing effects of SOE, serum levels of cholecystokinin (CCK) and glucose were evaluated on days 7 and 14 at various time periods following the onset of meals. The presence of 14 flavonoids in SOE was confirmed by HPTLC. When compared to the typical control rats, the rats treated with SOE and fluoxetine had a substantial decrease in intake of food and weight gain. Peak CCK levels were attained on the seventh day of treatment 30 minutes after the commencement of the meal in the fluoxetine-treated rats and 60 minutes later in the untreated animals. In the fluoxetine and SOE 400 mg/kg treated rats, CCK peaking was seen 30 minutes after the commencement of the meal on the 14th day. On both trial days, peak glucose levels were reached 60 minutes after the commencement of the meal in all treatment groups. It may be said that SOE showed a potential appetite-suppressing effect by causing a quicker-than-usual release of CCK, which caused rats to experience fullness earlier than usual. This impact might be attributed to the high flavonoid content (Panda & Shinde, 2017).

Panda et al. (2020) in their study examined the effects of aerobic exercise (AE) and a natural antioxidant-rich spinach extract (NAOE) on hyperlipidemia and obesity in rats administered with HFD (high-fat diet). They grouped the rats into seven groups (Control, HFD Control, Reference standard medication orlistat (10 mg/kg), NAOE (200 and 400 mg/kg), Only AE (swimming 20 minutes), and NAOEAE (NAOE 400 mg/kg plus AE) for 21 days with HFD. According to their findings, administering orlistat, NAOE, and NAOEAE to HFD-fed rats dramatically reduced food consumption, weight gain, pancreatic lipase activity, and lipid peroxidation while successfully reversing the lipid profile and antioxidant levels that had been impacted by the HFD. They came to the conclusion that NAOE's inhibition of pancreatic lipase resulted in a potential anti-hyperlipidemic impact. The greatest outcomes were from the NAOEAE combination therapy, demonstrating the critical impact that exercise and eating foods high in antioxidants have in preserving a normal lipid profile and managing obesity (Panda et al., 2020).

Celery (*Apium graveolens*), among other naturally occurring substances, is one of the most significant sources of phytochemicals, including phenolic acids, flavones, and flavonols, as well as antioxidants like vitamin C. Kim et al. (2021) conducted a study to verify celery seed's anti-obesity properties in 3T3-L1 adipocytes. Their research aimed to identify the chemical composition of celery seeds and assess the antioxidant and protective properties of celery seed fractions in an *in vitro* setting. Celery seeds were gradually fractionated using organic solvents, and the fractions were tested for antioxidant characteristics. After analyzing the metabolites of high antioxidative fractions, 3T3-L1 adipocytes were used to assess the anti-obesity characteristics and mechanisms of various fractions. *In vitro*, antioxidant capabilities such as radical scavenging and total phenolic content were greater in celery seed ethanol extract (CSE) and celery seed ethyl acetate fraction (CSEA) compared to hexane, butanol, and water fractions. A gas chromatography-mass selective detector was used to identify a total of 43 and 19 metabolites from CSE and CSEA, respectively. Only CSEA contained isoferulic acid and p-coumaric acid. By lowering adipogenic hormones including leptin and adiponectin, CSEA had stronger anti-adipogenesis in 3T3-L1 cells than CSE. Expression levels of genes and transcription factors associated with adipocytes, including C/EBP, PPAR, aP2, and FAS, dropped to levels similar to the control. CSEA has antioxidant and anti-obesity properties and might be utilized as a natural component (Kim et al., 2021).

Soy meals have gained a lot of attention because of their high protein content and unique isoflavone content. A possible mechanism by which isoflavones reduce fat formation and adipose tissue distribution is that they interact with intracellular estrogen receptors due to their structural similarity to endogenous estrogens (Kim et al., 2020). It was discussed in a study performed by Moriyasu et al. (2021) that Black Soybean Seed Coat Powder, which is suitable for use in food products, has anti-obesity effects comparable to those of traditional Yellow Soybean Seed Coat Powder. In this work, scientists assessed the anti-obesity benefits of feeding black soybean seed coat powder (BSCP) to obese model mice. As a control, regular yellow soybean seed coat powder (YSCP) was employed. A high-fat diet containing either BSCP or YSCP (20% fat) was given to the C57BL/6J mice model for obesity. The findings demonstrated that, compared to the YSCP group, the BSCP group saw a considerable reduction in weight gain and a significant decrease in the weight of white adipose tissue. Furthermore, it markedly boosted levels of antidiabetic adipocytokine and adiponectin while considerably reducing serum leptin levels, which were linked with visceral fat mass. These results indicate an anti-obesity impact for BSCP in obese model mice due to its pigmented components. Researchers believe that this substance, which can be made without the use of organic solvents and is safe for consumption, might be a functional food ingredient with anti-obesity properties that could be put into practice (Moriyasu et al., 2021).

A common dietary component is Rosmarinus officinalis (rosemary). Rosemary extract, which contains 40% carnosic acid (CA), displayed strong anti-obesity properties. It was assumed that rosemary exerts an anti-obesity effect by altering the gut microbiota. Therefore, He et al. (2022) studied the modulatory effect of CA on the gut microbiota of mice. For 10 weeks, C57BL/6 mice were fed either a standard diet, an HFD, or an HFD with 0.1 or 0.2% CA. In HFD-induced obese mice, CA showed potential anti-obesity benefits and significantly changed the gut microbiome. Proteobacteria and Firmicutes, as well as the useful bacteria *Akkermansia muciniphila, Muribaculaceae* unclassified, and *Clostridium innocuum* group, were more prevalent as a result of CA, which also reduced the growth of bacteria that cause diabetes. The Firmicutes to Bacteroidetes ratio was dose-dependently controlled by CA, falling from 13.22% to 2.42%. CA also inhibited the growth of bacteria that metabolize bile acids, including *Bilophila, Clostridium, Lactobacillus*, and *Leuconostoc.* The findings of the linear discriminant analysis and the examination of the effect magnitude suggested that CA reduced the microbial alterations brought on by HFD. The low CA (LCA) group (HFD containing 0.1% CA) showed an enormous amount of *Eisenbergiella, Intestinimonas,* and *Ruminococcaceae*, while the increased CA (HCA) group (HFD containing 0.2% CA) showed a greater proportion of *Verrucomicrobiae.* Their findings show that CA's prebiotic properties may be closely tied to its anti-obesity effects (He et al., 2022).

The fragrant flavor and advantageous health properties of blueberry (*Vaccinium ashei*) and blackberry (Rubus sp.) make them popular fruits. Anthocyanins, a particular class of polyphenol that aids in having an anti-obesity impact, are present in them. In C57BL/6 mice given a high-fat diet (HFD), Wu et al. (2018) examined the molecular mechanism behind the anti-obesity effects of eating blackberry anthocyanins (BLA) and blueberry anthocyanins (BBA). A low-fat diet (LFD), a high-fat diet (HFD), an HFD with orlistat, and BLA or BBA were given to 60 mice daily for 12 weeks. By preventing body weight increase by 40.5% and 55.4%, respectively, BLA and BBA ingestion reduced the body weight gain of mice given an HFD. In addition to considerably raising hepatic superoxide dismutase and glutathione peroxidase activities, the BLA and BBA treatments significantly decreased blood and hepatic lipid levels. The therapies also considerably reduced the expression of the genes for the inflammatory proteins' interleukin-6, nuclear factor-kappaB, and tumor necrosis factor TNF – while efficiently raising the levels of fecal acetate and butyrate. Furthermore, data from gas chromatography time-of-flight mass spectroscopy revealed that BLA and BBA profoundly impacted the hepato-lipidic and glucose metabolism pathways, together with glycerophospholipid, glutathione metabolism, and insulin-indicating systems. Therefore, BLA and BBA reduce oxidative stress and inflammation while increasing energy expenditure to counteract diet-induced obesity (Wu et al., 2018).

There are numerous health benefits associated with drinking tea and coffee, as well as the ability to prevent, mitigate, and treat a multitude of diseases. There is a possibility that caffeine present in both plants contributes to this ability. In tea and coffee, there are other molecules like polyphenols and theaflavins, catechins, their metabolites in tea, and polyphenol chlorogenic acid in coffee, which can explain physiological and medicinal effects (theaflavins, catechins, their metabolites, and polyphenols). Numerous metabolic disorders viz. metabolic syndrome, cardiovascular disease, type 2 diabetes, and obesity can be prevented and treated with plants and plant molecules. By suppressing adipocyte functions and promoting gut microbiota, plants and their constituents reduce fat storage. Through changes in fat metabolism, tea can also assist in preventing obesity by reducing appetite, consumption, and absorption of food in the gastrointestinal system (Sirotkin & Kolesárová, 2021). In order to fully understand how green tea extracts lower the body fat of rats, Xu et al. (2015) study focused on isolating the polyphenols, polysaccharides, and caffeine present in green tea to evaluate their effects on the onset of obesity. For 6 weeks, they tested total green tea extracts, polyphenols, polysaccharides, caffeine, and a complex of polysaccharides and polyphenols at a dose of 400 or 800 mg kg^{-1} in high-fat diet-fed rats to determine whether these compounds inhibit fat accumulation. Polyphenols and polysaccharides were found to play a role in the suppressive effect of green tea extract on fat accumulation and body weight gain. In addition to improving blood lipid and antioxidant levels, polyphenols, polysaccharides, and caffeine showed potential in reducing serum leptin levels systematically in an animal model, inhibiting fatty acid absorption, and significantly decreasing IL-6 and TNF-α gene expression. Furthermore, polysaccharides and polyphenols synergistically reduce serum leptin levels and inflammation. Based on these results, polysaccharides combined with polyphenols might be a viable treatment for obesity (Xu et al., 2015).

Another natural flavonoid substance that may be found in flaxseed and other plants is called herbacetin. Numerous medical effects of flaxseed have been noted, including anti-obesity, anti-diabetic, anti-hypertensive, anti-cancer, and antibacterial impacts. Therefore, Veeramani et al. (2018) examined the ameliorative impact of herbacetin in C57BL/6J mice with high-fat diet-induced hyperglycemia and hyperlipidemia. By continually giving the mice a high-fat diet for 10 weeks, obesity-related insulin resistance was developed. After that, mice were given daily intragastric injections of herbacetin (in varying dosages) combined with a high-fat diet for the following 5 weeks. Changes in body weight, lipid-regulating enzymes, HOMA-IR, blood glucose, insulin, and insulin resistance were assessed at the end of the 106th day. In mice with obesity-related insulin resistance, herbacetin dramatically decreased body mass, plasma glucose, serum insulin, and HOMA-IR activity (OIR). Additionally, the total cholesterol, triglycerides, and free fatty acids in the plasma and liver of OIR mice were considerably decreased after receiving herbacetin. Furthermore, when compared to OIR control mice, herbacetin significantly augmented the hepato-lipidic metabolizing and lipid-regulating enzymes, including SREBP-1c and 2, fatty acid synthase (FAS), fatty acid oxidation, malic enzyme, glucose 6-phosphate dehydrogenase (G6PD), and carnitine palmitoyltransferase (CPT). Herbacetin significantly lowers the number of lipid globules in the liver vicinity, according to histopathological analysis. Therefore, the observed results strongly suggest that herbacetin, owing to its anti-hyperglycemic and anti-hyperlipidemic characteristics through the regulation of hepatic lipid metabolizing and lipid-regulating enzymes, provides remarkable protection against the negative effects of chronic high-fat diet consumption (Veeramani et al., 2018).

The cranberry, a significant and beneficial source of phytochemicals with broad health advantages for humans, notably phenolic compounds mostly consisting of flavan-3-ols, A-type procyanidins, anthocyanins, benzoic acid, and ursolic acid, has excellent potential to prevent the onset of obesity and issues linked to obesity. Comparing cranberry fruits to other berries that are strong in B-type procyanidins, cranberry fruits have much greater A-type procyanidin levels. In a study by Peixoto et al. (2018), for 30 days, Wistar rats fed with HFD were given daily doses of 200 mg/kg body weight of cranberry extracts containing about 4 mg/kg of total polyphenol, 3 mg/kg body weight of proanthocyanidin, and 0.4 mg/kg body weight of anthocyanins to reduce oxidative stress and enhance metabolic profile, preventing the development of obesity and disorders associated with it (Peixoto et al., 2018). Additionally, it was shown that cranberry phenolic extracts with four primary anthocyanidins—cyanidin 3-galactoside, cyanidin 3-arabinoside, peonidin 3-galactoside, and peonidin 3-arabinoside—were capable of enhancing energy metabolism and reducing insulin resistance brought on by the HFD (Zhou et al., 2020).

Strawberries are another berry that may have anti-obesity properties. Numerous studies using cell or animal models have shown that strawberries' phenolic compositions may have anti-obesity properties. In 3T3-L1 cells, a strawberry extract including the bioactive compounds pelargonidin 3-glucoside, pelargonidin 3-malonyl glucoside, gallic acid derivatives, and flavonols was reported to enhance browning while decreasing pre-adipocyte differentiation and the gene expression of adipogenic transcription factors, such as C/EBP- and PPAR (Forbes-Hernández et al., 2020). In another research, it was shown that feeding rats strawberry powder rich in pelargonidin 3-glucoside prevented the development of obesity, heart disease, and hepatic inflammation while also reducing the buildup of fat in the liver (Ghattamaneni et al., 2019). Additionally, it has been shown that strawberry fruit extracts rich in ellagitannin can reduce the lipid peroxidation in the kidneys brought on by a diet rich in fructose while enhancing the lipid profile of the liver and serum (Fotschki et al., 2018).

Numerous studies have revealed that the pomegranate extract contains large amounts of hydrolyzable tannins including punicalin, pedunculagin, and punicalagin as well as anthocyanins like delphinidin, cyanidin, and pelargonidin (Al-Muammar & Khan, 2012). In an animal model (mice) of high-fat diet-induced obesity and hyperlipidemia, Lei et al. (2007) studied the anti-obesity benefits of pomegranate leaf extract (PLE). They used a high-fat diet (HFD) to make both male and female ICR mice obese. The animals were given 400/800 mg/kg of PLE every day over a period of 5 weeks once the weight of the HFD group reached a 20% higher level than the regular diet group. Throughout the experimental period, routine measurements of body weight and caloric consumption were made. After 5 weeks of therapy with PLE, the different adipose pads were weighed, and blood levels of total cholesterol (TC), triglycerides (TG), glucose, and high-density lipoprotein cholesterol (HDL-C) were assessed. In the experiment on fat absorption, 0.5 ml of lipid emulsion and 800 mg/kg of PLE were simultaneously administered to both control and obese groups. Serial measurements of blood TG levels were made at predetermined time slots (1, 2, 3, 4, and 6 hours) following the therapy. Following a peroral dose of lipoidal emulsion to the mice, TGs in fecal excretions were examined. On pancreatic lipase activity, the effects of PLE and its separated components (ellagic acid and tannic acid) were investigated *in vitro*. The findings showed that after 5 weeks of therapy, the PLE-treated groups significantly reduced their body weight, energy consumption, different adipose pad weight percentages, blood TC, TG, glucose levels, and TC/HDL-C ratio. In addition, when mice were administered an oral fat emulsion, PLE dramatically reduced the rise in blood TG levels and hindered intestinal fat absorption. In contrast to mice fed a regular diet, obese mice fed a high-fat diet exhibited no difference in their hunger reduction when given PLE. They concluded that PLE can prevent obesity and hyperlipidemia in mice that had been given a high-fat diet to make them obese. The effects seem to be partially mediated by lowering calorie intake and pancreatic lipase activity. PLE could be a cutting-edge appetite suppressant that solely treats obesity brought on by a high-fat diet (Lei et al., 2007).

11.6 CONCLUSION

Obesity poses serious risks to human health and is connected with numerous negative consequences. Diet and exercise are the most effective methods for both preventing and treating the condition; unfortunately, both demand a great deal of self-control and are challenging to maintain. The weight reduction only lasts as long as the medication is taken, and as soon as the treatment is discontinued, the weight is gained again. In addition, the usage of current drugs for treating obesity is ineffective due to adverse effects. As a result, it is currently required to develop alternative therapies using natural ingredients. The health advantages of naturally occurring plant polyphenols are becoming more well-known. To prevent or treat obesity, a widespread health issue, researchers and manufacturers are devoting time and money to the discovery and characterization of natural phenolic compounds. A vast family of phytochemicals known as polyphenols, which have a wide range of chemical properties, are recognized to be bioactive components of meals, animals, medicinal plants, and nutraceuticals. Fruits, vegetables, and items that are produced from them are the major sources of polyphenols. In addition to fruits and vegetables, consuming a diet that is abundant in plant-based goods such as beans, tea, and coffee may have a positive impact on one's overall health. Polyphenols have antioxidant, anti-inflammatory, and microbiota-modulating capabilities, which raises interest in these substances as an obesity therapy option. Although there is much knowledge about the biological processes that polyphenols participate in, there is still little proof that these processes have a definite impact on human health. Polyphenols in foods and beverages can be difficult to accurately measure because of the many different types, which makes it tedious and impractical to distinguish which molecule in a food or beverage is responsible for a given effect. Researchers also have little understanding of polyphenol absorption and metabolism. In light of this, the majority of the available evidence points to a mixture of phytochemicals rather than a single polyphenol as being the source of health benefits. There is a chance to boost the oral bioavailability of beneficial polyphenols by developing particular synergistic interactions. On the other hand, consideration should be given to how dietary supplements containing polyphenols affect the pharmacology and bioavailability of drugs. The wide inter-individual variance shown in polyphenol research might be due to variations in gut microbiota and how these phytochemicals are metabolized by microbes. As a result, it is anticipated that more thorough research, including human trials, would be required in order to offer evidence for the necessity of using natural phenolic compounds as functional foods or supplements to both prevent and treat human obesity.

ACKNOWLEDGMENTS

The authors express their sincere thanks to the administrative authority of Amity University Lucknow Campus, Teerthanker Mahaveer University, Moradabad, and IFTM University, Moradabad, Uttar Pradesh, for providing necessary facilities, especially the library during the preparation of this chapter.

KEYWORDS

- **adipocyte differentiation**
- **anti-obesity agent**
- **diet**
- **lipid metabolism**
- **microbiota**
- **obesity**
- **polyphenols**

REFERENCES

Adlercreutz, H. (2007). Lignans and human health. *Critical Reviews in Clinical Laboratory Sciences, 44*(5–6), 483–525.

Ali, A. T., Hochfeld, W. E., Myburgh, R., & Pepper, M. S. (2013). Adipocyte and adipogenesis. *European Journal of Cell Biology, 92*(6–7), 229–236.

Al-Muammar, M. N., & Khan, F. (2012). Obesity: The preventive role of the pomegranate (*Punica granatum*). *Nutrition, 28*(6), 595–604.

Ashrafi, K. (2007). Obesity and the regulation of fat metabolism. In WormBook: The Online Review of C. elegans Biology. Retrieved from: https://www.ncbi.nlm.nih.gov/books/NBK19757/ (accessed on 15 June 2024).

Bäckhed, F., Ding, H., Wang, T., Hooper, L. V., Koh, G. Y., Nagy, A., et al. (2004). The gut microbiota as an environmental factor that regulates fat storage. *Proceedings of the National Academy of Sciences of the United States of America, 101*, 15718–15723.

Balaji, M., Ganjayi, M. S., Hanuma Kumar, G. E., Parim, B. N., Mopuri, R., & Dasari, S. (2016). A review on possible therapeutic targets to contain obesity: The role of phytochemicals. *Obesity Research & Clinical Practice, 10*(4), 363–380.

Banerjee, M., Gupta, S., Sharma, P., Shekhawat, J., & Gauba, K. (2020). Obesity and COVID-19: A fatal alliance. *Indian Journal of Clinical Biochemistry, 35*(4), 410–417.

Bays, H. E. (2004). Current and investigational antiobesity agents and obesity therapeutic treatment targets. *Obesity Research, 12*, 1197–1211.

Bhardwaj, M., Yadav, P., Vashishth, D., Sharma, K., Kumar, A., Chahal, J., et al. (2021). A review on obesity management through natural compounds and a green nanomedicine-based approach. *Molecules, 26*(11), 3278.

Bhathena, S. J., & Velasquez, M. T. (2002). Beneficial role of dietary phytoestrogens in obesity and diabetes. *The American Journal of Clinical Nutrition, 76*(1), 191–201.

Bhuyan, D. J., & Basu, A. (2017). Phenolic compounds: Potential health benefits and toxicity. In Q. V. Vuong (Ed.), *Utilisation of Bioactive Compounds from Agricultural and Food Production Waste* (pp. 27–59). CRC Press, Taylor & Francis Group.

Birari, R. B., & Bhutani, K. K. (2007). Pancreatic lipase inhibitors from natural sources: Unexplored potential. *Drug Discovery Today, 12*(19–20), 879–889.

Boccellino, M., & D'Angelo, S. (2020). Anti-Obesity effects of polyphenol intake: Current status and future possibilities. *International Journal of Molecular Sciences, 21*(16), 5642.

Boccellino, M., Donniacuo, M., Bruno, F., Rinaldi, B., Quagliuolo, L., Ambruosi, M., et al. (2019). Protective effect of piceatannol and bioactive stilbene derivatives against hypoxia-induced toxicity in H9c2 cardiomyocytes and structural elucidation as 5-LOX inhibitors. *European Journal of Medicinal Chemistry, 180*, 637–647.

Borriello, S. P., Setchell, K. D. R., Axelson, M., & Lawson, A. M. (1985). Production and metabolism of lignans by the human faecal flora. *Journal of Applied Bacteriology, 58*(1), 37–43.

Bravo, L. (1998). Polyphenols: Chemistry, dietary sources, metabolism, and nutritional significance. *Nutrition Reviews, 56*, 317–333.

Brey, C. W., Nelder, M. P., Hailemariam, T., Gaugler, R., & Hashmi, S. (2009). Krüppel-like family of transcription factors: An emerging new frontier in fat biology. *International Journal of Biological Sciences, 5*(6), 622–636.

Buoncristiano, M., Williams, J., Simmonds, P., Nurk, E., Ahrens, W., Nardone, P., et al. (2021). Socioeconomic inequalities in overweight and obesity among 6- to 9-year-old children in 24 countries from the World Health Organization European region. *Obesity Reviews, 22*(Suppl 6), e13213.

Cannon, B., & Nedergaard, J. (2004). Brown adipose tissue: Function and physiological significance. *Physiological Reviews, 84*(1), 277–359.

Cawley, J., & Meyerhoefer, C. (2012). The medical care costs of obesity: An instrumental variables approach. *Journal of Health Economics, 31*(1), 219–230.

Chantre, P., & Lairon, D. (2002). Recent findings of green tea extract AR25 (exolise) and its activity for the treatment of obesity. *Phytomedicine, 9*(1), 3–8.

Chia, P. W., Lim, B. S., Tan, K. C., Yong, F. S., & Kan, S. Y. (2019). Water extract of onion peel for the synthesis of bisindolylmethanes. *Journal of King Saud University – Science, 31*, 642–647.

COVID-19andObesity:The2021Atlas.(n.d.).WorldObesityFederation.Retrievedfrom:https://www.worldobesity.org/resources/resource-library/covid-19-and-obesity-the-2021-atlas.

D'Angelo, S., Scafuro, M., & Meccariello, R. (2019). BPA and nutraceuticals, simultaneous effects on endocrine functions. *Endocrine, Metabolic & Immune Disorders – Drug Targets, 19*, 594—604.

Dahiya, D. K., Renuka, Puniya, M., Shandilya, U. K., Dhewa, T., et al. (2017). Gut microbiota modulation and its relationship with obesity using prebiotic fibers and probiotics: A review. *Frontiers in Microbiology, 8*, 563.

Dehghan, M., Akhtar-Danesh, N., & Merchant, A. (2005). Childhood obesity, prevalence and prevention. *Nutrition Journal, 2*(4), 24.

Flavonoids: Chemical structure, classification, and examples. (n.d.). Tuscany Diet. Retrieved from: https://www.tuscany-diet.net/2014/01/22/flavonoids-definition-structure-classification/ (accessed on 15 June 2024).

Flegal, K. M., Wei, R., Ogden, C. L., Freedman, D. S., Johnson, C. L., & Curtin, L. R. (2009). Characterizing extreme values of body mass index-for-age by using the 2000 Centers for Disease Control and Prevention growth charts. *American Journal of Clinical Nutrition, 90*(5), 1314–1320.

Forbes-Hernández, T. Y., Cianciosi, D., Ansary, J., Mezzetti, B., Bompadre, S., Quiles, J. L., et al. (2020). Strawberry (*Fragaria × ananassa* cv. Romina) methanolic extract promotes browning in 3T3-L1 cells. *Food & Function, 11*(1), 297–304.

Fotschki, B., Juśkiewicz, J., Kołodziejczyk, K., Jurgoński, A., Kosmala, M., Milala, J., et al. (2018). Protective effects of ellagitannin-rich strawberry extracts on biochemical and metabolic disturbances in rats fed a diet high in fructose. *Nutrients, 10*(4), 445.

Geoffroy, P., Ressault, B., Marchioni, E., & Miesch, M. (2011). Synthesis of Hoodigogenin A, aglycone of natural appetite suppressant glycosteroids extracted from *Hoodia gordonii*. *Steroids, 76*(7), 702–708.

Ghattamaneni, N. K., Sharma, A., Panchal, S. K., & Brown, L. (2020). Pelargonidin 3-glucoside-enriched strawberry attenuates symptoms of DSS-induced inflammatory bowel disease and diet-induced metabolic syndrome in rats. *European Journal of Nutrition, 59*(7), 2905–2918.

Giudice, A., Montella, M., Boccellino, M., Crispo, A., D'Arena, G., Bimonte, S., et al. (2017). Epigenetic changes induced by green tea catechins are associated with prostate cancer. *Current Molecular Medicine, 17*, 405–420.

Gong, D. W., He, Y., Karas, M., & Reitman, M. (1997). Uncoupling protein-3 is a mediator of thermogenesis regulated by thyroid hormone, β3-adrenergic agonists, and leptin. *Journal of Biological Chemistry, 272*(39), 24129–24132.

He, X., Zhang, M., Li, S. T., Li, X., Huang, Q., Zhang, K., et al. (2022). Alteration of gut microbiota in high-fat diet-induced obese mice using carnosic acid from rosemary. *Food Science & Nutrition, 10*(7), 2325–2332.

Herranz-López, M., Olivares-Vicente, M., Boix-Castejón, M., Caturla, N., Roche, E., & Micol, V. (2019). Differential effects of a combination of *Hibiscus sabdariffa* and *Lippia citriodora* polyphenols in overweight/obese subjects: A randomized controlled trial. *Scientific Reports, 9*(1), 2999.

Hostetler, G. L., Ralston, R. A., & Schwartz, S. J. (2017). Flavones: Food sources, bioavailability, metabolism, and bioactivity. *Advances in Nutrition, 8*(3), 423–435.

Hu, F. B. (2007). Obesity and mortality: Watch your waist, not just your weight. *Archives of Internal Medicine, 167*(9), 875–876.

Jiao, X., Wang, Y., Lin, Y., Lang, Y., Li, E., Zhang, X., et al. (2018). Blueberry polyphenols extract as a potential prebiotic with anti-obesity effects on C57BL/6 J mice by modulating the gut microbiota. *Journal of Nutritional Biochemistry, 64*, 88–100.

Kalupahana, N. S., Moustaid-Moussa, N., & Claycombe, K. J. (2012). Immunity as a link between obesity and insulin resistance. *Molecular Aspects of Medicine, 33*(1), 26–34.

Keservani, R. K., Sharma, A. K., & Kesharwani, R. K. (2014). Flavonoids: Emerging trends and potential health benefits. *Journal of Chinese Pharmaceutical Sciences, 23*(12), 815.

Keservani, R. K., Sharma, A. K., & Kesharwani, R. K. (2016a). Nutraceutical and functional foods for cardiovascular health. In A. K. Sharma (Ed.), *Food Process Engineering* (pp. 291–312). Apple Academic Press, CRC Press.

Keservani, R. K., Sharma, A. K., & Kesharwani, R. K. (2016b). Medicinal effect of nutraceutical fruits for the cognition and brain health. *Scientifica*, 2016. Article ID 3109254, 10 pages. doi:10.1155/2016/3109254.

Khan, M. K., Dangles, O., & Zill-E-Huma, D. O. (2014). A comprehensive review on flavanones, the major citrus polyphenols. *Journal of Food Composition and Analysis, 33*(1), 85–104.

Kim, M. A., Lee, H. J., Bae, H. G., Yang, S. O., Lee, H. J., & Kim, M. J. (2021). Metabolite analysis and anti-obesity effects of celery seed in 3T3-L1 adipocytes. *Food Science & Biotechnology, 30*, 277–286.

Kim, M., Im, S., Cho, Y. K., Choi, C., Son, Y., Kwon, D., et al. (2020). Anti-obesity effects of soybean embryo extract and enzymatically-modified isoquercitrin. *Biomolecules, 10*(10), 1394.

Kjær, T. N., Ornstrup, M. J., Poulsen, M. M., Stødkilde-Jørgensen, H., Jessen, N., Jørgensen, J. O. L., et al. (2017). No beneficial effects of resveratrol on the metabolic syndrome: A randomized placebo-controlled clinical trial. *Journal of Clinical Endocrinology & Metabolism, 102*, 1642–1651.

Korsholm, A., Kjær, T., Ornstrup, M., & Pedersen, S. (2017). Comprehensive metabolomic analysis in blood, urine, fat, and muscle in men with metabolic syndrome: A randomized, placebo-controlled clinical trial on the effects of resveratrol after four months' treatment. *International Journal of Molecular Sciences, 18*(3), 554.

Kumar Singh, A., Cabral, C., Kumar, R., Ganguly, R., Kumar Rana, H., Gupta, A., et al. (2019). Beneficial effects of dietary polyphenols on gut microbiota and strategies to improve delivery efficiency. *Nutrients, 11*(9), 2216. https://doi.org/10.3390/nu11092216.

Kumar, M., Barbhai, M. D., Hasan, M., Punia, S., Dhumal, S., Rais, N., et al. (2022). Onion (*Allium cepa* L.) peels: A review on bioactive compounds and biomedical activities. *Biomedicine & Pharmacotherapy, 146*, 112498. https://doi.org/10.1016/j.biopha.2022.112498.

Kumar, S., & Pandey, A. K. (2013). Chemistry and biological activities of flavonoids: An overview. *The Scientific World Journal, 2013*, Article 162750. https://doi.org/10.1155/2013/162750.

Lefterova, M. I., & Lazar, M. A. (2009). New developments in adipogenesis. *Trends in Endocrinology & Metabolism, 20*(3), 107–114. https://doi.org/10.1016/j.tem.2008.11.005.

Lei, F., Zhang, X. N., Wang, W., Xing, D. M., Xie, W. D., Su, H., et al. (2007). Evidence of anti-obesity effects of the pomegranate leaf extract in high-fat diet induced obese mice. *International Journal of Obesity, 31*(6), 1023–1029. https://doi.org/10.1038/sj.ijo.0803575.

Li, S., Tan, H. Y., Wang, N., Cheung, F., Hong, M., & Feng, Y. (2018). The potential and action mechanism of polyphenols in the treatment of liver diseases. *Oxidative Medicine and Cellular Longevity, 2018*, Article 8394818. https://doi.org/10.1155/2018/8394818.

Liu, P. K., Weng, Z. M., Ge, G. B., Li, H. L., Ding, L. L., Dai, Z. R., et al. (2018). Biflavones from *Ginkgo biloba* as novel pancreatic lipase inhibitors: Inhibition potentials and mechanism. *International Journal of Biological Macromolecules, 118*(Pt B), 2216–2223. https://doi.org/10.1016/j.ijbiomac.2018.06.010.

Liu, S., Li, D., Huang, B., Chen, Y., Lu, X., & Wang, Y. (2013). Inhibition of pancreatic lipase, alpha-glucosidase, alpha-amylase, and hypolipidemic effects of the total flavonoids from *Nelumbo nucifera* leaves. *Journal of Ethnopharmacology, 149*(1), 263–269. https://doi.org/10.1016/j.jep.2013.06.033.

Lowell, B. B., & Spiegelman, B. M. (2000). Towards a molecular understanding of adaptive thermogenesis. *Nature, 404*, 652. https://doi.org/10.1038/35007527.

Manach, C., Scalbert, A., Morand, C., Rémésy, C., & Jiménez, L. (2004). Polyphenols: Food sources and bioavailability. *American Journal of Clinical Nutrition, 79*, 727–747. https://doi.org/10.1093/ajcn/79.5.727.

Manach, C., Williamson, G., Morand, C., Scalbert, A., & Rémésy, C. (2005). Bioavailability and bioefficacy of polyphenols in humans. I. Review of 97 bioavailability studies. *American Journal of Clinical Nutrition, 81*, 230S–242S. https://doi.org/10.1093/ajcn/81.1.230S.

Matsumoto, H., Ikoma, Y., Sugiura, M., Yano, M., & Hasegawa, Y. (2004). Identification and quantification of the conjugated metabolites derived from orally administered hesperidin in rat plasma. *Journal of Agricultural and Food Chemistry, 52*(21), 6653–6659. https://doi.org/10.1021/jf049216f.

McDougall, G. J., Kulkarni, N. N., & Stewart, D. (2009). Berry polyphenols inhibit pancreatic lipase activity in vitro. *Food Chemistry, 115*(1), 193–199. https://doi.org/10.1016/j.foodchem.2008.12.088.

Mele, L., Bidault, G., Mena, P., Crozier, A., Brighenti, F., Vidal-Puig, A., & Del Rio, D. (2017). Dietary (Poly)phenols, brown adipose tissue activation, and energy expenditure: A narrative review. *Advances in Nutrition, 8*(5), 694–704. https://doi.org/10.3945/an.117.016535.

Mena, P., Domínguez-Perles, R., Gironés-Vilaplana, A., Baenas, N., García-Viguera, C., & Villaño, D. (2014). Flavan-3-ols, anthocyanins, and inflammation. *IUBMB Life, 66*(11), 745–758. https://doi.org/10.1002/iub.1334.

Mikulski, D., Górniak, R., & Molski, M. (2010). A theoretical study of the structure-radical scavenging activity of trans-resveratrol analogues and cis-resveratrol in gas phase and water environment. *European Journal of Medicinal Chemistry, 45*(3), 1015–1027. https://doi.org/10.1016/j.ejmech.2009.11.030.

Mohamed, G. A., Ibrahim, S. R. M., Elkhayat, E. S., & El Dine, R. S. (2014). Natural anti-obesity agents. *Bulletin of Faculty of Pharmacy, Cairo University, 52*(2), 269–284. https://sciencedirect.com/science/article/pii/S1110093114000179.

Moriyasu, Y., Fukumoto, C., Wada, M., Yano, E., Murase, H., Mizuno, M., et al. (2021). Validation of antiobesity effects of black soybean seed coat powder suitable as a food material: Comparisons with conventional yellow soybean seed coat powder. *Foods, 10*(4), 841. https://doi.org/10.3390/foods10040841.

Moser, J. S., Galindo-Fraga, A., Ortiz-Hernández, A. A., Gu, W., Hunsberger, S., Galán-Herrera, et al. (2019). Underweight, overweight, and obesity as independent risk factors for hospitalization in adults and children from influenza and other respiratory viruses. *Influenza and Other Respiratory Viruses, 13*(1), 3–9. https://doi.org/10.1111/irv.12603.

Motti, M. L., D'Angelo, S., & Meccariello, R. (2018). MicroRNAs, cancer and diet: Facts and new exciting perspectives. *Current Molecular Pharmacology, 11*, 90–96. https://doi.org/10.2174/1874467210666171107115246.

Mrduljaš, N., Krešić, G., & Bilušić, T. (2017). Polyphenols: Food sources and health benefits. In M. C. Hueda (Ed.), *Functional Food – Improve Health through Adequate Food* (pp. 257–278). IntechOpen. https://doi.org/10.5772/67687.

Naczk, M., & Shahidi, F. (2006). Phenolics in cereals, fruits and vegetables: Occurrence, extraction and analysis. *Journal of Pharmaceutical and Biomedical Analysis, 41*, 1523–1542. https://doi.org/10.1016/j.jpba.2006.04.002.

Nøhr, M. K., Dudele, A., Poulsen, M. M., Ebbesen, L. H., Radko, Y., Christensen, L. P., et al. (2016). LPS-enhanced glucose-stimulated insulin secretion is normalized by resveratrol. *PLoS ONE, 11*(1), e0146840. https://doi.org/10.1371/journal.pone.0146840.

Obesity rates by country 2022. (n.d.). World Population Review. Retrieved from: https://worldpopulationreview.com/country-rankings/obesity-rates-by-country (accessed on 15 June 2024).

Obesity. (n.d.). World Health Organization. Retrieved from: https://www.who.int/health-topics/obesity#tab=tab_1 (accessed on 15 June 2024).

Panda, V., & Shinde, P. (2017). Appetite suppressing effect of *Spinacia oleracea* in rats: Involvement of the short-term satiety signal cholecystokinin. *Appetite, 113*, 224–230. https://doi.org/10.1016/j.appet.2017.02.010.

Panda, V., Shinde, P., & Dande, P. (2020). Consumption of *Spinacia Oleracea* (spinach) and aerobic exercise controls obesity in rats by an inhibitory action on pancreatic lipase. *Archives of Physiology and Biochemistry, 126*(3), 187–195. https://doi.org/10.1080/13813455.2019.1582485.

Pandey, K. B., & Rizvi, S. I. (2009). Plant polyphenols as dietary antioxidants in human health and disease. *Oxidative Medicine and Cellular Longevity, 2*, 270–278. https://doi.org/10.4161/oxim.2.5.9498.

Park, E. J., & Pezzuto, J. M. (2015). The pharmacology of resveratrol in animals and humans. *Biochimica et Biophysica Acta (BBA) – General Subjects, 1852*(6), 1071–1113. https://doi.org/10.1016/j.bbagen.2015.01.004.

Pastor-Villaescusa, B., Rodriguez, E. S., & Rangel-Huerta, O. D. (2018). Polyphenols in obesity and metabolic syndrome. In *Obesity* (pp. 213–239). Academic Press. https://doi.org/10.1016/B978-0-12-812396-5.00015-7.

Peixoto, T. C., Moura, E. G., de Oliveira, E., Soares, P. N., Guarda, D. S., Bernardino, D. N., et al. (2018). Cranberry (*Vaccinium macrocarpon*) extract treatment improves triglyceridemia, liver cholesterol, liver steatosis, oxidative damage and corticosteronemia in rats rendered obese by high fat diet. *European Journal of Nutrition, 57*(5), 1829–1844. https://doi.org/10.1007/s00394-017-1444-2.

Peng, C. H., Cheng, J. J., Yu, M. H., Chung, D. J., Huang, C. N., & Wang, C. J. (2020). *Solanum nigrum* polyphenols reduce body weight and body fat by affecting adipocyte and lipid metabolism. *Food & Function, 11*(1), 483–492. https://doi.org/10.1039/C9FO01916E.

Piazzon, A., Vrhovsek, U., Masuero, D., Mattivi, F., Mandoj, F., & Nardini, M. (2012). Antioxidant activity of phenolic acids and their metabolites: Synthesis and antioxidant properties of the sulfate derivatives of ferulic and caffeic acids and of the acyl glucuronide of ferulic acid. *Journal of Agricultural and Food Chemistry, 60*(50), 12312–12323. https://doi.org/10.1021/jf3041252.

Ramli, F. N., Abu Bakar Sajak, A., Abas, F., Mat Daud, Z. A., & Azlan, A. (2020). Effect of saffron extract and crocin in serum metabolites of induced obesity rats. *BioMed Research International, 2020*, Article ID 1247946. https://doi.org/10.1155/2020/1247946.

Riaz, M., Zia-Ul-Haq, M., & Saad, B. (Eds.). (2016). *Anthocyanins and Human Health: Biomolecular and Therapeutic Aspects*. Springer.

Roh, E., Song, D. K., & Kim, M. S. (2016). Emerging role of the brain in the homeostatic regulation of energy and glucose metabolism. *Experimental & Molecular Medicine, 48*, e216. https://doi.org/10.1038/emm.2016.6.

Saberi-Karimian, M., Katsiki, N., Caraglia, M., Boccellino, M., Majeed, M., & Sahebkar, A. (2019). Vascular endothelial growth factor: An important molecular target of curcumin. *Critical Reviews in Food Science and Nutrition, 59*, 299–312. https://doi.org/10.1080/10408398.2017.1411976.

Sagar, N. A., Pareek, S., & Gonzalez-Aguilar, G. A. (2020). Quantification of flavonoids, total phenols and antioxidant properties of onion skin: A comparative study of fifteen Indian cultivars. *Journal of Food Science and Technology, 57*, 2423–2432. https://doi.org/10.1007/s13197-020-04216-3.

Scalbert, A., & Williamson, G. (2000). Dietary intake and bioavailability of polyphenols. *Journal of Nutrition, 130*(8S Suppl), 2073S–2085S. https://doi.org/10.1093/jn/130.8.2073S.

Schwartz, M. W., Woods, S. C., Porte, D., Seeley, R. J., & Baskin, D. G. (2000). Central nervous system control of food intake. *Nature, 404*(6778), 661–671. https://doi.org/10.1038/35007534.

Singh, M., Kaur, M., & Silakari, O. (2014). Flavones: An important scaffold for medicinal chemistry. *European Journal of Medicinal Chemistry, 84*, 206–239. https://doi.org/10.1016/j.ejmech.2014.07.076.

Singh, M., Thrimawithana, T., Shukla, R., & Adhikari, B. (2020). Managing obesity through natural polyphenols: A review. *Future Foods, 1*, 100002. https://doi.org/10.1016/j.fufo.2019.100002.

Sirotkin, A. V., & Kolesárová, A. (2021). The anti-obesity and health-promoting effects of tea and coffee. *Physiological Research, 70*(2), 161–168.

Song, H., & Seo, J. H. (2022). Anti-obesity effects of red onions extract. *Journal of Convergence Information Technology, 12*(3), 126–131. https://doi.org/10.6109/jcit.2022.12.3.126.

Srivastava, R. A., Pinkosky, S. L., Filippov, S., Hanselman, J. C., Cramer, C. T., & Newton, R. S. (2012). AMP-activated protein kinase: An emerging drug target to regulate imbalances in lipid and carbohydrate metabolism to treat cardio-metabolic diseases. *Journal of Lipid Research, 53*(12), 2490–2514. https://doi.org/10.1194/jlr.R027383.

Takei, K., Nakagawa, Y., Wang, Y., Han, S. I., Satoh, A., Sekiya, M., et al. (2017). Effects of K-877, a novel selective PPAR alpha modulator, on small intestine contribute to the amelioration of hyperlipidemia in low-density lipoprotein receptor knockout mice. *Journal of Pharmacological Sciences, 133*(4), 214–222. https://doi.org/10.1016/j.jphs.2017.11.005.

Tetens, I., Turrini, A., Tapanainen, H., Christensen, T., Lampe, J. W., Fagt, S., et al. (2013). Dietary intake and main sources of plant lignans in five European countries. *Food & Nutrition Research, 57*, 19805. https://doi.org/10.3402/fnr.v57i0.19805.

Tong, Q., & Hotamisligil, G. S. (2001). Molecular mechanisms of adipocyte differentiation. *Reviews in Endocrine & Metabolic Disorders, 2*(4), 349–355. https://doi.org/10.1023/A:1013174827209.

Torres-Fuentes, C., Schellekens, H., Dinan, T. G., & Cryan, J. F. (2015). A natural solution for obesity: Bioactives for the prevention and treatment of weight gain. A review. *Nutritional Neuroscience, 18*, 49–65. https://doi.org/10.1179/1476830514Y.0000000158.

Tsao, R. (2010). Chemistry and biochemistry of dietary polyphenols. *Nutrients, 2*(12), 1231–1246. https://doi.org/10.3390/nu2121231.

Upadhyay, J., Farr, O., Perakakis, N., Ghaly, W., & Mantzoros, C. (2018). Obesity as a Disease. *Medical Clinics of North America, 102*(1), 13–33. https://doi.org/10.1016/j.mcna.2017.08.008.

Veeramani, C., Alsaif, M. A., & Al-Numair, K. S. (2018). Herbacetin, a flaxseed flavonoid, ameliorates high percent dietary fat induced insulin resistance and lipid accumulation through the regulation of hepatic lipid metabolizing and lipid-regulating enzymes. *Chemico-Biological Interactions, 288*, 49–56. https://doi.org/10.1016/j.cbi.2018.04.013.

Vendrame, S., Del Bo' C., Ciappellano, S., Riso, P., & Klimis-Zacas, D. (2016). Berry fruit consumption and metabolic syndrome. *Antioxidants, 5*(4), 34. https://doi.org/10.3390/antiox5040034.

Wang, L., Zeng, B., Liu, Z., Liao, Z., Zhong, Q., Gu, L., et al. (2018). Green tea polyphenols modulate colonic microbiota diversity and lipid metabolism in high-fat diet treated HFA mice. *Journal of Food Science, 83*(3), 864–873. https://doi.org/10.1111/1750-3841.14066.

Wang, S., Moustaid-Moussa, N., Chen, L., Mo, H., Shastri, A., Su, R., et al. (2014). Novel insights of dietary polyphenols and obesity. *Journal of Nutritional Biochemistry, 25*(1), 1–18. https://doi.org/10.1016/j.jnutbio.2013.09.001.

Wang, Y., Chung, S., Song, W. O., & Chun, O. K. (2011). Estimation of daily proanthocyanidin intake and major food sources in the U. S. diet. *Journal of Nutrition, 141*, 447–452. https://doi.org/10.3945/jn.110.133199.

Wong, S. K., Chin, K. Y., Suhaimi, F. H., Fairus, A., & Ima-Nirwana, S. (2016). Animal models of metabolic syndrome: A review. *Nutrition & Metabolism, 13*, 65. https://doi.org/10.1186/s12986-016-0123-9.

Wood Dos Santos, T., Cristina Pereira, Q., Teixeira, L., Gambero, A., A Villena, J., & Lima Ribeiro, M. (2018). Effects of Polyphenols on thermogenesis and mitochondrial biogenesis. *International Journal of Molecular Sciences, 19*(9), 2757. https://doi.org/10.3390/ijms19092757.

Wu, T., Gao, Y., Guo, X., Zhang, M., & Gong, L. (2018). Blackberry and blueberry anthocyanin supplementation counteract high-fat-diet-induced obesity by alleviating oxidative stress and inflammation and accelerating energy expenditure. *Oxidative Medicine and Cellular Longevity, 2018*, Article ID 4051232. https://doi.org/10.1155/2018/4051232.

Xu, Y., Zhang, M., Wu, T., Dai, S., Xu, J., & Zhou, Z. (2015). The anti-obesity effect of green tea polysaccharides, polyphenols and caffeine in rats fed with a high-fat diet. *Food & Function, 6*(1), 297–304. https://doi.org/10.1039/C4FO00753H.

Yang, C. S., Landau, J. M., Huang, M. T., & Newmark, H. L. (2001). Inhibition of carcinogenesis by dietary polyphenolic compounds. *Annual Review of Nutrition, 21*, 381–406. https://doi.org/10.1146/annurev.nutr.21.1.381.

Yu, J. H., & Kim, M. S. (2012). Molecular mechanisms of appetite regulation. *Diabetes & Metabolism Journal, 36*(6), 391–398. https://doi.org/10.4093/dmj.2012.36.6.391.

Yu, S., Li, H., Cui, T., Cui, M., Piao, C., Wang, S., et al. (2021). Onion (*Allium cepa* L.) peel extract effects on 3T3-L1 adipocytes and high-fat diet-induced obese mice. *Food Bioscience, 41*, 101019. https://doi.org/10.1016/j.fbio.2021.101019.

Zhou, F., Guo, J., Han, X., Gao, Y., Chen, Q., Huang, W., et al. (2020). Cranberry polyphenolic extract exhibits an antiobesity effect on high-fat diet-fed mice through increased thermogenesis. *Journal of Nutrition, 150*(8), 2131–2138. https://doi.org/10.1093/jn/nxaa138.

CHAPTER 12

α-AMYLASE INHIBITORS: A SAFE NUTRACEUTICAL APPROACH FOR OBESITY MANAGEMENT

SNEHIL SINGH,[1] SAGAR PATNI,[1] AMRITA SINGH,[2] SONIA BHATT,[3] and SUMAN LATA MEHTA2

[1]*School of Pharmaceutical Sciences, C.S.J.M. University, Kanpur University, Uttar Pradesh, India*

[2]*Department of Pharmacy, IEC College of Engineering and Technology, Greater Noida, Uttar Pradesh, India*

[3]*Lingaya's Vidyapeeth, Nachauli, Old Faridabad, Haryana, India*

ABSTRACT

Enzymes are considered to be the most fundamental biocatalysts that catalyze various biological reactions. Amylases are among the most extensively investigated enzymes. The enzyme 4-α-D-glucan glucanohydrolase, also known as α-Amylase, hydrolyzes the bonds in big, α-linked polysaccharides like starch and glycogen to produce shorter chains of these compounds, dextrins, and maltose. Obesity and overweight are the fifth most occurring major concerns in the population nowadays, ultimately leading to mortality worldwide. In view of this, α-Amylase inhibitors (AIs) can serve as carbohydrate blockers by reducing the digestive capacity and intestinal absorption of carbohydrates. Changes in dietary strategies have been suggested as the method to tackle the issues affecting lipid and carbohydrate metabolism. The simplest way to reduce carbohydrate absorption is by introducing more dietary fibers into the diet. Another approach towards obesity is to reduce

Nutraceuticals in Obesity Management and Control. Raj K. Keservani & Alka Lohani (Eds.)

weight and slow down or inhibit the absorption of carbohydrates and sugar by giving α-amylase inhibitors, with proper physical activity and a fiber-rich diet simultaneously.

12.1 INTRODUCTION

Enzymes are considered to be the most fundamental biocatalysts that catalyze various biological reactions. They are large, globular proteins with a high molecular weight that, like other proteins, have a long linear chain of amino acids and unique capabilities that depend on the structure. A three-dimensional complex of polypeptide chains makes them up (Kermasha et al., 2021). Enzymes are employed in the textile and manufacturing industries as an alternative to harmful chemicals for many processing steps because they are available from a variety of sources including plants, animal tissues, and other microbes (Matamá et al., 2010). They are currently becoming increasingly significant in industries including medicine, green chemistry, and sustainable technology. The global market for enzymes was estimated to be worth USD 7.5 billion in 2020, and from 2016 to 2021, it is expected to expand by 8.2% annually (Roy et al., 2019; Rigoldi et al., 2018). A highly profitable expansion of enzymes in the detergent, pharmaceutical, and even chemical industries is anticipated worldwide. Enzymes are more susceptible to a wide range of variables; they become inactive in high temperatures, acids, and radiation, and they are also easily denatured by several biological stimuli (Silva et al., 2010).

Enzymes are potent biocatalysts. Raising the reaction rate at lower concentrations and carrying out the reaction without consumption or other modifications are both possible by lowering the activation energy (Robinson et al., 2015). Since each enzyme performs a different mechanism, such as covalent catalysis, acid-base, or electrostatic, they are distinct in their function and response (Kumar et al., 2020; Kani et al., 2020). Enzymes are used extensively in the pharmaceutical business to treat a wide range of diseases, including cancer (Kani et al., 2020). They have numerous uses outside of the pharmaceutical industry as well, including in industries like food processing, textile processing, paper manufacturing, etc.

Amylases are among the most extensively investigated enzymes (Noomen et al., 2009). In an effort to utilize their physiological and biotechnological implications, this enormous diversity of amylases has garnered attention on a global scale (San-Lang et al., 2011). Amylases are starch-degrading enzymes that maintain the alpha anomeric shape of the polysaccharides they produce while they hydrolyze internal alpha 1–4 glycosidic linkages (Takata et al., 1992). No matter the kingdom, they are present in all kinds of species. Amylases originating from plants and microorganisms have long been employed in the brewing industry. Fungus amylases are commonly used in the preparation of Asian cuisine (Mabel et al., 2006). Amylase from various sources has attracted worldwide attention and has become a topic of research as it holds a potential application in biotechnology and industries. Food, fermentation, and pharmaceutical sectors all use amylase in a variety of production processes. Amylase is a common ingredient in the creation of biofuel. The manufacture of bioethanol is the industry's second most prevalent use for amylase. The slurry was initially gelatinized using a jet cooker. The saccharification and release of fermentable sugars occur as a result of the liquefaction process using thermally stable α-amylase. Following fermentation, bioethanol is created (Cripwell et al., 2020). In the dry-grind process, replacing yeast with maize amylase minimizes the need for enzymes; the combined enzymes are then used to produce bioethanol (Kumar et al., 2016). By employing fermentation and saccharification techniques to treat enzymes like amylase with wheat bran, bioethanol can be generated from the waste stream of a bio-refinery (Wood et al., 2015).

12.2 CLASSIFICATION OF AMYLASE

Amylases are categorized based on their ability to hydrolyze starch into endoamylases and exoamylases, which depends on how they break the glycosidic linkage.

1. **Endoamylases:** Endoamylase randomly breaks down the α-1,4-D-glycosidic connection between adjacent glucose units in the polysaccharide chain while preserving the anomeric carbon structure (Sasi et al., 2008). Endoamylases, also known as α-amylases, are known for cleaving internal α-1,4 bonds to produce α-anomeric compounds (Sivaramakrishnan et al., 2006). Although some α-amylases have been identified to be intracellular, the majority are extracellular.
2. **Exoamylases:** These function at the non-reducing ends of polysaccharides to produce low molecular weight substances like glucose and maltose. These enzymes only cleave α-1,4-glycosidic bonds like β-amylase, or α-1,4 and α-1,6-glycosidic bonds like glucoamylase and α-glycosidase (Sivaramakrishnan et al., 2006). Glucoamylase and α-glucosidase only produce glucose, but β-amylase generates

maltose and β-limit dextrin in the starch hydrolysates. The released product's anomeric structure is also changed from α to β by glucoamylase and β-amylase (Pandey et al., 2000).

3. **α-Amylase:** Endoamylases have the ability to break down the 1-4-glycosidic linkages found in the endo-region of amylose or amylopectin chains. One well-known endoamylase is α-amylase. It can be present in a wide range of bacteria and archaea-related microorganisms (Pandey et al., 2000). As a result of α-amylase action, oligosaccharides are produced, which have a range of lengths and contain dextrins with a limit and configuration. In accordance with the degree of hydrolysis, they are frequently divided into two types. While liquefying only breaks down around 30 to 40% of the starch being hydrolyzed, α-amylases cause 50 to 60% of the hydrolysis through saccharification. They are calcium metalloenzymes, and they are dependent on calcium to function. Maltose and maltotriose are produced from amylose, while glucose, maltose, and limited dextrin are produced from amylopectin. These sugars are produced as a result of the enzyme α-amylase breaking down carbohydrates and starch. In humans, salivary and pancreatic amylases are the forms of α-amylases that can be obtained from plants, bacteria, and fungi sources.

4. **β-Amylase:** The second group of enzymes, known as exo amylases, either cleave 1-4-glycosidic bonds exclusively, like β-amylase, or both 1-4- and 1-6-glycosidic bonds, like amylo glucosidase, glucoamylase, and α-glucosidase. Exo amylases exclusively react with the outer glucose remaining part of amylopectin or amylose to produce glucose (glucoamylase and α-glucosidase) or maltose and β-limit dextrin. Additionally, the enzymes β α-amylase and glucoamylase convert the anomeric structure of the liberated maltose from α to β. In terms of substrate preference, α-glucosidase works better with short malto oligosaccharides and releases glucose with an α-configuration, whereas glucoamylase favors long-chain polysaccharides (Kim et al., 2004). Glucoamylases and α-amylases have also been known to be found in different microorganisms (Mabel et al., 2006).

5. **γ-Amylase:** It is also known to break down α-(1-6)-glycosidic linkages along with α-(1-4)-glycosidic linkages at the non-reducing end of amylopectin and amylose. It is known to work better in an acidic environment at an optimum pH of 3.

12.3 SOURCES OF ALFA-AMYLASE

12.3.1 PLANT SOURCES

The unicellular eukaryotes, bacteria, and archaea are among the organisms that include amylases, along with mammals, fungi, and plants (Lagea et al., 2007). Despite the fact that both plants and animals manufacture amylases, industrial processes typically require enzymes from microbial sources. This is caused by a variety of elements, such as productivity, the enzyme's thermostability, and the simplicity of microbe cultivation (Reddy et al., 1999). The selectivity with its corresponding high yield and exclusivity toward the targeted product is the main benefit of the enzymatic route (Kim et al., 2004). The *Bacillus* spp. are the bacteria employed in commercial manufacturing (Olafimihan et al., 1999; Gupta et al., 2003; Pandey et al., 2000). Others, including Escherichia spp., Pseudomonas, Proteus, Serratia, and Rhizobium also produce a sizable amount of the enzyme (Oliviera et al., 2007). Several fungi, including *Aspergillus, Rhizopus, Mucor, Neurospora, Penicillium,* and *Candida*, also produce extracellular amylases with a marketable value (Gupta et al., 2003). Plant sources had not yet been given enough weight as a potential source for these enzymes (Azad et al., 2009). Utilizing agricultural waste products has two advantages: it reduces pollution and improves the quality of the materials. In order to lower the price of fermentation media, agricultural wastes are employed for both liquid and solid fermentation. Amylases make up around 25–33% of the global enzyme industry and are manufactured commercially in large quantities from microorganisms (Nguyen et al., 2002). They were used in a wide range of contexts, such as the liquefaction of starch in traditional beverages, baking, and the textile industry for fabric desizing (Dauter et al., 1999; Pederson et al., 2000). Additionally, they have been used as detergent additives, digestives, and in the manufacturing of paper (Bruinenberg et al., 1996; Mitidieri et al., 2006).

12.3.2 MICROBIAL SOURCES

Despite their widespread availability, microorganism-derived amylases are employed on a large scale in a variety of industries because of their consistency, simplicity in process modification, cost-effectiveness, and ease of process optimization (Mamo et al., 1999; Burhan et al., 2003). Fungal amylase is used to create Asian cuisine. For use in industry, *Bacillus* sp. produces thermostable α-amylase. It has been determined that *B.*

stearothermophilus, *B. subtilis*, *B. amyloliquefaciens*, and *B. licheniformis* are excellent producers of α-amylase and are employed in industry (Kim et al., 1995). Similarly, filamentous fungi have created amylases for eons in huge amounts. The molds are frequently utilized to produce many enzymes, including α-amylase because they are known to be prolific extracellular protein producers. The most often used fungi for alpha-amylase synthesis are those in the genus *Aspergillus*. Using these molds to produce enzymes in solid-state fermentation has proven to be a more affordable method of manufacturing.

12.4 CARBOHYDRATE DIGESTION AND AMYLASE

Amylase is an important enzyme that acts on starch or glycogen and is found in animals, plants, bacteria, and fungi. Starch obtained from plants is a macromolecule polymer composed of amylopectin, a polymer with a branched chain linked at -1,4 points of 10^5 connected glucose units, and amylose, a straight-chain polymer with linkages at -1,4 points with approximately 10^6 units. Animal glycogen has a similar structure to amylopectin, although it has a lower molecular weight. The enzyme α-amylase breaks the -1,4 linkage if it is not close to a branch point or a terminal glucose residue, producing maltotriose (3 glucose residues), α-limit dextrins (containing 5 to 6 residues), and maltose (containing 5 residues).

Isomaltase and Glucoamylase are brush border enzymes that hydrolyze the -1,6 and -1,4 linkages, respectively, further cleaving them in vertebrates into monosaccharides (Alpers et al., 1994). Studies have shown that the rate-limiting stage in humans' ability to absorb complex carbohydrates is hydrolysis, not the absorption of monosaccharides (Hiele et al., 1989). The pancreas, liver, parotid, urine, serum, and other organs or tumors in animals sometimes contain small amounts of α-amylase; the salivary amylase and pancreatic amylase proteins are quite analogous to each other (Stiefel et al., 1973). Salivary amylase starts acting upon carbohydrates in the mouth itself while the pancreas acts upon them in the intestinal lumen. Despite being generated as a 57 kDa protein, human pancreatic α-amylase's cDNA predicts a protein with 512 amino acids (Whitcomb et al., 2007). This contains a signal sequence, and amylase with 496 amino acids was extracted from human pancreatic juice (Ferey-Roux et al., 1998). The analyzed molecular weight for amylase in different species is 50–57 kDa and it also contains a 7.1 isoelectric point. Its composition is made up of a single-chain protein with a single carbohydrate unit. Amylase from the human pancreas exists in two isoforms, HPA I and HPA II, with pI values of 7.2 and 6.6 and no sugar groups (Ferey-Roux et al., 1998). Porcine pancreatic amylase has five disulfide bridges described in it (Pasero et al., 1986).

The AMY1 gene codes for salivary amylase, the AMY2 gene for pancreatic amylase, and the AMY2B gene for a third form found in some tumors (Nakamura et al., 1984; Schibler et al., 1982; Wise et al., 1984; Yokouchi et al., 1990). By redirecting a pancreatic amylase gene's promoter to become a salivary gene, a retroviral insertion into the gene's promoter has been utilized to chart the evolution of the amylase gene family (Enclosures & Ting, 1993). Multiple genes and pseudogenes belonging to the amylase family are found on chromosomes 1 in humans and 3 in mice (Gumucio et al., 1988; Sugino, 2007). A/J, CE/J, and the majority of wild mice have multiple forms of amylase, whereas the majority of inbred mouse strains only express one species of the enzyme (Tosi et al., 1984). It's interesting to note that people from agricultural societies who eat high-starch diets have more copies of the salivary amylase genes (Perry et al., 2007) and more copies result in more protein and a stronger perception of oral starch (Santos et al., 2012; Mandel et al., 2010). Human amylase protein is assigned as A, B, and C, which is known as a three-domain structure that begins at the amino-terminal (Brayer et al., 1995). A domain active site may be stabilized by the Calcium binds to the B domain (Buisson et al., 1987). The C domain is a spheroid domain with an unspecified function. Chloride allosterically triggers the activity of a few amylases, including human pancreatic amylase, by adjusting the pH (D'Amico et al., 2000; Maurus et al., 2005). The amylase's active center has five subsites that enable it to bind different substrate glucose residues (Seigner et al., 2000). In a recent review, the enzymatic mechanism for glycosidases is described (Vasella et al., 2002).

According to kinetic authentication, there might be more carbohydrate binding sites (Alkazaz et al., 1996). Some of these are surface-bound sites that aid in amylase's attachment to the starch granules (Zhang et al., 2016). The structure of starch, which has been divided into three categories—rapidly digested, slowly digested, and resistant starch—influences the rate of starch digestion as well. Cooking, which converts starch granules to soluble starch, can also have an impact on starch digestion (Dhital et al., 2017). A large family of plant α-amylase inhibitory proteins has helped with studies of the enzymatic mechanism (Bompard-Gilles et al., 1996; Svensson et al., 2004; Williams, 2019). In the most thoroughly researched of these, the enzyme-inhibitor complex's structure has been established, which is from beans (Santimone et al., 2004). Pseudotetrasaccharides, of which acarbose, a Pseudotetrasaccharides, is one, have yielded more powerful inhibitors that have received clinical approval. Pig amylase complexed with acarbose's crystal structure has been reported (Gilles et al., 1996). In contrast to proteinaceous inhibitors, these pseudo-oligosaccharide inhibitors block intestinal brush border enzymes, amylase, and all glucosidases (Kumar Singla et al., 2016). Several pancreatic enzymes, together with amylase, are discovered to be absorbed on the surface of the duodenal mucosa despite the fact that high salt may be used to remove them (Alpers et al., 1994). However, it has been discovered that amylase binds to the specific N-linked oligosaccharides of brush border glycoproteins and that this binding increases amylase activity (Matsushita et al., 2002). Sucrase-isomaltase (SI) and SGLT1 have been identified as specific glycoproteins that bind amylase (Asanuma et al., 2012). This binding increases the activity of SI and amylase while decreasing the activity of SGLT1. According to the authors, this improves digestion while limiting excessively quick glucose absorption. Amylase is internalized into enterocytes after binding to brush border proteins, restoring glucose uptake (Date et al., 2015).

12.5 OBESITY AND ALPHA-AMYLASE

Obesity and overweight are the fifth most occurring major concerns in the population nowadays, ultimately leading to mortality worldwide (Peddio et al., 2022). Over 1.9 billion adults, including over 650 million obese individuals, were overweight in 2016, according to WHO. Overweight and obesity rates are expected to double globally over the next 10 years, with 2.3 billion adults expected to be overweight and over 700 million expected to be obese by 2015.

It can be seen in adolescents as well as in children, in which 340 million children and adolescents of age group 5–19 were found to be obese in 2016, a hike of 14% from 1975 can be seen (Barrett & Udani, 2011). The number of obese people underweight is greater in every region, globally excluding the sub-Saharan Africa and Asian region. The imbalance caused between energy expenditure and diet intake has been recognized as the origin of the condition, which occurs mainly due to the decline in physical activity and high sugar intake, fats rich diet, and a low amount of fibers and micronutrients (Meigs et al., 2006). Risks of VS disorders include hypertension, dyslipidemia, Type 2 DM (Taroeno-Hariadi et al., 2021), osteoarthritis affecting joints and cartilage (Mohammad et al., 2021), and several types of cancers (Raud et al., 2020). Currently, it has been found as a reason for poor clinical outcomes and risk of hospitalization during the COVID-19 pandemic (Grabitske & Slavin, 2009). Changes in dietary strategies have been suggested to address the issues related to lipid and carbohydrate metabolism. One simple way to reduce carbohydrate absorption is by adding more dietary fibers to your diet. Another approach to combat obesity and lose weight is to slow down or inhibit carbohydrate and sugar absorption by using α-amylase inhibitors, along with regular physical activity and a fiber-rich diet.

12.6 INHIBITORS OF ALPHA-AMYLASE

Inhibitors of amylase are also termed starch blockers because they contain substances that prevent the body's absorption of dietary starches. Complex carbohydrates, termed starches, must first be broken down by the digestive enzyme amylase and other secondary enzymes in order to be absorbed. Salivary α-amylase hydrolyzes the -1,4 bonds in starch to start the process of breaking down carbs in the mouth. The end products of this process are maltose, glucose, fructose, small dextrins, and maltriose. Pancreatic α-amylase continues the starch-digesting process in the small intestine. Maltase, sucrase, and lactase, also referred to as disaccharidases or α-glucosidases, are the digestive enzymes that finish the digestion process and produce the absorbable monosaccharides glucose, fructose, and galactose. Although a tiny part of monosaccharides can be passively absorbed, a carrier protein is necessary to absorb the quantity consumed in a typical diet (Truscheit et al., 2010).

It has been suggested that increased postprandial blood glucose is related to carbohydrate digestion. Limiting the activity of intestinal enzymes that break down carbohydrates is one method for lowering postprandial hyperglycemia. The primary enzyme, α-amylase, catalyzes the hydrolysis of α-1,4-glucan linkages found in starch, maltodextrins, and other similar carbohydrates to break down the polymeric substrate into shorter oligomers (Suetsugu et al., 1974).

This enzyme breaks down the 1,4-glycosidic link to release glucose from the polysaccharide and non-reducing end, contributing to the body's effective metabolism of carbohydrates. The digestive enzyme amylase and other secondary enzymes must first break down starches, which are complex carbohydrates before they can be absorbed (Pradeep & Sreerama, 2015).

Flavonoids, Tannins, Anthocyanins, and Phenolic acids have all been documented to be starch hydrolase inhibitors in cereals. The majority of the investigations that have been published have used crude phenolic extracts, both soluble and bound. Corn, Rice, barley, Sorghum, millet, and quinoa Phenolic compounds were found to be potent inhibitors of α-amylase (Rosén et al., 2011; Shukla et al., 2014; Horii et al., 1986).

12.7 TYPES OF ALPHA-AMYLASE INHIBITORS

Amylase inhibitors (AIs) can serve as carbohydrate blockers by reducing the digestive capacity and intestinal absorption of carbohydrates (Franco et al., 2002). According to their source of origin, there are two types of alpha-amylase inhibitors – proteinaceous and non-proteinaceous.

12.7.1 PROTEINACEOUS ALPHA-AMYLASE INHIBITORS

According to similarities in sequence and three-dimensional structures, there are seven different categories of proteinaceous alpha-amylase inhibitors in nature (Garcia-Olmedo et al., 1987; Ho & Whitaker, 1993; Lu et al., 1999; Chagolla et al., 1994; Bloch & Richardson, 1991). Six varieties are from higher plants (Garcia-Maroto et al., 1991), while the remaining kind is found in species of Streptomyces (Kamitori et al., 1999). Examples of proteinaceous alpha-amylase inhibitors are represented in Table 12.1.

TABLE 12.1 Examples of Proteinaceous Alpha-Amylase Inhibitors from Plant and Microbial Sources

Sl. No.	Inhibitor Type	Etymology	α-Amylase Target
1.	Microbial (Ho et al., 1994)	Streptomycin (Chagolla et al., 1994)	Bacteria, Mammalian
2.	Knottin like (Carugo et al., 2001)	Amaranth (Chagolla et al., 1994)	Insect
3.	γ-Theonine like	Sorghum (Bloch et al., 1991)	Insect (Mammalian)
4.	CM-Proteins (Franco et al., 2000, 2002; Ho et al., 1994)	Cereal seeds (Campos et al., 1983; Garcia et al., 1991; Barber et al., 1986)	Bacteria, Mammalian, Insect
5.	Thaumatin-like (Franco et al., 2002)	Maize (Schimolar et al., 2001)	Insect
6.	Legume-lectins like	Common bean (Marshall et al., 1975; Ho et al., 1993)	Mammalian, insect, fungi

12.7.2 NON-PROTEINACEOUS ALPHA-AMYLASE INHIBITORS

Due to their cyclic structures, which resemble amylase substrates, easily bind to α-amylase catalytic sites, and have an inhibitory effect against amylases. This class includes a variety of chemical compounds, including cyclodextrins, isoacarbose, acarbose, acarviosine-glucose, and hibiscus acid (Barrett & Udani, 2011; Yamagishi et al., 2009; Barbosa et al., 2010; Ho et al., 1994; Ve´rtesy et al., 1984).

12.8 ALPHA-AMYLASE INHIBITORS IN OBESITY MANAGEMENT

Amylase inhibitors are also termed starch blockers because they contain substances that inhibit dietary starches from being absorbed by the body. Starches are complex carbohydrates that cannot be absorbed unless they are first broken down by the digestive enzyme amylase and other secondary enzymes. Salivary amylase hydrolyzes the 1,4 bonds in starch to start the process of breaking down carbs in the mouth. The end products of this process are maltose, glucose, fructose, small dextrins, and maltriose. Pancreatic amylase continues the starch-digesting process in the small intestine. Maltase, sucrase, and lactase, also known as disaccharidases or glucosidases, are the digestive enzymes that complete the digestion process and produce the absorbable monosaccharides glucose, fructose, and galactose. While a small portion of monosaccharides can be absorbed passively, a carrier protein is needed to absorb the amount consumed in a typical diet (Grabitske et al., 2009). A different approach could involve the use of some phytochemicals to slow down carbohydrate absorption. By blocking the essential enzyme activity, specifically amylase, and glucosidase, this might be accomplished by preventing intestinal breakdown (Fukagawa et al., 1990).

A digesting enzyme called amylase is mainly secreted by the pancreas and salivary glands, while it is also found in very small levels in other organs. Early in the 1800s, amylase was first described, making it one of the first enzymes in human history to be the subject of scientific investigation. It was formerly known as diastase but in the early 20th century, the name was changed to amylase (Kandra et al., 2003). The 512 amino acids human isoform is a single peptide chain that weighs around 57 kDa and needs calcium ions to maintain structural integrity (Sabory et al., 2000; Whitcomb et al., 2007).

This is one of the primary secretory enzymes produced by the pancreas and salivary glands, and it is essential for the breakdown of starch and the absorption of derived simple sugars. Dextrins are shorter oligosaccharides that nonetheless retain the anomeric form. They are composed of maltose, maltotriose, and branched oligosaccharides of 6–8 glucose units with both 1,4 and 1,6 linkages. Dextrins are further hydrolyzed by other intestinal brush border enzymes (particularly glucosidase, maltase, and isomaltase), and the resultant sugars can then be absorbed. The action of amylase has little impact on terminal glucose or -D-(1–6) glycosidic linkages (de Sales et al., 2012).

Structurally, all α-amylases are usually folded into three domains: A, B, and C. Domain A consists of a (β/α)8-barrel, which is the core structure of the enzyme. Domain B is a sheet of four anti-parallel β-strands with a pair of anti-parallel β-strands. The binding site for calcium ions is located in this domain. Domain C consists of eight β-strands forming a Greek key motif. Thus, α-amylase represents the crucial step in the initiation of the process of digestion and absorption of dietary polysaccharides (Tangphatsornruang et al., 2005).

12.9 SOME EXAMPLES OF ALPHA-AMYLASE INHIBITORS FOR THE MANAGEMENT OF OBESITY

12.9.1 COMMON BEAN (PHASEOLUS VULGARIS L.)

In actuality, the common bean is cultivated widely throughout the world and has many beneficial nutritional qualities. Additionally, these inhibitors are typically regarded as safe (there were no negative effects reported as with other plants) (Kusaba-Nakayama et al., 2000). Lectins, which attach to carbohydrates and precipitate or agglutinate cells, glycoconjugates, including glycoproteins, are α-amylase inhibitors. *P. vulgaris* produces three different types of lectins: Artificial Immune Systems (AIs), phytohemagglutinin (PHA), and arcelins (ARL), as seed defense mechanisms against biotic (i.e., insect predation) and abiotic stress (i.e., drought, salinity, and wounding) (Mojica et al., 2015; Moreno et al., 1990). These substances are considered as antinutritional elements (Obiro et al., 2008). However, due to their high sulfur amino acid concentration, thermal denaturation (usually obtained during boiling) inactivates anti-nutrient agents, providing nutritious value (Mojica et al., 2015). Three main α-AIs can be found in common beans: isoform 1 (α-AI1), isoform 2 (α-AI2), and α-amylase inhibitor-like (α-AIL) (Keiko Ishimoto et al., 1995; Obiro et al., 2008).

All of these proteins have the ability to exclusively block animal α-amylases while having no effect on plant amylases (Moreno et al., 1990). These proteins have been suggested as pesticides for bruchid pests due to their activity against insect amylases (Le Berre et al., 2000). In order to give resistance to other insect pests, their genes have also been transgenically produced in other plants (such as tobacco and peas) (Altabella et al., 1990; Schroeder et al., 1995). On the other hand, only α-AI1 has an effect on human amylases, making it the target for nutraceuticals clinical studies. Heterologous expression of α-AI1 in yeasts has also been recently described to improve potential large-scale production.

Contrarily, only α-AI1 specifically affects mammalian (and thus human) amylases, making it the subject of clinical studies on nutraceuticals. Additionally, heterologous expression of α-AI1 in yeasts has recently been reported to enhance potential large-scale output (Brain-Isasi et al., 2017).

As indicated, there are seven different types of natural protein inhibitors of α-amylases (α-AIs) and six of them are:

- Knottin-like type (Bhide et al., 2017);
- γ-Thionin-like type (Mojica et al., 2017);
- Cereal type;
- Kunitz type;
- Thaumatin-like type; and
- Lectin-like type.

These are extracted from plants and others are extracted from bacteria (Sumitani et al., 2000). Only insects may produce amylase inhibitors of the knottin-like, Kunitz-type, and thaumatin-like varieties (Pereira et al., 1999). They were given their name due to the great degree of amino acid sequence homology they share with the highly produced lectin proteins in these plants. The diverse cultivars of the legume *P. vulgaris* include the currently recognized AI isoforms AI1 and AI2 (Berre-Anton et al., 1997; Hoffman et al., 1985).

The function of PHA in body WL is still up for question, though. In fact, the use of raw bean extract combined with a diet containing PHA at levels less than 0.2 g/kg results in a decrease in body weight and body fat in obese Zucker rats (Pusztai et al., 1998). Without losing any body proteins or skeletal muscle, this group dropped fatter than the control group. A greater lipid dose in the meal combined with a higher PHA concentration (0.4 g/kg) was tolerated. Bean lectin has been proposed as a dietary supplement to combat obesity in a safe and effective dose range based on these findings (Bardocz et al., 1996).

As a result, the preparation of *P. vulgaris* extract with an action inhibition of amylase produced by PHA has come to light (Fantini et al., 2009).

Numerous natural substances that can be recovered in large enough amounts from natural sources have the potential to be beneficial to human health. We can list the proteins that block the mammalian α-amylase enzyme among these compounds. Numerous research carried out over the past 20–30 years suggests the potential value of these inhibitors, derived from *P. vulgaris* seeds, in developing methods to limit the absorption of complex carbohydrates. Numerous clinical investigations have produced good results, leading the main American and European regulatory agencies to approve the marketing of medications based on common beans.

Today, we can say that these medications are safe for human health, albeit they may cause brief adverse effects depending on dosage. This review effort may inspire additional research to more thoroughly explore these problems, which may have an impact on the clinical effectiveness of commercial medicines. The majority of the world's bean output takes place in poorer nations (almost 90%). The challenge for us in the next years will be to choose *P. vulgaris* cultivars with the best inhibitor/anti-nutritional factor ratio and whose cultivation can adhere to the requirements of improved environmental sustainability. There are thousands of *P. vulgaris* cultivars existing in the world (Izzo et al., 2016).

12.9.2 PLANT-DERIVED POLYPHENOLS

In the previous 26 years, consumers, food scientists, and nutritionists have paid more attention to natural products isolated from plant origins, such as polyphenols (PPs), because of their importance to human health (Rasouli et al., 2016; Tsao et al., 2010; Morton et al., 2000; Akbari et al., 2012).

Foods derived from plants, especially fruits, seeds, and vegetables, are rich sources of PPs, which are reactive and secondary metabolites (Rasouli et al., 2016).

Numerous polyphenols (Keservani & Sharma, 2014; Keservani et al., 2016a, b) with more than two phenolic hydroxyl groups act as natural antioxidants and are advantageous to human health. According to the literature, PPs can be divided into four major groups: (i) phenolic acids; (ii) flavonoids; (iii) tannins; and (iv) stilbenes. There are numerous findings indicating that PPs can control or adjust blood glucose levels following a meal (Croft et al., 2016).

In *ex vivo* experiments, some of these substances can directly increase the release of insulin from pancreatic cells, but this effect may be insignificant due to their limited systemic bioavailability. For the treatment of diverse forms of diabetes mellitus, there are numerous therapeutic approaches (DM). A variety of metabolic disorders, including diabetes mellitus (DM), are characterized by blood glucose levels that are more than 200 mg/dL at any moment during the day or during a fast plasma glucose concentration that is higher than 126 mg/dL (Gundala et al., 201; Viswanath et al., 2017).

One of the therapeutic approaches is to lower postprandial glucose levels by preventing oligo- and disaccharide breakdown. This could be accomplished by inhibiting the vital enzymes for digesting starch and glycogen, α-amylase (A) and α-glucosidase (G), which are responsible for slowing the absorption of glucose (Sales et al., 2012).

These enzymes break down oligosaccharides and disaccharides into monosaccharides so that they are suitable for absorption. They are found in the small intestinal brush border (Rutten et al., 2005; Jhong et al., 2015). The digestion of sugar and carbohydrates is delayed by α-A and α-G enzyme inhibitors, such as PPs, which lowers the rate of glucose absorption and aids in weight loss and hyperglycemia (Tadera et al., 2006; Nyambe-Silavwe et al., 2015).

12.10 CONCLUSION

α-Amylase, a pancreatic or salivary enzyme, is crucial for the early conversion of complex carbohydrates into simple molecules. The breakdown of complex carbohydrates is significantly reduced when α-amylase activity is modulated, and this reduction is more pronounced the stronger the modulation. The majority of investigations have concentrated on phenolic chemicals that are anti-amylase. Amylase inhibitor's presence in the majority of *P. vulgaris* accessions, which are widely cultivated worldwide. The α-amylase inhibitor has been confirmed to be safe in more recent investigations. Further study is necessary for a number of the inhibitor's properties. These include more extensive clinical studies conducted over longer periods of time to confirm the inhibitor's efficacy and safety, the ingredient functionality of the inhibitor in different food systems, and further clarification of molecular-level binding interactions to enable the development of synthetic blockers based on the inhibitor. Numerous natural substances that can be recovered in large enough amounts from natural sources have the potential to be beneficial to human health. We could include the proteins that inhibit the mammalian-amylase enzyme in these compounds. Several studies conducted in the last

20–30 years indicate the promising potential of these inhibitors, extracted from *P. vulgaris* seeds, in creating approaches to reduce the absorption of complex carbohydrates. Several clinical studies have yielded positive results, prompting the main American and European regulatory authorities to approve the marketing of medications based on common beans. These preparations are currently considered safe for human health.

By inhibiting alpha-amylase, alpha-amylase inhibitors have the potential to support weight loss and reduce the fat mass induced by carbohydrates. This chapter provides detailed information for a thorough analysis and various uses of alpha-amylase inhibitors.

KEYWORDS

- **carbohydrate**
- **obesity**
- **pancreatic amylase**
- **pseudo-tetrasacharides**
- **α-amylase**
- **α-amylase inhibitors**

REFERENCES

Akbari, M., Rasouli, H., & Bahdor, T. (2012). Physiological and pharmaceutical effect of fenugreek: A review. *IOSR Journal of Pharmacy (IOSRPHR), 2*(4), 49–53.

Alkazaz, M., Desseaux, V., Marchis-Mouren, G., Payan, F., Forest, E., & Santimone, M. (1996). The Mechanism of Porcine Pancreatic α-Amylase: Kinetic Evidence for Two Additional Carbohydrate-Binding Sites. *European Journal of Biochemistry, 241*(3), 787–796. https://doi.org/10.1111/j.1432-1033.1996.00787.x.

Alpers, D. H. (1994). Digestion and absorption of carbohydrates and proteins. In L. R. Johnson (Ed.), *Physiology of the Gastrointestinal Tract* (3rd ed., pp. 1723–1756). Raven Press.

Altabella, T., & Chrispeels, M. J. (1990). Tobacco plants transformed with the bean α AI gene express an inhibitor of insect α-amylase in their seeds. *Plant Physiology, 93*(2), 805–810. https://doi.org/10.1104/pp.93.2.805.

Ankomah, A., Byaruhanga, J., Woolley, E., Boamah, S., & Akombi-Inyang, B. (2022). Double burden of malnutrition among migrants and refugees in developed countries: A mixed-methods systematic review. *PloS One, 17*(8), e0273382. https://doi.org/10.1371/journal.pone.0273382.

Asanuma-Date, K., Hirano, Y., Le, N., Sano, K., Kawasaki, N., Hashii, N., & Ogawa, H. (2012). Functional regulation of sugar assimilation by N-glycan-specific interaction of pancreatic α-amylase with glycoproteins of duodenal brush border membrane. *Journal of Biological Chemistry, 287*(27), 23104–23118. https://doi.org/10.1074/jbc.M112.343434.

Ashok, C., Palanimuthu, D., Selvadurai, S. D., & Varshini, R. (2021). An apodictic review on recent approaches in enzyme technology. *Biointerface Research in Applied Chemistry, 12*, 3446–3471. https://doi.org/10.33263/BRIAC121.34463471.

Azad, M. A. K., Bae, J. H., Kim, J. S., Lim, J. K., Song, K. S., Shin, B. S., & Kim, H. R. (2009). Isolation and characterization of a novel thermostable α-amylase from Korean pine seeds. *New Biotechnology, 26*(3–4), 143–149. https://doi.org/10.1016/j.nbt.2009.08.002.

Barber, D., Sanchez-Monge, R., Méndez, E., Lázaro, A., Garcia-Olmedo, F., & Salcedo, G. (1986). New α-amylase and trypsin inhibitors among the CM-proteins of barley (*Hordeum vulgare*). *Biochimica et Biophysica Acta (BBA) – Protein Structure and Molecular Enzymology, 869*(1), 115–118. https://doi.org/10.1016/0167-4838(86)90116-3.

Barbosa, A. E., Albuquerque, É. V., Silva, M., Souza, D. S., Oliveira-Neto, O. B., Valencia, A., & Grossi-de-Sa, M. F. (2010). α-Amylase inhibitor-1 gene from *Phaseolus vulgaris* expressed in *Coffea arabica* plants inhibits α-amylases from the coffee berry borer pest. *BMC Biotechnology, 10*, 1–8. https://doi.org/10.1186/1472-6750-10-1.

Bardocz, S., Grant, G., Pusztai, A., Franklin, M. F., & Carvalho, A. D. F. (1996). The effect of phytohaemagglutinin at different dietary concentrations on the growth, body composition and plasma insulin of the rat. *British Journal of Nutrition, 76*(4), 613–626. https://doi.org/10.1079/BJN19960066.

Barrett, M. L., & Udani, J. K. (2011). A proprietary alpha-amylase inhibitor from white bean (*Phaseolus vulgaris*): A review of clinical studies on weight loss and glycemic control. *Nutrition Journal, 10*, 24. https://doi.org/10.1186/1475-2891-10-24.

Bhide, A. J., Channale, S. M., Yadav, Y., Bhattacharjee, K., Pawar, P. K., Maheshwari, V. L., & Giri, A. P. (2017). Genomic and functional characterization of coleopteran insect-specific α-amylase inhibitor gene from *Amaranthus* species. *Plant Molecular Biology, 94*(3), 319–332. https://doi.org/10.1007/s11103-017-0616-7.

Blanco-Labra, A., & Iturbe-Chinas, F. A. (1981). Purification and characterization of an α-amylase inhibitor from maize (*Zea mays*). *Journal of Food Biochemistry, 5*(1), 1–17. https://doi.org/10.1111/j.1745-4514.1981.tb00314.x.

Bloch, C., & Richardson, M. (1991). A new family of small (5 kDa) protein inhibitors of insect α-amylases from seeds of sorghum (*Sorghum bicolor* (L.) Moench) have sequence homologies with wheat γ-purothionins. *FEBS Letters, 279*(1), 101–104. https://doi.org/10.1016/0014-5793(91)80188-4.

Bompard-Gilles, C., Rousseau, P., Rougé, P., & Payan, F. (1996). Substrate mimicry in the active center of a mammalian α-amylase: Structural analysis of an enzyme–inhibitor complex. *Structure, 4*(12), 1441–1452. https://doi.org/10.1016/S0969-2126(96)00152-7.

Brain-Isasi, S., Álvarez-Lueje, A., & Higgins, T. J. V. (2017). Heterologous expression of an α-amylase inhibitor from common bean (*Phaseolus vulgaris*) in *Kluyveromyces lactis* and *Saccharomyces cerevisiae*. *Microbial Cell Factories, 16*(1), 1–13. https://doi.org/10.1186/s12934-017-0808-0.

Brayer, G. D., Luo, Y., & Withers, S. G. (1995). The structure of human pancreatic α-amylase at 1.8 Å resolution and comparisons with related enzymes. *Protein Science, 4*(9), 1730–1742. https://doi.org/10.1002/pro.5560040902.

Bruinenberg, P. M., Hulst, A. C., Faber, A., & Voogd, R. H. (1996). A process for surface sizing or coating of paper. *European Patent Application, 690, A1*.
Buisson, G., Duee, E., Haser, R., & Payan, F. (1987). Three-dimensional structure of porcine pancreatic alpha-amylase at 2.9 A resolution. Role of calcium in structure and activity. The EMBO Journal, 6(13), 3909–3916. https://doi.org/10.1002/j.1460-2075.1987.tb02757.x.
Burhan, A., Nisa, U., Gökhan, C., Ömer, C., Ashabil, A., & Osman, G. (2003). Enzymatic properties of a novel thermostable, thermophilic, alkaline and chelator resistant amylase from an alkaliphilic Bacillus sp. isolate ANT-6. Process Biochemistry, 38(10), 1397–1403. https://doi.org/10.1016/S0032-9592(02)00207-5.
Campos, F. A. P., & Richardson, M. (1983). The complete amino acid sequence of the bifunctional alpha-amylase/trypsin inhibitor from seeds of ragi (Indian finger millet, Eleusine coracana Gaertn.). Febs Letters, 152(2), 300–304. https://doi.org/10.1016/0014-5793(83)80193-3.
Carugo, O., Lu, S., Luo, J., Gu, X., Liang, S., Strobl, S., & Pongor, S. (2001). Structural analysis of free and enzyme-bound amaranth alpha-amylase inhibitor: Classification within the knottin fold superfamily and analysis of its functional flexibility. Protein Engineering, 14(9), 639–646. https://doi.org/10.1093/protein/14.9.639.
Chagolla-Lopez, A., Blanco-Labra, A., Patthy, A., Sánchez, R., & Pongor, S. (1994). A novel alpha-amylase inhibitor from amaranth (Amaranthus hypocondriacus) seeds. Journal of Biological Chemistry, 269(38), 23675–23680. https://doi.org/10.1016/S0021-9258(18)39501-2.
Choudhury, A. K. R. (2020). Introduction to enzymes. In G. E. Rutten & C. Van Weel (Eds.), Sustainable Technologies for Fashion and Textiles (pp. 75–90). Woodhead Publishing.
Cripwell, R. A., van Zyl, W. H., & Viljoen-Bloom, M. (2021). Fungal biotechnology: Fungal amylases and their applications. In: Encyclopedia of Mycology, 326–336.
Croft, K. D. (2016). Dietary polyphenols: Antioxidants or not? Archives of Biochemistry and Biophysics, 595, 120–124. https://doi.org/10.1016/j.abb.2016.02.015.
D'Amico, S., Gerday, C., & Feller, G. (2000). Structural similarities and evolutionary relationships in chloride-dependent alpha-amylases. Gene, 253(1), 95–105. https://doi.org/10.1016/S0378-1119(00)00238-1.
Da Lage, J. L., Danchin, E. G., & Casane, D. (2007). Where do animal alpha-amylases come from? An interkingdom trip. FEBS Letters, 581(21), 3927–3935. https://doi.org/10.1016/j.febslet.2007.07.017.
Date, K., Satoh, A., Iida, K., & Ogawa, H. (2015). Pancreatic alpha-amylase controls glucose assimilation by duodenal retrieval through N-glycan-specific binding, endocytosis, and degradation. Journal of Biological Chemistry, 290(28), 17439–17450. https://doi.org/10.1074/jbc.M114.628246.
Dauter, Z., Dauter, M., Brzozowski, A. M., Christensen, S., Borchert, T. V., Beier, L., & Davies, G. J. (1999). X-ray structure of Novamyl, the five-domain "maltogenic" alpha-amylase from Bacillus stearothermophilus: Maltose and acarbose complexes at 1.7 Å resolution. Biochemistry, 38(26), 8385–8392. https://doi.org/10.1021/bi990371w.
Desmyter, A., Spinelli, S., Payan, F., Lauwereys, M., Wyns, L., Muyldermans, S., & Cambillau, C. (2002). Three camelid VHH domains in complex with porcine pancreatic alpha-amylase: Inhibition and versatility of binding topology. Journal of Biological Chemistry, 277(26), 23645–23650. https://doi.org/10.1074/jbc.M200876200.
Dhital, S., Warren, F. J., Butterworth, P. J., Ellis, P. R., & Gidley, M. J. (2017). Mechanisms of starch digestion by alpha-amylase—Structural basis for kinetic properties. Critical Reviews

in Food Science and Nutrition, 57(5), 875–892. https://doi.org/10.1080/10408398.2014.963667.

E. H. Lisdonk, G. E. Rutten & C. Van Weel, Rev. (2005). Alphaglucosidase inhibitors for type 2 diabetes mellitus. Cochrane Database Syst, 1(2), 1–184.

Fantini, N., Cabras, C., Lobina, C., Colombo, G., Gessa, G. L., Riva, A., & Carai, M. A. (2009). Reducing effect of a Phaseolus vulgaris dry extract on food intake, body weight, and glycemia in rats. Journal of Agricultural and Food Chemistry, 57(19), 9316–9323. https://doi.org/10.1021/jf901807y.

Ferey-Roux, G., Perrier, J., Forest, E., Marchis-Mouren, G., Puigserver, A., & Santimone, M. (1998). The human pancreatic alpha-amylase isoforms: Isolation, structural studies and kinetics of inhibition by acarbose. Biochimica et Biophysica Acta (BBA) – Protein Structure and Molecular Enzymology, 1388(1), 10–20. https://doi.org/10.1016/S0167-4838(97)00176-8.

Franco, O. L., Rigden, D. J., Melo, F. R., & Grossi-de-Sá, M. F. (2002). Plant alpha-amylase inhibitors and their interaction with insect alpha-amylases: Structure, function and potential for crop protection. European Journal of Biochemistry, 269(2), 397–412. https://doi.org/10.1046/j.0014-2956.2001.02615.x.

Franco, O. L., Rigden, D. J., Melo, F. R., Bloch Jr, C., Silva, C. P., & Grossi de Sá, M. F. (2000). Activity of wheat alpha-amylase inhibitors towards bruchid alpha-amylases and structural explanation of observed specificities. European Journal of Biochemistry, 267(8), 2166–2173. https://doi.org/10.1046/j.1432-1327.2000.01246.x.

Fukagawa, N. K., Anderson, J. W., Hageman, G., Young, V. R., & Minaker, K. L. (1990). High-carbohydrate, high-fiber diets increase peripheral insulin sensitivity in healthy young and old adults. The American Journal of Clinical Nutrition, 52(3), 524–528. https://doi.org/10.1093/ajcn/52.3.524.

García Olmedo, F., Salcedo Duran, G., Sánchez-Monge Laguna de Rins, R., Gómez, L., Royo, J., & Carbonero Zalduegui, P. (1987). Plant Proteinaceous Inhibitors of Proteinases and Alpha-Amylases, 4, 275–334.

García-Maroto, F., Carbonero, P., & García-Olmedo, F. (1991). Site-directed mutagenesis and expression in Escherichia coli of WMAI-1, a wheat monomeric inhibitor of insect alpha-amylase. Plant Molecular Biology, 17(5), 1005–1011. https://doi.org/10.1007/BF00037020.

Gilles, C., Astier, J. P., Marchis-Mouren, G., Cambillau, C., & Payan, F. (1996). Crystal structure of pig pancreatic alpha-amylase isoenzyme II, in complex with the carbohydrate inhibitor acarbose. European Journal of Biochemistry, 238(2), 561–569. https://doi.org/10.1111/j.1432-1033.1996.0561z.x.

Grabitske, H. A., & Slavin, J. L. (2009). Gastrointestinal effects of low-digestible carbohydrates. Critical Reviews in Food Science and Nutrition, 49(4), 327–360. https://doi.org/10.1080/10408390802067126.

Gumucio, D. L., Wiebauer, K., Caldwell, R. M., Samuelson, L. C., & Meisler, M. H. (1988). Concerted evolution of human amylase genes. Molecular and Cellular Biology, 8(3), 1197–1205. https://doi.org/10.1128/MCB.8.3.1197.

Gundala, N. K., Naidu, V. G., & Das, U. N. (2017). Arachidonic acid and lipoxin A4 attenuate alloxan-induced cytotoxicity to RIN5F cells in vitro and type 1 diabetes mellitus in vivo. BioFactors, 43(2), 251–271. https://doi.org/10.1002/biof.1324.

Gupta, R., Gigras, P., Mohapatra, H., Goswami, V. K., & Chauhan, B. (2003). Microbial alpha-amylases: A biotechnological perspective. Process Biochemistry, 38(11), 1599–1616. https://doi.org/10.1016/S0032-9592(03)00053-0.

Hernández, M. S., Rodríguez, M. R., Guerra, N. P., & Rosés, R. P. (2006). Amylase production by Aspergillus niger in submerged cultivation on two wastes from food industries. Journal of Food Engineering, 73(1), 93–100. https://doi.org/10.1016/j.jfoodeng.2005.01.009.

Hiele, M., Ghoos, Y., Rutgeerts, P., & Vantrappen, G. (1989). Starch digestion in normal subjects and patients with pancreatic disease, using a 13CO2 breath test. Gastroenterology, 96(2), 503–509. https://doi.org/10.1016/0016-5085(89)90534-2.

Hmidet, N., Ali, N. E. H., Haddar, A., Kanoun, S., Alya, S. K., & Nasri, M. (2009). Alkaline proteases and thermostable alpha-amylase co-produced by Bacillus licheniformis NH1: Characterization and potential application as detergent additive. Biochemical Engineering Journal, 47(1–3), 71–79. https://doi.org/10.1016/j.bej.2009.07.004.

Ho, M. F., & Whitaker, J. R. (1993). Purification and partial characterization of white kidney bean (Phaseolus vulgaris) beta-amylase inhibitors from two experimental cultivars. Journal of Food Biochemistry, 17(1), 15–33. https://doi.org/10.1111/j.1745-4514.1993.tb00441.x.

Ho, M. F., Yin, X., Lajolo, F., & Whitaker, J. R. (1994). Naturally occurring alpha-amylase inhibitors: Structure/function relationships. In J. R. Whitaker & F. Shahidi (Eds.), Protein Structure-Function Relationships in Foods (pp. 89–119). Springer.

Hoffman, L. M., Ma, Y., & Barker, R. F. (1982). Molecular cloning of Phaseolus vulgaris lectin mRNA and use of cDNA as a probe to estimate lectin transcript levels in various tissues. Nucleic Acids Research, 10(23), 7819–7828. https://doi.org/10.1093/nar/10.23.7819.

Horii, S., Fukase, H., Matsuo, T., Kameda, Y., Asano, N., & Matsui, K. (1986). Synthesis and alpha-D-glucosidase inhibitory activity of N-substituted valiolamine derivatives as potential oral antidiabetic agents. Journal of Medicinal Chemistry, 29(6), 1038–1046. https://doi.org/10.1021/jm00156a020.

Ishimoto, M., Suzuki, K., Iwanaga, M., Kikuchi, F., & Kitamura, K. (1995). Variation of seed alpha-amylase inhibitors in the common bean. Theoretical and Applied Genetics, 90(3), 425–429. https://doi.org/10.1007/BF00222190.

Izzo, A. A., Hoon-Kim, S., Radhakrishnan, R., & Williamson, E. M. (2016). A critical approach to evaluating clinical efficacy, adverse events and drug interactions of herbal remedies. Phytotherapy Research, 30(5), 691–700. https://doi.org/10.1002/ptr.5578.

Jhong, C. H., Riyaphan, J., Lin, S. H., Chia, Y. C., & Weng, C. F. (2015). Screening alpha-glucosidase and alpha-amylase inhibitors from natural compounds by molecular docking in silico. BioFactors, 41(4), 242–251. https://doi.org/10.1002/biof.1218.

Kamitori, S., Kondo, S., Okuyama, K., Yokota, T., Shimura, Y., Tonozuka, T., & Sakano, Y. (1999). Crystal structure of Thermoactinomyces vulgaris R-47 alpha-amylase II (TVAII) hydrolyzing cyclodextrins and pullulan at 2.6 Å resolution. Journal of Molecular Biology, 287(5), 907–921. https://doi.org/10.1006/jmbi.1999.2643.

Keservani, R. K., Sharma, A. K., & Kesharwani, R. K. (2014). Flavonoids: Emerging trends and potential health benefits. Journal of Chinese Pharmaceutical Sciences, 23(12), 815.

Keservani, R. K., Sharma, A. K., & Kesharwani, R. K. (2016a). Nutraceutical and Functional Foods for Cardiovascular Health. In R. K. Keservani & A. K. Sharma (Eds.), Food Process Engineering (pp. 291–312). Apple Academic Press, CRC Press.

Keservani, R. K., Sharma, A. K., & Kesharwani, R. K. (2016b). Medicinal effect of nutraceutical fruits for the cognition and brain health. Scientifica, 2016, Article ID 3109254, 10 pages. https://doi.org/10.1155/2016/3109254.

Kim, S., & Dale, B. E. (2004). Global potential bioethanol production from wasted crops and crop residues. Biomass and Bioenergy, 26(4), 361–375. https://doi.org/10.1016/j.biombioe.2003.08.002.

Kim, T. U., Gu, B. G., Jeong, J. Y., Byun, S. M., & Shin, Y. C. (1995). Purification and characterization of a maltotetraose-forming alkaline (alpha)-amylase from an alkalophilic Bacillus strain, GM8901. Applied and Environmental Microbiology, 61(8), 3105–3112. https://doi.org/10.1128/AEM.61.8.3105-3112.1995.

Kumar Singla, R., Singh, R., & Kumar Dubey, A. (2016). Important aspects of post-prandial antidiabetic drug, acarbose. Current Topics in Medicinal Chemistry, 16(23), 2625–2633. https://doi.org/10.2174/1568026616666160113145133.

Kumar, D., & Singh, V. (2016). Dry-grind processing using amylase corn and superior yeast to reduce the exogenous enzyme requirements in bioethanol production. Biotechnology for Biofuels, 9(1), 1–12. https://doi.org/10.1186/s13068-015-0423-8.

Kumar, J., Pandey, A., & Singh, S. P. (2020). An introduction to enzyme structure dynamics and enzyme catalysis. In A. Pandey, S. Negi, & C. R. Soccol (Eds.), Biomass, Biofuels, Biochemicals (pp. 3–10). Elsevier.

Le Berre-Anton, V., Bompard-Gilles, C., Payan, F., & Rougé, P. (1997). Characterization and functional properties of the α-amylase inhibitor (α-AI) from kidney bean (Phaseolus vulgaris) seeds. Biochimica et Biophysica Acta (BBA) – Protein Structure and Molecular Enzymology, 1343(1), 31–40. https://doi.org/10.1016/S0167-4838(96)00234-6.

Lehtiö, J., Teeri, T. T., & Nygren, P. Å. (2000). Alpha-amylase inhibitors selected from a combinatorial library of a cellulose binding domain scaffold. Proteins: Structure, Function, and Bioinformatics, 41(3), 316–322. https://doi.org/10.1002/1097-0134(20001115)41:3<316: AID-PROT90>3.0.CO;2-M.

Lu, S., Deng, P., Liu, X., Luo, J., Han, R., Gu, X., & Pongor, S. (1999). Solution structure of the major α-amylase inhibitor of the crop plant amaranth. Journal of Biological Chemistry, 274(29), 20473–20478. https://doi.org/10.1074/jbc.274.29.20473.

Mamo, G., & Gessesse, A. (1999). Effect of cultivation conditions on growth and α-amylase production by a thermophilic Bacillus sp. Letters in Applied Microbiology, 29(1), 61–65. https://doi.org/10.1046/j.1472-765x.1999.00586.x.

Mandel, A. L., Peyrot des Gachons, C., Plank, K. L., Alarcon, S., & Breslin, P. A. (2010). Individual differences in AMY1 gene copy number, salivary α-amylase levels, and the perception of oral starch. PloS One, 5(10), e13352. https://doi.org/10.1371/journal.pone.0013352.

Marshall, J. J., & Lauda, C. M. (1975). Purification and properties of phaseolamin, an inhibitor of alpha-amylase, from the kidney bean, Phaseolus vulgaris. Journal of Biological Chemistry, 250(20), 8030–8037.

Matama, T., & Cavaco-Paulo, A. (2010). Enzymatic modification of polyacrylonitrile and cellulose acetate fibers for textile and other applications. In G. K. E. Scobbie & C. M. Carr (Eds.), Advances in Textile Biotechnology (pp. 98–131). Woodhead Publishing.

Matsushita, H., Takenaka, M., & Ogawa, H. (2002). Porcine pancreatic α-amylase shows binding activity toward N-linked oligosaccharides of glycoproteins. Journal of Biological Chemistry, 277(7), 4680–4686. https://doi.org/10.1074/jbc.M110358200.

Maurus, R., Begum, A., Kuo, H. H., Racaza, A., Numao, S., Andersen, C., & Brayer, G. D. (2005). Structural and mechanistic studies of chloride induced activation of human pancreatic α-amylase. Protein Science, 14(3), 743–755. https://doi.org/10.1110/ps.041198105.

Meigs, J. B., Wilson, P. W., Fox, C. S., Vasan, R. S., Nathan, D. M., Sullivan, L. M., & D'Agostino, R. B. (2006). Body mass index, metabolic syndrome, and risk of type 2 diabetes or cardiovascular disease. The Journal of Clinical Endocrinology & Metabolism, 91(8), 2906–2912. https://doi.org/10.1210/jc.2005-2846.

Meisler, M. H., & Ting, C. N. (1993). The remarkable evolutionary history of the human amylase genes. Critical Reviews in Oral Biology & Medicine, 4(3), 503–509. https://doi.org/10.1177/10454411930040031101.

Mitidieri, S., Martinelli, A. H. S., Schrank, A., & Vainstein, M. H. (2006). Enzymatic detergent formulation containing amylase from Aspergillus niger: A comparative study with commercial detergent formulations. Bioresource Technology, 97(10), 1217–1224. https://doi.org/10.1016/j.biortech.2005.04.020.

Mohammad, S., Aziz, R., Al Mahri, S., Malik, S. S., Haji, E., Khan, A. H., & Bouchama, A. (2021). Obesity and COVID-19: What makes obese host so vulnerable? Immunity & Ageing, 18(1), 1–10. https://doi.org/10.1186/s12979-020-00205-1.

Mojica, L., & de Mejía, E. G. (2015). Characterization and comparison of protein and peptide profiles and their biological activities of improved common bean cultivars (Phaseolus vulgaris L.) from Mexico and Brazil. Plant Foods for Human Nutrition, 70(2), 105–112. https://doi.org/10.1007/s11130-015-0487-y.

Mojica, L., de Mejia, E. G., Granados-Silvestre, M. Á., & Menjivar, M. (2017). Evaluation of the hypoglycemic potential of a black bean hydrolyzed protein isolate and its pure peptides using in silico, in vitro and in vivo approaches. Journal of Functional Foods, 31, 274–286. https://doi.org/10.1016/j.jff.2017.01.002.

Morton, L. W., Caccetta, R. A. A., Puddey, I. B., & Croft, K. D. (2000). Chemistry and biological effects of dietary phenolic compounds: Relevance to cardiovascular disease. Clinical and Experimental Pharmacology and Physiology, 27(3), 152–159. https://doi.org/10.1046/j.1440-1681.2000.03218.x.

Mundy, J., Hejgaard, J., & Svendsen, I. (1984). Characterization of a bifunctional wheat inhibitor of endogenous α-amylase and subtilisin. FEBS Letters, 167(2), 210–214. https://doi.org/10.1016/0014-5793(84)80802-8.

Murao, S., Goto, A., Matsui, Y., & Ohyama, K. (1980). New proteinous inhibitor (Haim) of animal α-amylase from Streptomyces griseosporeus YM-25. Agricultural and Biological Chemistry, 44(7), 1679–1681. https://doi.org/10.1080/00021369.1980.10862795.

Murao, S., Oouchi, N., Goto, A., & ARAI, M. (1983). New proteinaceous α-amylase inhibitor (Paim) from Streptomyces corchorusii. Agricultural and Biological Chemistry, 47(2), 453–454. https://doi.org/10.1080/00021369.1983.10866430.

Nakamura, Y., Ogawa, M., Nishide, T., Emi, M., Kosaki, G., Himeno, S., & Matsubara, K. (1984). Sequences of cDNAs for human salivary and pancreatic α-amylases. *Gene, 28*(2), 263–270. https://doi.org/10.1016/0378-1119(84)90158-4.

Nguyen, Q. D., Rezessy-Szabó, J. M., Claeyssens, M., Stals, I., & Hoschke, Á. (2002). Purification and characterization of amylolytic enzymes from thermophilic fungus *Thermomyces lanuginosus* strain ATCC 34626. *Enzyme and Microbial Technology, 31*(3), 345–352. https://doi.org/10.1016/S0141-0229(02)00138-5.

Nyambe-Silavwe, H., Villa-Rodriguez, J. A., Ifie, I., Holmes, M., Aydin, E., Jensen, J. M., & Williamson, G. (2015). Inhibition of human α-amylase by dietary polyphenols. *Journal of Functional Foods, 19*, 723–732. https://doi.org/10.1016/j.jff.2015.10.024.

Obiro, W. C., Zhang, T., & Jiang, B. (2008). The nutraceutical role of the *Phaseolus vulgaris* α-amylase inhibitor. *British Journal of Nutrition, 100*(1), 1–12. https://doi.org/10.1017/S0007114507894437.

Ohtsubo, K. I., & Richardson, M. (1992). The amino acid sequence of a 20 kDa bifunctional subtilisin/α-amylase inhibitor from brain of rice (*Oryza saliva L.*) seeds. *FEBS Letters, 309*(1), 68–72. https://doi.org/10.1016/0014-5793(92)80757-9.

Olafimihan, C. A., & Akinyanju, J. A. (1999). Thermophilic amylase producers from the soil. *Nig. J. Pure Appl. Sci., 14*, 816–822.

Oliveira, A. N. D., Oliveira, L. A. D., Andrade, J. S., & Chagas Júnior, A. F. (2007). Rhizobia amylase production using various starchy substances as carbon substrates. *Brazilian Journal of Microbiology, 38*, 208–216. https://doi.org/10.1590/S1517-83822007000200007.

Pandey, A., Nigam, P., Soccol, C. R., Soccol, V. T., Singh, D., & Mohan, R. (2000). Advances in microbial amylases. *Biotechnology and Applied Biochemistry, 31*(2), 135–152. https://doi.org/10.1042/ba19990073.

Pasero, L., Mazzéi-Pierron, Y., Abadie, B., Chicheportiche, Y., & Marchis-Mouren, G. (1986). Complete amino acid sequence and location of the five disulfide bridges in porcine pancreatic α-amylase. *Biochimica et Biophysica Acta (BBA) – Protein Structure and Molecular Enzymology, 869*(2), 147–157. https://doi.org/10.1016/0167-4838(86)90040-5.

Peddio, S., Padiglia, A., Cannea, F. B., Crnjar, R., Zam, W., Sharifi-Rad, J., & Zucca, P. (2022). Common bean (*Phaseolus vulgaris* L.) α-amylase inhibitors as safe nutraceutical strategy against diabetes and obesity: An update review. *Phytotherapy Research*, 36, 2803–2823. Advance online publication. https://doi.org/10.1002/ptr.7328.

Pedersen, H., & Nielsen, J. (2000). The influence of nitrogen sources on the α-amylase productivity of *Aspergillus oryzae* in continuous cultures. *Applied Microbiology and Biotechnology, 53*(3), 278–281. https://doi.org/10.1007/s002530051624.

Pereira, P. J. B., Lozanov, V., Patthy, A., Huber, R., Bode, W., Pongor, S., & Strobl, S. (1999). Specific inhibition of insect α-amylases: Yellow meal worm α-amylase in complex with the Amaranth α-amylase inhibitor at 2.0 Å resolution. *Structure, 7*(9), 1079–1088. https://doi.org/10.1016/S0969-2126(99)80139-2.

Perry, G. H., Dominy, N. J., Claw, K. G., Lee, A. S., Fiegler, H., Redon, R., & Stone, A. C. (2007). Diet and the evolution of human amylase gene copy number variation. *Nature Genetics, 39*(10), 1256–1260. https://doi.org/10.1038/ng2123.

Petrovic, C. (2023). Enzyme dynamics and enzyme evolution. *Journal of the Royal Society Interface, 20*(15), 20230612. https://doi.org/10.1098/rsif.2023.0612.

Pradeep, P. M., & Sreerama, Y. N. (2015). Impact of processing on the phenolic profiles of small millets: Evaluation of their antioxidant and enzyme inhibitory properties associated with hyperglycemia. *Food Chemistry, 169*, 455–463. https://doi.org/10.1016/j.foodchem.2014.08.052.

Pusztai, A., Grant, G., Buchan, W. C., Bardocz, S., De Carvalho, A. F. F. U., & Ewen, S. W. B. (1998). Lipid accumulation in obese Zucker rats is reduced by inclusion of raw kidney bean (*Phaseolus vulgaris*) in the diet. *British Journal of Nutrition, 79*(2), 213–221. https://doi.org/10.1079/BJN19980029.

Rasouli, H., Farzaei, M. H., Mansouri, K., Mohammadzadeh, S., & Khodarahmi, R. (2016). Plant cell cancer: May natural phenolic compounds prevent onset and development of plant cell malignancy? A literature review. *Molecules, 21*(9), 1104. https://doi.org/10.3390/molecules21091104.

Raud, B., Gay, C., Guiguet-Auclair, C., Bonnin, A., Gerbaud, L., Pereira, B., & Coudeyre, E. (2020). Level of obesity is directly associated with the clinical and functional consequences of knee osteoarthritis. *Scientific Reports, 10*(1), 1–7. https://doi.org/10.1038/s41598-020-71958-1.

Reddy, R. M., Reddy, P. G., & Seenayya, G. (1999). Enhanced production of thermostable β-amylase and pullulanase in the presence of surfactants by *Clostridium thermosulfurogenes* SV2. *Process Biochemistry, 34*(1), 87–92. https://doi.org/10.1016/S0032-9592(98)00095-5.

Rigoldi, F., Donini, S., Redaelli, A., Parisini, E., & Gautieri, A. (2018). Review: Engineering of thermostable enzymes for industrial applications. *APL Bioengineering, 2*, 011501. https://doi.org/10.1063/1.4999055.

Robinson, P. K. (2015). Enzymes: Principles and biotechnological applications. *Essays in Biochemistry, 59*, 1. https://doi.org/10.1042/bse0590001.

Rosén, L. A., Östman, E. M., & Björck, I. M. (2011). Effects of cereal breakfasts on postprandial glucose, appetite regulation and voluntary energy intake at a subsequent standardized lunch; focusing on rye products. *Nutrition Journal, 10*(1), 1–11. https://doi.org/10.1186/1475-2891-10-7.

Saboury, A. A., & Karbassi, F. (2000). Thermodynamic studies on the interaction of calcium ions with alpha-amylase. *Thermochimica Acta, 362*(1–2), 121–129. https://doi.org/10.1016/S0040-6031(00)00585-0.

Sales, P. M., Souza, P. M., Simeoni, L. A., Magalhães, P. O., & Silveira, D. (2012). α-Amylase inhibitors: A review of raw material and isolated compounds from plant source. Journal of Pharmacy & Pharmaceutical Sciences, 15(1), 141–183. https://doi.org/10.18433/J3FC7P.

Santimone, M., Koukiekolo, R., Moreau, Y., Le Berre, V., Rougé, P., Marchis-Mouren, G., & Desseaux, V. (2004). Porcine pancreatic α-amylase inhibition by the kidney bean (Phaseolus vulgaris) inhibitor (α-AI1) and structural changes in the α-amylase inhibitor complex. Biochimica et Biophysica Acta (BBA) – Proteins and Proteomics, 1696(2), 181–190. https://doi.org/10.1016/j.bbapap.2003.11.026.

Santos, J. L., Saus, E., Smalley, S. V., Cataldo, L. R., Alberti, G., Parada, J., & & Estivill, X. (2012). Copy number polymorphism of the salivary amylase gene: Implications in human nutrition research. Lifestyle Genomics, 5(3), 117–131. https://doi.org/10.1159/000337133.

Sasi, A., Baghyaraj, R., Yogananth, N., Chanthuru, A., & Ravikumar, M. (2008). Production of α-amylase in submerged fermentation by using Bacillus sp. Research Journal of Biological Sciences, 1, 50–57.

Schibler, U., Pittet, A. C., Young, R. A., Hagenbüchle, O., Tosi, M., Gellman, S., & Wellauer, P. K. (1982). The mouse α-amylase multigene family: Sequence organization of members expressed in the pancreas, salivary gland and liver. Journal of Molecular Biology, 155(3), 247–266. https://doi.org/10.1016/0022-2836(82)90239-3.

Schimoler-O'Rourke, R., Richardson, M., & Selitrennikoff, C. P. (2001). Zeamatin inhibits trypsin and α-amylase activities. Applied and Environmental Microbiology, 67(5), 2365–2366. https://doi.org/10.1128/AEM.67.5.2365-2366.2001.

Schroeder, H. E., Gollasch, S., Moore, A., Tabe, L. M., Craig, S., Hardie, D. C., & Higgins, T. J. (1995). Bean α-amylase inhibitor confers resistance to the pea weevil (Bruchus pisorum) in transgenic peas (Pisum sativum L.). Plant Physiology, 107(4), 1233–1239. https://doi.org/10.1104/pp.107.4.1233.

Seigner, C., Prodanov, E., & Marchis-Mouren, G. (1987). The determination of subsite binding energies of porcine pancreatic α-amylase by comparing hydrolytic activity towards substrates. Biochimica et Biophysica Acta (BBA) – Protein Structure and Molecular Enzymology, 913(2), 200–209. https://doi.org/10.1016/0167-4838(87)90096-2.

Sharifi, M., Sohrabi, M. J., Hosseinali, S. H., Hasan, A., Kani, P. H., Talaei, A. J., & Falahati, M. (2020). Enzyme immobilization onto the nanomaterials: Application in enzyme stability and prodrug-activated cancer therapy. International Journal of Biological Macromolecules, 143, 665–676. https://doi.org/10.1016/j.ijbiomac.2019.12.235.

Shukla, K., & Srivastava, S. (2014). Evaluation of finger millet incorporated noodles for nutritive value and glycemic index. Journal of Food Science and Technology, 51(3), 527–534. https://doi.org/10.1007/s13197-011-0471-6.

Silva, C., Cavaco-Paulo, A., & Nierstrasz, V. A. (2010). Enzymatic hydrolysis and modification of core polymer fibres for textile and other applications. In A. Cavaco-Paulo & G. Gubitz (Eds.), Advances in Textile Biotechnology (pp. 77–97). Woodhead Publishing.

Sivaramakrishnan, S., Gangadharan, D., Nampoothiri, K. M., Soccol, C. R., & Pandey, A. (2006). α-Amylases from microbial sources – An overview on recent developments. Food Technology and Biotechnology, 44(2), 173–184.

Stiefel, D. J., & Keller, P. J. (1973). Preparation and some properties of human pancreatic amylase including a comparison with human parotid amylase. Biochimica et Biophysica Acta (BBA) – Enzymology, 302(2), 345–361. https://doi.org/10.1016/0005-2744(73)90183-8.

Suetsugu, N., Koyama, S., & Kuge, T. (1974). Kinetic studies on the hydrolyses of α-, β-, and γ-cyclodextrins by Taka-amylase A. The Journal of Biochemistry, 76(1), 57–63. https://doi.org/10.1093/oxfordjournals.jbchem.a130521.

Sugino, H. (2007). Comparative genomic analysis of the mouse and rat amylase multigene family. FEBS Letters, 581(3), 355–360. https://doi.org/10.1016/j.febslet.2007.01.030.

Sumitani, J. I., Tsujimoto, Y., Kawaguchi, T., & Arai, M. (2000). Cloning and secretive expression of the gene encoding the proteinaceous α-amylase inhibitor Paim from Streptomyces corchorusii. Journal of Bioscience and Bioengineering, 90(2), 214–216. https://doi.org/10.1016/S1389-1723(00)80191-7.

Svensson, B., Fukuda, K., Nielsen, P. K., & Bønsager, B. C. (2004). Proteinaceous α-amylase inhibitors. Biochimica et Biophysica Acta (BBA) – Proteins and Proteomics, 1696(2), 145–156. https://doi.org/10.1016/j.bbapap.2003.11.024.

Tadera, K., Minami, Y., Takamatsu, K., & Matsuoka, T. (2006). Inhibition of α-glucosidase and α-amylase by flavonoids. Journal of Nutritional Science and Vitaminology, 52(2), 149–153. https://doi.org/10.3177/jnsv.52.149.

Tangphatsornruang, S., Naconsie, M., Thammarongtham, C., & Narangajavana, J. (2005). Isolation and characterization of an α-amylase gene in cassava (Manihot esculenta). Plant Physiology and Biochemistry, 43(9), 821–827. https://doi.org/10.1016/j.plaphy.2005.07.009.

Taroeno-Hariadi, K. W., Hardianti, M. S., Sinorita, H., & Aryandono, T. (2021). Obesity, leptin, and deregulation of microRNA in lipid metabolisms: Their contribution to breast cancer prognosis. Diabetology & Metabolic Syndrome, 13(1), 1–10. https://doi.org/10.1186/s13098-020-00625-3.

Tosi, M., Bovey, R., Astolfi, S., Bodary, S., Meisler, M., & Wellauer, P. K. (1984). Multiple non-allelic genes encoding pancreatic alpha-amylase of mouse are expressed in a strain-specific fashion. The EMBO Journal, 3(12), 2809–2816. https://doi.org/10.1002/j.1460-2075.1984.tb02276.x.

Truscheit, E., Frommer, W., Junge, B., Müller, L., Schmidt, D. D., & Wingender, W. (1981). Chemistry and biochemistry of microbial α-glucosidase inhibitors. Angewandte Chemie International Edition in English, 20(9), 744–761. https://doi.org/10.1002/anie.198107441.

Tsao, R. (2010). Chemistry and biochemistry of dietary polyphenols. Nutrients, 2(12), 1231–1246. https://doi.org/10.3390/nu2121231.

Vasella, A., Davies, G. J., & Böhm, M. (2002). Glycosidase mechanisms. Current Opinion in Chemical Biology, 6(5), 619–629. https://doi.org/10.1016/S1367-5931(02)00369-0.

Vértesy, L., Oeding, V., Bender, R., Zepf, K., & Nesemann, G. (1984). Tendamistat (HOE 467), a tight-binding α-amylase inhibitor from Streptomyces tendae 4158: Isolation, biochemical properties. European Journal of Biochemistry, 141(3), 505–512. https://doi.org/10.1111/j.1432-1033.1984.tb08231.x.

Viswanath, B., Choi, C. S., Lee, K., & Kim, S. (2017). Recent trends in the development of diagnostic tools for diabetes mellitus using patient saliva. TrAC Trends in Analytical Chemistry, 89, 60–67. https://doi.org/10.1016/j.trac.2017.02.009.

Wang, S. L., Liang, Y. C., & Liang, T. W. (2011). Purification and characterization of a novel alkali-stable α-amylase from Chryseobacterium taeanense TKU001, and application in antioxidant and prebiotic. Process Biochemistry, 46(3), 745–750. https://doi.org/10.1016/j.procbio.2010.11.011.

Whitcomb, D. C., & Lowe, M. E. (2007). Human pancreatic digestive enzymes. Digestive Diseases and Sciences, 52(1), 1–17. https://doi.org/10.1007/s10620-006-9581-0.

Williams, J. A. (2019). Amylase. Pancreapedia: The Exocrine Pancreas Knowledge Base. Retrieved from: https://www.pancreapedia.org/reviews/amylase (accessed on 15 June 2024).

Wise, R. J., Karn, R. C., Larsen, S. H., Hodes, M. E., Gardell, S. J., & Rutter, W. J. (1984). A complementary DNA sequence that predicts a human pancreatic amylase primary structure consistent with the electrophoretic mobility of the common isozyme, Amy2 A. Molecular Biology & Medicine, 2(5), 307–322. https://doi.org/10.1002/j.1522-2586.1984.tb00709.x.

Wood, I. P., Cook, N. M., Wilson, D. R., Ryden, P., Robertson, J. A., & Waldron, K. W. (2016). Ethanol from a biorefinery waste stream: Saccharification of amylase, protease and xylanase treated wheat bran. Food Chemistry, 198, 125–131. https://doi.org/10.1016/j.foodchem.2015.11.003.

Yamagishi, S. I., Matsui, T., Ueda, S., Fukami, K., & Okuda, S. (2009). Clinical utility of acarbose, an α-glucosidase inhibitor in cardiometabolic disorders. Current Drug Metabolism, 10(2), 159–163. https://doi.org/10.2174/138920009787048382.

Yokouchi, H., Horii, A., Emi, M., Tomita, N., Doi, S., Ogawa, M., & Matsubara, K. (1990). Cloning and characterization of a third type of human α-amylase gene, AMY2B. Gene, 90(2), 281–286. https://doi.org/10.1016/0378-1119(90)90411-5.

Zhang, X., Caner, S., Kwan, E., Li, C., Brayer, G. D., & Withers, S. G. (2016). Evaluation of the significance of starch surface binding sites on human pancreatic α-amylase. Biochemistry, 55(43), 6000–6009. https://doi.org/10.1021/acs.biochem.6b00888.

CHAPTER 13

MARINE NUTRACEUTICALS: A POTENTIAL SOURCE FOR THE MANAGEMENT OF OBESITY

GARIMA RAJ,[1] NIHARIKA LAL,[2] NEERAJ KUMAR,[1] NITIN KUMAR,[1] and PRIYANKA ARYA[1]

[1]*Galgotias College of Pharmacy, Knowledge Park II, Greater Noida, Uttar Pradesh, India*

[2]*Metro College of Pharmacy, Knowledge Park III, Greater Noida, Uttar Pradesh, India*

ABSTRACT

Due to metabolic syndrome, type 2 diabetes, and cardiovascular disease, obesity is a serious problem that threatens human health on a global scale. One possibility for the treatment and management of obesity is therapeutic intervention using weight loss medications, along with diet and exercise. However, orlistat, a synthetic pancreatic lipase inhibitor, is the only approved anti-obesity medication currently on the market. While several anti-obesity medications have been discontinued due to severe side effects, other anti-obesity medications are still under investigation at various levels of clinical studies. Therefore, new anti-obesity medications are needed, especially those derived from biological sources. Seaweeds, in particular, are a promising source of marine algae with anti-obesity properties. Fucoxanthin, alginates, fucoidans, and phlorotannins are the four main bioactive substances found in seaweeds that have the potential to be used as anti-obesity treatments. Fucoxanthin and fucoidans, which impact satiety among other things, alginates, and the prevention of adipocyte development are just a few ways

Nutraceuticals in Obesity Management and Control. Raj K. Keservani & Alka Lohani (Eds.)

these substances exhibit anti-obesity properties (e.g., fucoxanthin). Before any novel anti-obesity medications based on algal products can be developed, more research is needed, particularly testing bioactive chemicals in extensive human trials.

13.1 INTRODUCTION

Over the past few years, research and the creation of new functional foods have been sparked by growing consumer awareness of the connection between diet, health, and the prevention of disease. Stephen DeFelice coined the term "nutraceutical" in 1989 by fusing the words "nutrition" and "pharmaceutical." Bioactive molecules, also known as bioactive compounds, are physiologically active chemicals that have health benefits above and beyond those of basic nutrition (Suleria et al., 2016). They can be found in raw foods, fortified foods, or dietary supplements. The aging of the population, the decline in quality of life brought on by stress, and the high prevalence of lifestyle diseases (such as cardiovascular disease, obesity, cancer, diabetes, and allergies) serve as the impetus behind the search for new foods and diets that support healthy active aging, enhance well-being, and reduce the risk of contracting numerous diseases (Thorpe et al., 2000). In the prevention, initiation, and progression of chronic diseases such as atherosclerosis, obesity, diabetes, hypertension, osteoporosis, cancer, and cardiovascular disease, food is known to play a significant influence.

Compared to terrestrial ecosystems, marine ecosystems have a higher diversity of living things, which offer a variety of supplies for human nutrition and health. A diverse group of organisms, marine invertebrates can be found in all ocean ecosystems, from the aquatic environment to the deep ocean. The various taxonomic groups that make up marine invertebrates can be divided into several major phyla, including Porifera (sponges), Cnidaria (corals, sea anemones, hydrozoans, jellyfish), Annelida (Polychaetes, marine worms), Bryozoa (moss animals or sea mats), Mollusca (oysters, abalone, clams, mussels, squid, cuttlefish, octopuses), Arthropoda (lobsters, crabs, shrimps, prawns, crayfish), and Echinodermata (sea stars, sea cucumbers, sea urchins) (Keith, 2000; Hill et al., 2010). This varied category also includes crustaceans, fish species, bacteria, cyanobacteria, macroalgae, and microalgae that create secondary metabolites to survive in the harsh maritime environment. The maritime environment provides a great source of nutritious food, and seaweed is one of many marine organisms that contain a variety of chemicals, many of which have biological capabilities known as "bioactive substances." New functional foods can be created by extracting these compounds and incorporating them into various food substrates (Hu et al., 2016).

The Food and Agriculture Organization (FAO) defines functional foods as those that look like traditional food, are meant to be consumed as a regular component of a diet, and include biologically active substances that have the potential to improve health or lower the risk of disease (Bakshi et al., 2018). Functional foods are those that, in addition to their nutritional impacts, have been shown to enhance health or well-being, lower the risk of disease, and help one or more bodily processes in humans. Functionality may be intrinsic to a feature added to the food matrix that improves health or lessens any unfavorable effects on health, such as:

- Elimination of a toxic component or encouragement of a chemical change.
- The addition of fresh, health-promoting dietary components or probiotic bacteria in a potent concentration.
- Increasing the concentration of an existing dietary element that promotes health by adding more of it.
- Increasing the ingredient in the diet that promotes health's bioavailability or stability.

The properties of the marine environment, such as temperature, salinity, light, pressure, and nutrients, are particularly significant since marine species have had to develop defense mechanisms and metabolites in response to their diverse range of values. Many marine organisms, including seaweed, contain a variety of chemicals, many of which have biological qualities known as bioactive compounds. The marine environment provides a major source of healthful food (Hamed et al., 2020; Liu, 2003). These substances can be isolated and added to various food matrices, resulting in the development of new functional foods.

Recent research on molecules derived from marine sources has revealed new bioactive compounds with significant capabilities, enhancing their usability as nutraceuticals (Keservani et al., 2010a, b, 2017, 2020) in the food and supplement industries (Voultsiadou, 2010). Marine sources have garnered a lot of attention. The "father of modern medicine," Hippocrates is known for explaining the beneficial effects of several marine invertebrates and their constituents on human health. Nearly 40% of all fisheries in the world come from marine invertebrates, and seafood from these sources is highly regarded for its beneficial effects on health due to its higher content of polyunsaturated fatty acids, different peptides, minerals (selenium and iodine), and other bioactive substances like carotenoids and taurine. The marine ecosystems also provide many compounds with biological properties that are employed as pharmaceuticals (Borresen, 2009; Rovira et al., 2013).

The marine nutraceutical market is booming and quickly expanding. Instead of treating and managing diseases, preventive healthcare practices are more in line with current market trends in healthcare. This trend is expected to intensify as healthcare expenses rise in both developed and emerging nations (Gahche, 2011). An increase in the prevalence of chronic diseases and the high expense of healthcare interventions are driving increased demand for customized nutrition. Those sources, as well as the constituent bioactive compounds, are discussed in the sections that follow and are enumerated in Table 13.1.

TABLE 13.1 Marine-Derived Bioactive Components

Derivative	Source	Activity
Protein and peptides	Fish (albacore tuna, silver-line grunt, brown-backed toadfish, hake, trout, lingcod, catfish, rainbow trout, yellow sea bream, common horse mackerel, etc.).	Antioxidant, anti-hypertensive, and anti-skin-aging activities.
Polysaccharides	Macroalgae, e.g., K. alvarezii, E. denticulatum and B. gelatinum.	Anticoagulant and antioxidant properties.
	Red alga is a main source of agar-agar like Gelidium, Gracilaria, Hypnea, and Gigartina.	Increase dietary fiber, reduce lipid absorption, antitumor, bactericidal, and fungicidal activities.
Fatty acids	Almost all marine sources.	Numerous health benefits (e.g., visual and neurodevelopment, reduced risk of cardiovascular problems, ameliorated diseases such as arthritis and hypertension).
Vitamins and minerals	Almost all marine sources. Seaweeds are rich sources of vitamins and minerals.	Vitamins and minerals perform many essential functions in the body, for example, they provide transport inside cells and also serve as cofactors during metabolic processes.
Phenolic compounds and other pigments	marine brown algae, Dunaliella salina, Sarcina maxima, Chlorella protothecoides, Chlorella vulgaris, and Haematococcus pluvialis.	Vitamin A precursors, antioxidants, anti-carcinogenic and anti-inflammatory.

13.2 MARINE SOURCES OF BIOACTIVE MOLECULES

Marine lipids (of both animal and microalgal origin), macroalgal polysaccharides, marine probiotics, marine natural colors, chitin, and other related products, bioactive marine peptides/enzymes, and vitamins are the major categories into which marine nutraceuticals fall (Anraku, 2011). These organisms produce compounds that are highly specific for their target molecules, typically an enzyme, and are effective as treatments for both infectious and non-infectious disorders.

13.2.1 MARINE ALGAE

The most common type of algae in the nutraceutical sector is macroalgae, often known as seaweed, which offers a wide range of food and food ingredients, particularly in Asian nations like Korea, Japan, and China.

Microalgae, also known as phytoplankton, are tiny marine organisms that are present in benthic and littoral habitats in the ocean. They include blue-green algae (phylum *Cyanobacteria,* class *Cyanophyceae*), diatoms (phylum *Ochrophyta,* class *Bacillariophyceae*), dinoflagellates (phylum *Myzozoa,* class *Dinophyceae*), as well as green and yellow-brown flagella. Microalgae are essential producers of several highly bioactive substances and play a significant role in the productivity of oceans, forming the foundation of the marine food chain (Kraan, 2013). One of the main products of macroalgae is agarose; however, macroalgae are also sources of metabolites and organic materials with distinct medicinal and nutritional qualities. PUFAs and pigments like carotenoids and chlorophylls are abundant in microalgae; the pigments of interest found in blue-green algae are chlorophyll a, phycocyanins, and phycoerythrin (phycobilins) (Biris-Dorhoi et al., 2020).

These substances have biological traits like anti-tumor, anti-bacterial, anti-fungal, and immuno-suppressive characteristics. Diatoms are photosynthetic organisms that predominate in cold, nutrient-rich seas' phytoplankton. They also generate the antioxidants fucoxanthin and chlorophyll, as well as PUFAs including eicosapentaenoic acid (EPA), docosahexaenoic acid (DHA), and other omega-3 FAs. Dinoflagellates are eukaryotic primary producers that are abundant in PUFAs, carotenoids, and chlorophyll (Udayangani et al., 2020).

Marine algae are employed as food sources and food additives in the nutraceutical industry. The two primary types of algae are microalgae and macroalgae, and both have uses in nutraceuticals. The most fundamental and uncomplicated marine plant life form, microalgae, is a rich source of nutrients including beta-carotene, vitamins C, A, E, H, B1, B2, B6, and B12, astaxanthin, polysaccharides, and polyunsaturated fatty acids. As a result, bioactive compounds from microalgae are synthesized commercially and added to foods, newborn milk formulas, and dietary supplements (Biris-Dorhoi et al., 2020; Anraku, 2011).

13.2.2 MARINE FISH

Fish are the most consumed marine animals and have a significant impact on the global economy. The most frequently consumed fish species are herring, salmon, cod, flounder, tuna, mullet, and anchovies, which together account for over 16% of the world's protein needs in 2012 (Charu et al., 2015). However, fish and fish byproducts are known sources of potentially active ingredients, such as fish oils rich in polyunsaturated fatty acids (PUFAs) from fish livers, calcium from fish bones, protein hydrolysates of high biological value, peptides with biological properties like antihypertensive activity, amino acids like taurine, which have antioxidant activity. A variety of substances found in fish heads, viscera, skin tails, blood, and seafood shells have the potential to be employed as functional food ingredients (Noitup et al., 2005). By-products of marine processing can be used to extract bioactive chemicals, allowing for the isolation of bioactive peptides, oligosaccharides, and FAs ideal for biotechnological applications, and favorable effects on the cardiovascular system, as well as vitamins and minerals.

The proteins, unsaturated essential fatty acids, minerals (such as calcium, iron, selenium, and zinc), and vitamins—specifically Vitamins A, B3, B6, B12, E, and D—present in fish are what give it its nutritional advantages. Additionally, studies have indicated that peptides made from fermented fish after being treated with enzymes may be effective therapies for the management of a variety of prevalent acute and chronic disorders, including cancer, hypertension, and Alzheimer's disease (Aneiros et al., 2004). In place of mammalian collagen, which is known to be immunogenic, fish collagen may potentially be used to treat bones.

13.2.3 MARINE FUNGI AND BACTERIA

Researchers from all around the world are paying more and more attention to marine bacteria and fungi because they are thought to be sources of novel marine natural chemicals. Since they have metabolic pathways tailored to a variety of harsh marine settings, marine extremophilic bacteria, for instance, are of great interest. Exopolysaccharides and microbial enzymes from extremophiles have special qualities (Luiten et al., 2003). Interest has also been shown in the study of bacteria isolated from the intestines of marine species like fish, as these strains may represent new probiotics or possess additional properties like antibiotic activity. In contrast to those obtained from a cheese starter, it has been observed that Lactococcus lactis isolates from the digestive system of freshwater fish have different phenotypic characteristics (Suleria et al., 2016). Also receiving a lot of attention are marine fungi, which have had their metabolites researched. A marine unicellular fungus that contains a significant amount of GABA, a potential functional and beneficial dietary element. Additionally, marine fungi are a possible source of novel bioactive substances with antiviral, antibacterial, anticancer, and antiplasmodial effects (Luiten et al., 2003).

13.2.4 CRUSTACEANS, MOLLUSKS, AND ECHINODERMS

Together with echinoderms, mollusks have long been popular marine diets and are regarded as natural functional foods. Numerous studies on bioactive compounds from various sources have produced several important results. Ground abalone and its shells are used to cure eye problems, whereas bioactive peptides derived from fermented blue mussel and oyster sauces considerably lower hypertension (Nagappan et al., 2017). Due to their medicinal properties, many Asian communities eat cuttlefish, squid, octopus, and nautiloids. For instance, cuttlefish bones can treat rickets, gastrointestinal ailments, and ear infections.

The second most common natural polymer, chitin, may be extracted from the shells of crustaceans. A friendly and biodegradable polymer chitin derivative is chitosan. As an anticholesterol agent, it makes use of its capacity to absorb fat. Due to their purported biological properties (antioxidant, antitumor, anticancer, hypocholesterolemic, immunity-enhancing, and antibacterial), chitosan and chito-oligosaccharides are used in the food and healthcare industries (Ngamwonglumler et al., 2019). When the nutritional makeup of marine crustaceans like shrimp and krill was analyzed, it was discovered that eating them reduced overall blood lipid levels in people and increased levels of vitamin A, certain proteins, and the omega-3 fatty acid eicosapentaenoic acid. Due to their enhanced nutritional content, these are recommended for use in the creation of value-added health food items and for human consumption (Thakur, 2020).

13.2.5 SPONGES

Sponges are the most basic type of multicellular organisms. They are sessile metazoans made of a gelatinous substance called mesohyl. Spicules, a silica, or calcium structure resembling tiny needles, and spongin, or collagen fibers, support their hollow pitcher-like body (Naczk et al., 2004). Alkaloids, terpenoids, polyketides, macrolides, polyphenolic chemicals, peptides, and sterols are just a few of the chemically varied substances recovered from sponges that have the potential to treat a wide range of diseases.

13.3 MARINE-DERIVED BIOACTIVE COMPONENTS

Differently structured marine-derived chemicals provide a wealth of bioactive core skeletons for brand-new lead molecules in medicine. The various structural types of these substances, such as azaphilones, dioxopiperazines, indole alkaloids, cytochalasans, and other xanthone derivatives, are known as the biggest primitive photoautotrophic and polyphyletic group of eukaryotes. Algae are responsible for more than 50% of the photosynthesis on Earth (Menaa et al., 2022). They are primarily categorized as either macroalgae or microalgae depending on their physical characteristics, such as whether they are unicellular (like diatoms) or multicellular (sometimes referred to as seaweeds). Based on the existence of particular pigments, marine algae are divided into three main types. As a result, algae can be brown (Phaeophyta/Phaeophyceae, such as *Sargassum polycystum, Padina pavonica,* and *Cystophora moniliformis),* blue-green (Cyanophyta/Cyanophyceae, such as *Spirulina platensis, Chlorococcum humicola,* and *Chlorella vulgaris*), or green (Chlorophyta) (Nasab et al., 2022). Marine algae are abundant in bioactive substances like carbohydrates, proteins, minerals, polyunsaturated fatty acids (PUFAs), fatty acids (FAs), amines, and amides as well as antioxidants (like polyphenols and tocopherols) and pigments like carotenoids, chlorophylls, xanthophylls, and phycobilins (phycocyanin (PC) and phycoerythrin (PE), which act as reducing, stabilizing, and capping agents to create natural phytoconstituents that are thermodynamically stable. It is significant to note that both biotic (i.e., type of algal species) and abiotic factors (e.g., temperature, pH, salinity, inorganic carbon (C), oxygen (O_2), light intensity, and carbon dioxide (CO_2), as well as the dynamic algal-associated halobionts) all have an impact on the quality of biological moieties (Miazek et al., 2015).

Marine algae-derived bioactive compounds are potential sources for a variety of physiologically active components. A substantial source of new chemicals with significant pharmacological and therapeutic significance is marine fungi and bacteria (Debbab et al., 2010). Examples of high-value-added compounds with nutraceutical potential that can be used as functional additives include omega-3 oils, chitin, chitosan, algal components, carotenoids, and other bioactive ingredients. The use of polysaccharides like chitin and chitosan is expanding. They are believed to be a fantastic source of lipids, high in unsaturated fatty acids and high-quality protein, and perhaps improve human health by reducing the risks of cardiovascular disease (Grienke et al., 2014). A possible source of bio-products with interesting biotechnological applications is marine bioactive compounds. It is necessary to assess a variety of biological processes in order to find and classify emerging marine natural products. The increased sensitivity of omics technologies, notably next-generation high-throughput sequencing combined with liquid chromatography-mass spectrometry and nuclear magnetic resonance, has hastened the discovery of novel bioactive compounds. Mycosporine-like amino acids (MAAs), which have been derived from a range of marine microorganisms with UV absorption capabilities, are the most promising emerging marine natural products (Rosic, 2021). A significant source of nutritious foods comes from bioactive compounds and secondary metabolites produced by sponges, crabs, seaweed, algae, fungi, fish, bacteria, and other marine organisms. The main biologically active components used as functional foods that come from marine sources are pigments, polysaccharides, proteins, lipids, vitamins, and phenolic compounds. Seaweeds are a potential product because of their antioxidant, anticancer, anti-inflammatory, anticoagulant, anti-obesity, and antibacterial properties. Microalgae and fish oils high in polyunsaturated fatty acids can help to enhance the nutritional profile of food (Prabha et al., 2019). *Rhodophyceae, Phaeophyceae,* and *Chlorophyceae* are the three families of photosynthetic polyphyletic algae. Macroalgae grow quickly in the open ocean, producing a lot of biomasses. In addition to having a higher rate of photosynthetic activity than terrestrial biomass, macroalgae also have the advantage of not needing land or water. The multicellular eukaryotic cells known as red algae include chlorophyll and phycobiliproteins. They have a characteristic red color due to the high phycoerythrin concentration. Red seaweed may metabolize Floridian starch, which is identical to amylose, as a food reserve. A variety of sizes and shapes of multicellular algae, including brown algae, can be found in the water. Some can grow to a length of 60 meters, while others are only a few millimeters long. With more than half of the dry biomass made up of carbohydrates, brown algae have a high carbohydrate content. For the production of alginate and as a food source, brown algae are produced extensively (Centella et al., 2017; Romano et al., 2017).

13.3.1 PROTEINS

The genetic code determines the order of the 20 amino acids that make up proteins, along with a range of other amino acids. In biological and dietary systems, proteins act as hormones (insulin), antibodies, and transport proteins (hemoglobin), in addition to being important nutrients (immunoglobulins). Seaweeds have long been used as food or herbal medicine to treat or prevent a wide range of illnesses and disorders because of their strong nutritional and therapeutic capabilities. Additionally, they are used as food supplements, fungicides, herbicides, animal feed, and a source of agar, alginate, and carrageenan for a variety of industrial and pharmaceutical applications. It is widely accepted that seaweeds have been effectively used as a source of protein for many decades (Pooja et al., 2020).

13.3.2 PEPTIDES

There has been a lot of interest in using protein hydrolysis to create bioactive peptides, particularly peptides made from marine proteins. These peptides have been isolated from marine fish, algae, and crustaceans. Depending on the composition and sequencing of the amino acids, bioactive peptides can contain anywhere between 3 and 20 amino acid residues. They possess biological characteristics including, among others, anti-inflammatory, immunostimulatory, anti-cancer, antithrombotic, anti-hypertensive, and antioxidant capabilities (Hamed et al., 2015). It may be advantageous to use peptides made from marine protein sources as essential antihypertensive ingredients in functional meals (Norris et al., 2013).

13.3.3 AMINO ACIDS

In shellfish muscles, the water-soluble amino acids taurine, Pro, Gln, Ala, Gly, and Arg are widely distributed. It is anticipated that when seafood is gently prepared, the beneficial properties of the water-soluble components will be more pronounced because they are lost during cooking or thermal processing. Children's diets commonly lack sulfur-containing, Lys- and Thr-containing amino acids, especially when they are based on cereals. It is therefore believed that eating fish muscle proteins, which are rich in specific amino acids, may enhance human nutrition by increasing the nutritional content of foods (Romano et al., 2017).

13.3.4 LIPIDS AND FATTY ACIDS

The two most prevalent omega-3 polyunsaturated fatty acids (PUFAs), derived from aquatic sources, are eicosapentaenoic acid (EPA) and docosahexaenoic acid (DHA). Linolenic acid can elongate and desaturate to EPA and DHA in small amounts in humans. The only way to get these PUFAs is through seafood and supplements. Compared to EPA and DHA, DPA is present in fish oils in incredibly low amounts. However, it is virtually as important in seal blubber oil as either EPA or DHA. Phytoplankton, algae, and other multicellular and unicellular sea plants all produce EPA and DHA. They ascend the food chain and eventually end up in aquatic creatures like fish and marine mammals' lipids. Omega-3 fatty acids have been demonstrated in animal and *in vitro* studies to modify blood lipid profiles, gene expression, cardiovascular health, eicosanoid synthesis, and membrane lipid composition. According to epidemiological studies, consuming fatty acids from natural sources may affect the onset and course of a variety of disease states, including cancer, autoimmune disease, and cardiovascular disease (Shahidi & Ambigaipalan, 2015). Low levels of saturated fatty acids are frequently present in the fatty acid composition of seafood and saturated fatty acids (SFAs). A decrease in SFA intake is advised because it has long been believed that eating them increases the risk of developing cardiovascular disease. However, a recent study challenges this notion. Seafood contains a lot of monounsaturated fatty acids (MUFAs) and polyunsaturated fatty acids (PUFAs), both of which are thought to be beneficial if not oxidized (Hoffman et al., 2009).

13.3.5 CARBOHYDRATES AND DIETARY FIBER

Carbohydrates, important substances in marine life obtained from marine organisms, have shown antioxidant and immune-enhancing functions that play an important role in anti-aging. Most of the natural carbohydrates found in marine organisms are polysaccharides, with a small number being mono- or oligosaccharides. Trehalose is a disaccharide found in seaweed and shrimp that has an anti-aging effect by regulating the Nrf2 and insulin signaling pathways (Wang et al., 2021). Brown algae mainly contain three crucial forms of soluble dietary fiber polysaccharides, including alginate, fucoidan, and laminaran. Cellulose makes up the majority of the insoluble fiber. Alginate, the main polymer of brown algae, is composed of polymannuronic acid, polyguluronic acid, and a linear mixture of polymannuronic acid and polyguluronic acid. Alginate is present in multiple forms of acid and salt because it is considered an important part of the cell wall. Depending on the type of brown algae, fucoidan is a sulfated polysaccharide rich in fucose sugars with other monosaccharides (such as glucose, glucuronic acid, mannose, xylose, and galactose present in small amounts) (Gurpilhares et al., 2019). Laminaran, fucoidan, and alginate are the three most common types of soluble fiber polysaccharides produced by brown algae. Polysaccharides are also obtained from brown algae. Alginate is the main polymer present in brown algae, which consists of polymannuronic acid, polyguluronic acid, and a linear mixture of polymannuronic acid and polyguluronic acid (Jin et al., 2015). Brown seaweed polysaccharides have a complicated structure that inhibits them from being broken down by natural enzymes in the human colon. Fucoidan, laminaran, and alginate all include dietary fiber. In order to boost fiber bioavailability (both soluble and insoluble), a significant amount of effort has gone into developing effective methods for extracting, purifying, and elucidating the structural properties of algal prebiotics (Gurpilhares et al., 2019). Natural aminopolysaccharides like chitin and chitosan have unique architectural structures and multimodal properties. Over the past decade, chitin and chitosan derivatives have attracted much attention in industrial fields such as food, biomedical, culinary, and biopharmaceutical, with applications like tissue engineering and wound healing biomaterials. Chitin can be partially deacetylated to produce glucosamine, chitosan, and chitosan oligosaccharides, among other things (Pati et al., 2020). These chitosan derivatives are more beneficial as nutraceutical ingredients than the fully acetylated, insoluble kind of chitin because of their improved water solubility. Even though chitosan's effectiveness in reducing fat absorption has been questioned, multiple chitosan products on the market nowadays are promoted as cholesterol and fat burners. Commercial interest in chitosan and its derivatives has been ignited by the variety of biological properties of chitosan and its derivatives, including biodegradability, biocompatibility, and non-toxicity (Gurpilhares et al., 2019; Nagaoka et al., 2011; Zhang et al., 2012). Alginate, fucoidan, and laminaran are three varieties of soluble dietary fiber polysaccharides found in brown algae. Most insoluble fiber is made up of cellulose. Laminaran, an α-glucan used by algae as their main storage carbohydrate, is predominantly made up of 1,3-D-glucopyranose residue that is branched with 1,6-D-glucopyranose (Gurpilhares et al., 2019). Marine polysaccharides generated from seaweeds, such as agar, alginate, carrageenan, and fucoidan, have a wide range of physiological qualities and are frequently utilized in food, agriculture, and healthcare. However, their low solubility and poor absorption have severely restricted their use. Marine oligosaccharides have attracted much interest as degradation products of these polysaccharides due to their distinct biological activities, enhanced solubility, and excellent bioavailability (Zhu et al., 2021).

13.3.6 PIGMENTS

Up to 8% of phycobiliproteins can be produced by the marine red algae *Porphyridium cruentum* and *A. platensis*, which are used as fluorescent markers when covalently bonded to hormones, lectins, biotin, A-proteins, antibodies, and other molecules. Phycobiliproteins are composed of a protein and the chromophore phycobilin (connected by covalent bonds). The two most well-known phycobiliproteins are phycocyanin and phycoerythrin from *Arthrospira* and *Porphyridium*, respectively. They can be employed as non-radioactive markers in DNA, microscopy, and fluorescence-based immunology investigations (De Jesus Raposo et al., 2013).

The yellow, orange, and red colors of the aquatic species' skin, shells, and exoskeletons are caused by the presence of carotenoids. They exist in algal species as well. Mammals use carotenoids (particularly β-carotene) as precursors for vitamin A, which is one of their most crucial physiological functions. α-carotene, cryptoxanthin, canthaxanthin, 3,4-dehydro-β-carotene, β-apo-8′-carotenoic acid ethyl ester, and echinenone have all been shown to have vitamin A activity. According to studies, marine carotenoids in the gastrointestinal lumen can decrease lipase activity and lessen the absorption of triacylglycerol. Brown seaweeds are a rich source of the marine carotenoid fucoxanthin, which has been linked to cancer (Matsumoto et al., 2010; Manivasagan et al., 2018). Yeast and algae from the ocean, such as *Chlorella zofingiensis, Chlorococcum,* and *Haematococcus,* create natural astaxanthin (e.g., *Phaffia rhodozyma*) (Khoo et al., 2019).

13.3.7 ENZYMES, VITAMINS, AND MINERALS

Enzymes can be used in the food and nutraceutical industries to convert other molecules into vital biotechnological processes. Enzymes can have an impact on food safety, processing, storage, and spoiling. All of the red algal enzymes needed to break down starch, including -1,4-glucanase, lipase, transglutamase, chitinolytic enzymes, polyphenol oxidase, and others, come from marine sources. They have better catalytic, physical, and chemical properties than their terrestrial counterparts. At a comfortable temperature, they can also be rendered inactive. Additionally, these enzymes are used as flavorings in food. Extremophiles are typically believed to have a significant potential to be profitable resources for biotechnological applications due to their distinctive activity under abnormal conditions, which makes biomolecules extracted from extremophiles, such as enzymes, particularly valuable in the food industry. The body uses vitamins and minerals for a variety of functions, such as providing intracellular transportation and acting as cofactors in metabolic processes. Seaweeds are a great source of vitamins and minerals including iron (Suleria et al., 2015). A group of enzymes called xylanases catalyze the production of xylose from hemicellulose. A crucial carbon source for bacteria, xylose is also a factor in the infection of plants by pathogens. Among the organisms that produce xylanases are gastropods, arthropods, bacteria, fungi, and algae. Despite this, microorganisms are preferred over plant and animal sources for the production of xylanase because they are more readily available, produce more xylanase per unit of time, are structurally stable, and are easier to manipulate genetically. Actinomycetes, in particular, and fungi have been used to identify the bulk of marine xylanases. There have been found to be microbial sources of marine xylanases (Izadpanah et al., 2020). Chitinolytic enzymes are capable of catalyzing chitin hydrolysis. The usage of chitinolytic enzymes in biotechnology and medicine has attracted a lot of attention. Recently, marine organisms have emerged as a novel source for the commercial separation of enzymes and the production of numerous special valuable compounds. Because the sea environment is so varied, we could find microorganisms suited to various extreme circumstances (halophiles, psychrophiles, thermophiles, and so on) that could be helpful in a variety of sectors (Beygmoradi et al., 2018). Because of the polysaccharides on the cell surface, which can make up to 36% of the dry mass in some species, seaweeds are noted for having high mineral (Na, Ca, Mg, P, and K) and trace element (Zn, I, and Mn) contents. This is related to their capacity to retain inorganic sea chemicals. Due to their high calcium and potassium content, many different species of seaweed are suggested as food supplements to meet daily mineral and trace element requirements. Selenium, iodine, zinc, magnesium, and calcium are additional minerals that are present in some shellfish at higher concentrations than, say, beef. A lower risk of cancer has been linked to increased dietary selenium intake. In certain nations with low iodine intake, seaweeds are an alternative to fortified salt as a means of providing iodine through diet. Seaweed is one of the most promising natural iodine sources.

13.3.8 PROBIOTICS

More than 100 trillion bacteria reside in the gastrointestinal tract as part of the gut flora, which is a collection of microorganisms. The most prevalent intestinal microbial species, including *Eubacterium, Bacteroides, Enterococcus, Prevotella, Clostridium, Staphylococcus, Streptococcus,* and *Enterobacter*, carry out a number of beneficial tasks for the host in the exploitation of underutilized energy sources. Numerous strains can turn pathogenic in a healthy gut under specific conditions. As a result, it has been discovered that fostering a favorable habitat while reducing the number of dangerous species. Numerous strategies for boosting the beneficial effects of intestinal microbiota have been put forth in this field. One of the best methods to encourage healthy microbes in the gut is using probiotic strains, which are living microbes that are good for gut flora and may be able to lessen the activity of bacteria that cause disease. Prebiotics eventually enable specific modifications to the gastrointestinal microflora's structure and functioning, which improves the host's overall health and well-being. Live strains of *Lactobacillus* and *Bifidobacterium* are routinely used to create probiotics. Particularly fermented dairy products include yogurts.

13.3.9 MISCELLANEOUS BIOACTIVE COMPOUNDS FROM MARINE ORGANISMS

Around 30% of the waste produced during the cooking of seafood is rich in collagen. Marine collagen has the potential to take the role of mammalian collagen in a number of uses, such as dressings for wounds. Additionally, collagen peptides have been demonstrated by numerous researchers to support bone preservation as people age and promote wound healing (Hosseini et al., 2020). For the development of useful biomaterials, collagen is also a promising material. Using electrospun collagen scaffolds made from tilapia fish skin, researchers were able to accelerate *in vivo* wound healing and reepithelialization (Ganesan et al., 2020a). Marine gelatin is made from the collagen found in aquatic animals' skin and bones. It is an essential biopolymer that gels and provides meals their flexibility, viscosity, and stability. Fish waste, most frequently fish skin and bones, is used to create fish gelatin, a high-protein raw material. It has 27–49% protein by dry weight. Gelatin can produce high-quality films because of its monomer makeup and linear structure. Gelatin films have been used as packaging or encasing materials due to the properties of low oxygen permeability and high UV light barrier that have been demonstrated in prior studies (Uranga et al., 2016). The oligomeric sterol or triterpene glycosides known as saponins can be found in a broad variety of plants and animals, such as sea cucumbers and starfish. Sea cucumbers contain saponin in their triterpene form, whereas starfish contain saponin in their steroidal form. Sea cucumber saponins have been proven to be pancreatic lipase inhibitors in *in-vitro* experiments. Researchers looked at the anti-obesity characteristics of two sulfated triterpene saponins derived from sea cucumbers (*Pearsonothuria graeffei*), echinoside A and holothurin A (Wang et al., 2018). Water-soluble pigments called phycobiliproteins (PBPs) are found in the stroma and cytoplasm of chloroplasts. Only red seaweeds have phycoerythrin, a reddish-pink pigment that serves as a major light-harvesting pigment by transferring light energy to chlorophyll. PBPs such as phycocyanin (blue color), allophycocyanin (blue color), and phycoerythrin emit red and yellow fluorescence. One instance of how these pigments have been utilized in culinary preparations as natural colorants is phycocyanin, which is extracted from spirulina (Sudhakar et al., 2019).

13.4 MARINE-DERIVED BIOACTIVE COMPONENTS IN OBESITY

13.4.1 SEAWEEDS AS FOOD AND THEIR POTENTIAL ANTI-OBESITY EFFECTS

Some of the potentially beneficial chemicals found in seaweeds are not found in terrestrial plants. Proteins like lectins or phycobiliproteins, carotenoids, pigments, polyphenols, phlorotannins, and certain polysaccharides are a few examples of these substances. They might influence chronic disease and have health-promoting qualities (Brown et al., 2014). In nations like Japan and Korea, seaweed is an essential part of the diet. For instance, about 21% of meals in Japan include seaweed (Yoshinaga et al., 2001), and between 1955 (4.3 g/day) and 1995 (5.3 g/day), the daily consumption per person remained largely stable (Matsumura et al., 2001). The most commonly used seaweeds include Wakame (*Undaria*), Nori (*Porphyra*), Konbu (*Laminaria)*, and Hijiki (*Hizikia*) (Phang et al., 2010).

Seaweed consumption has been linked to a lower prevalence of chronic diseases like cancer, hyperlipidemia, and cardiovascular disease in epidemiological studies comparing Southeast Asian and Western-style diets (Cavalli-Sforza et al., 1996; Drewnowski et al., 1997).

A diet high in fiber has been shown to slow down the gastric emptying process, boosting satiety and lowering food intake (Kristensen et al., 2011). Given that seaweeds are an excellent source of dietary fiber, numerous studies have evaluated the potential medical advantages of eating seaweed for the control of body weight and obesity (Lange et al., 2015). Although there have been an increasing number of human trials, studies on the anti-obesity effects of seaweeds have primarily used cell-based and animal models. These studies have used whole seaweed meal, seaweed extracts, or seaweed bioactives. Some of such studies are mentioned here. Like eating *Sargassum polycystum* seaweed powder prevented weight gain in rats given a high-fat diet and decreased cholesterol as well as triacylglycerols levels in the blood (Awang et al., 2014). Another study includes where diet-induced obese mice, eating the brown seaweed *Undaria pinnatifida* had favorable effects on body weight growth, energy consumption, and blood levels of glucose and insulin (Grasa-López et al., 2016). Furthermore, there were more and smaller adipocytes in the retroperitoneal tissue due to decreased lipogenesis, higher energy expenditure, and lower expression of the inflammatory marker interleukin-6 (IL-6). The researchers hypothesized that additional algal constituents, such as eicosapentaenoic acid (EPA) and fiber, along with fucoxanthin were also responsible for the decrease in body weight.

More studies like those mentioned above were also conducted involving human trials where energy consumption of 12 healthy, overweight, and obese men was compared regarding their calorie intake during a test meal four hours after consuming bread enriched with the brown seaweed *Ascophyllum nodosum* (4% per 400 g whole meal loaf) with those men who had bread without *Ascophyllum nodosum*. In the 24 hours following the test meal, those who received the seaweed-enriched bread significantly reduced their energy intake (16.4%). According to the author's hypothesis, the effects of stomach stretching brought on by the bulking caused by the presence of alginates in the seaweed-enriched bread may be linked to reduced energy intake. However, there were no appreciable variations in blood sugar and cholesterol levels (Hall et al., 2012).

The effectiveness of seaweed extract was also demonstrated by a study based on *in vitro* and *in vivo* models. For example, the anti-obesity properties of ethanol extracts from Jeju Island seaweeds in Korea were demonstrated. The red seaweed *Plocamium telfairiae* extract was discovered to have the highest inhibitory effect among the tested extracts on lipogenesis in adipocytes, particularly in reducing the expression of the adipogenic-specific proteins peroxisome proliferator-activated receptor (PPAR) and CCAAT/

enhancer-binding protein (C/EBP). In another study, mice fed a high-fat diet experienced a decrease in body weight after receiving extracts from the edible red seaweed *Gelidium amansii*. This outcome was associated with a reduction in the expression of adipogenic genes in adipocytes. The treated mice also exhibited a significant reduction in their levels of blood sugar, insulin, triacylglycerol, and total cholesterol (Kang et al., 2016).

13.4.2 MARINE ALGAE AS A SOURCE OF ANTI-PANCREATIC LIPASE AGENT

One of the primary therapeutic goals of anti-obesity medications is the inhibition of lipases, particularly pancreatic lipase. Orlistat, a currently available and licensed anti-obesity medication, works in this manner. Pancreatic and stomach lipases are effectively inhibited by the synthetic, hydrogenated derivative of lipstatin known as orlistat (Kakkar et al., 2015). Lipstatin was shown to be an extremely powerful, selective, and irreversible inhibitor of pancreatic lipase through target-directed screening of microbial broths from soil organisms (Hadvary et al., 1985). Similar to esterastin, the lipstatin molecule features a unique β-lactone structure integrated into a hydrocarbon backbone (Puls et al., 1985). In one study to determine the anti-lipase activity, 54 marine algae were examined for the potential presence of triacylglycerol acylhydrolase, an inhibitor of pancreatic lipase. Caulerpenyne, an active inhibitor, was isolated from a *Caulerpa taxifolia* extract using ethyl acetate extraction and subsequent chromatographic studies on ODS and silica gel columns (Bitou et al., 1999).

Furthermore, studies were performed in order to identify the anti-lipase activity of marine algae. Like in another study, the effectiveness of ethanol extracts made from various marine algae collected on the Tunisian coast to inhibit lipase was investigated. Using TC4 as a short-chain triacylglycerol substrate and olive oil as a long-chain triacylglycerol substrate, the results showed that only *C. prolifera* extract inhibited both gastric and pancreatic lipases. The inhibition is often influenced by the substrate type and lipase type. Studies revealed that the presence of *C. prolifera* extract significantly reduces the activities of pancreatic and gastric lipases (Rebah et al., 2008). More studies were also performed like using an *in vitro* simulation of the upper digestive tract and a turbidimetric lipase activity assay, the impact of three Hebridean brown seaweeds on lipase activity was evaluated. In this study, the whole seaweed homogenate, sodium carbonate extract, and ethanol extracts of *Ascophyllum nodosum, Fucus vesiculosus,* and *Pelvetia canaliculata* were tested as the preparations (pellet and supernatant were tested separately). All extracts significantly inhibited lipase, indicating the presence of numerous bioactive substances, possibly including alginates, fucoidans, and polyphenols. The most effective lipase inhibitor was *F. vesiculosus* whole homogenate extract. The ethanol pellet provided the most effective suppression for *A. nodosum* and *P. canaliculata* (Chater et al., 2016).

Alginates are a different category of seaweed substances that have been demonstrated to have pancreatic lipase-inhibitory activity. Depending on the compound's source and chemical forms, the inhibitory activity may change. The study performed by (Wilcox et al., 2014) showed that pancreatic lipase was much more inhibited by High-G alginates from *Laminaria hyperborea* seaweed than by High-M alginates from *Lessonia nigrescens*, indicating a relationship between inhibition and alginate structure. The molecular weight of the alginates does not, however, influence how inhibitory they are. When alginates were put into a bread vehicle and cooked at temperatures up to 200°C or digested in a model gut, the pancreatic lipase inhibitory action remained unaffected, and this was explained by Houghton et al. (2015). The hydroxyl group of alginates is thought to interact with the enzyme by hydrogen bonding, while the carboxyl groups and the alginate's negatively charged COO-group may also interact with the enzyme through charge-charge interactions. Alginates have the potential to be used as an anti-obesity treatment because the technology to use them as a pancreatic lipase inhibitor has been patented by Richardson et al. (2010).

Recent research has discovered that fucoxanthin, a compound derived from edible seaweeds, and its metabolite fucoxanthinol have anti-obesity properties. The researchers examined how different carotenoids affected the absorption of triglycerides in conscious rats implanted with cannulae into the portal or jugular vein and a lymph duct. Their findings demonstrate that these two marine carotenoids reduce triglyceride absorption and inhibit lipase activity in the gastrointestinal lumen. Fucoxanthin was also transformed into fucoxanthinol in the intestine and discharged into the lymph (Matsumoto et al., 2010).

13.4.3 ALGAL COMPOUNDS WITH ANTI-OBESITY EFFECT

Seaweeds are a nutritionally undervalued resource that could not only enhance the standard Western diet but also possibly provide extra health advantages beyond just their nutritional value. Green algae (*Chlorophyceae*), red algae (*Rhodophyceae*), blue-green algae (*Cyanophyceae*), and brown algae are the four different families of seaweed algae (*Phaeophyceae*). Polysaccharides and polyphenols are just two of the many bioactive substances found in seaweeds. Brown seaweeds are a source of polyphenols such as phenolic acids, flavonoids (Keservani & Sharma, 2014; Keservani et al., 2016a, b), phlorotannin, stilbenes, and lignans as well as polysaccharides like fucoidan, laminarin, and alginate. These substances have been demonstrated to decrease the activity of digestive enzymes, regulating enzymes like pepsin, lipase, α-amylase, and β-glucosidase.

13.4.3.1 FUCOXANTHIN

Fucoxanthin, a marine carotenoid that makes up more than 10% of all naturally occurring carotenoids, is mostly found in brown seaweeds and diatoms (Maeda et al., 2008). In edible seaweeds like *Undaria pinnatifida, Laminaria digitata,* and *Hijikia fusiformis,* it is widely distributed. Additionally, because their concentrations of the pigment are substantially higher than those of brown seaweeds, marine microalgae like *Phaeodactylum tricornutum* and *Isochrysis galbana* have been identified as prospective fucoxanthin producers for the commercial market (Kim et al., 2012). A powerful antioxidant, fucoxanthin has the potential used in the creation of nutritious foods (Chu et al., 2011; Mise et al., 2011). Regarding its anti-obesity impact, this carotenoid is also one of the most researched algae compounds (Gammone et al., 2015; Miyashita et al., 2011). Fucoxanthin's polyene chromophore, which has an allenic link and two hydroxyl groups, is what's responsible for its bioactivity (Miyashita et al., 2011). In an obese mouse model, consumption of the fucoxanthin-rich food Wakame has been demonstrated to have anti-diabetic and anti-obesity effects (Maeda et al., 2009). Mice fed a high-fat diet followed by a diet high in fucoxanthin experienced reduced weight growth and modified blood glucose and insulin levels. When fucoxanthin and fish oil were given to KK-Ay mice, the weight gain of white adipose tissue (WAT) was shown to be less than when fucoxanthin was given to the mice alone (Maeda et al., 2007). A diet high in fucoxanthin also reduced MCP-1 mRNA expression in WAT, which reduced inflammatory responses in those tissues. In a different investigation, Tan & Hou (2014) showed that feeding fucoxanthin to an obese mice model decreased the levels of inflammatory markers such as interleukin-1ß (IL-1ß), TNF-, inducible nitric oxide synthase (iNOS), and cyclooxygenase-2 (COX-2) (Tan et al., 2014). In a co-culture of adipocytes and macrophage cells, fucoxanthinol, a metabolite of fucoxanthin, was found to reduce TNF- and MCP-1 mRNA suppression, supporting the claim that it suppresses low-grade inflammation in adipocytes (Maeda et al., 2015). Fucoxanthin lowered WAT mass, and decreased blood triacylglycerols, but increased serum HDL cholesterol, according to a more recent study by Grasa-Lopez et al. (2016) utilizing a mouse model (Grasa-López et al., 2016). Other positive outcomes included better insulin resistance, decreased adiponectin serum levels, lowered blood pressure, enhanced expression, and reduced resistance and a decline in leptin expression. Additionally, the higher oxidation resulted from Uncoupling protein 1 expression (UCP-1). Numerous studies have demonstrated that fucoxanthin reduces obesity by altering lipid levels and metabolism. For example, feeding seaweed extract with fucoxanthin was discovered to improve oxidation and lower lipogenesis in a mouse model of obesity (Kang et al., 2012). Additionally, in epididymal adipose tissue, fucoxanthin boosted the activity of two crucial enzymes involved in lipid metabolism: AMP-activated protein kinase (AMPK) and acetyl-CoA carboxylase (ACC). Fucoxanthin and conjugated linoleic acid have been demonstrated to lower triacylglycerols, glucose, and leptin levels in the serum of diet-induced obese rats (Hu et al., 2012). The trans-10, cis-12 isomer of conjugated linoleic acid, a category of isomers of linoleic acid, is known to have an anti-obesity effect. Rats administered fucoxanthin with conjugated linoleic acid experienced a decrease in WAT weight increase; however, rats fed fucoxanthin alone did not. In the rats' WAT, it was discovered that the combination controlled the mRNA expression of several lipid metabolism-related enzymes, including carnitine palmitoyl transferase 1A. By controlling metabolic enzyme activity and promoting fatty oxidation activity, fucoxanthin also affects the amount of lipids in the liver (Woo et al., 2010).

A mouse model showed that this impact was caused by increased β-oxidation and decreased activity of the hepatic lipogenic enzymes glucose-6-phosphate dehydrogenase, malic enzyme, fatty acid synthase, and phosphatidate phosphohydrolase. Fucoxanthin's anti-obesity properties are also a result of its increase of UCP1 expression in WAT, which improves energy loss through fatty acid oxidation and heat production (Maeda et al., 2015). Before being absorbed in the gut, dietary fucoxanthin is changed to fucoxanthinol in the digestive system. This is then transformed into amarouciaxanthin A in the mouse liver (Asai et al., 2004). In the adipose tissue of mice, fucoxanthin, fucoxanthinol, and amarouciaxanthin were accumulated to varying degrees (13%, 32%, and 55%, respectively) (Hashimoto et al., 2009). A number of toxicity studies have been carried out as part of the examination of fucoxanthin's safety in light of its prospective usage as a nutraceutical, particularly for its anti-obesity activity. In one study, rats were given Fucoxanthin (95% purity) orally repeatedly for 4 weeks without exhibiting any discernible harm (Kadekaru et al., 2008). After a 4-week daily treatment, another study found that rats fed extracts containing 0.0012% fucoxanthin showed no acute toxicity (Zaragoza et al., 2008). In a different investigation, fucoxanthin toxicity tests in mice at single (1,000 and 2,000 mg/kg body weight) and recurrent doses (500 and 1,000 mg/kg body weight, 30 days) revealed no fatalities or gross abnormalities. However, mice fed fucoxanthin showed a substantial increase in plasma total cholesterol (Beppu et al., 2009). Fucoxanthin has already been commercially formulated as a nutraceutical with anti-obesity properties available in stores. Fucoxanthin and other ingredients are found in the commercial product Xanthigen and the fatty acid punicic acid, which is found in pomegranate oil (Abidov et al., 2010).

13.4.3.2 ALGINATES

Due in part to their high dietary fiber content, which is not greatly processed in the gut, seaweeds may have health benefits (MacArtain et al., 2007). These fibers' capacity to bulk up can promote satiety and facilitate digestive transit. Among the seaweed fibers with established anti-obesity properties are alginates. Alginates are compounds made from alginic acid, a polymer that gels and is a structural element of brown seaweeds (Draget et al., 2011). Up to 40% of the dry weight of brown seaweeds is made up of alginates (Stiger-Pouvreau et al., 2016). The majority of the alginates that are utilized commercially come from brown seaweeds belonging to the genera *Laminaria, Macrocystis, Ascophyllum*, and *Lessonia*. With Laminaria and Lessonia species accounting for 81% of the seaweed harvests, they are the main sources of alginates. Alginates are frequently utilized in food items as a thickening or emulsification stabilizer. The most prevalent type of alginate used in the food sector is sodium alginate (Bixler et al., 2011). Supplementing with dietary alginate has been found to improve satiety, lower energy consumption, and help weight loss (Lange et al., 2015). One study found that obese and overweight women with poor rigid restraint levels consumed less energy after consuming a calcium-gelled fiber beverage twice daily (Pelkman et al., 2007). Delay in stomach emptying, stimulation of gastric stretch receptors, and reduced food absorption are some of the mechanisms causing the impact. The majority of studies on alginates were carried out using ready-to-drink alginate formulations. When chocolate milk with 2.5% alginate was provided to study participants, it was discovered that this lowered mean appetite by 13% when compared to chocolate milk alone (El-Khoury et al., 2014).

Alginates' anti-obesity properties may be regulated by the polysaccharide's conformational shape. A study conducted on mice given a high-fat diet investigated the anti-obesity effects of dietary acid-hydrolyzed (A-AO) and enzymatic-digested (E-AO) alginate oligomers. E-AO had more potent anti-obesity benefits than A-AO in terms of weight loss in the body and adipose tissue. Additionally, *in vitro* research demonstrated that E-AO, but not the entire polymer, prevented lipid buildup in differentiated 3T3-L1 adipocytes (Nakazono et al., 2016).

Alginate ingestion has been demonstrated to have positive effects on postprandial glucose absorption and insulin response in both animal and human investigations (Jensen et al., 2013). There have been suggestions that the outcome is due to the viscosity and gelling characteristics of alginates, which are comparable to those of other dietary fibers including ß-glucans and pectin (Kristensen et al., 2011). Additionally, it has been demonstrated that giving rats a high-cholesterol diet will lower their blood cholesterol levels (Idota et al., 2016).

13.4.3.3 FUCOIDANS

A class of highly sulfated polysaccharides called fucoidans contains large levels of fucose, detected primarily in brown seaweeds' extracellular matrix. These polysaccharides additionally include one or more minute amounts of glucose, L-rhamnose, arabinose, D-xylose, D-mannose, D-galactose, D-glucuronic acid, and acetyl groups that differ amongst various species of seaweed. Most articles on fucoidan bioactivity and anti-tumor activity are connected (Wu et al., 2016). There were research studies that show fucoidans do, nevertheless, have anti-obesity properties. Fucoidans from *Undaria pinnatifida,* for instance, have been demonstrated to have an anti-adipogenic effect by decreasing key adipogenic markers, such as adipocyte protein 2, and the expression of genes related to inflammation in adipocytes during adipogenesis. Fucoidans also prevent lipids and ROS from building up in adipocytes. Additionally, it was discovered that fucoidans reduce lipid synthesis in differentiated 3T3-L1 adipocytes (Park et al., 2011). Animal model studies have also shown that fucoidans have anti-obesity properties. For instance, research revealed that mice on high-fat diets fed fucoidans had less body weight growth, a lower food-efficiency ratio, and less relative liver and epididymal fat content than mice on high-fat diets alone (Kim et al., 2014). Additionally, there was a decline in the plasma levels in the mice fed fucoidans, triacylglycerols, total cholesterol, and low-density lipoprotein (LDL) were measured. The genes encoding aP2, ACC, and PPAR in the epididymal adipose tissue were also downregulated. Fucoidans from *Sargassum henslowianum* were reported to reduce blood cholesterol, triacylglycerol, and LDL-cholesterol levels in obese mice in a different study (Cuong et al., 2015).

13.4.3.4 PHLOROTANNINS

Brown seaweeds frequently contain phlorotannins, which are polyphenols based on phloroglucinol. They are made up of phloroglucinol monomers with molecular weights ranging from 126 to 650 Da and are produced via the polyketide pathway. There are numerous ways the phloroglucinol units can be joined together, leading to a wide range of compounds.

Based on the kind of linkage, phlorotannins can be divided into four subclasses: Eckols (with a dibenzodioxin linkage), fucols (with a phenyl linkage), fucophloroethols (with an ether and phenyl linkage), and fuhalols and phlorethols (phlorotannins with ether and phenyl (La Barre et al., 2010). Through a number of methods, including inhibition of pancreatic lipase and restriction of adipocyte development, phlorotannins reduce obesity and the problems associated with it. Phlorotannins from *E. cava* and *E. stolonifera*, for example, reduced lipid accumulation during adipogenesis while having no negative effects on cell survival. Phloroglucinol, eckol, and dieckol inhibited PPAR and C/EBP, respectively, to reduce adipogenesis. Phloroglucinol and eckol also downregulated C/EBP. Preadipocytes underwent apoptosis when exposed to the phlorotannin diphlorethohydroxycarmalol (DPHC) from Ishigeo Kamurae. On the other hand, there are no reports of research on mature adipocytes (Park et al., 2013). Due to its various inhibitions of pancreatic lipase, adipogenesis, and PTP1B, eckol appears to be the most attractive target chemical among the phlorotannins for the development of anti-obesity drugs. However, the majority of phlorotannin investigations were conducted *in vitro* (cell lines and enzyme inhibitory assay). The effectiveness of phlorotannins as anti-obesity drugs merits further research utilizing both human and animal models (Hu et al., 2016).

13.5 COMMERCIAL PRODUCTS OF MARINE NUTRACEUTICALS

Commercial products of marine nutraceuticals are listed in Table 13.2.

TABLE 13.2 Commercial Products of Marine Nutraceuticals

Category	Product Name	Obtained From	Mechanism	References
Seaweeds	CadalminTM	*Green mussel Perna viridis*	Reduces cholesterol and inhibits adipocyte differentiation and lipid absorption.	https://icar.org.in/node/8097
Algae	Xanthigen	*Undaria pinnatifida (BSE) and pomegranate seed oil.*	Increased weight loss, reduced body, and liver fat content, and improved liver function tests in obese non-diabetic women.	Abidov et al. (2010)
Microalgae	FucoVital	*Phaeodactylum tricornutum microalgae.*	It inhibited the lipase activity in the gastrointestinal tract resulting in decreased triglyceride absorption.	https://www.nature.com/articles/d41586-017-06926-1; Younossi et al. (2018)
Microalgae	Spirulina	Spiral blue-green microalgae and filamentous cyanobacterium.	It affects appetite, food absorption, gut microbiota, insulin resistance, oxidative stress, and inflammation.	Moradi et al. (2019)
Fish	Omega-3	Fish	Increased adiponectin and decreased leptin levels.	Gray et al. (2013)
Fish	Collagen	Skin and bones of fish and sharks.	It suppressed the fat accumulation and regulation of lipid metabolism.	Woo et al. (2018)
Algae	Chitozin	*Shells of shrimp* the cell walls of fungi and the exoskeleton of crustaceans. Deacetylation of chitin to varying degrees.	It attenuates obesity by modifying the intestinal microbiota and increasing serum leptin levels.	Tang et al. (2020)

13.6 CONCLUSION

Seaweeds, in particular, as a dietary component, are advantageous in the control of body weight and obesity. Algal substances including fucoxanthin, alginates, fucoidans, and phlorotannins may be used as anti-obesity medications. These substances may be useful for nutritional supplements or nutraceuticals for controlling body weight and obesity. To evaluate the effectiveness of these substances as anti-obesity treatments, further extensive human trials are still required. Further research is needed to identify new pharmacological leads based on algal products in order to create new anti-obesity medications, particularly pancreatic lipase inhibitors.

KEYWORDS

- **alginates**
- **anti-obesity medication**
- **fucoidans**
- **fucoxanthin**
- **marine algae**
- **obesity**
- **phlorotannins**
- **seaweeds**

REFERENCES

Abidov, M., Ramazanov, Z., Seifulla, R., & Grachev, S. (2010). The effects of Xanthigen™ in the weight management of obese premenopausal women with non-alcoholic fatty liver disease and normal liver fat. Diabetes, Obesity & Metabolism, 12(1), 72–81. https://doi.org/10.1111/j.1463-1326.2009.01132.x.

Anraku, M., Fujii, T., Kondo, Y., Kojima, E., Hata, T., Tabuchi, N., & Tsutsumi, H. (2011). Antioxidant properties of high molecular weight dietary chitosan in vitro and in vivo. Carbohydrate Polymers, 83, 501–505. https://doi.org/10.1016/j.carbpol.2010.08.005.

Asai, A., Sugawara, T., Ono, H., & Nagao, A. (2004). Biotransformation of fucoxanthinol in amarouciaxanthin A in mice and Hep-G2 cells: Formation and cytotoxicity of fucoxanthin metabolites. Drug Metabolism and Disposition, 32(2), 205–211. https://doi.org/10.1124/dmd.32.2.205.

Awang, A. N., Ng, J. L., Matanjun, P., Sulaiman, M. R., Tan, T. S., & Ooi, Y. B. (2014). Anti-obesity property of the brown seaweed, Sargassum polycystum using an in vivo animal model. Journal of Applied Phycology, 26(2), 1043–1048. https://doi.org/10.1007/s10811-013-0133-6.

Bakshi, P. S., Selvakumar, D., Kadirvelu, K., & Kumar, N. S. (2018). Comparative study on antimicrobial activity and biocompatibility of N-selective chitosan derivatives. Reactive and Functional Polymers, 124, 149–155. https://doi.org/10.1016/j.reactfunctpolym.2018.01.002.

Beppu, F., Niwano, Y., Tsukui, T., Hosokawa, M., & Miyashita, K. (2009). Single and repeated oral dose toxicity study of fucoxanthin (FX), a marine carotenoid, in mice. Journal of Toxicological Sciences, 34(5), 501–510. https://doi.org/10.2131/jts.34.501.

Beygmoradi, A., Homaei, A., Hemmati, R., Santos-Moriano, P., Hormigo, D., & Fernández-Lucas, J. (2018). Marine chitinolytic enzymes, a biotechnological treasure hidden in the ocean? Applied Microbiology and Biotechnology, 102(22), 9937–9948. https://doi.org/10.1007/s00253-018-9303-y.

Biris-Dorhoi, E. S., Michiu, D., Pop, C. R., Rotar, A. M., Tofana, M., Pop, O. L., & Farcas, A. C. (2020). Macroalgae—A sustainable source of chemical compounds with biological activities. Nutrients, 12(10), 3085. https://doi.org/10.3390/nu12103085.

Bitou, N., Ninomiya, M., Tsujita, T., & Okuda, H. (1999). Screening of lipase inhibitors from marine algae. Lipids, 34(4), 441–445. https://doi.org/10.1007/s11745-999-0383-6.

Bixler, H. J., & Porse, H. (2011). A decade of change in the seaweed hydrocolloids industry. Journal of Applied Phycology, 23(3), 321–335. https://doi.org/10.1007/s10811-010-9567-6.

Brown, E. S., Allsopp, P. J., Magee, P. J., Gill, C. I., Nitecki, S., Strain, C. R., & McSorley, E. M. (2014). Seaweed and human health. Nutrition Reviews, 72(3), 205–216. https://doi.org/10.1111/nure.12091.

Cavalli-Sforza, L. T., Rosman, A., de Boer, A. S., & Darnton-Hill, I. (1996). Nutritional aspects of changes in disease patterns in the Western Pacific region. *Bulletin of the World Health Organization, 74*(3), 307–318.

Centella, M. H., Arévalo-Gallegos, A., Parra-Saldivar, R., & Iqbal, H. M. N. (2017). Marine-derived bioactive compounds for value-added applications in bio- and non-bio sectors. Journal of Cleaner Production, 168, 1559–1565. https://doi.org/10.1016/j.jclepro.2017.09.162.

Charu, G., & Dhan, P. (2015). Nutraceuticals for geriatrics. Journal of Traditional and Complementary Medicine, 5(1), 5–14. https://doi.org/10.1016/j.jtcme.2014.10.005.

Chater, P. I., Wilcox, M. D., Houghton, D., & Pearson, J. P. (2015). The role of seaweed bioactives in the control of digestion: Implications for obesity treatments. Food & Function, 6(11), 3420–3427. https://doi.org/10.1039/C5FO00720F.

Chater, P. I., Wilcox, M., Cherry, P., Herford, A., Mustar, S., Wheater, H., & Pearson, J. (2016). Inhibitory activity of extracts of Hebridean brown seaweeds on lipase activity. Journal of Applied Phycology, 28(2), 1303–1313. https://doi.org/10.1007/s10811-015-0631-7.

Chu, W. L. (2011). Potential applications of antioxidant compounds derived from algae. Current Topics in Nutraceutical Research, 9, 83.

Cuong, H. D., Thuy, T. T., Huong, T. T., Ly, B. M., & Van, T. T. (2015). Structure and hypolipidaemic activity of fucoidan extracted from brown seaweed Sargassum henslowianum. Natural Product Research, 29(5), 411–415. https://doi.org/10.1080/14786419.2014.922495.

De Jesus Raposo, M. F., De Morais, R. M. S. C., & De Morais, A. M. M. B. (2013). Health applications of bioactive compounds from marine microalgae. Life Sciences, 93(14–16), 479–486. https://doi.org/10.1016/j.lfs.2013.06.001.

Debbab, A., Aly, A. H., Lin, W. H., & Proksch, P. (2010). Bioactive compounds from marine bacteria and fungi: Minireview. Microbial Biotechnology, 3(5), 544–563. https://doi.org/10.1111/j.1751-7915.2010.00192.x.

Draget, K. I., & Taylor, C. (2011). Chemical, physical and biological properties of alginates and their biomedical implications. Food Hydrocolloids, 25(2), 251–256. https://doi.org/10.1016/j.foodhyd.2010.06.005.

Drewnowski, A., & Popkin, B. M. (1997). The nutrition transition: New trends in the global diet. Nutrition Reviews, 55(1), 31–43. https://doi.org/10.1111/j.1753-4887.1997.tb01593.x.

El Khoury, D., Goff, H. D., Berengut, S., Kubant, R., & Anderson, G. H. (2014). Effect of sodium alginate addition to chocolate milk on glycemia, insulin, appetite and food intake in healthy adult men. *European Journal of Clinical Nutrition, 68*(5), 613–618. https://doi.org/10.1038/ejcn.2014.8.

Gammone, M. A., & D'Orazio, N. (2015). Anti-obesity activity of the marine carotenoid fucoxanthin. *Marine Drugs, 13*(4), 2196–2214. https://doi.org/10.3390/md13042196.

Ganesan, A. R., Saravana Guru, M., Balasubramanian, B., Mohan, K., Chao Liu, W., Valan Arasu, M., et al. (2020). Biopolymer from edible marine invertebrates: A potential functional food. *Journal of King Saud University – Science, 32*(4), 1772–1777. https://doi.org/10.1016/j.jksus.2020.01.036.

Grasa-López, A., Miliar-García, A., Quevedo-Corona, L., Paniagua-Castro, N., Escalona-Cardoso, G., Reyes-Maldonado, E., & Jaramillo-Flores, M. (2016). Undaria pinnatifida and fucoxanthin ameliorate lipogenesis and markers of both inflammation and cardiovascular dysfunction in an animal model of diet-induced obesity. *Marine Drugs, 14*(8), 148. https://doi.org/10.3390/md14080148.

Grienke, U., Silke, J., & Tasdemir, D. (2014). Bioactive compounds from marine mussels and their effects on human health. *Food Chemistry, 142*, 48–60. https://doi.org/10.1016/j.foodchem.2013.07.077.

Gurpilhares, D. D. B., Cinelli, L. P., Simas, N. K., Pessoa, A., & Sette, L. D. (2019). Marine prebiotics: Polysaccharides and oligosaccharides obtained by using microbial enzymes. *Food Chemistry, 280*, 175–186. https://doi.org/10.1016/j.foodchem.2018.12.092.

Hamed, A. A., Abdelhamid, I. A., Saad, G. R., Elkady, N. A., & Elsabee, M. Z. (2020). Synthesis, characterization and antimicrobial activity of a novel chitosan Schiff bases based on heterocyclic moieties. *International Journal of Biological Macromolecules, 153*, 492–501. https://doi.org/10.1016/j.ijbiomac.2020.02.038.

Hamed, I., Özogul, F., Özogul, Y., & Regenstein, J. M. (2015). Marine bioactive compounds and their health benefits: A review. *Comprehensive Reviews in Food Science and Food Safety, 14*(4), 446–465. https://doi.org/10.1111/1541-4337.12151.

Hashimoto, T., Ozaki, Y., Taminato, M., Das, S. K., Mizuno, M., Yoshimura, K., Maoka, T., & Kanazawa, K. (2009). The distribution and accumulation of fucoxanthin and its metabolites after oral administration in mice. *British Journal of Nutrition, 102*(2), 242–248. https://doi.org/10.1017/S0007114508163457.

Hill, R. T., & Fenical, W. (2010). Pharmaceuticals from marine natural products: Surge or ebb? *Current Opinion in Biotechnology, 21*(6), 777–779. https://doi.org/10.1016/j.copbio.2010.09.010.

Hoffman, D. R., Boettcher, J. A., & Diersen-Schade, D. A. (2009). Toward optimizing vision and cognition in term infants by dietary docosahexaenoic and arachidonic acid supplementation: A review of randomized controlled trials. *Prostaglandins, Leukotrienes and Essential Fatty Acids, 81*(2–3), 151–158. https://doi.org/10.1016/j.plefa.2009.05.003.

Hosseini, S. F., Rezaei, M., & Mcclements, D. J. (2020). Bioactive functional ingredients from aquatic origin: A review of recent progress in marine-derived nutraceuticals. *Critical Reviews in Food Science and Nutrition*, 1242–1269. Advance online publication. https://doi.org/10.1080/10408398.2020.1817096.

Houghton, D., Wilcox, M. D., Chater, P. I., Brownlee, I. A., Seal, C. J., & Pearson, J. P. (2015). Biological activity of alginate and its effect on pancreatic lipase inhibition as a potential treatment for obesity. *Food Hydrocolloids, 49*, 18–24. https://doi.org/10.1016/j.foodhyd.2015.02.014.

Hu, X., Tao, N., Wang, X., Xiao, J., & Wang, M. (2016). Marine-derived bioactive compounds with anti-obesity effect: A review. *Journal of Functional Foods, 21*, 372–387. https://doi.org/10.1016/j.jff.2015.12.022.

Idota, Y., Kogure, Y., Kato, T., Ogawa, M., Kobayashi, S., Kakinuma, C., Yano, K., Arakawa, H., Miyajima, C., Kasahara, F., et al. (2016). Cholesterol-lowering effect of calcium alginate in rats. *Biological and Pharmaceutical Bulletin, 39*(1), 62–67. https://doi.org/10.1248/bpb.b15-00587.

Izadpanah, F., Homaei, A., Fernandes, P., & Javadpour, S. (2018). Marine microbial L-asparaginase: Biochemistry, molecular approaches and applications in tumor therapy and in food industry. *Microbiological Research, 208*, 99–112. https://doi.org/10.1016/j.micres.2018.04.004.

Jensen, M. G., Pedersen, C., Kristensen, M., Frost, G., & Astrup, A. (2013). Efficacy of alginate supplementation in relation to appetite regulation and metabolic risk factors: Evidence from animal and human studies. *Obesity Reviews, 14*(2), 129–144. https://doi.org/10.1111/obr.12044.

Jin, W., Zhang, W., Liang, H., & Zhang, Q. (2015). The structure-activity relationship between marine algae polysaccharides and anti-complement activity. *Marine Drugs, 13*(1), 1–15. https://doi.org/10.3390/md13010001.

Kadekaru, T., Toyama, H., & Yasumoto, T. (2008). Safety evaluation of fucoxanthin purified from Undaria pinnatifida. *Nippon Shokuhin Kagaku Kogaku Kaishi, 55*(7), 304–308. https://doi.org/10.3136/nskkk.55.304.

Kakkar, A. K., & Dahiya, N. (2015). Drug treatment of obesity: Current status and future prospects. *European Journal of Internal Medicine, 26*, 89–94. https://doi.org/10.1016/j.ejim.2014.12.015.

Kang, M. C., Kang, N., Kim, S. Y., Lima, I. S., Ko, S. C., Kim, Y. T., & Jeon, Y. J. (2016). Popular edible seaweed, Gelidium amansii prevents against diet-induced obesity. *Food and Chemical Toxicology, 90*, 181–187. https://doi.org/10.1016/j.fct.2016.02.024.

Kang, S. I., Shin, H. S., Kim, H. M., Yoon, S. A., Kang, S. W., Kim, J. H., & Kim, S. J. (2012). Petalonia binghamiae extract and its constituent fucoxanthin ameliorate high-fat diet-induced obesity by activating AMP-activated protein kinase. *Journal of Agricultural and Food Chemistry, 60*(14), 3389–3395. https://doi.org/10.1021/jf3002412.

Keith, W. G. (2009). *Marine Products for Healthcare: Functional and Bioactive Nutraceutical Compounds from the Ocean.* CRC Press Taylor and Francis Group.

Keservani, R. K., & Sharma, A. K. (2014). Flavonoids: Emerging trends and potential health benefits. *Journal of Chinese Pharmaceutical Sciences, 23*(12), 815.

Keservani, R. K., Kesharwani, R. K., Sharma, A. K., Vyas, N., & Chadoker, A. (2010b). Nutritional supplements: An overview. *International Journal of Current Pharmaceutical Review and Research, 1*(1), 59–75.

Keservani, R. K., Kesharwani, R. K., Vyas, N., Jain, S., Raghuvanshi, R., & Sharma, A. K. (2010a). Nutraceutical and functional food as future food: A review. *Der Pharmacia Lettre, 2*(1), 106–116.

Keservani, R. K., Sharma, A. K., & Kesharwani, R. K. (2016a). Nutraceutical and functional foods for cardiovascular health. In R. K. Keservani, A. K. Sharma, & R. K. Kesharwani (Eds.), *Food process engineering* (pp. 257–278). Apple Academic Press, CRC Press. ISBN: 9781771884020.

Keservani, R. K., Sharma, A. K., & Kesharwani, R. K. (2016b). Medicinal effect of nutraceutical fruits for cognition and brain health. *Scientifica,* 2016. *Article ID 3109254*, 10 pages. https://doi.org/10.1155/2016/3109254.

Keservani, R. K., Sharma, A. K., & Kesharwani, R. K. (2017). An overview and therapeutic applications of nutraceutical and functional foods. In *Recent advances in drug delivery technology* (pp. 160–201). ISBN: 9781522507543.

Keservani, R. K., Sharma, A. K., & Kesharwani, R. K. (Eds.). (2020). *Nutraceuticals and Dietary Supplements: Applications in Health Improvement and Disease Management*, 1–15. CRC Press. ISBN: 9781771888738.

Khoo, K. S., Chew, K. W., Yew, G. Y., Leong, W. H., Chai, Y. H., Show, P. L., et al. (2020). Recent advances in downstream processing of microalgae lipid recovery for biofuel production. *Bioresource Technology, 304*, 122996. https://doi.org/10.1016/j.biortech.2020.122996.

Kim, M. J., Jeon, J., & Lee, J. S. (2014). Fucoidan prevents high-fat diet-induced obesity in animals by suppression of fat accumulation. *Phytotherapy Research, 28*(1), 137–143. https://doi.org/10.1002/ptr.4965.

Kim, S. M., Jung, Y. J., Kwon, O. N., Cha, K. H., Um, B. H., Chung, C. D., & Pan, C. H. (2012). A potential commercial source of fucoxanthin extracted from the microalga Phaeodactylum tricornutum. *Applied Biochemistry and Biotechnology, 166*(7), 1843–1855. https://doi.org/10.1007/s12010-011-9530-3.

Kim, S. M., Kang, S. W., Kwon, O. N., Chung, C. D., & Pan, C. H. (2012). Fucoxanthin as a major carotenoid in Isochrysis aff. galbana: Characterization of extraction for commercial application. *Journal of the Korean Society of Applied Biological Chemistry, 55*(5), 477–483. https://doi.org/10.1007/s13765-012-2121-0.

Kraan, S. (2013). *Pigments and Minor Compounds in Algae*. Woodhead Publishing Limited.

Kristensen, M., & Jensen, M. G. (2011). Dietary fibres in the regulation of appetite and food intake: Importance of viscosity. *Appetite, 56*(1), 65–70. https://doi.org/10.1016/j.appet.2010.11.147.

La Barre, S., Potin, P., Leblanc, C., & Delage, L. (2010). The halogenated metabolism of brown algae (Phaeophyta), its biological importance and its environmental significance. *Marine Drugs, 8*(4), 988–1010. https://doi.org/10.3390/md8040988.

Lange, K. W., Hauser, J., Nakamura, Y., & Kanaya, S. (2015). Dietary seaweeds and obesity. *Food Science & Human Wellness, 4*(2), 87–96. https://doi.org/10.1016/j.fshw.2015.07.001.

Liu, R. H. (2003). Health benefits of fruit and vegetables are from additive and synergistic combinations of phytochemicals. *American Journal of Clinical Nutrition, 78*(3), 517S–520S. https://doi.org/10.1093/ajcn/78.3.517S.

Luiten, E. E., Akkerman, I., Koulman, A., Kamermans, P., Reith, H., Barbosa, M. J., & Wijffels, R. H. (2003). Realizing the promises of marine biotechnology. *Biomolecular Engineering, 20*(4–6), 429–439. https://doi.org/10.1016/S1389-0344(03)00084-6.

MacArtain, P., Gill, C. I., Brooks, M., Campbell, R., & Rowland, I. R. (2007). Nutritional value of edible seaweeds. *Nutrition Reviews, 65*(12), 535–543. https://doi.org/10.1111/j.1753-4887.2007.tb00325.x.

Maeda, H. (2015). Nutraceutical effects of fucoxanthin for obesity and diabetes therapy: A review. *Journal of Oleo Science, 64*(3), 125–132. https://doi.org/10.5650/jos.ess14221.

Maeda, H., Hosokawa, M., Sashima, T., & Miyashita, K. (2007). Dietary combination of fucoxanthin and fish oil attenuates the weight gain of white adipose tissue and decreases blood glucose in obese/diabetic KK-Ay mice. *Journal of Agricultural and Food Chemistry, 55*(19), 7701–7706. https://doi.org/10.1021/jf071569n.

Maeda, H., Hosokawa, M., Sashima, T., Murakami-Funayama, K., & Miyashita, K. (2009). Anti-obesity and anti-diabetic effects of fucoxanthin on diet-induced obesity conditions in a murine model. *Molecular Medicine Reports, 2*(6), 897–902. https://doi.org/10.3892/mmr_00000189.

Maeda, H., Kanno, S., Kodate, M., Hosokawa, M., & Miyashita, K. (2015). Fucoxanthinol, metabolite of fucoxanthin, improves obesity-induced inflammation in adipocyte cells. *Marine Drugs, 13*(8), 4799–4813. https://doi.org/10.3390/md13084799.

Maeda, H., Tsukui, T., Sashima, T., Hosokawa, M., & Miyashita, K. (2008). Seaweed carotenoid, fucoxanthin, as a multi-functional nutrient. *Asia Pacific Journal of Clinical Nutrition, 17*(S1), 196–199.

Matsumoto, M., Hosokawa, M., Matsukawa, N., Hagio, M., Shinoki, A., Nishimukai, M., et al. (2010). Suppressive effects of the marine carotenoids, fucoxanthin and fucoxanthinol on triglyceride absorption in lymph duct-cannulated rats. *European Journal of Nutrition, 49*(4), 243–249. https://doi.org/10.1007/s00394-009-0078-1.

Matsumura, Y. (2001). Nutrition trends in Japan. *Asia Pacific Journal of Clinical Nutrition, 10*(S1), S40–S47. https://doi.org/10.1046/j.1440-6047.2001.00123.x.

Matsuno, T. (2001). Aquatic animal carotenoids. *Fisheries Science, 67*(5), 771–783. https://doi.org/10.1046/j.1444-2906.2001.00320.x.

Menaa, F., Wijesinghe, P. A. U. I., Thiripuranathar, G., Uzair, B., Iqbal, H., Khan, B. A., & Menaa, B. (2020). Ecological and industrial implications of dynamic seaweed-associated microbiota interactions. *Marine Drugs, 18*(12), 641. https://doi.org/10.3390/md18120641.

Mise, T., Ueda, M., & Yasumoto, T. (2011). Production of fucoxanthin-rich powder from Cladophora okamuranus. *Advance Journal of Food Science and Technology, 3*(2), 73–76.

Miyashita, K., Nishikawa, S., Beppu, F., Tsukui, T., Abe, M., & Hosokawa, M. (2011). The allenic carotenoid fucoxanthin, a novel marine nutraceutical from brown seaweeds. *Journal of the Science of Food and Agriculture, 91*(7), 1166–1174. https://doi.org/10.1002/jsfa.4326.

Naczk, M., & Shahidi, F. (2004). *Phenolics in Food and Nutraceuticals*. CRC Press. ISBN: 9780849316721.

Nagaoka, I., Igarashi, M., Hua, J., Ju, Y., Yomogida, S., & Sakamoto, K. (2011). Recent aspects of the anti-inflammatory actions of glucosamine. *Carbohydrate Polymers, 84*(2), 825–830. https://doi.org/10.1016/j.carbpol.2010.12.030.

Nakazono, S., Cho, K., Isaka, S., Abu, R., Yokose, T., Murata, M., Ueno, M., Tachibana, K., Hirasaka, K., Kim, D., et al. (2016). Anti-obesity effects of enzymatically-digested alginate oligomer in mice model fed a high-fat diet. *Bioactive Carbohydrates and Dietary Fibre, 7*(1), 1–8. https://doi.org/10.1016/j.bcdf.2016.04.002.

Nasab, S. B., Homaei, A., Pletschke, B. I., Salinas-Salazar, C., Castillo-Zacarias, C., & Parra-Saldívar, R. (2020). Marine resources effective in controlling and treating diabetes and its associated complications. *Process Biochemistry, 92*, 313–342. https://doi.org/10.1016/j.procbio.2019.11.018.

Ngamwonglumlert, L., & Devahastin, S. (2019). Carotenoids. In L. Melton, F. Shahidi, & P. Varelis (Eds.), *Encyclopedia of Food Chemistry* (pp. 485–495). Elsevier. https://doi.org/10.1016/B978-0-08-100596-5.22320-6.

Noitup, P., Garnjanagoonchorn, W., & Morrissey, M. T. (2005). Fish skin type I collagen. *Journal of Aquatic Food Product Technology, 14*(1), 17–28. https://doi.org/10.1300/J030v14n01_03.

Norris, R., Harnedy, P. A., & FitzGerald, R. J. (2013). Antihypertensive peptides from marine sources. In *Bioactive Compounds from Marine Foods: Plant and Animal Sources* (pp. 506–517). John Wiley & Sons, Ltd. https://doi.org/10.1002/9781118412893.ch22.

Park, M. H., Jeon, Y. J., Kim, H. J., & Han, J. S. (2013). Effect of diphlorethohydroxycarmalol isolated from Ishige okamurae on apoptosis in 3T3-L1 preadipocytes. *Phytotherapy Research, 27*(6), 931–936. https://doi.org/10.1002/ptr.4818.

Park, M. K., Jung, U., & Roh, C. (2011). Fucoidan from marine brown algae inhibits lipid accumulation. *Marine Drugs, 9*(8), 1359–1367. https://doi.org/10.3390/md9081359.

Pelkman, C. L., Navia, J. L., Miller, A. E., & Pohle, R. J. (2007). Novel calcium gelled, alginate-pectin beverage reduced energy intake in non-dieting overweight and obese women: Interactions with restraint status. *American Journal of Clinical Nutrition, 86*(5), 1595–1602. https://doi.org/10.1093/ajcn/86.5.1595.

Phang, S. M. (2010). Potential products from tropical algae and seaweeds, especially with reference to Malaysia. *Malaysian Journal of Science, 29*(3), 160–166. https://doi.org/10.22452/mjs.vol29no3.5.

Pooja, K., Rani, S., Rana, V., & Pal, G. K. (2022). Aquatic plants as a natural source of antimicrobial and functional ingredients. Elsevier. ISBN: 9780323994914.

Prabha, S. P., Nagappan, S., Rathna, R., Viveka, R., & Nakkeeran, E. (2019). Blue biotechnology: A vision for future marine biorefineries. Elsevier. ISBN: 9780128176634.

Puls, W., Krause, H. P., Muller, L., Schutt, H., Sitt, R., & Thomas, G. (1985). Inhibitors of the rate of carbohydrate and lipid absorption by the intestine. In A. C. Sullivan & S. Garattini (Eds.), *Novel Approaches and Drugs for Obesity* (pp. 181–190). John Libbey & Co., Ltd.

Rebah, F. B., Smaoui, S., Frikha, F., Gargouri, Y., & Miled, N. (2008). Inhibitory effects of Tunisian marine algal extracts on digestive lipases. *Applied Biochemistry and Biotechnology, 151*(1), 71–79. https://doi.org/10.1007/s12010-008-8173-5.

Richardson, J. C., Dettmar, P. W., Wilcox, M. D., Brownlee, I. A., & Pearson, J. P. (2010). Inhibition of pancreatic lipase. U.S. Patent No. 8,084,054. U.S. Patent and Trademark Office.

Romano, G., Costantini, M., Sansone, C., Lauritano, C., Ruocco, N., & Ianora, A. (2017). Marine microorganisms as a promising and sustainable source of bioactive molecules. Marine Environmental Research, 128, 58–69. https://doi.org/10.1016/j.marenvres.2016.05.002.

Rosic, N. N. (2021). Recent advances in the discovery of novel marine natural products and mycosporine-like amino acid UV-absorbing compounds. Applied Microbiology and Biotechnology, 105, 7053–7067. https://doi.org/10.1007/s00253-021-11583-5.

Shahidi, F., & Ambigaipalan, P. (2015). Novel functional food ingredients from marine sources. Current Opinion in Food Science, 2, 123–129. https://doi.org/10.1016/j.cofs.2015.03.008.

Stiger-Pouvreau, V., Bourgougnon, N., & Deslandes, E. (2016). Carbohydrates from seaweeds. In J. Fleurence & I. Levine (Eds.), Seaweeds in Health and Disease Prevention (pp. 223–274). Academic Press.

Sudhakar, M. P., Kumar, B. R., Mathimani, T., & Arunkumar, K. (2019). A review on bioenergy and bioactive compounds from microalgae and macroalgae—Sustainable energy perspective. Journal of Cleaner Production, 228, 1320–1333. https://doi.org/10.1016/j.jclepro.2019.04.161.

Suleria, H. A. R., Gobe, G., Masci, P., & Osborne, S. A. (2016). Marine bioactive compounds and health promoting perspectives: Innovation pathways for drug discovery. Trends in Food Science & Technology, 50, 44–55. https://doi.org/10.1016/j.tifs.2015.10.015.

Suleria, H. A. R., Osborne, S., Masci, P., & Gobe, G. (2015). Marine-based nutraceuticals: An innovative trend in the food and supplement industries. Marine Drugs, 13(10), 6336–6351. https://doi.org/10.3390/md13106336.

Tan, C. P., & Hou, Y. H. (2014). First evidence for the anti-inflammatory activity of fucoxanthin in high-fat-diet-induced obesity in mice and the antioxidant functions in PC12 cells. Inflammation, 37(2), 443–449. https://doi.org/10.1007/s10753-013-9766-5.

Thakur, M. (2020). Marine Bioactive Components: Sources, Health Benefits, and Future Prospects. In Technological Processes for Marine Foods-from Water to Fork: Bioactive Compounds, Industrial Applications and Genomics (pp. 61–72). Apple Academic Press.

Thorpe, J. P., Sole-Cava, A. M., & Watts, P. C. (2000). Exploited marine invertebrates: Genetics and fisheries. Hydrobiologia, 420, 165–184. https://doi.org/10.1023/A:1003980114143.

Udayangani, R. M. A. C., Somasiri, G. D. P., Wickramasinghe, I., & Kim, S. (2020). Potential health benefits of sulfated polysaccharides from marine algae. In Encyclopedia of Marine Biotechnology (pp. 629–635). Wiley-Blackwell.

Uranga, J., Leceta, I., Etxabide, A., Guerrero, P., & Caba, K. D. (2016). Crosslinking of fish gelatins to develop sustainable films with enhanced properties. European Polymer Journal, 78, 82–90. https://doi.org/10.1016/j.eurpolymj.2016.03.031.

Voultsiadou, E. (2010). Therapeutic properties and uses of marine invertebrates in the ancient Greek world and early Byzantium. Journal of Ethnopharmacology, 130(2), 237–247. https://doi.org/10.1016/j.jep.2010.05.038.

Wang, T., Jónsdóttir, R., & Ólafsdóttir, G. (2009). Total phenolic compounds, radical scavenging and metal chelation of extracts from Icelandic seaweeds. Food Chemistry, 116(1), 240–248. https://doi.org/10.1016/j.foodchem.2009.01.051.

Wilcox, M. D., Brownlee, I. A., Richardson, J. C., Dettmar, P. W., & Pearson, J. P. (2014). The modulation of pancreatic lipase activity by alginates. Food Chemistry, 146, 479–484. https://doi.org/10.1016/j.foodchem.2013.09.080.

Woo, M. N., Jeon, S. M., Kim, H. J., Lee, M. K., Shin, S. K., Shin, Y. C., Park, Y. B., & Choi, M. S. (2010). Fucoxanthin supplementation improves plasma and hepatic lipid metabolism and blood glucose concentration in high-fat fed C57BL/6N mice. Chemico-Biological Interactions, 186(3), 316–322. https://doi.org/10.1016/j.cbi.2010.04.012.

Wu, L., Sun, J., Su, X., Yu, Q., Yu, Q., & Zhang, P. (2016). A review about the development of fucoidan in antitumor activity: Progress and challenges. Carbohydrate Polymers, 15, 96–111. https://doi.org/10.1016/j.carbpol.2015.11.020.

Yoshinaga, J., Morita, M., Yukawa, M., Shiraishi, K., & Kawamura, H. (2001). Certified reference material for analytical quality assurance of minor and trace elements in food and related matrixes based on a typical Japanese diet: Interlaboratory study. Journal of AOAC International, 84(4), 1202–1208. https://doi.org/10.1093/jaoac/84.4.1202.

Zaragoza, M. C., López, D., Sáiz, M. P., Poquet, M., Pérez, J., Puig-Parellada, P., Marmol, F., Simonetti, P., Gardana, C., Lerat, Y., et al. (2008). Toxicity and antioxidant activity in vitro and in vivo of two Fucus vesiculosus extracts. Journal of Agricultural and Food Chemistry, 56(16), 7773–7780. https://doi.org/10.1021/jf8003086.

Zhu, B., Ni, F., Xiong, Q., & Yao, Z. (2011). Marine oligosaccharides originated from seaweeds: Source, preparation, structure, physiological activity and applications. Critical Reviews in Food Science and Nutrition, 61, 60–74. https://doi.org/10.1080/10408398.2018.1540895.

CHAPTER 14

THE ROLE OF FUNCTIONAL FOODS TO COMBAT WEIGHT GAIN AND OBESITY

EKNATH D. AHIRE,[1] RAHUL LAXMAN JADHAV,[2] MANISHA VYANKATRAO PATIL,[3] and RAJ K. KESERVANI[4]

[1]*Department of Pharmaceutics, METs, Institute of Pharmacy, BKC, SPPU, Adgoan, Nashik, Maharashtra, India*

[2]*Principal, Shivraj College of Pharmacy, Gadhinglaj, Kolhapur, Maharashtra, India*

[3]*Professor, Adarsh College of Pharmacy, Vita, Sangli, Maharashtra, India*

[4]*Associate Professor, Faculty of B. Pharmacy, CSM Group of Institutions, Prayagraj, Uttar Pradesh, India*

ABSTRACT

Obesity is an increasing public health concern, especially in underdeveloped countries. Weight management and obesity prevention are emphasized to reduce metabolic disorders. New eating behaviors, production, and consumption trends contribute to the global obesity crisis. Dietary and lifestyle changes are important for managing obesity, but functional foods may also help with weight loss and prevention. Diet and exercise are key to preventing and treating obesity. Because of the potential side effects of obesity medicines, natural components, and functional diets are gaining popularity for treating obesity. Functional foods seem like conventional foods but are healthier. Functional meals can help healthy adults maintain a

Nutraceuticals in Obesity Management and Control. Raj K. Keservani & Alka Lohani (Eds.)

healthy weight, according to studies. Functional foods that reduce appetite and enhance happiness and those that speed up the body's metabolism have been examined as obesity therapies. Nutraceutical therapy for obesity and weight loss is under investigation. Low-glycemic index foods, chromium, green tea extract, and 5-hydroxytryptophan promote weight loss. Each component boosts weight loss in clinical experiments.

14.1 INTRODUCTION

According to the World Health Organization, obesity is a severe problem that has far-reaching repercussions on people's social, physiological, and mental health (World Health Organization). A body mass index (BMI) of 30 kg/m^2 is used to define obesity, which is associated with an elevated risk of chronic diseases, morbidity, and mortality (Wollner et al., 2017). Studies conducted in Europe show that childhood obesity is rapidly becoming a serious health problem, especially in Mediterranean countries where obesity rates are already rather high (Farajian et al., 2011). Occupying a prominent place on the obesity scale is a complex issue. Genetic factors, diseases, lifestyle, medications, inflammation, and food diet are examples of both causal and reactive factors.

Instructing people to eat less of all meals may not be effective for weight loss since high-energy-dense foods increase energy intake more than foods with lower energy density (Konstantinidi & Koutelidakis, 2019). Methods that promote a healthy diet (like the Mediterranean diet) and regular physical activity may be more effective in the long run because they help people eat more foods that are low in energy density (Rolls, 2014). There are a variety of definitions for "functional foods" used by various groups and agencies (Bigliardi & Galati, 2013). In the 1980s, Japan's Ministry of Health and Welfare established a regulating framework for foods with potential health advantages, which led to the first definition of functional foods (FFs). Besides its nutritional value, food can be considered "functional" if it significantly affects specific bodily functions with the intention of enhancing health and well-being and/or decreasing the prevalence of chronic diseases. As stated in The IFT Expert Panel Report, Functional Foods Opportunities and Challenges (for the intended population), "functional foods" are defined as foods and food components that deliver a health benefit beyond basic nutrition (IFT, 2005). In addition to the essential nutrients needed for proper maintenance, growth, and development, these compounds also provide a variety of other biologically active components that have been shown to have positive impacts on health. The use of functional foods in people's diets is rapidly growing in popularity (Brown et al., 2015). The term "functional foods" refers to foods that have been formulated to perform a specific function, as opposed to merely satisfying hunger. In addition to their nutritional value, foods are considered "functional" when there is evidence that they may also improve the performance of specific bodily processes, leading to enhanced health and/or a reduced risk of developing a chronic disease (Brown et al., 2018; Martirosyan & Singh, 2015). However, statements about the nutritional value and health benefits of functional meals for the purpose of disease prevention have only been validated under specific conditions where there is sufficient scientific evidence to back up the claimed properties of the food. In addition, there is mounting evidence that functional foods, like those included in the Mediterranean diet, may improve human health, but only when they are part of a comprehensively healthy eating plan (Ntrigiou et al., 2018; Elmaliklis et al., 2019; Koutelidakis & Dimou, 2016). Figure 14.1 shows the relationship between energy expenditure (EE) and energy intake (EI) in maintaining a constant body weight. Over time, even a small disruption in this energy balance can result in significant weight gain or loss and contribute to obesity.

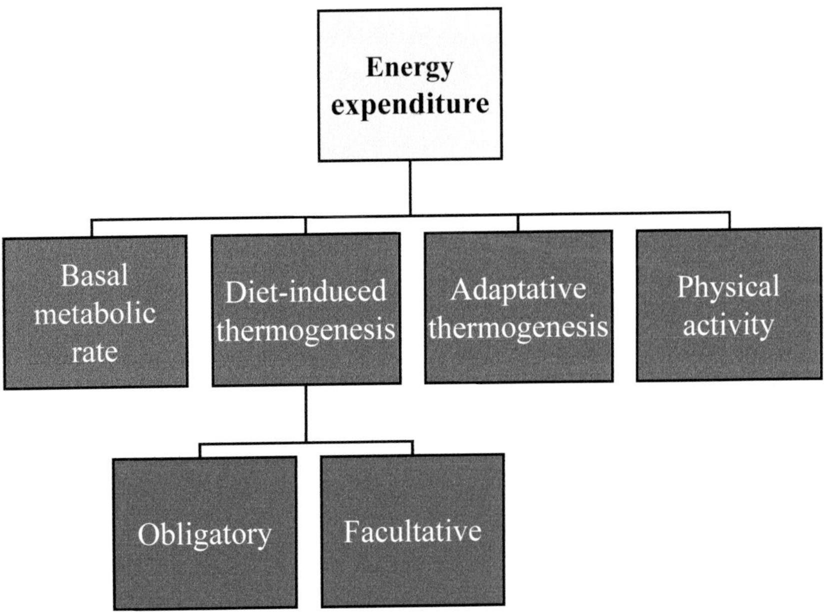

FIGURE 14.1 Primary drivers of energy costs.

In addition to being associated with other chronic diseases, obesity ranks high on the list of global health concerns. Minor dietary adjustments, such as the addition of functional foods for weight management, can help people avoid gaining weight due to subtle shifts in their energy balance (Koutelidakis & Dimou, 2016). It's been shown that cutting calories and boosting activity can lead to weight loss, but these changes can be hard to make and keep up with (Anderson et al., 2001). One of the goals of including functional meals in weight management is to reduce appetite. It stands to reason that this would lead to less hunger and, ultimately, a slimmer you. Therefore, a weight-loss diet may benefit from the inclusion of functional foods that influence metabolic activity and fat partitioning. Among the categories of foods that could serve a functional purpose are dietary fats. Many studies have shown that increasing dietary fiber intake can help dieters lose weight and keep it off. The following are some examples of functional foods that have antiobese properties: capsaicin, conjugated linoleic acid (CLA), *Momordica charantia* (MC), and psyllium fiber (Kasbia, 2005). Food supplements containing chitosan, glucomannan, G sylvestre, fenugreek, and vitamin C have been shown to reduce body fat and weight in obese patients. Some bioactive components in these foods, such as caffeine, gallic acid, catechins, anthocyanins, polyphenols, ascorbic acid, oleuropein, quercetin, and capsaicin, have been linked to weight loss, prevention of obesity, and amelioration of obesity's metabolic consequences (Kasbia, 2005). Consequently, this chapter provides a comprehensive analysis of all conceivable types of functional foods, as shown in Figure 14.2.

14.2 NUTRIENTS WITH CARBOHYDRATES

Fiber in the diet aids in the prevention of chronic diseases in a number of ways. To some extent, weight growth is related to the glycemic index (GI) of carbohydrates and the fiber content of diets. Hunger levels could be affected by dietary fiber, both because of the qualities it lends to food and because of the physiological impact it has on the consumer. It's possible that high-fiber diets, by providing bulk and leading to abdominal distention, can help you feel full faster (Kasbia, 2005). The majority of research into this effect has indicated that it leads to feelings of fullness and reduced hunger (Dikeman & Fahey Jr, 2006). To achieve satiety and appetite suppression, the macronutrient content of one's diet is paramount (Larsen et al., 2010). Kozuka et al. studied the effects of brown rice and oryzanol on mice's aversion to dietary fat (2012). -Oryzanol, found in brown rice bran, is a mixture of ferulic acid esters. Mice

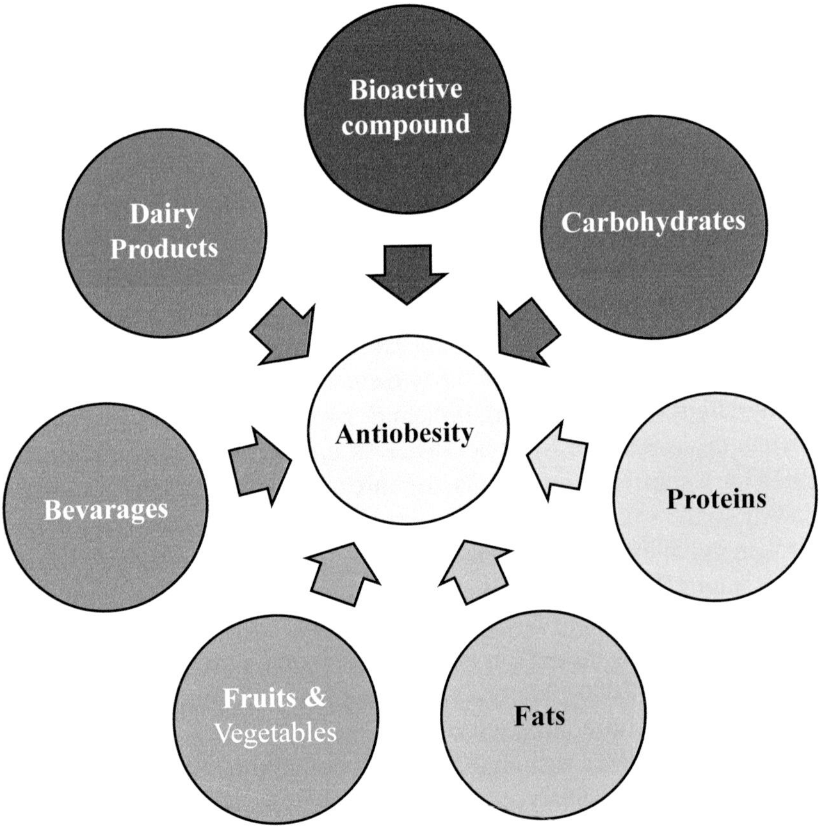

FIGURE 14.2 Several weight loss functional foods.

fed brown rice or oryzanol showed a preference for the low-fat control diet over the high-fat diet (Kozuka et al., 2012). Fiber in the diet has been shown to reduce appetite and promote satiety; however, this is not always associated with reduced calorie consumption. Studies primarily included people of ordinary or slightly above-average weight. Well-designed randomized, controlled clinical trials in overweight and/or obese people are necessary to assess the efficacy of dietary fiber as a method for weight loss (Surana et al., 2021).

14.3 PROTEIN AND FAT-RICH NUTRIENTS

It has been demonstrated that diets high in protein can promote satiety, decrease appetite, and reduce overall food consumption (Anderson & Moore, 2004). Protein has a greater satiety and thermogenic effect than its macronutrient equivalents, carbohydrates, and lipids, due to the higher energy expenditure associated with catabolism and protein synthesis. This is because protein synthesis and catabolism both require more energy. In human participants, the consumption of protein-rich legumes such as lentils, peas, peanuts, chickpeas, beans, soybeans, and Faba beans resulted in a 49% increase in the amount of energy expended (Iwashita et al., 2006).

Potential functional foods include but are not limited to, dietary fats like medium-chain triacylglycerols (MCTs), diacylglycerols, and beverages like tea, milk, and almonds. Medium-chain triglycerides (MCTs) are triacylglycerols derived from fatty acids ranging in carbon number from 6 to 12. Triacylglycerols with a longer chain length are referred to as LCTs. The content and mode of transport of the two are distinctively different. Medium- and long-chain triglycerides are broken down into fatty acids with different chain lengths in the digestive tract (MCFAs and LCFAs, respectively). Since MCFAs have shorter chain lengths, they are able to skip peripheral tissues on their way to the liver via the portal circulation, where they are less likely to be broken down by hormone-sensitive lipase and deposited as fat in adipose tissue storage (Bach & Babayan, 1982). Liquid oil produced from coconuts is high in medium-chain triglycerides (MCTs), which have the ability to boost thermogenesis more than triacylglycerols do and hence aid in weight loss (Nagao et al., 2000). Many different cooking oils contain trace levels of diacylglycerols, with cottonseed oil having one of the highest proportions (9.5%). There is now a diacylglycerol-rich cooking oil available that tastes and looks just like ordinary oil but has 80% more of these beneficial fats. Programs that aim to reduce body fat often recommend eating fish high in saturated fat. A better plasma lipid profile was also seen when salmon was included in a low-calorie diet (Mori et al., 2004).

14.4 VEGETABLES AND FRUITS AS NUTRACEUTICALS

Consuming a diet rich in fruits and vegetables may help prevent the development of chronic diseases. Apples, mangoes, bilberries, and sea buckthorn all helped people lose weight, grow less muscle mass, and produce less glucose, according to a 2013 study (Boqué et al., 2013). Studies have shown that vegetables like bitter gourd, green tomatoes, onion peel tea, and piper sarmentosum (a medicinal plant) reduce the risk of gaining weight (Boqué et al., 2013; Chaturvedi, 2012; Choi et al., 2013). It is possible that the synergistic and cumulative effect of eating a variety of berries, such as blackberry, blueberry, strawberry, and others, can help promote human health and avoid obesity. Incorporating more berries into your diet may be an effective option for making other dietary modifications to ward off metabolic syndrome (Choi et al., 2013; Matsunaga et al., 2014).

Avocados are high in fats and contain provitamin A carotenoids, and they resemble berries in appearance. Since about 80% of an avocado's edible portion is composed of 72% water and 6.8% dietary fiber, they are a good source of lutein and have a moderate calorie density. The avocado, like other low-fat fruits and vegetables, has been found to aid in weight loss (Kopec et al., 2014).

The antioxidant content of the pomegranate fruit is particularly high. Many bioactive compounds, including tannins, ellagitannins, procyanidins, flavonoids, and others, are concentrated in pomegranates and may contribute to their health benefits. The pomegranate skin, which accounts for 30–40% of the fruit, is typically thrown away as surplus (Fischer et al., 2011).

14.5 BEVERAGES, DIARY PRODUCTS IN OBESITY

The plant Camellia sinensis, which is used to make tea, is consumed widely all over the globe. Caffeine, which is found in tea, has been shown to stimulate thermogenesis and increase energy expenditure. Caffeine and polyphenols in tea both contribute to increased fat burning. Green tea, unlike black and oolong teas, has not been fermented, thus it retains many of its healthy polyphenolic constituents. Fermented black tea is rich in theaflavins and polyphenols. The polyphenols in black tea have been shown to alter lipid metabolism by inhibiting pancreatic lipase (Yuda et al., 2012; Chaloupka et al., 2011).

Coffee's antioxidant potential as an anti-obesity beverage has been studied (Zemel et al., 2000). Multiple studies found that green coffee bean extract, likely due to its high chlorogenic acid content, was more effective at reducing body weight and fat in the epididymis and perineum than roasted coffee and caffeine (Pan et al., 2016). Finally, there are indications that coffee may play a role in weight loss. Researchers looked into the effects of two high-anthocyanin juices on weight loss: mulberry (MBJ) and blueberry (BBJ) (Wu et al., 2013; Bukowiecki et al., 1983). Adiposity is inversely connected to a low intake of dairy products and calcium. Dietary calcium is crucial in the regulation of energy metabolism and the risk of obesity (Ackley et al., 1983). Calcium is mostly obtained through dairy products, and various theories for understanding calcium's role have been postulated (Zemel et al., 2000; Barba & Russo, 2006).

14.6 BIOACTIVE COMPOUNDS AND OBESITY

Many researchers have spent time and energy in recent years looking for bioactive components in foods and herbs that can help with obesity and its accompanying complications. Many different types of fruits, vegetables, and herbs include polyphenols, which are a very important chemical class of bioactives. Triglyceride levels were found to be significantly lower in those who consumed Indian gooseberry (Patil et al., 2009). A natural flavonoid called kaempferol was also investigated for its potential to combat obesity. In addition, synergistic effects may be seen when many bioactive substances are combined. It has been shown that a combination of crocin, chlorogenic acid, geniposide, and quercetin can reduce the buildup of triglycerides and cholesterol in human beings. Researchers discovered that extracts of ginseng green leaf, ginseng dry leaf, and ginseng seed oil were all effective at reducing triglyceride and cholesterol levels. When diallyl disulfide, a major organosulfur present in garlic, is added to green tea extract, the effects on adipogenesis and triglyceride synthesis are enhanced. The daily required amount can be obtained by consuming one cup of green tea and two cloves of garlic (Sandner et al., 2020; Bernhoft, 2010; Ahire et al., 2021).

14.7 NUTS AND OBESITY

The high levels of energy, proteins, and fiber in nuts may contribute to their ability to curb hunger (Neale et al., 2017). Nuts are high in energy, and some studies have suggested that this makes them a good meal to swap out for others in an effort to reduce overall caloric intake and keep weight gain to a minimum. Almonds were included in the low-calorie diet of 62% of the study participants, leading to greater weight loss, smaller waist circumference, and more fat mass loss, as well as better glycemic control than the carbohydrate-low-calorie diet group (Kranz et al., 2014; Bitok et al., 2017).

14.8 CONCLUSION

When consumed as part of a healthy, well-balanced diet, certain functional foods have been proposed as a potential alternative strategy for controlling one's weight and warding off obesity. The progression of obesity is caused by the combination of a number of different systems that are quite complex. Instead of focusing on a single process, it is necessary to target multiple processes. Even if there is evidence that functional foods have a significant amount of potential to be produced, the real challenge for the food industry is to create products that are successful through a variety of different procedures. Another challenge in the process of producing functional foods for obesity is the lack of available biomarkers that can be used to evaluate the ingredients. Long-term research ought to center on determining the optimum amount of an item that can be safely ingested without compromising its efficiency or safety. Obesity can only be significantly reduced by making significant changes to one's lifestyle, such as one's food and level of physical activity, which can only be accomplished with the application of a multidisciplinary approach.

KEYWORDS

- **diet**
- **food industry**
- **functional foods**
- **health**
- **nutrition**
- **obesity**

REFERENCES

Ackley, S., Barrett-Connor, E., & Suarez, L. (1983). Dairy products, calcium, and blood pressure. The American Journal of Clinical Nutrition, 38(4), 457–461.

Ahire, E., Sonawane, V., Surana, K., & Talele, G. (2021). Drug Discovery, Drug-Likeness Screening, and Bioavailability: Development of Drug-Likeness Rule for Natural Products. Applied Pharmaceutical Practice and Nutraceuticals, 191–208. Apple Academic Press.

Anderson, G. H., & Moore, S. E. (2004). Dietary proteins in the regulation of food intake and body weight in humans. The Journal of Nutrition, 134(4), 974S–979S.

Anderson, J. W., Konz, E. C., Frederich, R. C., & Wood, C. L. (2001). Long-term weight-loss maintenance: a meta-analysis of US studies. *The American Journal of Clinical Nutrition, 74*(5), 579–584.

Bach, A., & Babayan, V. (1982). Medium-chain triglycerides: an update. The American Journal of Clinical Nutrition, 36(5), 950–962.

Barba, G., & Russo, P. (2006). Dairy foods, dietary calcium and obesity: a short review of the evidence. Nutrition, Metabolism and Cardiovascular Diseases, 16(6), 445–451.
Bernhoft, A. (2010). A brief review on bioactive compounds in plants. Bioactive Compounds in Plants-Benefits and Risks for Man and Animals, 50, 11–17.
Bigliardi, B., & Galati, F. (2013). Innovation trends in the food industry: The case of functional foods. Trends in Food Science & Technology, 31(2), 118–129.
Bitok, E., Jaceldo-Siegl, K., Rajaram, S., Serra-Mir, M., Roth, I., Feitas-Simoes, T., Ros, E., & Sabaté, J. (2017). Favorable nutrient intake and displacement with long-term walnut supplementation among elderly: results of a randomized trial. British Journal of Nutrition, 118(3), 201–209.
Blades, M. (2000). Functional foods or nutraceuticals. Nutrition & Food Science. 1, 30(2), 73–76.
Boqué, N., De la Iglesia, R., De la Garza, A. L., Milagro, F. I., Olivares, M., Bañuelos, Ó., Soria, A. C., Rodríguez-Sánchez, S., Martínez, J. A., & Campión, J. (2013). Prevention of diet-induced obesity by apple polyphenols in Wistar rats through regulation of adipocyte gene expression and DNA methylation patterns. Molecular Nutrition & Food Research, 57(8), 1473–1478.
Brown, L., Caligiuri, S. P., Brown, D., & Pierce, G. N. (2018). Clinical trials using functional foods provide unique challenges. Journal of Functional Foods, 45, 233–238.
Brown, L., Poudyal, H., & Panchal, S. K. (2015). Functional foods as potential therapeutic options for metabolic syndrome. Obesity Reviews, 16(11), 914–941.
Bukowiecki, L. J., Lupien, J., Follea, N., & Jahjah, L. (1983). Effects of sucrose, caffeine, and cola beverages on obesity, cold resistance, and adipose tissue cellularity. American Journal of Physiology-Regulatory, Integrative and Comparative Physiology, 244(5), R500–R507.
Chaloupka, F. J., Powell, L. M., & Chriqui, J. F. (2011). Sugar-sweetened beverages and obesity prevention: Policy recommendations. Journal of Policy Analysis and Management, 30(3), 662–664.
Chaturvedi, P. (2012). Antidiabetic potentials of Momordica charantia: multiple mechanisms behind the effects. Journal of Medicinal Food, 15(2), 101–107.
Choi, K. M., Lee, Y. S., Shin, D. M., Lee, S., Yoo, K. S., Lee, M. K., Lee, J. H., Kim, S. Y., Dikeman, C. L., & Fahey Jr, G. C. (2006). Viscosity as related to dietary fiber: a review. Critical Reviews in Food Science and Nutrition, 46(6), 649–663.
Elmaliklis, I.-N., Liveri, A., Ntelis, B., Paraskeva, K., Goulis, I., & Koutelidakis, A. E. (2019). Increased functional foods' consumption and Mediterranean diet adherence may have a protective effect in the appearance of gastrointestinal diseases: a case–control study. Medicines, 6(2), 50.
Farajian, P., Risvas, G., Karasouli, K., Pounis, G. D., Kastorini, C. M., Panagiotakos, D. B., & Zampelas, A. (2011). Very high childhood obesity prevalence and low adherence rates to the Mediterranean diet in Greek children: the GRECO study. Atherosclerosis, 217(2), 525–530.
Fischer, U. A., Carle, R., & Kammerer, D. R. (2011). Identification and quantification of phenolic compounds from pomegranate (Punica granatum L.) peel, mesocarp, aril and differently produced juices by HPLC-DAD–ESI/MSn. Food Chemistry, 127(2), 807–821.
Iwashita, S., Mikus, C., Baier, S., & Flakoll, P. J. (2006). Glutamine supplementation increases postprandial energy expenditure and fat oxidation in humans. Journal of Parenteral and Enteral Nutrition, 30(1), 76–80.

Kasbia, G. S. (2005). Functional foods and nutraceuticals in the management of obesity. Nutrition & Food Science, 35(5), 344–349.

Konstantinidi, M., & Koutelidakis, A. E. (2019). Functional foods and bioactive compounds: A review of its possible role on weight management and obesity's metabolic consequences. Medicines, 6(3), 94.

Kopec, R. E., Cooperstone, J. L., Schweiggert, R. M., Young, G. S., Harrison, E. H., Francis, D. M., Clinton, S. K., & Schwartz, S. J. (2014). Avocado consumption enhances human postprandial provitamin A absorption and conversion from a novel high–β-carotene tomato sauce and from carrots. The Journal of Nutrition, 144(8), 1158–1166.

Koutelidakis, A., & Dimou, C. (2016). The effects of functional food and bioactive compounds on biomarkers of cardiovascular diseases. Functional Foods Text Book, 1st ed.; Martirosyan, D., Ed, 89–117.

Kozuka, C., Yabiku, K., Sunagawa, S., Ueda, R., Taira, S.-I., Ohshiro, H., Ikema, T., Yamakawa, K., Higa, M., & Tanaka, H. (2012). Brown rice and its component, γ-oryzanol, attenuate the preference for high-fat diet by decreasing hypothalamic endoplasmic reticulum stress in mice. Diabetes, 61(12), 3084–3093.

Kranz, S., Hill, A., Fleming, J., Hartman, T., West, S., & Kris-Etherton, P. (2014). Nutrient displacement associated with walnut supplementation in men. Journal of Human Nutrition and Dietetics, 27(3), 247–254.

Larsen, T. M., Dalskov, S.-M., van Baak, M., Jebb, S. A., Papadaki, A., Pfeiffer, A. F., Martinez, J. A., Handjieva-Darlenska, T., Kunešová, M., & Pihlsgaard, M. (2010). Diets with high or low protein content and glycemic index for weight-loss maintenance. New England Journal of Medicine, 363(22), 2102–2113.

Lee, Y. M., & Hong, J. T. (2013). Green tomato extract attenuates high-fat-diet-induced obesity through activation of the AMPK pathway in C57BL/6 mice. The Journal of Nutritional Biochemistry, 24(2), 335–342.

Martirosyan, D. M., & Singh, J. (2015). A new definition of functional food by FFC: what makes a new definition unique? Functional Foods in Health and Disease, 5(6), 209–223.

Matsunaga, S., Azuma, K., Watanabe, M., Tsuka, T., Imagawa, T., Osaki, T., & Okamoto, Y. (2014). Onion peel tea ameliorates obesity and affects blood parameters in a mouse model of high-fat-diet-induced obesity. Experimental and Therapeutic Medicine, 7(2), 379–382.

Mori, T. A., Burke, V., Puddey, I. B., Shaw, J. E., & Beilin, L. J. (2004). Effect of fish diets and weight loss on serum leptin concentration in overweight, treated-hypertensive subjects. Journal of Hypertension, 22(10), 1983–1990.

Nagao, T., Watanabe, H., Goto, N., Onizawa, K., Taguchi, H., Matsuo, N., Yasukawa, T., Tsushima, R., Shimasaki, H., & Itakura, H. (2000). Dietary diacylglycerol suppresses accumulation of body fat compared to triacylglycerol in men in a double-blind controlled trial. The Journal of Nutrition, 130(4), 792–797.

Neale, E. P., Tapsell, L. C., Martin, A., Batterham, M. J., Wibisono, C., & Probst, Y. C. (2017). Impact of providing walnut samples in a lifestyle intervention for weight loss: a secondary analysis of the HealthTrack trial. Food & Nutrition Research, 61(1), 1344522.

Ntrigiou, V., Ntrigios, I., Rigopoulos, N., Dimou, C., & Koutelidakis, A. E. (2018). Functional food consumption correlates with anthropometric characteristics and body composition in healthy adults. *Current Topics in Nutraceutical Research, 16*(3), 279–285.

Pan, M. H., Tung, Y. C., Yang, G., Li, S., & Ho, C. T. (2016). Molecular mechanisms of the anti-obesity effect of bioactive compounds in tea and coffee. *Food & Function, 7*(11), 4481–4491.

Patil, B. S., Jayaprakasha, G. K., Chidambara Murthy, K., & Vikram, A. (2009). Bioactive compounds: historical perspectives, opportunities, and challenges. *Journal of Agricultural and Food Chemistry, 57*(18), 8142–8160.

Rolls, B. (2014). What is the role of portion control in weight management? *International Journal of Obesity, 38*(S1), S1–S8.

Sandner, G., König, A., Wallner, M., & Weghuber, J. (2020). Functional foods-dietary or herbal products on obesity: application of selected bioactive compounds to target lipid metabolism. *Current Opinion in Food Science, 34*(June), 9–20.

Surana, K. R., Ahire, E. D., Sonawane, V. N., Talele, S. G., & Talele, G. (2021). Informatics and Methods in Nutrition Design and Development. In *Natural Food Products and Waste Recovery: Healthy Foods, Nutrition Design, and Extraction of Valuable Compounds* (pp. 33).

Wollner, M., Roberto, B.-B. P., Roncally, S. C. A., Jurandir, N., & Edil, L. S. (2017). Accuracy of the WHO's body mass index cut-off points to measure gender-and age-specific obesity in middle-aged adults living in the city of Rio de Janeiro, Brazil. *Journal of Public Health Research, 6*(1), 108–112.

Wu, T., Qi, X., Liu, Y., Guo, J., Zhu, R., Chen, W., Zheng, X., & Yu, T. (2013). Dietary supplementation with purified mulberry (Morus australis Poir) anthocyanins suppresses body weight gain in high-fat diet fed C57BL/6 mice. *Food Chemistry, 141*(1), 482–487.

Yuda, N., Tanaka, M., Suzuki, M., Asano, Y., Ochi, H., & Iwatsuki, K. (2012). Polyphenols extracted from black tea (Camellia sinensis) residue by hot-compressed water and their inhibitory effect on pancreatic lipase in vitro. *Journal of Food Science, 77*(9), H254–H261.

Zemel, M. B., Shi, H., Greer, B., Dirienzo, D., & Zemel, P. C. (2000). Regulation of adiposity by dietary calcium. *The FASEB Journal, 14*(9), 1132–1138.

INDEX

B

C

G

H

M

For Product Safety Concerns and Information please contact our EU representative GPSR@taylorandfrancis.com Taylor & Francis Verlag GmbH, Kaufingerstraße 24, 80331 München, Germany